Surgical
Anatomy and Physiology
for the
Surgical Technologist

Surgical
Anatomy and Physiology
for the
Surgical Technologist

Kevin B. Frey, CST, MA
Paul Price, CST/CFA, MBA

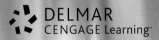

DELMAR
CENGAGE Learning

Australia • Brazil • Japan • Korea • Mexico • Singapore • Spain • United Kingdom • United States

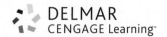
DELMAR
CENGAGE Learning™

Surgical Anatomy and Physiology for the Surgical Technologist
Kevin B. Frey, Paul Price

Vice President, Health Care Business Unit:
William Brottmiller

Editorial Director: Matthew Kane

Acquisitions Editor: Rhonda Dearborn

Developmental Editor: Sherry Conners

Editorial Assistant: Debra Gorgos

Marketing Director: Jennifer McAvey

Marketing Channel Manager: Tamara Caruso

Marketing Coordinator: Christopher Manion

Production Director: Carolyn Miller

Senior Production Editor: James Zayicek

Project Editor: Natalie Pashoukos

Library of Congress Control Number: 2005048624

ISBN-13: 978-0-7668-4113-0

ISBN-10: 0-7668-4113-8

Delmar
Executive Woods
5 Maxwell Drive
Clifton Park, NY 12065
USA

Cengage Learning is a leading provider of customized learning solutions with office locations around the globe, including Singapore, the United Kingdom, Australia, Mexico, Brazil, and Japan. Locate your local office at **www.cengage.com/global**

Cengage Learning products are represented in Canada by Nelson Education, Ltd.

To learn more about Delmar, visit **www.cengage.com/delmar**

Purchase any of our products at your local bookstore or at our preferred online store **www.cengagebrain.com**

Notice to the Reader

Printed in China
4 5 6 7 17 16 15 14

CONTENTS

PREFACE

An understanding of the anatomic systems and structures of the human body, and the physiology associated with them, is essential to proper training and practice for the surgical technologist. This knowledge is applied to every procedure in the operating room; in fact, patient outcomes for intraoperative care can be negatively affected by the surgical technologist who does not understand anatomy. It is especially important that the practitioner of intraoperative care understand the distinction between general and surgical anatomy. For the surgical technology student to function effectively in the operating room, an accurate view of the human body is necessary, with emphasis placed on the application of this science to practical surgery. The anatomy observed during didactic or laboratory instruction or even cadaveric dissection is very different from the anatomy observed on a living patient during an actual procedure. Therefore, the purpose of a surgical anatomy and physiology textbook is to provide general information combined with correlating surgical information, including basic pathophysiology, so that the student of surgical technology can best apply that knowledge to what is actually encountered during the procedure.

FEATURES

Surgical Anatomy and Physiology for the Surgical Technologist contains the following features:

- It meets the content requirements of the fifth edition of the *Core Curriculum for Surgical Technology*, mandated by the Accreditation Review Committee on Education in Surgical Technology (ARC-ST) for compliance with accreditation Standards. This edition of the core curriculum provides more detail for proper instruction than have previous editions, and places an emphasis on surgical anatomy and physiology. This textbook is designed to help the instructor fulfill that requirement.
- In addition to surgical applications for anatomy and physiology, specific information related to surgical practice is included in boxes interspersed throughout the chapters.
- Case studies and corresponding review questions are included at the beginning and end of each chapter to further relate chapter information to surgical practice. It is essential that the instructor understand that these cases studies require higher levels of critical thinking and further review with other instructional resources for proper solution. They are also intended to stimulate classroom discussion about what will eventually be encountered during clinical components of the curriculum.
- At the end of the chapter, a section titled "Implications for the Surgical Technologist" correlates the specific chapter content to the practice of surgical technology.
- Questions for further review at the end of each chapter are designed to stimulate critical thinking skills specific to the practice of surgical technology. Again, resources for further review should be made available to the student for proper solution. Furthermore, the development of critical thinking skills is essential for proper surgical practice, and these skills are best honed through techniques that require thought and research, rather than passive memorization or answers that are easily found within the text itself.
- Full-color illustrations provide important tools for understanding complex anatomic or surgical elements.
- A comprehensive glossary is located at the end of the book, listing definitions of key terms.

1

ORGANIZATION OF THE HUMAN BODY

CHAPTER OBJECTIVES

After completing the study of this chapter, you should be able to:

1. Describe the body planes and directional terms.
2. Describe the quadrants and regions of the abdomen.
3. List the cavities of the body and the organs contained within each cavity.
4. Locate the surgical anatomic points of reference.
5. List the body systems, the organs contained within each system, and the general functions of each system.
6. Define homeostasis.
7. Describe how the body maintains homeostasis.

KEY TERMS

abdominal cavity	condyle	fibrous pericardium	iliac regions (right and left)
abdominopelvic cavity	coronal plane (frontal plane)	foramen	inferior (caudal)
anatomic position	cranial cavity	fossa	integumentary system
anatomy	cross section	genitourinary system	lateral
anterior (ventral)	diaphragm	hepatic flexure	left lower quadrant (LLQ)
autonomic nervous system (ANS)	digestive system	Hesselbach's triangle	left upper quadrant (LUQ)
	distal	homeostasis	ligament of Treitz
cardiac muscle	dorsal cavity	hormones	lumbar regions (right and left)
cardiovascular system	endocrine system	hypochondriac regions (right and left)	lymphatic system
central nervous system (CNS)	epicondyle		lymphocytes
circulatory system	epigastric region	hypogastric region	medial

KEY TERMS (Continued)

mediastinum	pelvic cavity	right lower quadrant (RLQ)	sympathetic division
meninges	pericardial sac	right upper quadrant (RUQ)	target tissue
mesentery	peripheral nervous system	sagittal plane	thoracic cavity
midsagittal plane (median	(PNS)	skeletal muscles (voluntary;	transverse plane (horizontal
plane)	peripheral vascular system	striated)	plane)
negative feedback mechanism	peritoneal cavity	skeletal system	triangle of Calot
nervous system	peritoneal space	smooth muscles (involuntary;	trigone of bladder
normal ranges	physiology	nonstriated)	trochanter
omentum	posterior (dorsal)	somatic nervous system	umbilical region
parasympathetic division	proximal	(SNS)	ventral cavity
parietal pericardium	quadrants	spermatozoa	viscera
parietal peritoneum	regions	spinal cavity	visceral pericardium
parietal pleura	reproductive system	splenic flexure	visceral peritoneum
pathophysiology	respiratory system	superior (cephalad)	visceral pleura

Case Study 1

A patient is scheduled for a left-lung lobectomy, the removal of a lobe of the lung. The surgeon indicates that the patient is to be placed on the operating room table in the lateral position with the affected side up in order to make an incision that goes from lateral to posterior. The inferior lobe of the lung will be removed.

1. The lungs are located in what body cavity?

2. Define the term *lateral* and how it relates to positioning of the patient.

3. Describe the lateral to posterior incision.

4. The inferior lobe refers to which lobe of the left lung?

AN INTRODUCTION TO ANATOMY AND PHYSIOLOGY

The study of anatomy and physiology has paralleled the development of cultures, religion, and technology. Based on examinations of skeletons, it has been hypothesized that some ancient civilizations such as the Maya and Incas performed surgery, including craniotomies. Many ancient civilizations also relied on a primary healer, who had assistants, to treat various disorders and diseases. They often used herbs, roots, leaves, and other plants as cures, based on knowledge passed down through the years. Considering the recent resurgence of holistic medicine and use of natural substances to heal individuals, these practices cannot be dismissed.

During the period from 2500 BC to 500 BC the Greeks and Egyptians made significant contributions to the advancement of medicine and study of anatomy. Some of the contributors are included in the following:

1. Imhotep, 2500 BC: recorded some of the earliest information on surgery

2. Aristotle, 500 BC: the founder of comparative anatomy

3. Herophilus, 500 BC: known as the "Father of Anatomy"; developed the Doctrine of Pulse, which describes the diagnostic values of the pulse

4. Erasistratos, 500 BC: contributed to the understanding of brain anatomy and noted the difference between motor and sensory nerves.

However, the biggest influence on the study of anatomy and physiology came from two individuals: Galen and Andreas Vesalius. Galen, beginning in the year 0, was the first great anatomist, and his writings remained unchallenged for 1500 years. His contributions were highly significant, but contained many mistakes, which stemmed from his religious faith. In order to serve the church and not break its laws, Galen conformed his anatomic findings to theological principles, which included not dissecting dead human bodies. Many of his findings, therefore, were based on dissections of animals, and his writings assumed that the anatomy of the animals was comparable to human anatomy. Then, in 1500, Andreas Vesalius, the "Father of Modern Anatomy," changed everything. He broke from Galen, challenging his writings and correcting his mistakes. He accomplished this by first dissecting human cadavers himself and then hiring the best illustrator of that time to draw his findings. Vesalius eventually wrote the most important anatomic textbook of its time, *De Humani Corporis Fabrica Libri Septem*.

At the same time, in 1500, Ambroise Paré, who was from France, established himself as the greatest surgeon of the sixteenth century. He was the first to ligate bleeding vessels with clamps or ties, or by pinching the vessels with forceps to control bleeding after amputations. He also advocated not using hot irons or oils to stop the bleeding, thereby lowering the morbidity and mortality rates of soldiers.

These are just a few examples of the individuals who have contributed to the advancement of medicine, surgery, and the study of anatomy and physiology. The student is encouraged to learn more about the extensive history of medicine and surgery by exploring a book that covers the subject.

Anatomy and physiology are closely linked. Each complements the other, and, therefore, it is hard to separate the two. **Anatomy** is the study of the structure and morphology of the body and its systems. **Physiology** is the study of the functions of the cells, tissue, and organs of the body. To understand the physiology of an organ, one must first understand its anatomy.

Pathophysiology is the study of disease and disorders of the human body. The knowledge of normal anatomy and physiology makes it easier to understand these disorders. For example, multiple sclerosis is a disease in which the myelin sheath of neurons in the **central nervous system (CNS)** deteriorates, leading to muscle weakness, paralysis, and many other neurological deficits. Knowledge about the normal anatomy and physiology of the central nervous system aids in understanding a disease like multiple sclerosis, and underscores the intimate relationship between anatomy, physiology, and pathophysiology.

As has been discussed, the study of anatomy and physiology is an ancient one—but it is also an ever ongoing field. There is still much to learn about the human body. Research continues to better understand the physiological processes of the body, and the discoveries that result (e.g., gene mapping and greater knowledge of the physiology of the brain) aid health care providers in developing better treatments of pathologies.

DIRECTIONAL TERMS AND BODY PLANES

To effectively communicate with one another, medical professionals have developed a universal anatomic terminology consisting of several terms that are used on a daily basis in medicine and, in particular, surgery. These terms are used to describe directions, body planes, quadrants, regions, cavities, and levels of body organization. The terms are defined in reference to the body in **anatomic position**, which means the human body is standing erect, facing forward, with arms at the sides and the palms of the hands and feet facing forward (Figure 1-1).

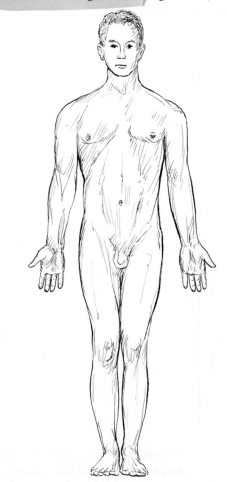

FIGURE 1-1 Anatomic Position

Directional Terms

The following are the most common directional terms (Figure 1-2), and are used to describe a part of the body in relation to the whole body:

1. **Superior**: The synonymous term is **cephalad**, and refers to above or toward the head. Example: The lung is superior to the diaphragm.
2. **Inferior**: The synonymous term is **caudal**, and refers to being below, underneath, or toward the feet. Example: The cecum is inferior to the transverse colon.
3. **Anterior**: The synonymous term is **ventral**, and means toward the front. Example: The trachea is anterior to the esophagus.
4. **Posterior**: The synonymous term is **dorsal**, and refers to the back; opposite of anterior. Example: The spinal cord is posterior to the small intestine and colon.
5. **Medial**: Means toward the middle of the body. It also relates to an imaginary midline that divides the body into equal left and right halves. Example: The ulna is medial to the radius in the forearm.

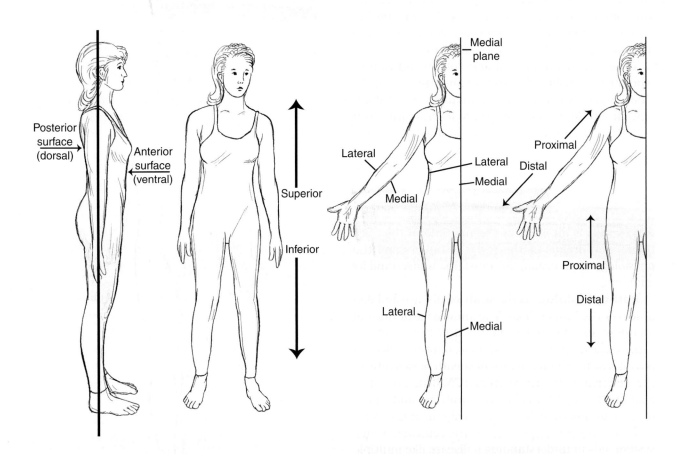

FIGURE 1-2   Directional Terminology: anterior/posterior, inferior/superior, lateral/medial, distal/proximal

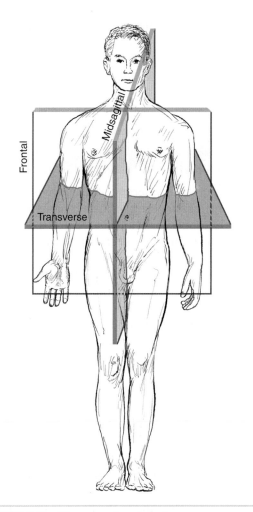

FIGURE 1-3   Planes—frontal view

procedure. These are just two of an endless number of surgical examples, emphasizing that mastering surgical terminology is essential both to communicating in the operating room and to providing quality patient care.

Body Planes

In conjunction with the directional terms, the body is also sectioned into various imaginary geometric planes (Figures 1-3 and 1-4). The planes are used most often when dissecting organs and when viewing x-rays or other types of diagnostic images. The **midsagittal plane**, also called **median plane**, refers to vertically dividing the body into equal left and right portions. **Sagittal plane** refers to any plane that is parallel to the median plane vertically dividing the body in unequal left and right halves.

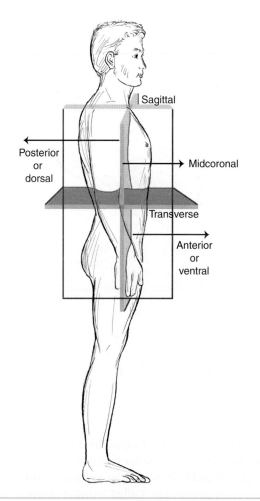

FIGURE 1-4   Planes—side view

6. **Lateral**: Means toward the side of the body or away from the midline. Example: Lateral position means the patient is lying on their side.
7. **Proximal**: Means closer to the origin. Example: The elbow joint is proximal to the wrist joint.
8. **Distal**: Means away from the origin; opposite of proximal. Example: The elbow joint is distal to the shoulder joint.

Because these terms are frequently used in surgery, the surgical technologist must know their precise meaning. For example, the surgeon might ask the surgical technologist to relocate the retractors to expose a wound in a cephalad direction. This means the surgical technologist should move the retractors upward or in a superior direction. Or, the surgeon might ask the surgical technologist to reposition a leg laterally during a knee arthroscopy

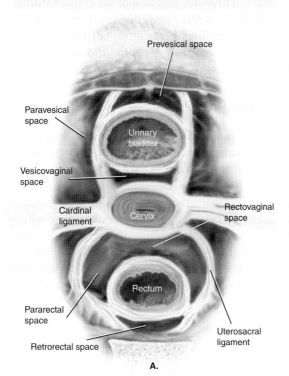

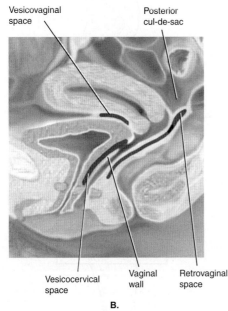

FIGURE 1-5 Cleavage Planes: A) cross section and B) sagittal

The **transverse plane**, also called **horizontal plane**, refers to any plane that divides the body into superior and inferior portions, equal or unequal. The **coronal plane**, also called **frontal plane**, is a plane that divides the body into anterior and posterior

sections that are at a right angle to the sagittal plane. Another commonly used term when dissecting a body organ is **cross section**, which refers to a transverse cut that is at right angles to the long axis of the organ (Figure 1-5).

SURGICAL ANATOMIC POINTS OF REFERENCE

Anatomic points of reference that have been established over the years are used by surgeons to identify key anatomic landmarks and features. For example, if a particular pathology such as a tumor of the abdomen has caused the normal anatomy to become difficult to determine, the surgeon will use anatomic points of reference to identify the sections of the small intestine and colon. A discussion of all the anatomic points of reference is beyond the scope of this book; however, the following are some of the more well-known and important points used in surgery (Figures 1-6 and 1-7):

1. **Epicondyle**: Projection on the surface of bone located just superior to the condyle.
2. **Condyle**: Projection on the surface of bone located at the epiphysis that articulates with another bone and serves as the site of attachment of ligaments.
3. **Foramen**: Opening in the bone or tissue for the passage of blood vessels, ligaments, or nerves. Two examples of important foramen are (a) foramen magnum, an opening in the occipital bone of the skull through which the spinal cord enters the spinal column, and (b) foramen of Munro, a passage through the lateral and third ventricles of the brain.
4. **Fossa**: A slight depression on the end of a bone such as the olecranon fossa.
5. **Trochanter**: A large process on a bone, in particular the lesser and greater trochanters on the femur, which serves as sites for the attachment of muscles.
6. **Triangle of Calot**: Anatomic triangle formed by the cystic duct, common hepatic duct, and inferior border of the liver. Used to locate the cystic artery, which is often within the triangle.
7. **Hesselbach's triangle**: Anatomic triangle that is important in the identification of direct hernias. It is formed inferiorly by the epigastric artery, laterally by the rectus abdominus muscle, and bounded by the inguinal ligament.

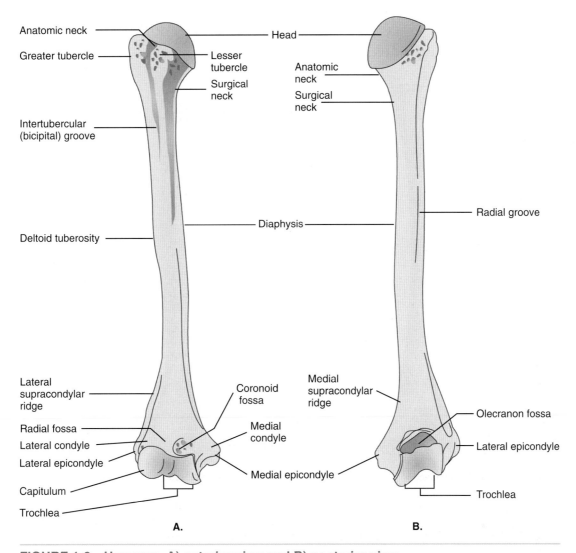

FIGURE 1-6   Humerus, A) anterior view and B) posterior view

8. **Trigone of bladder**: An important clinical landmark formed by the two posterolateral openings of the ureters into the bladder, with the apex formed by the urethral opening.
9. **Ligament of Treitz**: A ligament that attaches the end of the duodenum to the posterior abdominal wall and marks the beginning of the jejunum.
10. **Hepatic flexure**: The point where the ascending colon ends; forms a gentle curve to begin the transverse colon.
11. **Splenic flexure**: The point where the transverse colon ends; forms a gentle curve to begin the descending colon.

BODY REGIONS

To aid surgeons in making a diagnosis, the abdomen is divided into **quadrants** and **regions**. The surgical technologist should be familiar with these divisions for the following reasons:

1. The location of surgical incisions is often indicated according to the quadrant or region.
2. The location of the organ or portion of the organ to be operated upon will be indicated by the quadrant or region.

Clinically, quadrants are the division used most frequently. A transverse plane and a midsagittal plane

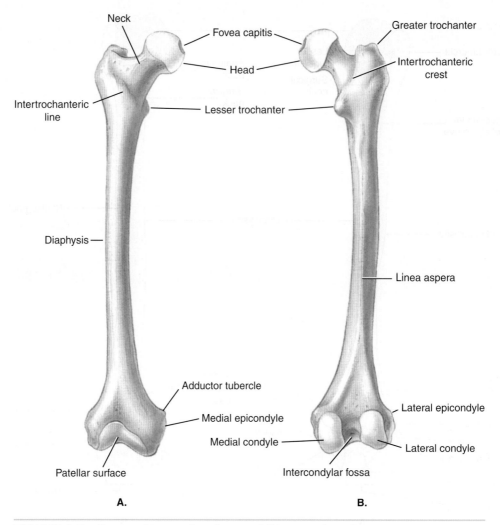

FIGURE 1-7 Femur, A) anterior view and B) posterior view

divide the abdomen into equal quadrants (Figure 1-8):

1. **Right upper quadrant (RUQ)**
2. **Right lower quadrant (RLQ)**
3. **Left upper quadrant (LUQ)**
4. **Left lower quadrant (LLQ)**

Following are two clinical examples:

1. A patient is admitted to the emergency department complaining of right lower quadrant pain. Often this pain indicates appendicitis. If it is a female patient, it can indicate either appendicitis or ovarian cyst.
2. A patient visits a general surgeon with a primary complaint of pain in the right upper quadrant with pain radiating laterally and to the back. Gallstones are frequently the cause of this type of pain.

Two sagittal planes and two transverse planes divide the abdomen into nine regions (Figure 1-9), as follows:

1. **Epigastric region**: Superior middle region
2. **Right and left hypochondriac regions**: Each side of the epigastric region
3. **Umbilical region**: Central middle region
4. **Right and left lumbar regions**: On each side of the umbilical region
5. **Hypogastric region**: Lower middle region
6. **Right and left iliac regions**: On each side of the hypogastric region

BODY ORGANIZATION AND CAVITIES

The body is divided into two major cavities: **dorsal cavity** and **ventral cavity** (Figure 1-10). The dorsal cavity is further divided into the **cranial cavity**,

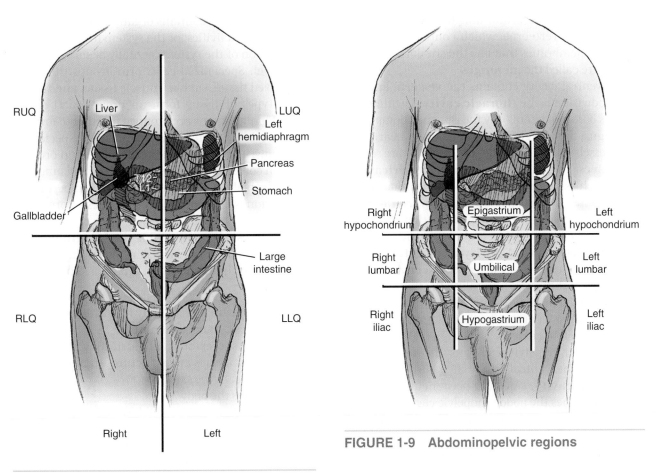

FIGURE 1-8   Abdominopelvic quadrants

FIGURE 1-9   Abdominopelvic regions

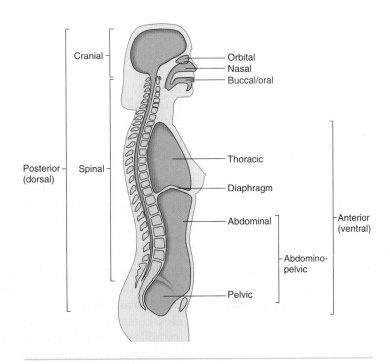

FIGURE 1-10   Cavities of the body

which contains the brain, and the **spinal cavity**, formed by the vertebrae, which contains the spinal cord. The membranes that line the cranial and spinal cavities are called the **meninges**.

The ventral cavity contains the **viscera**, and the first subdivision is the **thoracic cavity**. The thoracic cavity is bordered laterally by the ribs and contains the esophagus, thymus gland, trachea, lungs, heart, and great vessels. The membranes of the cavity are serous membranes. The heart is contained in the **pericardial sac**, which is composed of three pericardial membranes: outer **fibrous pericardium**, **parietal pericardium**, and **visceral pericardium**, that covers the surface of the heart. The pleural membrane that lines the cavity is composed of two layers: **parietal pleura**, which lines the cavity wall, and **visceral pleura**, which covers the lungs. Separating the two lungs is a space called the **mediastinum**. A special muscle called the **diaphragm** separates the thoracic cavity from the **abdominopelvic cavity**.

The abdominopelvic cavity is the second subdivision of the ventral cavity. It is also called the **peritoneal cavity**, since the peritoneum, a serous membrane, lines the abdominopelvic cavity. The peritoneal membrane is divided into the **parietal peritoneum**, which lines the wall of the abdominopelvic cavity, and the **visceral peritoneum**, which covers the organs in the cavity. The small space between the two layers of peritoneum is called the **peritoneal space** and contains a serous fluid that aids in lubrication to decrease friction when organs rub against each other. A fold of peritoneum that invests the intestines and attaches them to the posterior abdominal wall for support is called the **mesentery**. Another fold of peritoneum is the **omentum**. It is a double fold of peritoneum and is divided into the greater omentum and the lesser omentum. The greater omentum is attached to the greater curvature of the stomach and hangs loosely downward covering the intestines. It is actually a double sheet of peritoneum folded over on itself, thereby creating four layers. The lesser omentum is a continuous layer with the peritoneal covering of the surface of the stomach and first portion of the duodenum. It is attached to the lesser curvature of the stomach and duodenum.

The first subdivision of the abdominopelvic cavity is the **abdominal cavity**. It contains the stomach, liver, kidneys, gallbladder, spleen, small intestine, and colon. The other subdivision is the **pelvic cavity**, which is enclosed by the bony pelvis. It contains the sigmoid, rectum, urinary bladder, and internal reproductive organs.

The human body is further divided into organ systems; each system contains organs that together perform mutual activities for the system to function. The organization of the systems actually begins at the cellular level. Specialized cells form groups that form specialized tissue, such as muscle tissue, and the different types of tissue form an organ, such as the heart. Finally, organs are grouped together to form an organ or body system that performs a specialized function. The systems are interdependent in order to function correctly and maintain the normal functioning of the body. A good method for remembering the progression is as follows: cells → tissues → organs → systems.

The largest organ system is the **integumentary system**, which includes the skin, sweat glands, sebaceous glands, hair, and nails. Functions include the following:

1. Aids in regulation of body temperature
2. Provides cutaneous sensation
3. Contains receptor sites for detecting pressure
4. Protects tissues and structures that are located underneath the skin
5. Insulates the body
6. Is first line of defense against infection causes by microbes
7. Contains accessory structures such as sweat glands and sebaceous glands
8. Plays a role in the manufacture of vitamin D
9. Facilitates drug absorption such as nicotine patches that help individuals to stop smoking

The **skeletal system** includes the skeleton composed of bones and the muscles, ligaments, cartilage, and tendons. The functions of the system include supporting, giving shape to, and aiding in movement of the body. The bone tissue is also a source of erythrocytes and stores fat in the yellow bone marrow. The skeleton also serves to protect the internal organs. Ligaments, tendons, and cartilage bind the bones together and attach muscle to bone.

Muscles help in maintaining body posture and are a source of body heat. **Skeletal muscles**, also called **voluntary muscles** and **striated muscles**, are attached to the bones; they contract and relax to aid in moving the body. The contraction of the skeletal muscle also helps in pushing blood through the veins back to the heart by "squeezing" the veins and therefore fighting the forces of gravity. **Smooth muscles**, also called **involuntary muscles** and **nonstriated muscles**, comprise one of the layers of the wall of the intestinal tract and blood vessels to help in pushing food through the gastrointestinal tract and blood through the circulatory system. The heart is composed of cardiac muscle and is the only organ that contains both striated and nonstriated muscle.

The **nervous system** consists of the brain, spinal cord, cranial nerves, and peripheral nerves. The main functions of the nervous system include:

1. Sensory: Detecting alterations in external and internal stimuli.
2. Motor: Appropriate behaviors and reactions are initiated.
3. Integrative: Sensory information is analyzed and appropriate behaviors are initiated in response. This includes memory; when a certain stimulus has been previously experienced, it is likely the individual will respond in the same way. It also controls the input from the special senses of sight, hearing, taste, touch, and smell.

The nervous system is subdivided into the **central nervous system (CNS)** and **peripheral nervous system (PNS)**. The CNS consists of the brain and spinal cord. The PNS comprises the nerves that connect the various portions of the body to the CNS. The PNS is further subdivided into the **somatic nervous system (SNS)** and the **autonomic nervous system (ANS)**. The SNS is responsible for connecting the CNS to the skin and skeletal muscles via the cranial and spinal nerves to initiate voluntary movements and responses. The ANS connects the CNS to the visceral organs via the cranial and spinal nerves in order to initiate involuntary responses. The ANS is subdivided into the **sympathetic** and **parasympathetic** divisions. The sympathetic response initiates the "fight or flight" response, whereas the parasympathetic division acts to calm the body, conserve energy, and restore the homeostatic balance.

The **endocrine system** is intimately involved with the nervous system. It consists of the pituitary gland, thyroid, parathyroid glands, pancreas, thymus, adrenal glands, testes, and ovaries. These glands secrete **hormones**, which are responsible for chemically affecting the metabolism and functions of the body. Some of the hormones are very powerful. When a hormone is released it enters the circulatory system to travel toward the group of cells to be affected, which is called **target tissue**. The pituitary gland is called the "master gland," since it has primary control over most of the endocrine glands. The hypothalamus of the brain signals the pituitary to release a hormone that will target one of the other endocrine glands to stimulate the release of its hormone.

The **circulatory system** is divided into two subsystems: (a) the **cardiovascular system**, which consists of the heart, coronary arteries, and great vessels (which include the aorta, pulmonary arteries and veins, and superior and inferior vena cava); and (b) the **peripheral vascular system**, which includes all the arteries, veins, and capillaries outside of the heart. The functions of the circulatory system include:

1. The heart begins the process of pumping oxygenated blood through the vessels of the body.
2. Blood transports the oxygen to the tissues and cells of the body.
3. Deoxygenated blood travels back to the heart and then to the lungs to be reoxygenated.
4. Blood transports wastes to be eliminated by the body.
5. Blood transports hormones.
6. Blood flow aids in maintaining normal body temperature.

The **lymphatic system**, also called the immune system, is composed of the lymph fluid, lymph nodes, lymphatic vessels, spleen, and thymus gland. It is responsible for draining the spaces between cells and tissues, called interstitial space, of excess interstitial fluid to prevent edema, and absorbing fats from the intestinal tract and carrying them to the circulatory system. The cells of the lymphatic system are called **lymphocytes**. They either travel through the system or are fixed and work with the lymph nodes to protect the body from disease by filtering out and destroying disease-causing microorganisms and other foreign-body substances.

The **digestive system** breaks down food particles into simpler forms that can be used for energy by the cells of the body. Indigestible material is transported to the outside of the body. The system includes the mouth, teeth, tongue, salivary glands, pharynx, esophagus, stomach, liver, gallbladder, biliary duct system, pancreas, small intestine, and colon.

The **respiratory system** is responsible for the exchange of oxygen and carbon dioxide between the blood and inhaled air. When a person breathes in air, oxygen is taken into the lungs and the capillaries absorb the oxygen for transport in the blood. In exchange, carbon dioxide leaves the blood to be exhaled by the person. The system consists of the nasal cavity, pharynx, larynx, trachea, bronchi, bronchioles, alveoli, and lungs.

The **genitourinary system**, also referred to as the urinary system, consists of the two kidneys, two ureters, the urinary bladder, and urethra. The kidneys are the filters of the body; they are responsible for removing wastes from the blood, forming urine for elimination of the waste and excess fluid, and maintaining homeostasis by balancing the body's water and electrolyte levels, thereby maintaining the normal pH level within the body.

The **reproductive system** is subdivided into the male reproductive system and the female reproductive system. The male system consists of the scrotum, testes, epididymides, vas deferens, seminal vesicles, prostate gland, bulbourethral glands, urethra, and penis. These structures work together to produce and maintain **spermatozoa**, the sex cells of the male. Some of the structures, such as the urethra and penis, are responsible for transporting the spermatozoa into the female reproductive tract.

The female system consists of the ovaries, fallopian tubes, uterus, vagina, clitoris and external genitalia (collectively called the vulva), and the breasts. These structures work together to produce the ova, (the female sex cells), transport the fertilized egg to the uterus, receive the spermatozoa, support the development of a fertilized ova now called an embryo, and serve during the labor process. The breasts contain the mammary glands that supply colostrums and milk to the infant. Additionally, the organs function in the menstrual cycle when the ova has not been fertilized. As part of the endocrine system, both the male and female reproductive systems function to begin the formation of sexual characteristics and maintenance of these characteristics.

HOMEOSTASIS

Homeostasis is the coordination of all the various functions of the body to maintain a normal internal environment. If an organ is malfunctioning due to disease or injury, a state of imbalance will occur; the body will attempt to correct the situation to reestablish homeostasis or the person may be forced to seek medical help.

The maintenance of life and homeostasis are dependent on many factors to ensure survival; however, the basic requirements for the maintenance of homeostasis are water, food, oxygen, and heat. Obviously food is a necessity, since it provides the chemical substances required for energy, a source of vitamins, and materials needed to maintain and build tissue. The body consists primarily of water; therefore, the need for daily replenishment cannot be overemphasized. The cells and tissues of the body require water to carry out the variety of metabolic processes, regulate body temperature, and transport substances. Humans can live for a short period without water, but that is not the case with oxygen. If a person is de-

prived of oxygen for several minutes, irreversible brain tissue damage or death can occur. Oxygen is essential for use by the cells of the body to stimulate and push forward the metabolic processes, such as contraction of the muscles during exercise. Heat is a form of energy and is a by-product of the metabolic processes. It also contributes to the metabolic rate: less heat, slower rate; more heat, faster rate. Heat affects the temperature of the body.

These factors in coordination with the functioning of the organs of the body work on a constant, daily basis to maintain homeostasis. An example of a homeostatic mechanism is the regulation of the level of glucose in the bloodstream. After an individual eats a meal that has carbohydrates such as vegetables and fruits, the blood glucose level increases due to the breakdown of carbohydrates into the sugar, glucose. Cells use the glucose; however, the excess glucose stimulates the pancreas to release the hormone called insulin. In turn, insulin stimulates the storage of the excess glucose in the liver where is it converted to glycogen. As the excess glucose is stored, the glucose level in the bloodstream returns to normal and the pancreas senses that insulin no longer needs to be excreted. Thus homeostasis is reestablished. However, between meals or if the individual goes for a lengthy period without eating, the blood glucose level decreases below normal. Now the pancreas is stimulated to release glucagon, which breaks down the glycogen in the liver into glucose for release back into the bloodstream. Again, homeostasis is maintained by the return of the blood glucose to a normal level. This example is just one of many homeostatic mechanisms that represent what is called the **negative feedback mechanism**, by which the body's response reverses the stimulus and keeps the organ systems of the body within the **normal ranges** of functioning.

The negative feedback mechanism works by receiving signals or feedback on changes in the internal environment of the body. This initiates a response that reverses the changes in the opposite or negative direction back to the normal level. Although homeostatic mechanisms work at maintaining a constant internal environment, it is understood that each person's physiological values will vary. For example, the normal ranges for adult blood pressure are 100/60 to 140/90. However, a professional triathlete who trains in high altitude could have a blood pressure of 90/50, which is normal for that individual, and a base level (consistent blood pressure reading) is established to demonstrate that normalcy.

The hman body is complex and the organ systems work together to maintain homeostasis. The urinary

Case Study 2

A patient was involved in a motor vehicle accident (MVA) while sitting in the front seat passenger side and wearing a seat belt. When the patient arrived at the Emergency Room the physician noted bruising in the left upper quadrant. The physician quickly inserted a needle with syringe in the umbilical region and withdrew 10 mL of blood. The patient's vital signs were decreasing. The Emergency Room physician immediately called the Surgery Department to notify them that a patient would soon be arriving.

1. What is the most likely diagnosis?

2. What other organs are located in the left upper quadrant?

3. What organs are located in the umbilical region that the doctor would need to ensure were not penetrated by the needle?

4. What type of surgical incisions might be used by the surgeon?

system filters the blood of waste products so a buildup of the waste does not occur in the circulatory system, allowing it to deliver the nutrients obtained from the digestive system and oxygen from the respiratory system to the cells and tissues of the body. If one or more organ systems fails to contribute to maintaining homeostasis, the individual will experience complications, disease, and possibly death if the internal environment cannot be corrected.

CHAPTER SUMMARY

- The study of anatomy and physiology has paralleled the development of cultures, religion, and technology.

- The Greeks and Egyptians made significant contributions to the advancement of medicine and understanding the anatomy of the human body.

- Galen and Andreas Vesalius were two individuals who greatly influenced the study of anatomy and physiology. Vesalius corrected many of Galen's previous findings.

- Anatomy is the study of the structure and morphology of the body and its systems.

- Physiology is the study of the functions of the cells, tissues, and organs of the body.

- Pathophysiology is the study of disease and disorders of the human body. Knowledge of anatomy and physiology is essential to understanding these disorders.

- In the anatomic position, the body is erect and facing forward with arms at the sides and palms of the hands and the feet facing forward.

- Directional terms include superior and inferior, anterior and posterior, medial and lateral, and proximal and distal. These terms are frequently used in surgery.

- The body is sectioned into imaginary geometric planes. The planes are midsagittal plane, sagittal plane, transverse plane, coronal plane, and cross section.

- Reference points are used to identify key anatomic landmarks and features that are often used by the surgeon.

- Some of the more commonly used points of reference include epicondyle, condyle, foramen, fossa, trochanter, triangle of Calot, Hesselbach's triangle, trigone of bladder, ligament of Treitz, and hepatic and splenic flexures.

- The abdomen is divided into quadrants and nine regions.

- When making clinical diagnoses surgeons frequently use quadrants to indicate the area of bodily pain.

- Surgical incisions and location of organ(s) to be operated upon will be indicated by the quadrant or region.

- A transverse plane and a midsagittal plane divide the abdomen into quadrants: right upper quadrant (RUQ), right lower quadrant (RLQ), left upper quadrant (LUQ), and left lower quadrant (LLQ).

- Two sagittal planes and two transverse planes divide the abdomen into nine regions.

- The body is divided into two major cavities: dorsal and ventral.

- The dorsal cavity is subdivided into the cranial cavity and spinal cavity. The membranes that line these two cavities are called meninges.

- The ventral cavity contains the viscera. It is subdivided into the thoracic cavity and abdominopelvic cavity.

- The heart, which is in the thoracic cavity, is contained in the pericardial sac. The pleural membrane that lines the thoracic cavity consists of the parietal pleura and visceral pleura. Separating the two lungs is the mediastinum.

- The diaphragm separates the thoracic cavity from the abdominopelvic cavity, the second subdivision of the ventral cavity.

- The peritoneum lines the abdominopelvic cavity and is divided into the parietal peritoneum and visceral peritoneum. Between the two layers is the peritoneal space, which contains serous fluid.

- The mesentery is a fold of peritoneum that invests the intestines and attaches them to the posterior abdominal wall for support.

- The abdominal cavity is the first subdivision of the abdominopelvic cavity. The second subdivision is the pelvic cavity.

- The human body is further divided into systems. Each system contains organs that work together to make the system function. The organization of the systems is as follows: specialized cells form specialized tissue, which forms an organ, and the organs are grouped together to form a body system that performs a specialized function.

- The integumentary system consists of skin, sweat glands, sebaceous glands, hair, and nails. It is the largest organ system. It regulates body temperature, provides receptor sites for detecting pressure, protects tissues and underlying structures, and insulates the body.

- The skeletal system comprises bones, muscles, ligaments, cartilage, and tendons. It supports and gives shape to the body, aids in movement, is a source of erythrocytes, stores fat in the yellow bone marrow, protects internal organs, binds bones together, and binds muscle to bone.

- There are two types of muscles. Skeletal muscles are attached to bones to aid in moving the body and pushing blood through the veins. Smooth muscles aid in pushing food through the gastrointestinal tract and blood through the vessels. The heart is the only muscle composed of both striated and nonstriated muscle.

- The nervous system consists of the brain, spinal cord, cranial nerves, and peripheral nerves, and is responsible for the sensory, motor, and integrative functions. It is subdivided into the central nervous system and peripheral nervous system. The peripheral nervous system is further subdivided into the somatic nervous system and autonomic nervous system. The autonomic nervous system is subdivided into two divisions: sympathetic and parasympathetic.

- The endocrine system comprises the following: pituitary gland, thyroid, parathyroid glands, thymus, pancreas, adrenal glands, ovaries, and testes. Glands secrete hormones, which are chemically responsible for affecting the metabolism and functions of the body.

- The circulatory system comprises (a) the cardiovascular system—heart, coronary arteries, and great vessels—(b) the peripheral vascular system—arteries, veins, and capillaries outside of the heart. It functions as follows: the heart pumps oxygenated blood into the great vessels for delivery to the rest of the body; blood transports oxygen and nutrients to the tissues and cells of the body; blood transports wastes to be eliminated from the body; and blood transports hormones.

- The lymphatic system consists of lymph fluid, lymph nodes, lymphatic vessels, spleen, and thymus gland. Cells of the lymphatic system are called lymphocytes and coordinate with the lymph nodes in protecting the body from disease by filtering out microorganisms and other foreign-body substances. The system also drains the interstitial space of excess interstitial fluid to prevent edema, and absorbs fats from the intestinal tract and carries them to the circulatory system.

- The digestive system comprises the mouth, teeth, tongue, salivary glands, pharynx, esophagus, stomach, liver, gallbladder, biliary duct system, pancreas, small intestine, and colon. It receives food to be broken down into molecules that can be used by the cells of the body. It also transports the indigestible material for elimination.

- The respiratory system consists of the nasal cavity, pharynx, larynx, trachea, bronchi, bronchioles, alveoli, and lungs. It is responsible for the exchange of oxygen and carbon dioxide between the blood and outside air.

- The genitourinary system comprises two kidneys, two ureters, the urinary bladder, and urethra. The kidneys filter wastes from the blood and form urine to be eliminated from the body.

- The reproductive system is different for the two genders. The male reproductive system comprises scrotum, testes, epididymides, vas deferens, seminal vesicles, prostate gland, bulbourethral glands, urethra, and penis. It produces and maintains spermatozoa; transports spermatozoa into the female reproductive tract; and produces secondary male sexual characteristics by secretion of hormones. The female reproductive system consists of ovaries, fallopian tubes, uterus, vagina, clitoris, vulva, and breasts. It produces the ova; transports the ova to the uterus; receives the spermatozoa; supports the fertilized ova; participates in the menstrual cycle; and produces secondary female sexual characteristics by secretion of hormones.

- Homeostasis is the coordination of all the various functions of the body to maintain a normal internal environment.

- Homeostasis is an indication that a person is healthy, such as a normal blood pressure, normal pulse rate, and normal laboratory results.

- The basic ingredients of life are water, food, oxygen, and heat. These factors along with the functioning of the organs work together to maintain homeostasis on a daily basis.

- The maintenance of a normal level of blood glucose is an example of homeostasis and represents what is called a negative feedback mechanism.

CRITICAL THINKING QUESTIONS

1. List the quadrants of the abdomen and name one body organ located in each quadrant.
2. What is the function of the mesentery?
3. Describe the functions of the three types of muscles.
4. Discuss how the body maintains homeostasis in relation to maintaining normal body temperature.
5. How does the parietal peritoneum differ from the visceral peritoneum?

2

CHEMISTRY, CELLULAR STRUCTURE, AND FUNCTION

CHAPTER OUTLINE

CHAPTER OBJECTIVES

After completing the study of this chapter, you should be able to:

1. Describe the basic concepts of chemistry.
2. Compare and contrast the structures and functions of the cell.
3. Evaluate the importance of cell movement and responsiveness.
4. Compare and contrast the elements of cell reproduction.
5. Compare and contrast glycolysis and the Krebs cycle.

KEY TERMS

acids	cilia	facilitated diffusion	Krebs cycle
active transport	citric acid	flagella	lipids
adenosine triphosphate (ATP)	compounds	genes	lysosomes
anaphase	cytoplasm	glycolysis	matter
bases	cytoplasmic membrane	Golgi apparatus	meiosis
carbohydrates	electrolytes	group translocation	messenger RNA
cellular respiration	elements	heterochromatin	metaphase
centrioles	endoplasmic reticulum (ER)	interphase	microtubules
centromere	energy	ionization	mitochondria
chromatin	euchromatin	ions	mitosis
chromosomes	eukaryotic	kinetic energy	molecules

Case Study 1

Gene is a surgical assistant with a group of plastic surgeons. Today, Gene and Dr. Michaels are removing a basal cell carcinoma from the forehead of a 39-year-old woman under local anesthesia. Dr. Michaels hands the specimen to Gene and instructs him to send it to the lab. The pathologist will look at the specimen's borders to ensure that the "borders are clean."

1. What does "borders are clean" refer to?

2. What would happen if a few cancerous cells were allowed to remain?

3. What would Gene and Dr. Michaels do if the pathologist continued to report that the borders were not clean, and a large portion of skin had to be removed from the forehead?

INTRODUCTION

The surgical technologist must have a solid understanding of the chemistry that makes up life processes because this understanding is the foundation for all basic sciences that follow in the education of the surgical technologist. Without this knowledge, the student cannot fully grasp the complex functions of the cell, and therefore cannot fully grasp the tissues that are made of cells, the organs that are made of tissues, and the systems that are made of organs. In other words, without the foundation of chemistry, proper descriptions cannot be made for all the systems that follow.

We begin the description of anatomic structures and systems with the chemistry of life, and follow it with the details of the structures and processes associated with the human cell. Surgical technologists deal with cells in everything that they do, from learning to destroy cells for sterility, to preserving them for laboratory analysis. Cancerous cells are dealt with daily as well, and many of the newest minimally invasive techniques for surgical procedures, such as sterotactic craniotomies, are designed to preserve normal cells while targeting those with disease.

CHEMISTRY OF LIFE

Chemistry is the science of matter; that is, the branch of the natural sciences that deals with the composition of substances and their properties and reactions. Because body functions are intimately involved with chemical reactions within cells, basic concepts of chemistry are introduced before those related to cell structure and function. In fact, a basic knowledge of chemistry is essential to the understanding of physiology.

Matter

Objects that have mass and take up space are referred to as **matter**. It is important to note that weight and mass are different; weight represents the pull that the Earth's gravity has on an object (an object has weight relative to its distance to a large object), and mass is the amount of matter an object contains.

All matter is the same in that it is all made up of atoms, but different types of atoms make up different types of matter. It is essentially the properties of the atoms that give matter its individual, distinct properties.

Matter is constantly in a state of flux given the conditions that surround it (usually a change in temperature). Physical changes in matter allow it to change states but retain its identifying characteristics. For example, ice is water in the solid state, but if the ice is dropped into a liquid, it begins to melt because the temperature is higher than that of the ice. If the water is heated, it changes to a gas form (steam).

Energy

Light, electricity, sound, and heat are not forms of matter, but are actually forms of **energy** that produce changes in matter. The most common form of energy is mechanical energy, the type of energy that makes objects move or change course. The mechanical energy of an object is measured by the amount of work it can do.

An object can store energy as the result of its position. For example, a cart poised at the top of a hill stores energy as a result of its position. This stored energy of position is referred to as **potential energy**. The cart would not have potential energy if it were sitting at the base of the hill. A firecracker has chemical potential energy, as does the battery of a car. Elastic potential energy is the energy stored in elastic materials as the result of stretching or compressing, as in a rubber band or bungee cord.

Kinetic energy is the energy of motion. The cart at the top of the hill expends its potential energy as it speeds down the hill. Just before it began to move, the cart had only potential energy; just before it reached the bottom of the hill, it had only kinetic energy.

The mechanical energy of an object can be the result of its motion (e.g., kinetic energy) or the result of its stored energy of position (e.g., potential energy). The total amount of mechanical energy is merely the sum of the potential energy and the kinetic energy. This sum is simply referred to as the total mechanical energy (TME). Therefore, TME = PE + KE.

Atoms

The Bohr model of the atom describes its structure as electrons circling the nucleus at different levels, or orbitals, much like planets circle the sun. This model was proposed by Niels Bohr in 1915; it is not completely correct, but is an approximate representation close to the one described by the theory of quantum mechanics, which more accurately describes the atomic model. This similarity between a planetary model and the Bohr model of the atom ultimately arises because the attractive gravitational force in a solar system and the attractive Coulomb (electrical) force between the positively charged nucleus and the negatively charged electrons in an atom are mathematically of the same form.

Atoms are composed of three types of particles: protons, neutrons, and electrons. Protons and neutrons are responsible for most of the atomic mass because the mass of an electron is very small. Figure 2-1 reveals the structure of the atom.

Both the protons and neutrons reside in the nucleus of the atom, but protons have a positive charge, whereas neutrons have no charge. The orbiting electrons are negatively charged. For any element, the electrons in the outermost energy level (shell) are the most important. Called valence electrons, these determine an element's chemical properties—how it will react in a chemical reaction.

The number of protons determines the atomic number of the atom, and is typically equal to the number of orbiting electrons. The number of protons in an element is constant (e.g., H = 1, Ur = 92) but the neutron number may vary, so mass number (protons + neutrons) may vary. Varying numbers of neutrons within an element form elements called isotopes. An isotope consists of two nuclei of the same element that have

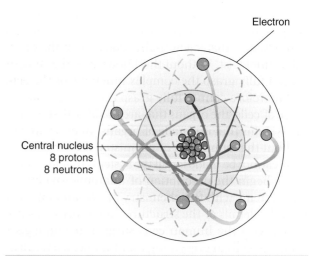

FIGURE 2-1 The structure of an atom. Eight protons and eight neutrons are tightly bound in the central nucleus, around which the eight electrons revolve

the same atomic number but different masses. For example, Uranium-238 contains 92 protons and 146 neutrons, whereas the isotope U-235 contains 92 protons and 143 neutrons. Oxygen has an atomic number of 8 but may have 8, 9, or 10 neutrons. The chemical properties of isotopes are the same, although the physical properties may differ.

Elements

All matter is made up of fundamental **elements** that cannot be broken down by chemical means. There are 92 elements that occur naturally (and a few more synthetic varieties). Hydrogen, carbon, nitrogen, and oxygen are the elements that make up most living organisms. Other elements found in living organisms include calcium, magnesium, sodium, phosphorus, and potassium.

Elements are sorted according to their chemical properties, listed horizontally in order by atomic number on the Periodic Table of Elements. Living organisms require chemically reactive gases; therefore, the noble gases, such as helium, are not found in living organisms. Atoms constantly seek stable electron configurations, like the noble gases, and can obtain stability by losing, sharing, or gaining electrons. For a stable configuration, each atom must fill its outer energy level, but the maximum number that can exist at any level is strictly limited:

- First level: two electrons
- Second level: eight electrons
- Third level: eight electrons
- Fourth level: eight electrons

Atoms that have one, two, or three electrons in their outer levels will tend to lose them in interactions with atoms that have five, six, or seven electrons in their outer levels. Atoms that have five, six, or seven electrons in their outer levels will tend to gain electrons from atoms with one, two, or three electrons in their outer levels. Atoms that have four electrons in the outermost energy level will neither totally lose nor totally gain electrons during interactions. **Ionization** is the gain or loss of electrons. The loss of electrons converts an atom into a positively charged ion, whereas the gain of electrons converts an atom into a negatively charged ion.

Compounds

A **compound** is a substance that can be broken down into two or more other substances by chemical means. Certain elements can combine in specific proportions to form a compound, but the compound has different properties than the separate elements comprising them. For example, H_2O is made of oxygen and hydrogen, both gaseous elements. But combined, they form a compound that is liquid in nature.

Compounds are represented by formulas that describe the elements that combine to form them. The formula also describes the proportion of each element within the compound by weight. Common formulas include table salt (NaCl), baking powder ($NaHCO_3$), glucose ($C_6H_{12}O_6$), carbon dioxide (CO_2), and carbon monoxide (CO).

Molecules

Molecules are groups of atoms joined by chemical bonds (created by electron attraction and interaction). For example, 12 carbon atoms, 22 hydrogen atoms, and 6 oxygen atoms combine to form one sugar molecule ($C_6H_{12}O_6$).

Molecular weight equals the sum of the atomic weights of the atoms in the molecule. A salt molecule (NaCl) contains one sodium and one chlorine atom. The atomic weight of sodium is 23 and the weight of chlorine is 35; therefore, $23 + 35 = 58$, the molecular weight of NaCl.

Inorganic and Organic Compounds

Most of the body's chemicals exist in the form of compounds that can be divided into two primary classes. Inorganic compounds are made of molecules that do not contain the element carbon. They include oxygen, carbon dioxide, water, and many **salts**, acids, and bases.

An organic compound is any of a large class of chemical compounds the molecules of which contain carbon, with the exception of carbides, carbonates, and carbon oxides. Organic compounds are studied in organic chemistry; many of them, such as proteins, fats, and carbohydrates, are also of prime importance in biochemistry (described in detail later in this chapter). The dividing line between organic and inorganic is somewhat arbitrary, but, generally speaking, organic compounds have carbon-hydrogen bonds, and inorganic compounds do not.

Ions and Electrolytes

The electrons of atoms can be shared with other atoms to form chemical bonds. If an atom gives up an electron to another atom, it will have more protons than electrons, and therefore a positive charge. The atom that received the electron will have more electrons than protons and will therefore have a negative charge.

A positively or negatively charged atom is referred to as an **ion**. Ions make it possible for compounds to recombine into new and different compounds.

A compound that disassociates into positive and negative ions in a solution is called an **electrolyte,** so named because it can conduct an electric current. For body functions, electrolytes play important roles. For example, they serve as cofactors for enzyme activity and production. Certain ions control the osmosis of water between body compartments, and help maintain the acid–base balance required for cellular activities. Because they carry an electric current, ions can control production of action potentials, allow for secretion of neurotransmitters, and control hormone secretions.

Acids, Bases, and Salts

In the seventeenth century, the English writer and amateur chemist Robert Boyle first labeled substances as either **acids** or **bases** by noting that acids have a sour taste, are corrosive to metals, and become less acidic when mixed with bases. Bases, he noted, feel slippery and become less basic when mixed with acids. He also noted that acids change litmus (a dye extracted from lichens) red, whereas bases change litmus blue.

In the late 1800s Swedish scientist Svante Arrhenius suggested that acids are compounds that contain hydrogen and can dissolve in water to release hydrogen ions into solution. Arrhenius defined bases as substances that dissolve in water to release hydroxide ions (OH$^-$) into solution.

In 1923, Johannes Bronsted and Thomas Lowry refined Arrhenius's theory by stating that acids and bases are substances that are capable of splitting off or taking up hydrogen ions, respectively. Although the Bronsted–Lowry definition of acids is very similar to the Arrhenius definition (in that any substance that can donate a hydrogen ion is an acid), the Bronsted definition of bases is completely different from the Arrhenius definition. The Bronsted base is defined as any substance that can accept a hydrogen ion, meaning that a base is the exact opposite of an acid, explaining why substances that do not contain OH$^-$ can act like bases.

We know now that both acids and bases are related to the concentration of hydrogen ions present in a dissolved solution. Acids increase the concentration of hydrogen ions, whereas bases decrease the concentration of hydrogen ions by accepting them. Therefore, the acidity or alkalinity (basicity) of something can be measured by its hydrogen ion concentration.

For homeostasis, there must be a relatively equal balance between the amounts of acids and bases in the body. Chemical reactions are sensitive to small changes in this balance. A solution's acidity or alkalinity is expressed by the **pH scale**.

pH Scale

In 1909, the Danish biochemist Sören Sörensen invented the pH scale for measuring acidity; the scale ranges from 0 to 14. Substances with a pH between 0 and less than 7 are acids, whereas substances with a pH greater than 7 and up to 14 are bases (the higher the pH, the stronger the base). Right in the middle, at pH = 7, are neutral substances (e.g., pure water). Figure 2-2 shows the color changes that occur on a pH strip, and also shows the pH values of some common acids, bases, and human body fluids.

Homeostatic mechanisms maintain the pH of blood between 7.35 and 7.45, which is slightly more basic than pure water. Urine can be acidic because the kidneys remove excess acid from the blood. Buffer systems in the body convert strong acids or bases (which are unstable and ionize rather easily) into weaker acids or bases.

INTRODUCTION TO AND HISTORY OF CELLS

The smallest living units of the human body are cells, some 75 trillion to 100 trillion of them that fall into more than 100 different types. The health of the body is directly related to the health of its cells, and, in fact, many diseases, such as cancer, can be traced directly to malfunctioning cells.

The development of the microscope opened up new doors in the field of biology by allowing scientists to observe the cellular world. Zacharias Jansen, of Middleburg, Holland, developed the first compound microscope in the year 1595. Other microscope pioneers included Athanasius Kircher and Anton von Leeuwenhoek.

Robert Hooke was an English naturalist who, in the year 1663, coined the term *cell* after viewing slices of cork through a microscope. The term came from the Latin word *cella*, which means "storeroom" or "small compartment." He documented his work in the book *Micrographia: Physiological Descriptions of Minute Bodies made by Magnifying Glasses*, written in 1665.

In 1824, Rene Dutrochet stated that "the cell is the fundamental element in the structure of living bodies, forming both animals and plants through juxta-

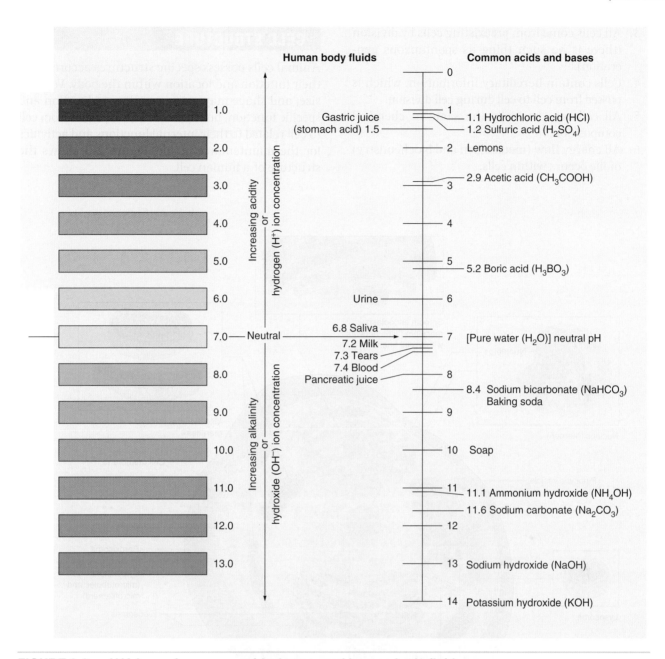

FIGURE 2-2   pH Values of common acids, bases, and human body fluids

position." However, the first sightings of the internal action of the cell were made by Robert Brown.

Matthias Schleiden and Theodor Schwann proposed the cell theory in 1838, which stated the following:

1. The cell is the unit of structure, physiology, and organization in living things.
2. The cell retains a dual existence as a distinct entity and a building block in the construction of organisms.
3. Cells form by free-cell formation, similar to the formation of crystals (spontaneous generation).

We now know that the first two tenets are correct and that the third is wrong. The correct interpretation of cell formation by division was finally enunciated by Rudolph Virchow's powerful dictum, "Omnis cellula e cellula," which means "all cells only arise from preexisting cells."

The modern tenets of the cell theory are as follows:

1. All known living things are made up of cells.
2. The cell is the structural and functional unit of all living things.

3. All cells come from preexisting cells by division (there is no such thing as spontaneous generation).
4. Cells contain hereditary information, which is passed from cell to cell during cell division.
5. All cells are basically the same in chemical composition.
6. All energy flow (metabolism and biochemistry) of life occurs within cells.

CELL STRUCTURE

Animal cells possess specific structures according to their function and location within the body. Volume, size, and shape may vary according to location and specific function, but there are consistencies from cell to cell related to their internal functions and activities for the maintenance of life. Figure 2-3 shows the structure of a human cell.

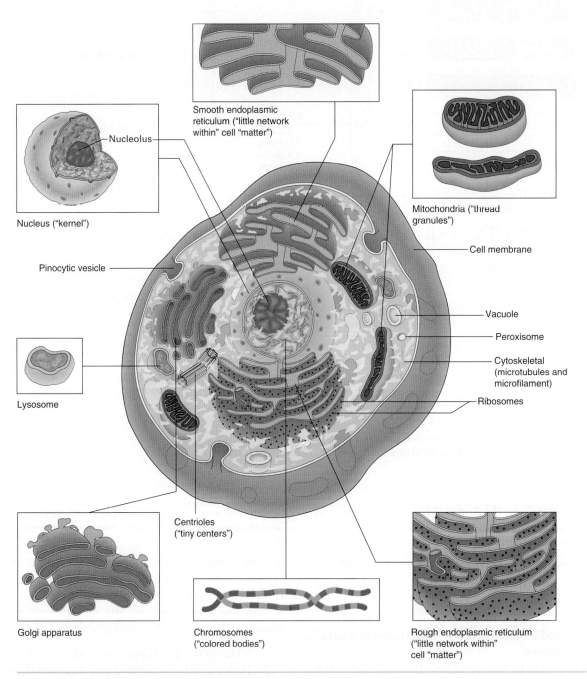

Smooth endoplasmic reticulum ("little network within" cell "matter")

Nucleolus

Nucleus ("kernel")

Mitochondria ("thread granules")

Pinocytic vesicle

Cell membrane

Vacuole

Peroxisome

Cytoskeletal (microtubules and microfilament)

Ribosomes

Lysosome

Golgi apparatus

Centrioles ("tiny centers")

Chromosomes ("colored bodies")

Rough endoplasmic reticulum ("little network within" cell "matter")

FIGURE 2-3 **The structure of a human cell**

Size and Shape

Cell shape is controlled by the extracellular matrix and the cytoskeletal structure within the cell. The shape of the cell depends partly on the surface tension and viscosity of the cytoplasm, the mechanical action that the adjoining cells exert, and the rigidity of the membrane. Many cells have a polyhedral shape, which is determined principally by pressure from adjacent cells. In these cases, the original spherical form is modified by contact with the other cells.

Some cells, such as leukocytes, have a variable shape, while others are relatively stable (such as erythrocytes, epithelial cells, muscle cells, and nerve cells). These cells have a fixed shape with a specific characteristic for each cell type. When isolated in a liquid medium, many cells tend to take on a spherical form, obeying the laws of surface tension. For example, leukocytes in circulating blood are spherical, but by the influence of adequate stimuli can resemble ameboid movement and become completely irregular in shape. When fixed cells are removed from the body and placed into culture dishes, they form distinct shapes: nerve cells produce axon processes, muscle cells produce contractile proteins, and epithelial cells form sheets of continuous cells.

With the exception of the nerve cells, cell volume varies between 200 cubic microns and 15,000 cubic microns. In general, the volume of the cell is fairly constant for any one cell type and independent of the size of the individual. The differences in the total mass of any body organ are due to the number and not to the volume of the cells.

Composition

As described earlier, these organic compounds always contain the element carbon (C) combined with hydrogen or other elements. There are four primary groups of organic compounds, and all cells are composed of these four types of macromolecules (biological building blocks): carbohydrates, proteins, lipids (fats), and nucleic acids.

Carbohydrates

Carbohydrates, also referred to as sugars, are composed of chains of carbon atoms with hydrogen and oxygen atoms attached in the C:H:O ratio of 1:2:1. Carbohydrates are the molecules from which all other biomolecules are derived. They can exist as single-sugar units (called monosaccharides), as two-sugar units (called disaccharides), or as long chains or polymers of sugar units (called polysaccharides). Monosaccharides can exist as a linear or ring-shaped molecule.

Proteins

Proteins are composed of building blocks called amino acids. This name is derived from the fact that amino acids contain an amine (NH_2) group on one end and a carboxylic acid (COOH) on the other end, separated by a carbon in the center. Amino acids are attached together into chains called **peptides** by covalent peptide bonds between the NH_2 of one and the COOH of the next. Long chains of amino acids are called polypeptides or proteins. There are 20 types of amino acids found in proteins, each differing only by the side chain ("R" group) attached to the central carbon.

Lipids

Lipids, or simple fats, are composed of chains of molecules called triglycerides. Each triglyceride contains a molecule of glycerol (a hydrophilic 3-carbon molecule) and three fatty acids (long hydrophobic hydrocarbon chains) joined to the three carbons of the glycerol by covalent ester or ether bonds.

Nucleic Acids

Nucleic acids, RNA (ribonucleic acid) and DNA (deoxyribonucleic acid), are long linear polymers of smaller subunits called nucleotides. Each nucleotide is composed of a nitrogenous base, a pentose sugar (ribose for RNA or deoxyribose for DNA), and a phosphate. In RNA nucleotides, the bases are adenine, guanine, cytosine, or uracil. In DNA nucleotides, the bases are adenine, guanine, cytosine, and thymine. Nitrogenous bases are cyclic molecules composed of both carbon and nitrogen in the ring structure.

Cytoplasm

Cytoplasm is defined as the material that lies within the cytoplasmic membrane, (the membrane that surrounds a cell). Although it contains none of a cell's genetic material, it does contain a lot of water and the cell's organelles. It is made up of proteins, vitamins, ions, nucleic acids, amino acids, sugars, carbohydrates, and fatty acids. All of the functions for cell expansion, growth, and replication are carried out in the cytoplasm of a cell.

Cell (Cytoplasmic) Membrane

The **cytoplasmic membrane** is that area of the cell immediately surrounding the cytoplasm. Membranes are thin structures, measuring 8 nm thick. They are the major barrier in the cell, separating the inside of the cell from the outside. It is this structure that allows cells to selectively interact with their environment. Membranes are highly organized and are also dynamic, constantly adapting to changing environmental conditions.

Membranes are composed of **phospholipids** and proteins. Phospholipids contain a charged or polar group (often a phosphate, hence the name) attached to a 3-carbon glycerol backbone. There are also two fatty acid chains dangling from the other carbons of glycerol. The phosphate end of the molecule is hydrophilic and is attracted to water. The fatty acids are hydrophobic and are driven away from water.

Because phospholipids have hydrophobic and hydrophilic portions, they do remarkable things. When placed in an aqueous environment, the hydrophobic portions stick together, as do the hydrophilic. A very stable form of this arrangement is the lipid bilayer, in which the hydrophobic parts of the molecule form one layer, as do the hydrophilic. Lipid bilayers form spontaneously if phospholipids are placed in an aqueous environment. These are known as membrane vesicles and are used to study membrane properties experimentally.

Typically, 20%–30% of membrane proteins are soluble in water and loosely associated. The other 70%–80% are tightly bound to the membrane, often spanning both sides. These proteins are also often amphipathic molecules (contain both hydrophobic and hydrophilic portions) with stretches of both hydrophilic and hydrophobic amino acids. Most of them are situated within the membranes so that the hydrophobic amino acids associate with the lipids in the membrane and the hydrophilic amino acids are outside the membrane interacting with the cytoplasm.

Functions of the Cell Membrane

The cell membrane retains the cytoplasm. The concentration of solutes, sugars, ions, and so on, are much higher within the cell than outside. A fundamental principle of nature, however, is that solute concentrations tend to equilibrate, causing water to flow into the cell (a process known as osmosis) and the solutes to flow out. Therefore, nutrients can come in and wastes can go out. The cell membrane prevents free flow of material and thus serves as an osmotic, selective barrier. Figure 2-4 illustrates the process of osmosis.

Some molecules can cross the membrane without assistance, but most cannot. Water, nonpolar molecules, and some small polar molecules can cross. Nonpolar molecules penetrate by actually dissolving into the lipid bilayer. Most polar compounds, such as amino acids, organic acids, and inorganic salts, are not allowed entry, and must be specifically transported across the membrane by proteins.

Many of the proteins in the membrane function to help carry out selective transport. These proteins typically span the whole membrane, making contact with the outside environment and the cytoplasm. They often require the expenditure of energy to help compounds move across the membrane.

There are four basic types of transport systems:

- **Passive diffusion**
- **Facilitated diffusion**
- **Group translocation**
- **Active transport**

During passive diffusion, molecular transport is directed by laws of simple diffusion. There is no transport protein, it is nonspecific, and energy is not required. A concentration gradient of these molecules cannot be generated. Compounds capable of

Initial stage

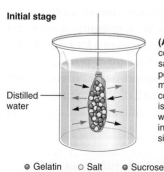

Distilled water

• Gelatin ○ Salt • Sucrose

(A) Initially, the sausage casing contains a solution of gelatin, salt, and sucrose. The casing is permeable to water and salt molecules only. Because the concentration of water molecules is greater outside the casing, water molecules will diffuse into the casing. The opposite situation exists for the salt.

10-12 hours later

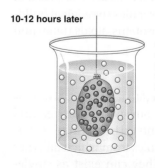

(B) The sausage casing swells due to the net movement of water molecules inward. However, the volume of distilled water in the beaker remains constant.

FIGURE 2-4   Osmosis: the diffusion of water through a semipermeable membrane (a sausage casing is an example of a semipermeable membrane)

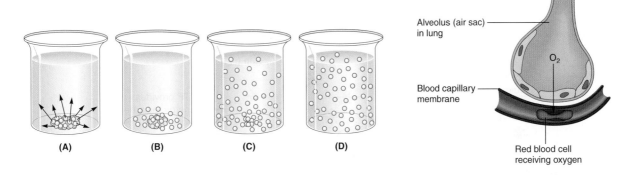

FIGURE 2-5   Diffusion: (A) A small lump of sugar is placed into a beaker of water; its molecules dissolve and begin to move outward. (B and C) The sugar molecules continue to diffuse through the water from an area of greater concentration to an area of lesser concentration. (D) Over time, the sugar molecules are evenly distributed throughout the water, reaching a state of equilibrium.

Example of diffusion in the human body: oxygen diffuses from an alveolus in a lung where it is in greater concentration, across the blood capillary membrane, into a red blood cell where it is in lesser concentration.

passive diffusion must be soluble both in the lipid membrane and in the cytoplasm outside of the cell. Figure 2-5 reveals the process of diffusion.

Facilitated diffusion involves a protein that binds a molecule for transport across the cell membrane, and is, therefore, specific. However, solutes are neither concentrated against a gradient, nor is energy required.

During group translocation, a protein specifically binds the target molecule and during transport a chemical modification takes place. No actual concentration of the transported substance takes place because it is chemically different as it enters the cell. Most group translocation requires energy.

In active transport, the target is not altered and a significant accumulation occurs in the cytoplasm, with the inside concentration reaching many times its external concentration. Active transport proteins are molecular pumps that pump their substrates against a concentration gradient. As in all pumps, fuel is necessary and in the case of cells, this fuel comes in two forms, **adenosine triphosphate (ATP)** or the proton motive force (PMF). Figure 2-6 illustrates the process of active transport.

Membranes also contain specialized enzymes that carry out many biosynthetic functions. These functions include:

1. Membrane synthesis
2. Cell wall assembly
3. Secretion of many proteins

Nucleus

The **nucleus** is the largest, most prominent structure within a cell and its presence within a cell distinguishes the cell as being **eukaryotic**, meaning "possessing a true nucleus," versus being **prokaryotic**, meaning "lacking a true nucleus." Eukaryotic nuclear materials are bound by a membrane (called the nuclear membrane), but prokaryotic nuclear materials are not.

The cell nucleus is a remarkable organelle because it forms the package for our genes and their controlling factors, and guides the life processes of the cell. The nucleus houses the DNA, which stores genetic information for a cell. The DNA contains instructions for the production of the cell's proteins and for reproduction.

Structurally, the nucleus is composed of three main parts: the nucleolus, the nuclear envelope, and the chromatin (described later). The nucleus functions to:

1. Direct cellular reproduction, where a cell divides into two new cells.
2. Control a cell's differentiation during the development of the organism.
3. Regulate the metabolic activities of the cell.
4. Produce messages with messenger ribonucleic acid or mRNA (described later) that code for proteins.
5. Produce ribosomes in the nucleolus.
6. Organize the uncoiling of DNA to replicate key genes.

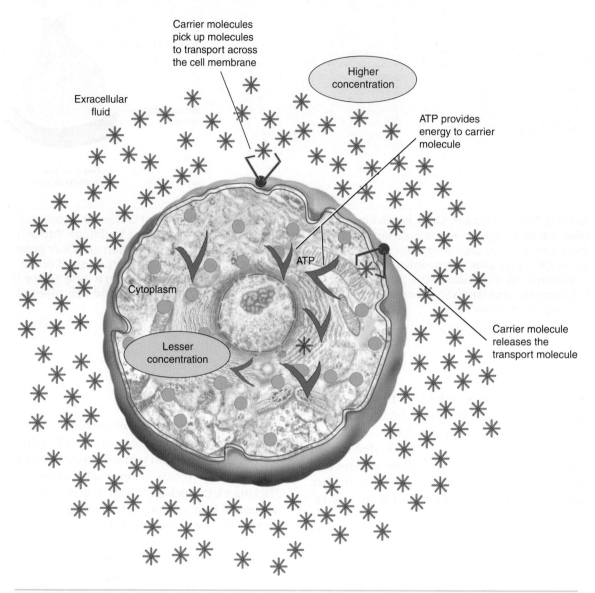

Carrier molecules pick up molecules to transport across the cell membrane

Higher concentration

Exracellular fluid

ATP provides energy to carrier molecule

ATP

Cytoplasm

Lesser concentration

Carrier molecule releases the transport molecule

FIGURE 2-6   Active transport of molecules from an area of lesser concentration to an area of greater concentration

Nuclear Membrane

The nucleus is enveloped by a pair of membranes enclosing a lumen that is continuous with that of the endoplasmic reticulum (ER; described later in the chapter). The nucleus is surrounded by a membrane, called the **nuclear envelope**, which is similar to the cell membrane that encloses the entire cell. The envelope is riddled with holes, called nuclear pores, which allow specific materials to pass in and out of the nucleus (much like proteins in the cell membrane regulate the movement of molecules in and out of the cell itself). Attached to the nuclear envelope is the ER. The nucleus is surrounded by the cytoplasm inside a cell.

The nuclear envelope is important because it allows the nucleus to control the rest of the cell, such as by sending out ATP. The envelope will let molecules like ATP through but will keep other things in or out, so the nucleus is isolated from the cytoplasm.

Nucleolus

The **nucleolus** contains ribosomes, RNA, DNA, and proteins, and is the site where ribosomal RNA (rRNA) is transcribed, processed, and assembled into ribosome subunits. The ribosomes can pass from the nucleus through the nuclear pores into the cytoplasm, where they aid in protein synthesis. In recent years, the nucleolus has been implicated in many aspects of cell biology, and now includes functions such as gene silencing and cell cycle regulation.

Chromatin and Chromosomes

Chromatin (meaning "colored substance") is the name that describes nuclear material that contains the genetic code. In fact, the code is stored in individual units called **chromosomes** (described in detail later). As we shall see in subsequent text, these are highly ordered, organized packages designed for the storage of genetic material, its condensation during cell division (when the cell divides, the chromosomes fold up on themselves, getting wider), and regulation of gene expression.

Two types of chromatin can be described as follows:

1. **Heterochromatin** is the condensed form of chromatin organization, and is seen under a microscope as dense patches of chromatin. Sometimes it lines the nuclear membrane, but it is broken by clear areas at the pores so that transport is allowed. Abundant heterochromatin is seen in resting or reserve cells, such as lymphocyte memory cells that are waiting for exposure to a foreign antigen.
2. **Euchromatin** is threadlike and delicate, and is most abundant in active, transcribing cells. Its presence is significant because the regions of DNA to be transcribed or duplicated must uncoil before the genetic code can be read.

Just before cell division (and after DNA synthesis), the chromatin condenses further into individual metaphase chromosomes. The dividing chromosomes appear as two chromatids (described later in the chapter).

Organelles

Organelles are highly specialized structures that are designed for specific cellular activities. These structures include lysosomes, vacuoles, the endoplasmic reticulum, mitochondria, the Golgi apparatus, ribosomes, centrioles, cilia, and flagella. Each organelle's function is described in Table 2-1.

Lysosomes

Lysosomes digest waste materials and food within the cell, breaking down molecules into their base components with strong digestive enzymes. The presence of these structures illustrates the advantage of the compartmentalization of the eukaryotic cell: the cell could not support such destructive enzymes if they were not contained in a membrane-bound lysosome.

TABLE 2-1	Functions of Cell Organelles
ORGANELLE	**FUNCTION**
Cell membrane	Regulates transport of substances into and out of the cell.
Cytoplasm	Provides an organized watery environment in which life functions take place by the activities of the organelles contained in the cytoplasm.
Nucleus	Serves as the "brain" for the control of the cell's metabolic activities and cell division.
Nuclear membrane	Regulates transport of substances into and out of the nucleus.
Nucleoplasm	A clear, semifluid medium that fills the spaces around the chromatin and the nucleoli.
Nucleolus	Functions as a reservoir for RNA.
Ribosomes	Serve as sites for protein synthesis.
Endoplasmic reticulum	Provides passages through which transport of substances occurs in cytoplasm.
Mitochondria	Serves as sites of cellular respiration and energy production; stores ATP.
Golgi apparatus	Manufactures carbohydrates and packages secretions for discharge from the cell.
Lysosomes	Serve as centers for cellular digestion.
Peroxisome	Enzymes oxidize cell substances.
Centrosome and centrioles	Contains two centrioles that are functional during animal cell division.
Cytoskeleton	Forms internal framework.

Vacuoles

Vacuoles are membranous sacs that are formed when a portion of the cell membrane folds inward and pinches off, bringing with it a piece of substance from outside of the cell to the inside.

Endoplasmic Reticulum

The **endoplasmic reticulum (ER)** is the transport network for molecules targeted for certain modifications and specific final destinations, as opposed to molecules that are destined to float freely in the cytoplasm. There are two types of ER, rough and smooth. Rough ER has ribosomes attached to it, and smooth ER does not.

Mitochondria

Mitochondria are membrane-enclosed organelles distributed throughout the cytosol of most eukaryotic cells. They are the sites of aerobic respiration, and generally are the major energy production center in eukaryotes. In fact, their main function is the conversion of the potential energy of food molecules into ATP.

Mitochondria have two membranes, an inner and an outer. This configuration serves to increase the surface area of membrane on which membrane-bound reactions can take place. The existence of this double membrane has led many biologists to theorize that mitochondria are the descendants of some bacteria that was endocytosed, but not digested by a larger cell billions of years ago. This fascinating theory of symbiosis, which might lend an explanation to the development of eukaryotic cells, has additional supporting evidence. Mitochondria have their own DNA and their own ribosomes; and those ribosomes are more similar to bacterial ribosomes than to eukaryotic ribosomes.

A cell may have hundreds or even thousands of mitochondria depending on the particular cell's need for energy. (For example, the average human liver cell contains more than a thousand mitochondria.)

Of interest to the genealogist (among others) is the fact that all of an individual's mitochondria are derived from his or her mother. Although the sperm cell tail is packed with mitochondria to power its long journey to the egg cell, the tail and mitochondria drop off the sperm at fertilization and never enter the egg cell. Consequently, all of the mitochondria in the fertilized egg come from an individual's mother.

Golgi Apparatus

The **Golgi apparatus**, located near the nucleus, is composed of stacks of flattened membranous sacs. It modifies and refines proteins synthesized by the endoplasmic reticulum and packages them into small membrane-bound sacs called **vesicles**. The proteins arrive with a sugar molecule attached and are referred to as glycoproteins. The glycoproteins pass from layer after layer of the stacks, where they are modified chemically before passing into the cell membrane and outside of the cell, or into the cytoplasmic organelles.

Ribosomes

Ribosomes are the sites of protein synthesis where RNA is translated into protein. Protein synthesis is extremely important to cells, and so large numbers of ribosomes are found throughout cells (often numbering in the hundreds or thousands). Ribosomes exist floating freely in the cytoplasm, and also bound to the ER. ER bound to ribosomes is called rough ER because the ribosomes appear as black dots on the ER in electron microscope photos, giving the ER a rough texture.

Free ribosomes are found in the cytosol, and are responsible for proteins that go into solution in the cytoplasm or form important cytoplasmic structural or motile elements.

Bound ribosomes are bound to the exterior of the ER, and occur in greater number than free ribosomes in cells that secrete their manufactured proteins (e.g., pancreatic cells, producers of digestive enzymes). They are responsible for proteins that become a part of membranes or packaged into vesicles for storage in the cytoplasm or export to the cell exterior.

The main function of ribosomes is to serve as the site of **messenger RNA** (mRNA) translation (protein synthesis, the assembly of amino acids into proteins); once the two (large and small) subunits are joined by the mRNA from the nucleus, the ribosome translates the mRNA into a specific sequence of amino acids, or a polypeptide chain.

Centrioles, Cilia, and Flagella

Centrioles are cylindrical structures that are composed of groupings of microtubules arranged in a 9 + 3 pattern. The pattern is so named because a ring of nine microtubule "triplets" are arranged at right angles to one another. Centrioles are found in animal cells and play a role in cell division. Centrioles replicate in the interphase stage of mitosis and they help to organize the assembly of microtubules during cell division. Centrioles called "basal bodies" form **cilia** and **flagella**. A basal body is like a centriole except that it is found at the base of a cilium or flagellum. Both centrioles and basal bodies are similar in that they consist of an outer ring of nine paired tubulin tubes.

There are pairs of centrioles near the nucleus in eukaryote cells. They are involved in cell division (mitosis and meiosis). Each centriole consists of a bundle of nine filaments. At the beginning of cell division the centrioles move to opposite ends of the cell.

During the final stage of mitosis (telophase), two new nuclei are formed. By the end of cell division the centrioles are replicated, so that each new nucleus now has two centrioles rather than one.

Cilia and flagella move in a whiplike fashion, which is accomplished using a separate set of proteins that form arms attached to the tubulin. These protein arms allow neighboring tubulin tubes to slide past each other and bend the cilium. Cilia and flagella are similar but cilia tend to be much shorter than the length of the cell. Also cilia have a power stroke much like a swimmer would have, whereas flagella tend to pull the organism through water as a propeller pulls an airplane through the air.

Cilia function to move fluid or materials past an immobile cell as well as moving a cell or group of cells. The respiratory tract in humans is lined with cilia that keep inhaled dust, smog, and potentially harmful microorganisms from entering the lungs.

Cilia and flagella are used for cellular propulsion (e.g., sperm) or for transporting extracellular substances (e.g., embryonic fluid, oviduct and tracheal contents, and cerebrospinal fluid). Nonmotile cilia function in sensory cells, for example, in retinal photoreceptors and olfactory neurons. Human diseases and conditions in which cilia are affected include infertility, respiratory disorders, polycystic kidney disease, and situs inversus (left–right reversal of organs).

CELL MOVEMENT AND RESPONSIVENESS

Many cells are not stationary but can travel from one place to another. If cells could not move, embryos would not develop, wounds would never heal, and many tumors could not send off cells to colonize other parts of the body. Cells are complex and dynamic machines that can generate force along their own skeletons to move and to divide. Examples of cell movement include ciliary and flagellar propulsion and muscle contraction. White blood cells move into surrounding tissues and seek invaders. Cell movement also occurs in loose connective tissue, as fibroblasts that secrete a collagen matrix migrate to areas that have become wounded. Deep wounds stimulate a number of cells to divide and move.

Internal cellular movement is controlled by structures formed by the cellular cytoskeleton. These movements control DNA replication and cytokinesis and internal transport mechanisms such as vesicle movement.

Basic research into cell locomotion is very important because it helps us to understand wound healing, the movement of cancer cells, our immune system, and the development of human and animal embryos.

Scientists discovered several years ago that certain cells glide forward in a microscopic version of "moon walking." They have recently discovered that calcium channels (which function when cells stretch) help regulate cell movement. This finding of calcium channels may one day have profound clinical implications in wound healing and cancer treatment, the researchers say.

When cells are stretched, such as when they are going forward and their back end gets stuck, calcium channels along the sides open to admit more calcium ions. This boosts the cell's motility so that the back end is pulled away from whatever it has been stuck on, and it can move forward again.

BOX 2-1

Cancer Cell Movement

Cancer would not be the killer that it is if it did not have the capability to move and it did not know where to go. Better understanding of cancer cell movement could lead to steps both to inhibit tumor cell migration in the body and to prevent invasion of cancer cells into tissues. Active tumor cell movement highlights cancer's invasion into other parts of the body and its routing in previously unaffected tissues. The cells move in two stages by temporarily projecting their protoplasm forward (called pseudopod protrusion) in response to chemical attractants in the body. Each phase is regulated by separate signals within the cell.

In the initial phase, a cancer cell swells to form a convex, outward-reaching pouch. The activity is regulated by osmotic pressure, which developed because solutions of different solute concentrations were separated by the cell's semipermeable membrane. The semipermeable cell membrane allows only water molecules to pass, and the water moves into the solution containing the higher concentration of solute molecules (osmosis).

During the second phase, the cancer cell extends in an irregular shape and proteins in the pseudopod combine to form larger molecules. These molecules line up into rigid needle-like structures (similar to a metal rod reinforcement in a concrete block) that aid the cell extension.

Researchers have found that cell surface texture influences cancer cell movement. They have observed that perfectly round cells with smooth surfaces never protrude pseudopods, but cells with rougher surfaces do.

The entire movement process involves protrusion, attachment, adhesion, release of adhesion, and traction. Researchers believe that one way to inhibit the entire process of cancer cell movement is to inhibit the initial protrusion process. Because pseudopod protrusion is a prominent feature of cell migration, understanding biochemical mechanisms that regulate the assembly of the cell's needlelike structure is very important, and may lead to development of therapeutic agents to block this component of cancer spread.

CELL REPRODUCTION AND HEREDITY

Nucleic Acids

Inside the nucleus are 46 threadlike structures known as chromosomes, and contained in each chromosome are thousands of **genes**. Chromosomes and genes are made of DNA, which transfers the hereditary material from generation to generation. The nucleic acids, RNA and DNA, serve as storage units for our hereditary information. DNA can be thought of as a large cookbook with recipes for making every protein in the cell. RNA helps the ribosome translate the information in DNA into protein.

Despite the importance of nucleic acids in cellular function, nucleic acid structure is surprisingly simple. RNA and DNA are long polymers of only four nucleotides: adenine, guanine, cytosine, and thymine (or uracil for RNA).

The nucleotide structure can be broken down into two parts: the sugar–phosphate backbone and the base. All nucleotides share the sugar–phosphate backbone. Nucleotide polymers are formed by linking the monomer units together using an oxygen atom on the phosphate, and a hydroxyl group on the sugar.

The base on each nucleotide is different, but they still show similarities. Adenine (A) and guanine (G) are purines (with a two-ring structure), with the differences in the molecules coming in the groups attached to the ring. Likewise, cytosine (C), thymine (T), and uracil (U) are pyrimidines and share a similar structure, but differ in their side groups.

Base Pairing

If two strands of nucleic acid are adjacent to one another, the bases along the polymer can interact with complementary bases in the other strand. Adenine is capable of forming hydrogen bonds with thymine and cytosine can base pair with guanine. Adenine forms two hydrogen bonds with thymine; cytosine forms three with guanine. The G to C pair is 33% stronger than the A to T pair due to the extra hydrogen bond.

DNA

Cells contain two strands of DNA that are mirror images of each other. As mentioned earlier, A can pair with T and G can pair with C when correctly aligned. Because these strands are mirrors of each other, the amount of A is equal to the amount of T and the amount of C is equal to the amount of G in any double-stranded DNA molecule. In solution, the two strands will usually find each other and form a double helix, a favorable reaction because of the numerous hydrogen bonds that can be formed between the complementary bases. The DNA molecule can stretch for millions of base pairs and the size of DNA can vary greatly among organisms. *Figure 2-7 illustrates the schematic of DNA.*

RNA

RNA is similar in structure to DNA, except that uracil (U) takes the place of thymine in the molecule, and the ribose unit on each sugar contains a hydroxyl group. RNA functions to translate the genetic information in DNA into protein.

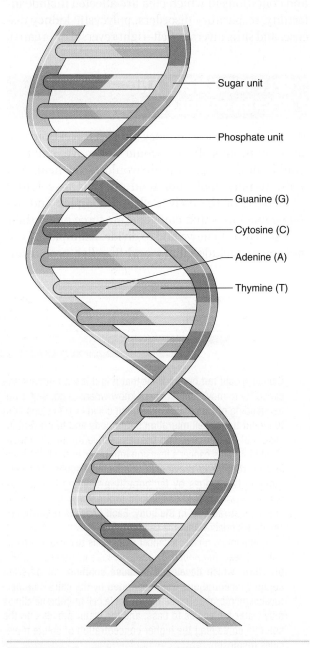

Sugar unit

Phosphate unit

Guanine (G)

Cytosine (C)

Adenine (A)

Thymine (T)

FIGURE 2-7 Schematic of DNA

TABLE 2-2   Differences Between DNA and RNA Molecules

TYPE OF NUCLEIC ACID	TYPE OF SUGAR PRESENT	TYPES OF BASES PRESENT	PHOSPHATE GROUP	LOCATION	NUMBER OF STRANDS PRESENT
DNA	Deoxyribose	A, T, G, C	Same as RNA	Cell nucleus, chromosomes	2
RNA	Ribose	A, U, G, C	Same as DNA	Cytoplasm, nucleoli, ribosomes	1

When a protein is to be made, the hydrogen bonds between the base pairs of the DNA segment break, nucleotides of RNA (A,C,G, and U) use enzymes to construct a single strand of nucleotides that is a complementary copy of half the DNA gene (with uracil in place of thymine). This copy of the gene is messenger RNA (mRNA). This copy separates from the DNA and leaves the nucleus and enters the cytoplasm. There it attaches itself to the ribosomes.

As a copy of the gene, mRNA is a series of triplets of bases. Each triplet is a code for one amino acid. Another type of RNA called **transfer RNA** (tRNA) resides in the cytoplasm. Each tRNA has an anticodon that is a triplet that is complementary to a triplet on the mRNA. The tRNA molecules pick up the amino acids and bring them to the corresponding triplets on the mRNA. The ribosomes contain enzymes to catalyze the formation of peptide bonds between the amino acids. When the amino acid has been brought to each triplet on the mRNA and all peptide bonds have been formed, the protein is complete. Table 2-2 describes the basic differences between DNA and RNA molecules.

DNA Replication

The DNA of a cell is like a single massive book. But the book cannot be torn in half and roughly distributed between the two dividing cell halves. Instead, each new cell needs its own complete copy. Therefore, before a cell can divide, it must duplicate its entire DNA, and each of the two new cells must receive a complete copy of the original DNA.

Replication is surprisingly simple, and is accomplished by the coordinated efforts of many cellular enzymes. Because DNA is double stranded, the two strands separate and each one serves as a template to make another complementary strand, a process known as semiconservative replication. At each cell division, each cell gets one old strand and one new strand.

Cell Division

All cells reproduce by dividing: one cell becomes two. When a cell divides, it divides roughly in half. The di-

vision of water and proteins between the dividing cell halves does not have to be exactly even. Instead, a roughly even distribution of the cellular material is acceptable.

Mitosis   All multicellular organisms are made of eucaryotic cells (cells that are characterized by having a well-defined cellular nucleus that contains the entire cell's DNA). Cell division for eucaryotic cells is called **mitosis** and has five primary steps:

1. **Prophase**: The chromosomes condense into clearly distinct and separate groupings of DNA (during the normal life of a cell, the chromosomes in the nucleus are sufficiently de-condensed so that they are not easily seen as being separate from each other). During cell division, each condensed chromosome that forms consists of two equal-length strands that are joined (the place where the two strands are joined is called a **centromere**). For each chromosome, each of the two strands is a duplicate of the other, coming from the preceding duplication of DNA. For a human cell there are a total of 92 strands comprising 46 chromosomes. The 46 chromosomes comprise two copies of all the information coded in the cell's DNA. One copy will go to one half of the dividing cell, and the other copy will go to the other half.

   During prophase, the chromosomal DNA is distributed between the two halves of the cell. The membrane of the nucleus disintegrates and simultaneously a spindle forms. The spindle is composed of **microtubules**, which are long, thin rods made of chained proteins. The spindle can have several thousand of these microtubules. Many of the microtubules extend from one half of the cell to the chromosomes, and a roughly equal number of microtubules extends from the opposite half of the cell to the chromosomes. Each chromosome's centromere becomes attached to microtubules from both halves of the cell.

2. **Metaphase**: When the spindle is complete, and all the centromeres are attached to microtubules, the chromosomes are aligned together. The alignment places all the centromeres in a plane that is oriented at a right angle to the spindle. The chromosomes are at their maximum contraction. The entire DNA is tightly bound so that none will break off during the actual separation of each chromosome. The separation itself is caused by a shortening of the microtubules. In addition, in some cases the separation is caused by the two bundles of microtubules moving away from each other.

3. **Anaphase**: The centromere, which held together the two strands of each chromosome, is pulled apart into two pieces. One piece of the centromere, attached to one chromosome strand, is pulled into one half of the cell. And the other centromere piece, attached to the other chromosome strand, is pulled into the opposite half of the cell. Therefore, the DNA is divided equally between the two halves of the dividing cell.

4. **Telophase**: Each chromatid is now considered a separate chromosome (there are two complete and separate sets). Once the divided DNA has reached the two respective cell halves, a normal-looking nucleus forms in each cell half. At least some of the spindle's microtubules first disintegrate, and a new nuclear membrane assembles around the DNA. The chromosomes become de-condensed within the new nucleus. Once the two new nuclei are established, a new cell membrane is built in the middle of the cell, dividing the cell in two. Depending on the type of cell, the new cell membrane may be a shared membrane. Or the new cell membrane may be two separate cell membranes, with each membrane facing the other. Once the membranes are completed, and the two new cells are truly divided, the remains of the spindle disintegrate.

5. **Interphase**: After new cells are formed, they must obtain nutrients for the manufacture of new living materials and the synthesis of many vital compounds. Chromosomes begin to double in the nucleus, and new ribosomes, lysosomes, mitochondria, and membranes begin to form in the cytoplasm. The interphase stage of the cell life cycle lasts until the cell begins mitosis. The five phases of mitosis are illustrated in Figure 2–8.

Meiosis   Meiosis results in the formation of gametes (egg and sperm cells). One cell with the diploid number of chromosomes (46) divides twice to form four cells, each with the haploid number (half the usual number) of chromosomes (23). Therefore, the result of meiosis is that the resulting chromosome numbers of the resulting sex cells are reduced by one-half. In males, meiosis takes place in the testes and is called **spermatogenesis**. In females, meiosis takes place in the ovaries and is called **oogenesis**.

Meiosis involves two successive divisions called the first and second meiotic divisions. The phases of these two divisions are first and second meiotic prophase, first and second meiotic metaphase, first and second meiotic anaphase, and first and second meiotic telophase, defined as follows:

1. First meiotic prophase: First meiotic prophase resembles prophase in mitosis, in which individual chromosomes appear as thin threads within the nucleus. The threads shorten and thicken, and the nucleoli disappear. Spindle fibers begin to organize and the nuclear membrane begins to disappear. During this phase, individual chromosomes (which became duplicated in the previous interphase stage) are composed of two identical chromatids held together by a central centromere.

   As prophase continues, homologous chromosomes approach each other and become tightly intertwined (a process called synapsis). The chromatids may break in a few places and exchange parts, forming chromatids with new combinations of genetic material. During this process, bits of the paternal chromatid mix with bits of the maternal source (referred to as "crossing over").

2. First meiotic metaphase: The synaptic pair of chromosomes becomes lined up about midway between the poles of the developing spindle. Each pair (consisting of two chromosomes and four chromatids) becomes associated with a spindle fiber.

3. First meiotic anaphase: The centromeres do not separate in this phase (like they do in mitotic anaphase), and as a result, the homologous chromosomes become separated and the chromatids of each chromosome move together to one end of the spindle. Therefore, each daughter cell receives only one member of a homologous pair of chromosomes (reducing the chromosome number by half).

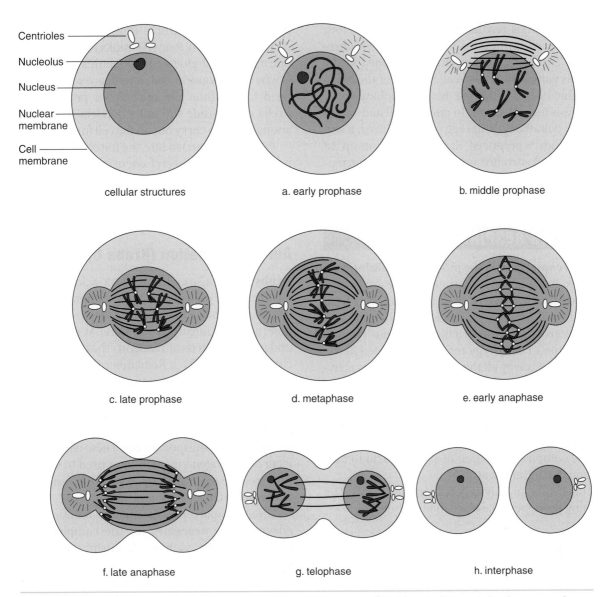

Centrioles
Nucleolus
Nucleus
Nuclear membrane
Cell membrane

cellular structures   a. early prophase   b. middle prophase

c. late prophase   d. metaphase   e. early anaphase

f. late anaphase   g. telophase   h. interphase

FIGURE 2-8   The five phases of mitosis: prophase, metaphase, anaphase, telophase, and interphase

4. First meiotic telophase: This phase is similar to mitotic telophase in that the parent cell divides into two daughter cells. Nuclear membranes appear around the chromosome sets, the nucleoli reappear, and the spindle fibers fade away.

After the first meiotic telophase, a short interphase ensues and lasts until the beginning of the second meiotic division:

1. Second meiotic prophase: Chromosomes reappear, with their chromatids held together by a centromere. The chromosomes move into

positions midway between the poles of the developing spindle.
2. Second meiotic metaphase: Double-stranded chromosomes become attached to spindle fibers.
3. Second meiotic anaphase: Centromeres separate so that chromatids are free to move to opposite poles of the spindle.
4. Second meiotic telophase: The cell divides into two daughter cells, and the new nuclei are organized around the sets of single-stranded chromosomes.

Spermatogenesis results in the formation of four sperm cells, each containing 23 single-stranded chromosomes. The genetic information contained in the sperm cells varies from cell to cell because of the crossing over that occurs in the first meiotic prophase.

Oogenesis meiosis results in one egg cell and a nonfunctional polar body. If the egg cell is fertilized, a second polar body is produced. Egg cells also contain 23 single-stranded chromosomes with genetic information varying from cell to cell.

CELLULAR RESPIRATION

Cellular respiration is the process of oxidizing food molecules, like glucose, to carbon dioxide and water. (When you take hydrogen ions or electrons away from a molecule, you "oxidize" that molecule; when you give hydrogen ions or electrons to a molecule, you "reduce" that molecule.) The energy released is trapped in the form of ATP for use by all the energy-consuming activities of the cell.

The process occurs in two phases:

- glycolysis, the breakdown of glucose to pyruvic acid
- the complete oxidation of pyruvic acid to carbon dioxide and water

In eukaryotes, glycolysis occurs in the cytosol. The remaining processes take place in mitochondria.

Glycolysis

For use as energy, the food we eat must first be converted to basic chemicals that the cell can use. During this process, the food is oxidized to produce high-energy electrons that are converted to stored energy. This energy is stored in high-energy phosphate bonds in ATP (ATP is converted from adenosine diphosphate by adding the phosphate group with the high-energy bond).

Some of the best energy-supplying foods contain sugars or carbohydrates (e.g., bread or pasta). The sugars are broken down by enzymes that split them into the simplest form of sugar (called glucose), which enters the cell with the help of special molecules in the membrane called glucose transporters.

Once inside the cell, glucose is broken down to make ATP in two pathways. The first pathway requires no oxygen and is called anaerobic metabolism, or **glycolysis**. During glycolysis (which occurs in the cytoplasm outside the mitochondria), glucose is broken down into pyruvate. Each reaction is designed to produce some

hydrogen ions (electrons) that can be used to make ATP. However, only four ATP molecules can be made by one molecule of glucose through this pathway, which is why mitochondria and oxygen are so important: we need to continue the breakdown process with the Krebs cycle inside the mitochondria in order to get enough ATP to carry out all the cell functions.

Pyruvate is carried into the mitochondria, where it is converted into acetyl coenzyme A (acetyl CoA), which enters the Krebs cycle. This first reaction produces carbon dioxide because it involves the removal of one carbon from the pyruvate.

Aerobic Oxidation (Krebs Cycle)

Krebs cycle (also called the citric acid cycle or tricarboxylic acid cycle) occurs in mitochondria and is the common pathway to completely oxidize molecules for fuel (which is mostly acetyl CoA). It enters the cycle and passes 10 steps of reactions that yield energy and carbon dioxide (CO_2). Remember that when you take hydrogen ions or electrons away from a molecule, you "oxidize" that molecule.

The whole idea behind respiration in the mitochondria is to use the Krebs cycle to get as many electrons as possible out of the food we eat. These electrons (in the form of hydrogen ions) are then used to drive pumps that produce the ATP that fuels cellular functions such as movement, transport, and division.

Several important molecules (in addition to all the enzymes) are necessary for the completion of the Krebs cycle: pyruvate (made during glycolysis from glucose) and special carrier molecules for the electrons. There are two types of these carrier molecules: nicotinamide adenine dinucleotide (NAD+) and flavin adenine dinucleotide (FAD+). The third molecule, of course, is oxygen.

Pyruvate is a 3-carbon molecule that, after entering the mitochondria, is broken down to a 2-carbon molecule by a special enzyme. This breaking down of pyruvate releases carbon dioxide. The two-carbon molecule is called acetyl CoA, and it enters the Krebs cycle by joining to a four-carbon molecule called oxaloacetate. Once the two molecules are joined, they make a six-carbon molecule called **citric acid** (2 carbons + 4 carbons = 6 carbons), hence the name "citric acid cycle." Citric acid is then broken down and modified, and, as this happens, carbon molecules and hydrogen ions are released. The carbon molecules are used to make more carbon dioxide and the hydrogen ions are picked up by NAD+ and FAD+. Eventually, the process produces the four-carbon oxaloacetate again, which is why the process is called a cycle: it always ends up where it started, with oxaloacetate available to combine with more acetyl CoA. Figure 2-9 illustrates the Krebs cycle.

In summary: pyruvate in the cytosol has to enter the mitochondria by transport through the outer and inner mitochondrial membranes. When this transport occurs, energy is used and carbon dioxide is released as a result. In reality, only two of the three carbons that make up the pyruvate molecule actually enter the cycle in the mitochondria. The transport "shuttle" that brings this two-carbon molecule (acetate) into the cycle is called coenzyme A, and it grabs the two carbons to become acetyl coenzyme A (acetyl CoA). The two carbons are then released to join with oxaloacetate to form citrate. This completes the first step of the Krebs cycle. The enzymes of the Krebs cycle then release the two carbons as carbon dioxide and retrieve energy from bonds as ATP and NADH.

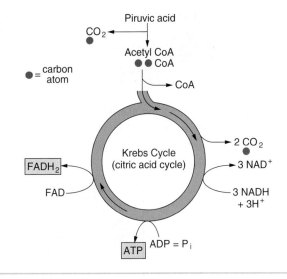

FIGURE 2-9 **A summary diagram of the Krebs cycle**

BOX 2-2

Complete Blood Count (CBC)

A complete blood count (CBC) provides important information about the kinds and numbers of cells in the blood: red blood cells (RBCs), white blood cells (WBCs), and platelets. A CBC can help a health professional evaluate symptoms and diagnose conditions. A CBC test usually includes:

- WBC count. WBCs attack and destroy invading foreign bacteria, viruses, or other organisms that can cause infection. When a person has a bacterial infection, the number of WBCs can increase dramatically as they rise to attack the invader, and the count can be analyzed in a blood sample. WBC count is also used to monitor the body's response to cancer treatments.

- RBC count. RBCs deliver oxygen from the lungs to the tissues of the body, and also assist in carrying carbon dioxide back to the lungs for exhalation from the body. The RBC count can help health specialists identify a lower than normal number of RBCs (which can indicate that tissues are not getting enough oxygen), or a higher than normal number (which can lead to the formation of life-threatening blood clots).

- WBC types (WBC differential). Each of the five major types of WBCs of the body plays a different, important role in immunity. The WBC types include the neutrophils, lymphocytes, monocytes, eosinophils, and basophils (immature neutrophils, called band neutrophils, are also included). An increase or decrease in the numbers of these different types of WBCs can help identify an infection, an allergic reaction to certain substances, and certain types of diseases (especially the leukemias).

- Hematocrit (HCT; also called packed cell volume [PCV]) measures the volume of RBCs in the blood (given as a percentage of RBCs in a volume of blood; e.g., an HCT of 42 indicates that 42% of the volume of blood examined is composed of RBCs).

- Hemoglobin (Hgb) is a carrier of oxygen and is the substance that gives blood its red color. Its measurement indicates the body's ability to deliver oxygen to tissues.

- RBC indices (used to diagnose anemia) are the mean corpuscular volume (MCV), which indicates the size of RBCs; mean corpuscular hemoglobin (MCH), which indicates the amount of Hgb in the average RBC; and mean corpuscular hemoglobin concentration (MCHC), which measures the concentration of Hgb in the average RBC.

- RBC distribution width (RDW), used to classify types of anemia, indicates if all the RBCs are about the same width, size, and shape.

- Platelet (thrombocyte) count. Platelets play a major role in the clotting of blood by clumping together and plugging areas of hemorrhage. Too few platelets can lead to uncontrolled bleeding, while too many can cause blood clots to form.

- Blood smear. For this test, a drop of blood is smeared on a slide and stained with a special dye, and then examined under a microscope to identify unusual numbers, sizes, or shapes of red blood cells; white blood cells; and platelets.

BOX 2-3

Microscopic Appearance of Cancer Cells

In addition to a large number of dividing cells, cancerous cells have a distinctive appearance under the microscope: variation in the size and shape of the nucleus and in the cell itself, a loss of specialized cell features, and a poorly defined tumor boundary. Figure 2-10 compares normal cells to cancerous cells.

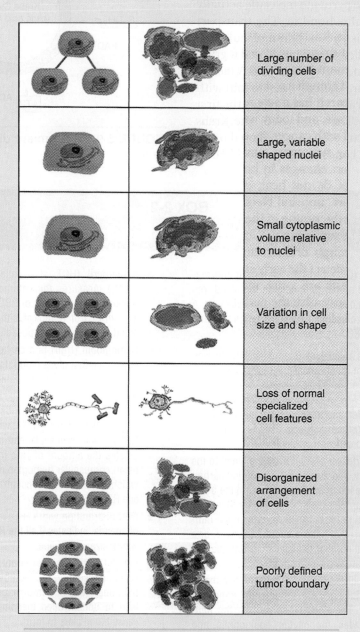

		Large number of dividing cells
		Large, variable shaped nuclei
		Small cytoplasmic volume relative to nuclei
		Variation in cell size and shape
		Loss of normal specialized cell features
		Disorganized arrangement of cells
		Poorly defined tumor boundary

FIGURE 2-10 Comparison of normal cells to cancerous cells *(Courtesy of National Cancer Society)*

Case Study 2

James is a surgical technologist on the cardiovascular team at St. Francis Memorial Hospital. The cardiovascular team is preparing for an off-pump beating heart coronary bypass procedure in which stem cells will be injected into the damaged myocardium of the left ventricle after the bypass is completed.

1. Why would stem cells help a damaged myocardium?

2. What are stem cells and how are they gathered for this type of procedure?

3. What does *off-pump beating heart* refer to?

CHAPTER SUMMARY

- Chemistry is the branch of the natural sciences that deals with the composition of substances and their properties and reactions.

- Entities that have mass and take up space are referred to as matter.

- An object can store energy as the result of its position (potential energy). Kinetic energy is the energy of motion. The total amount of mechanical energy is merely the sum of the potential energy and the kinetic energy.

- The Bohr model of the atom describes its structure as electrons circling the nucleus at different levels, or orbitals, much like planets circle the sun.

- Both the protons and neutrons reside in the nucleus of the atom, but protons have a positive charge, whereas neutrons have no charge. The orbiting electrons are negatively charged.

- The number of protons determines the atomic number of the atom, and is typically equal to the number of orbiting electrons.

- All matter is made up of fundamental elements that cannot be broken down by chemical means. There are 92 elements that occur naturally.

- Hydrogen, carbon, nitrogen, and oxygen are the elements that make up most living organisms.

- Atoms constantly seek stable electron configurations and can obtain stability by losing, sharing, or gaining electrons. For a stable configuration, each atom must fill its outer energy level, but the maximum number that can exist at any level is strictly limited.

- A compound is a substance that can be broken down into two or more other substances by chemical means.

- Molecules are groups of atoms joined by chemical bonds (created by electron attraction and interaction). Molecular weight equals the sum of the atomic weights of the atoms in the molecule.

- An organic compound is any of a large class of chemical compounds the molecules of which contain carbon.

- A positively or negatively charged atom is referred to as an ion.

- A compound that disassociates into positive and negative ions in a solution is called an electrolyte, so named because it can conduct an electric current.

- Acids and bases are related to the concentration of hydrogen ions present in a dissolved solution.

- Substances with a pH between 0 and less than 7 are acids, whereas substances with a pH greater than 7 and up to 14 are bases (the higher the pH, the stronger the base).

- The smallest living units of the human body are cells.

- Robert Hooke coined the term *cell* after viewing slices of cork through a microscope.

- Cell shape is controlled by the extracellular matrix and the cytoskeletal structure within the cell.

- There are four primary groups of organic compounds: carbohydrates, lipids (fats), proteins, and nucleic acids.

- Carbohydrates, also referred to as sugars, are composed of chains of carbon atoms with hydrogen and oxygen atoms attached in the C:H:O ratio of 1:2:1.

- Proteins are composed of building blocks called amino acids.

- Lipids, or simple fats, are composed of chains of molecules called triglycerides.

- Nucleic acids, RNA (ribonucleic acid) and DNA (deoxyribonucleic acid), are long linear polymers of smaller subunits called nucleotides. Each nucleotide is composed of a nitrogenous base, a pentose sugar (ribose for RNA or deoxyribose for DNA), and a phosphate.

- Cytoplasm is defined as the material that lies within the cytoplasmic membrane.

- All of the functions for cell expansion, growth, and replication are carried out in the cytoplasm of a cell.

- The cytoplasmic membrane is that area of the cell immediately surrounding the cytoplasm. It is structured to allow cells to selectively interact with their environment.

- Membranes are composed of phospholipids and proteins. Phospholipids contain a charged or polar group attached to a 3-carbon glycerol backbone.

- The cell membrane retains the cytoplasm, but solute concentrations tend to equilibrate, causing water to flow into the cell (osmosis) and the solutes to flow out.

- There are four basic types of transport systems: passive diffusion, facilitated diffusion, group translocation, and active transport.

- During passive diffusion, molecular transport is directed by laws of simple diffusion (no transport protein and energy is not required).

- Facilitated diffusion involves a protein that binds the molecule for transport across the cell membrane, and is therefore specific. Energy is not required.

- During group translocation, a protein specifically binds the target molecule and during transport a chemical modification takes place.

- Active transport proteins are molecular pumps that pump their substrates against a concentration gradient, requiring energy.

- Eukaryotic nuclear materials are bound by a membrane but prokaryotic nuclear materials are not.

- The nucleus forms the package for our genes and guides the life processes of the cell. It houses DNA, which contains instructions for the production of the cell's proteins and for reproduction.

- The nucleolus is the site where ribosomal RNA (rRNA) is transcribed, processed, and assembled into ribosome subunits.

- Chromatin are organized packages designed for the storage of genetic material, its condensation during cell division, and regulation of gene expression.

- Organelles are highly specialized structures that are designed for specific cellular activities. They include lysosomes, vacuoles, the endoplasmic reticulum, mitochondria, the Golgi apparatus, ribosomes, centrioles, cilia, and flagella.

- Lysosomes digest waste materials and food within the cell.

- Vacuoles are membranous sacs that are formed when a portion of the cell membrane folds inward and pinches off.

- The endoplasmic reticulum (ER) is the transport network for molecules targeted for certain modifications and specific final destinations. There are two types of ER: rough ER has attached ribosomes and smooth ER does not.

- Mitochondria are the sites of aerobic respiration, and are the major energy production center in eukaryotes. They convert the potential energy of food molecules into ATP.

- The Golgi apparatus modifies and refines proteins synthesized by the endoplasmic reticulum and packages them into small membranc-bound sacs called vesicles.

- Ribosomes are the sites of protein synthesis, where RNA is translated into protein.

- Centrioles are cylindrical structures that replicate in interphase stage of mitosis and help to organize the assembly of microtubules during cell division.

- Centrioles called basal bodies form cilia and flagella that function to move fluid or materials past an immobile cell, and are used for cellular propulsion or for transporting extracellular substances.

- Examples of cell movement include ciliary and flagellar propulsion, muscle contraction, and white blood cells that move into surrounding tissues and seek invaders.

- Inside the nucleus are 46 threadlike structures known as chromosomes, and contained in each chromosome are thousands of genes.

- Chromosomes and genes are made of DNA, which transfers the hereditary material from generation to generation.

- The nucleic acids, RNA and DNA, serve as storage units for our hereditary information.

- RNA and DNA are long polymers of only four nucleotides, adenine, guanine, cytosine and thymine (or uracil for RNA).

- Cells contain two strands of DNA that are mirror images of each other and will form a double helix.

- RNA is similar in structure to DNA, except that uracil (U) takes the place of thymine in the molecule, and the ribose unit on each sugar contains a hydroxyl group. RNA functions to translate the genetic information in DNA into protein.

- Before a cell can divide, it must duplicate its entire DNA, and each of the two new cells must receive a complete copy of the original DNA. The two strands separate and each one serves as a template to make another complementary strand, a process known as semiconservative replication.

- Cell division for eucaryotic cells is called mitosis and has four primary steps: prophase, metaphase, anaphase, and telophase.

- Meiosis results in the formation of gametes (egg and sperm cells). Meiosis involves two successive divisions called the first and second meiotic divisions.

- The phases of these two divisions are first and second meiotic prophase, first and second meiotic metaphase, first and second meiotic anaphase, and first and second meiotic telophase.

- Cellular respiration is the process of oxidizing food molecules, such as glucose, to carbon dioxide and water. The process occurs in two phases: glycolysis, the breakdown of glucose to pyruvic acid, and the complete oxidation of pyruvic acid to carbon dioxide and water.

- The whole idea behind respiration in the mitochondria is to use the Krebs cycle to get as many electrons as possible from the food we eat. These electrons (in the form of hydrogen ions) are then used to drive pumps that produce the ATP that fuels cellular functions such as movement, transport, and division.

CRITICAL THINKING QUESTIONS

1. The surgical technologist directly encounters cells on a daily basis. How many examples can you give?
2. How does an understanding of cell function help in sterilization or disinfection of operative items?
3. How does stereotactic neurosurgery minimize cell damage?
4. If cell division is necessary for survival, what do you think causes a cell to divide uncontrollably, leading to tumor formation?
5. How does cell movement contribute to metastasis?

BIBLIOGRAPHY

Afanas'ev, I, & Nozdrin, V. I. (1977). Regulation of cell structure and function. *Uspekhi Sovremennoi Biologii, 83*(3), 400–418.

Association of Surgical Technologists. (2003). *Surgical technology for the surgical technologist: A positive care approach* (2nd ed.). Clifton Park NY: Thomson Delmar Learning.

Bray, D., Lewis, J., Raff, M., Roberts, K., Watson, J. D. Alberts, B., (1994). *Molecular biology of the cell* (3rd ed.). New York: Garland Science.

Audesirk, G., & Audesirk, T. (1999). *Biology: Life on earth.* Upper Saddle River, NJ: Prentice Hall.

Baker, J. J., & Allen, G. E. (1981). *Matter, energy, and life* (4th ed.). Palo Alto, CA: Addison-Wesley.

Banyard, J., & Zetter, B. R. (1998). The role of cell motility in prostate cancer. *Cancer Metastasis Reviews, 17*(4), 449–458.

Carpi, A. (2003). *Acids & bases: An introduction.* Retrieved April 28, 2005, from http://www.visionlearning.com/library/module_viewer.php?mid=58

Chicurel, M. (2002). Cell biology: Cell migration research is on the move. *Science, 295,* 606–609.

Childs, G. V. (1996). *Mitochondria: Architecture dictates function.* Retrieved April 28, 2005, from http://cellbio.utmb.edu/cellbio/mitoch1.htm

Hole, J. W. Jr., (1987). *Human anatomy and physiology* (4th ed.). Dubuque, IA: W. C. Brown.

Paustian, T. (2003). *Nucleic acid structure.* Retrieved April 28, 2005, from http://lecturer.ukdw.ac.id/dhira/BacterialStructure/NucleicAcids. html

Paustian, T. (2003). *Cellular membrane.* Retrieved, May 16, 2005, from http://lecturer.ukdw.ac.id/dhira/BacterialStructure/MembraneGen.html

Preston-Martin, S., Pike, M. C., Ross, R. K., Jones, P. A., & Henderson, B. E. (1990). Increased cell division as a cause of human cancer. *Cancer Research, 50,* 7415–7421.

Rahn, H., & Howell, B. J. (1978) The OH-/H+ concept of acid-base balance: Historical development. *Respiratory Physiology, 33*(1), 91–97.

Scott, A. S., & Fong, E. (1998). *Body structures and functions* (9th ed.). Clifton Park, NY: Thomson Delmar Learning.

Spengler, R. (2003). *Topic: Complete blood count (CBC).* Retrieved May 16, 2005, from http://www.questdiagnostic.com/kbase/topic/medtest/hw4260/credits.html

Tortora, G. J., & Grabowski, S. R. (1996). *Principles of anatomy and physiology* (8th ed.). New York: HarperCollins.

Turner, S., & Fong, V. (1994). *Study describes actions of cancer cell movement.* Retrieved April 28, 2005, from http://www.engr.psu.edu/news/News/1994%20Press%20Releases/July/cancercell.html

Williamson, D. (1999). *Study: calcium channels regulate cell movement.* Retrieved April 28, 2005, www.unc.edu/news/archives/jul99/jacobson072199.htm

Wolfe, S. L. (1981). *Biology of the cell* (2nd ed.). Belmont, CA: Wadsworth.

3

TISSUES AND MEMBRANES

CHAPTER OBJECTIVES

After completing the study of this chapter, you should be able to:

1. Compare and contrast the types of epithelial tissue.
2. Compare and contrast the types of connective tissue.
3. Compare and contrast smooth, skeletal, and cardiac muscle tissue.
4. Evaluate the tissue that makes up the nervous system.
5. Compare and contrast serous, mucous, cutaneous, and synovial membranes.
6. Describe the classification of surgical wounds.
7. Evaluate the types of wound healing.
8. Describe the complications of the healing wound.
9. Describe the techniques of tissue typing, and explain the importance of DNA testing.
10. Describe the methods for specimen preparation and study.

KEY TERMS

basement membrane	fasciculi	lacunae	parietal layer
canaliculi	fibroblasts	lamellae	peritoneum
compound gland	goblet cells	macrophages	pleura
dehiscence	haversian canals	major histocompatibility	sarcolemma
endocrine glands	histiocytes	complex	sarcoplasm
epineurium	human leukocyte antigens	mast cells	simple gland
excision	incision	mucus	tissues
exocrine glands	keratinized	neurons	visceral layer

Case Study 1

John is a surgical technologist employed by a hospital that specializes in treating burn victims. He has been called out to do a procedure on a 34-year-old man who sustained severe burns during a house fire in the middle of the night. The surgeon has used the Rule of Nines to calculate that 36% of the patient's body has been burned. He also diagnoses the burns as third degree in nature. John has been asked to prepare for a debridement with skin grafting.

1. What is the Rule of Nines used for burn victims?

2. What are the differences between first-, second-, third-, and fourth-degree burns? What tissues are affected by each?

3. What is a debridement and how will skin be grafted?

INTRODUCTION

When groups of cells that have similar function and structure are grouped together, they form **tissues**. The classification of tissues is related to their function, arrangement, and type and amount of substance that lies between the cells of the tissue. This intercellular material is secreted by the cell, and may be a solid, semisolid, or liquid, depending upon the nature of the tissue.

There are four major types of tissue in the human body: epithelial, connective, muscle, and nervous. These tissues combine to form organs with specific functions (to be discussed in the following chapter).

EPITHELIAL TISSUE

Epithelial tissues are found throughout the body, and cover all body surfaces, both inside and out. Because they cover organs, form inner linings of body cavities, and line hollow organs, they always have a free surface. These tissues are made of rapidly dividing cells; therefore, injuries to their cells, such as those that line the intestinal tract and the skin, heal quickly as damaged cells are rapidly replaced by newer ones.

Epithelial tissues typically lack blood vessels, but receive nourishment from underlying connective tissues that are bound to the upper layers by a thin layer of tissue called the **basement membrane**, or basement lamina. The basement membrane provides structural support for the epithelium and also binds it to neighboring structures.

Epithelial tissues serve the body in the following ways:

1. Protection: They protect underlying tissues because their cells are tightly packed together, with little intercellular material; for example, epithelial cells from the skin prevent damaging ultraviolet rays from reaching the delicate tissues underneath. In addition, these cells protect underlying tissue from mechanical injury, harmful chemicals, invading bacteria, and excessive loss of water.

2. Excretion and secretion: Glands made of epithelial tissue secrete hormones (endocrine glands), mucous (mucous glands), and digestive enzymes. Epithelial tissues in the kidney excrete waste products from the body and reabsorb needed materials from the urine. In glands, epithelial tissue is specialized to secrete specific chemical substances such as enzymes, hormones, and lubricating fluids. Sweat is also excreted from the body by epithelial cells in the sweat glands.

3. Diffusion: Simple epithelium promotes the diffusion of gases, liquids, and nutrients. For example, the epithelial tissue that makes up the alveolar wall of the lungs is ideal for exchange of carbon dioxide and oxygen because of its single-layer design.

4. Cleaning: Ciliated epithelium assists in removing dust particles and foreign bodies that have entered the air passages.

5. Absorption: The epithelial lining of the intestinal tract absorbs nutrients from food.

6. Sensation: Specialized epithelial tissue containing sensory nerve endings is found in the skin, eyes, ears, nose, and on the tongue.

Types of Epithelial Tissue

Epithelial tissue is classified according to the shape, arrangements, and functions of its cells. Epithelial tissue with a single layer of cells is said to be simple, and with multiple layers it is called stratified. Cells that are thin, flattened, and slightly irregular in shape are called squamous, whereas cells with a cubelike appearance are called cuboidal. Cells with an elongated, rectangular appearance are referred to as columnar. The following describes these classifications.

Simple Squamous Epithelium

The cells of simple squamous epithelium have the appearance of thin, flat plates. The shape of the cell's nucleus usually corresponds to the cell form and helps to identify the type of epithelium. These cells form the lining of cavities such as the mouth, blood vessels, heart, and lungs, and make up the outer layers of the skin.

Simple Cuboidal Epithelium

The cells of simple cuboidal epithelium are shaped like cubes, and each cell has a spherical nucleus in the center. Simple cuboidal epithelium is found in glands, gland ducts, and the lining of the kidney tubules. In addition, cuboidal epithelium makes up the germinal epithelium that produces egg cells in the ovary and sperm cells in the testes.

Simple Columnar Epithelium

The cells of simple columnar epithelium are elongated and column-shaped, with nuclei that are elongated and located at the base of the cells near the basement membrane. These cells form the lining of the uterus, stomach, and intestines. Some columnar cells are specialized for sensory reception such as in the nose, ears, and the taste buds of the tongue. **Goblet cells**, which produce mucus to lubricate the intestinal wall, are found between the columnar epithelial cells of the duodenum.

Ciliated Columnar Epithelium

Ciliated columnar epithelium is composed of simple columnar epithelial cells that possess fine, hairlike cilia on their free surfaces. These cilia produce rapid, wavelike motions that direct mucus (secreted by the goblet cells) to flow in a specific direction. For example, cilia deep within the lung passages move fine particles embedded in mucus away from the lungs into the upper airway for removal. Cilia within the fallopian tubes move the ovum toward the uterus.

The cells of pseudostratified columnar epithelium only appear to be stratified (layered) because their nuclei are located at different sites within the cell and their shape is variable. However, each cell reaches down to the basement membrane.

Glandular Epithelium

Columnar epithelium with mucus-producing goblet cells is called glandular epithelium. In addition, columnar and cuboidal epithelial cells often become specialized as gland cells that synthesize and secrete enzymes, hormones, milk, sweat, wax, and saliva. Glands that secrete their substances into ducts are called **exocrine glands**, and those that secrete their products into tissue fluid or blood are called **endocrine glands**. Exocrine glands may be unicellular or multicellular. Multicellular glands may be classified as a **simple gland** (one that communicates with the surface through an unbranched duct) or a **compound gland** (multilobed gland, with a branched duct arising from each lobe). Most of the glands of the digestive tract are simple exocrine glands, as are sweat and sebaceous glands. Mammary glands are an example of compound exocrine glands.

Stratified Squamous Epithelium

Where the body is exposed to conditions that cause wear and tear, the epithelia located there are composed of several layers of cells, and are called stratified squamous epithelia. The top cells are flattened and may be **keratinized** (meaning that they are composed of a tough, resistant protein called keratin). The skin is an example of dry, keratinized, stratified epithelium, and the lining of the mouth cavity is an example of a nonkeratinized, stratified epithelium.

Transitional Epithelium

Transitional epithelium is designed to handle tension in tissues, and lines the walls of the urinary bladder, urethra, and ureters. This type of tissue is thin when the wall is stretched and thick when the wall is contracted. Although it is fairly malleable, transitional epithelium is designed to form a barrier that prevents the contents of the urinary passageways from diffusing into adjacent areas. Refer to Table 3-1 for a description of the different types of human tissue.

CONNECTIVE TISSUE

Connective tissue, the most varied and abundant tissue of the body, functions to support the body and to bind together all types of tissue. It also provides a mechanical framework (the skeleton), which plays an important role in locomotion. Unlike epithelial tissue, connective tissue is characterized by the large amounts of intercellular substance (matrix) secreted by relatively few, widely separated cells. The matrix is a nonliving material that may be liquid (blood), semisolid

TABLE 3-1 Different Types of Human Tissue

TYPE OF TISSUE	FUNCTION	CHARACTERISTICS AND LOCATION	MORPHOLOGY
I. EPITHELIAL	Cells form a continuous layer covering internal and external body surfaces, provide protection, produce secretions (digestive juices, hormones, and perspiration), and regulate the passage of materials across their cell membranes. **A. Covering and lining tissue** These cells can be stratified (layered), ciliated, or keratinized (hard, nonliving substance).	**1. Squamous epithelial cells** These are flat, irregularly shaped cells. They line the heart, blood and lymphatic vessels, body cavities, and alveoli (air sacs) of lungs. The outer layer of the skin consists of stratified and keratinized squamous epithelial cells. The stratified squamous epithelial cells on the outer skin layer protect the body against microbial invasion. **2. Cuboidal epithelial cells** These cube-shaped cells line the kidney tubules and cover the ovaries and secretory parts of certain glands. **3. Columnar epithelial cells** These cells are elongated, with the nucleus generally near the bottom and often ciliated on the outer surface. They line the ducts, digestive tract (especially the intestinal and stomach lining), parts of the respiratory tract, and glands.	

TABLE 3-1 *(continued)*

TYPE OF TISSUE	FUNCTION	CHARACTERISTICS AND LOCATION	MORPHOLOGY
I. EPITHELIAL (continued)	**B. Glandular or secretory tissue** These cells are specialized to secrete materials such as digestive juices, hormones, milk, perspiration, and wax. They are columnar or cuboidal shaped.	**1. Endocrine gland cells** These cells form ductless glands that secrete their substances (hormones) directly into the bloodstream. For instance, the thyroid gland secretes thyroxin, and adrenal glands secrete adrenaline. **2. Exocrine gland cells** These cells secrete their substances into ducts. The mammary glands, sweat glands, and salivary glands are examples.	Duct (where secretions leave); Secretory cells; Exocrine (duct) gland cell (e.g., sweat and mammary glands)
II. CONNECTIVE	Cells the intercellular secretions (matrix) of which support and connect the organs and tissues of the body.	Connective tissue is found almost everywhere within the body: bones, cartilage, mucous membranes, muscles, nerves, skin, and all internal organs.	
	A. Adipose tissue This tissue stores lipid (fat); acts as filler tissue; and cushions, supports, and insulates the body.	Adipose tissue is a type of loose, connective tissue composed of saclike adipose cells; they are specialized for the storage of fat. Adipose cells are found throughout the body: in the subcutaneous skin layer, around the kidneys, within padding around joints, and in the marrow of long bones.	Cytoplasm; Collagen fibers; Nucleus; Vacuole (for fat storage)
	B. Areolar (loose) tissue This tissue surrounds various organs and supports both nerve cells and blood vessels that transport nutrient materials (to cells) and wastes (away from cells). Areolar tissue also (temporarily) stores glucose, salts, and water.	Areolar tissue is composed of a large, semifluid matrix, with many different types of cells and fibers embedded in it. These include fibroblasts (fibrocytes), plasma cells, macrophages, mast cells, and various white blood cells. The fibers are bundles of strong, flexible, white fibrous protein called collagen, and elastic single fibers of elastin. Areolar tissue is found in the epidermis of the skin and in the tissue subcutaneous layer with adipose cells.	Mast cell; Reticular fibers; Collagen fibers; Fibroblast cell; Plasma cell; Elastic fiber; Matrix; Macrophage cell

(continues)

TABLE 3-1 *(continued)*

TYPE OF TISSUE	FUNCTION	CHARACTERISTICS AND LOCATION	MORPHOLOGY
II. CONNECTIVE (continued)	**C. Dense fibrous tissue** This tissue forms ligaments, tendons, and aponeuroses. **Ligaments** are strong, flexible bands (or cords) that hold bones firmly together at the joints. **Tendons** are white, glistening bands attaching skeletal muscles to the bones. **Aponeuroses** are flat, wide bands of tissue holding one muscle to another or to the periosteum (bone covering). **Fasciae** are fibrous connective tissue sheets that wrap around muscle bundles to hold them in place.	Dense fibrous tissue is also called white fibrous tissue because it is made from closely packed white collagen fibers. Fibrous tissue is flexible, but not elastic. This tissue has a poor blood supply and heals slowly.	Fibroblast / Closely packed collagen fibers
	D. Supportive tissue **1. Osseous (bone) tissue** Comprises the skeleton of the body, which supports and protects underlying soft-tissue parts and organs, and also serves as attachments for skeletal muscles.	This connective tissue's intercellular matrix is **calcified** by the deposition of mineral salts (like calcium carbonate and calcium phosphate). Calcification of bone imparts great strength. The entire skeleton is composed of bone tissue.	Bone lacunae / Bone cell / Cytoplasm / Nucleus
	2. Cartilage Provides firm but flexible support for the embryonic skeleton and part of the adult skeleton. **a. Hyaline** Forms the skeleton of the embryo.	Hyaline cartilage is found on articular bone surfaces, and also at the nose tip, bronchi, and bronchial tubes. Ribs are joined to the sternum (breastbone) by the costal cartilage. It is also found in the larynx and the rings in the trachea.	Cells (chondrocytes) / Matrix
	b. Fibrocartilage A strong, flexible, supportive substance, found between bones and wherever great strength (and a degree of rigidity) is needed.	Fibrocartilage is located within intervertebral discs and public symphysis between the pubic bones.	Lacuna (space enclosing cells) / Chondrocytes / Dense white fibers

(continues)

TABLE 3-1 *(continued)*

TYPE OF TISSUE	FUNCTION	CHARACTERISTICS AND LOCATION	MORPHOLOGY
II. CONNECTIVE (continued)	**D. Supportive tissue** (continued) **c. Elastic cartilage** The intercellular matrix is embedded with a network of elastic fibers and is firm but flexible.	Elastic cartilage is located inside the auditory ear tube, external ear, epiglottis, and larynx.	Elastic fibers / Chondrocyte / Nucleus
	E. Vascular (liquid blood tissue) **1. Blood** Transports nutrient and oxygen molecules to cells, and metabolic wastes away from cells (can be considered as a liquid tissue). Contains cells that function in the body's defense and in blood clotting.	Blood consists of two major parts: a liquid called plasma, and a solid cellular portion known as blood cells (or corpuscles). The plasma suspends corpuscles, of which there are two major types: red blood cells (erythrocytes) and white blood cells (leukocytes). A third cellular component (actually a cell fragment) is platelets (thrombocytes). Blood circulates within the blood vessels (arteries, veins, and capillaries) and through the heart.	Thrombocytes (platelets) / Erythrocytes / Neutrophil / Lymphocyte / Monocyte / Basophil / Eosinophil
	2. Lymph Transports tissue fluid, proteins, fats, and other materials from the tissues to the circulatory system. This occurs through a series of tubes called the lymphatic vessels.	Lymph fluid consists of water, glucose, protein, fats, and salt. The cellular components are lymphocytes and granulocytes. They flow in tubes called lymphatic vessels, which closely parallel the veins and bathe the tissue spaces between cells.	Red blood cells / White blood cell / Lymph / Cells / Blood capillary / Lymph capillary

(continues)

TABLE 3-1 *(continued)*

TYPE OF TISSUE	FUNCTION	CHARACTERISTICS AND LOCATION	MORPHOLOGY
III. MUSCLE	**A. Cardiac muscle** These cells help the heart contract in order to pump blood through and out of the heart.	Cardiac muscle is a striated (having a cross-banding pattern), involuntary (not under conscious control) muscle. It makes up the walls of the heart.	Centrally located nucleus; Striations; Branching of cell; Intercalated disc
	B. Skeletal (striated voluntary) muscle These muscles are attached to the movable parts of the skeleton. They are capable of rapid, powerful contractions and long states of partially sustained contractions, allowing for voluntary movement.	Skeletal muscle is striated (having transverse bands that run down the length of muscle fiber), voluntary because the muscle is under conscious control, and skeletal because these muscles attach to the skeleton (bones, tendons, and other muscles).	Nucleus; Myofibrils
	C. Smooth (nonstriated involuntary) These provide for involuntary movement. Examples include the movement of materials along the digestive tract, and controlling the diameter of blood vessels and the pupils of the eyes.	Smooth muscle is nonstriated because it lacks the striations (bands) of skeletal muscles; its movement is involuntary. It makes up the walls of the digestive tract, genitourinary tract, respiratory tract, blood vessels, and lymphatic vessels.	Spindle-shaped cell; Cells separated from each other; Nucleus
IV. NERVE	**Neurons (nerve cells)** These cells have the ability to react to stimuli. **1. Irritability** Ability of nerve tissue to respond to environmental changes. **2. Conductivity** Ability to carry a nerve impulse (message).	Nerve tissue consists of neurons (nerve cells). Neurons have branches through which various parts of the body are connected and their activities coordinated. They are found in the brain, spinal cord, and nerves.	Spindle-shaped cell; Cells separated from each other; Nucleus

(connective tissue), or solid (bone). Embedded in the matrix are a variety of connecting and supporting fibers, such as collagen fibers and elastic fibers. Connective tissue can be classified according to three subgroups: loose, dense, and specialized connective tissue.

Loose Connective Tissue

The fibers of loose connective tissue are delicate and loosely woven together, and serve to fill spaces between organs. There are three main types: areolar, adipose, and reticular. The cells that make up loose connective tissue are mainly fibroblasts, located a good distance apart and separated by a matrix that is made up of collagenous and elastic fibers.

Collagenous fibers, sometimes referred to as white fibers, are thick, tough fibers that are composed of the protein collagen. These flexible fibers are important in keeping separate structures together, primarily because of their tensile strength. This type of fiber is found frequently in dense connective tissue (described later).

Elastic fibers, sometimes referred to as yellow fibers, are made of the protein elastin. They are not as strong as collagenous fibers but are elastic; therefore, they are found in body areas that require a good amount of stretching for proper function.

Areolar tissue is the most widely distributed of the three types of connective tissue. It surrounds various organs, and lies beneath the layers of the epithelium, where it provides support for the various nerves and blood vessels necessary for transport of nutrients to the epithelial cells. Its delicate fibers are constructed of three types of cells: fibroblasts, histiocytes (macrophages), and mast cells.

Fibroblasts are the most common cell types in connective tissue. These are large, flattened cells with reduced cytoplasm, and are shaped somewhat like starfish. These cells form fibrils made of protein for the construction of the intercellular matrix.

Histiocytes, also known as macrophages, are mobile when not attached to fibers, and are designed to carry out phagocytosis, a major function of the immune system that scavenges foreign particles from tissues to prevent infection.

Mast cells are usually located near blood vessels, and are designed to manufacture heparin (a blood thinner) and histamine (an important agent in the inflammatory process and allergies).

Adipose tissue is often referred to as "fat," and is constructed of specialized cells called adipocytes that store fat droplets within their cytoplasm. This type of tissue is found beneath the skin and between the muscles, around the kidneys and the heart, behind the eyeballs, and within joint spaces. It serves to insulate (fat is a poor heat conductor), cushion (especially the kidneys), and store energy.

Reticular tissue consists of a network of delicate collagenous fibers that mechanically support the liver, bone marrow, spleen, and lymphoid organs.

Dense Connective Tissue

Dense connective tissue forms tendons, ligaments, and aponeuroses. It is composed primarily of tightly bound protein fibers, and can be further classified as either fibrous or elastic connective tissue.

Fibrous connective tissue is made of dense, thick collagenous fibers and a network of delicate elastic fibers. Fibrous connective tissue is strong and elastic, and functions to bind separate structures together. For example, tendons are composed primarily of collagenous fibers (with few elastic fibers), and are used to connect bone to muscles. Ligaments are strong elastic bands composed of a combination of collagenous and elastic fibers used to connect one bone to another. Structures made of fibrous connective tissue typically have a limited blood supply, which slows healing after injury. This is the reason that a sprained ankle (usually a result of overstretched ligaments around the ankle joint) is notorious for delayed healing.

Elastic connective tissue is made up of yellow, elastic fibers that are either branched or run in parallel strands. It makes up the ligamenta flava, which binds adjacent vertebra together, and also occurs in the walls of hollow organs, arteries, and airways.

Specialized Connective Tissue

Specialized connective tissue consists of cartilage, bone, blood and hematopoietic tissues, and reticuloendothelial tissue. Cartilage is made of cells called chondrocytes, found in cavities within cartilage called **lacunae**. Lacunae are surrounded by matrix. Cartilage structures are enclosed in perichondrium, which is a covering of fibrous connective tissue that supplies the cartilage with nutrients from a small blood supply (cartilage itself has no blood vessels).

There are three types of cartilage found in the body, each with a different type of matrix. Their strength and flexibility depend upon the amount of collagen and elastin embedded in their matrix. The three main types of cartilage are hyaline, fibrous, and elastic.

Hyaline cartilage has a matrix of delicate collagenous fibers, and it occurs at the ends of bones in many joints, in the supporting rings of the respiratory airways, and in the soft portion of the nose. The skeletal system of a fetus is made up completely of hyaline cartilage, which is eventually replaced by bone after six months in a process called ossification.

Elastic cartilage has a matrix of dense elastic fibers, and is therefore more flexible than hyaline cartilage. It provides the framework for the external ear, the auditory tubes, and the epiglottis.

Fibrocartilage is a dense, tough tissue with many collagenous fibers embedded within its matrix. It forms the intervertebral disks, which act as shock absorbers for the individual bones of the spine, and it connects the two pelvic bones at the pubic symphysis. It also acts as a shock absorber for the bones of the knee.

Bone

Bone (osseous tissue) is the hardest of the connective tissues because it contains mineral salts such as calcium phosphate and calcium carbonate, with a large amount of collagen serving as its intercellular matrix. The skeleton, in serving as the anchoring points for muscles and tendons, enables support and movement. In addition, bones are protective structures for critical organs like the brain, spinal cord, heart, and lungs. It also contains red marrow, necessary for the formation of new red blood cells. Bone also stores various inorganic salts.

Bone matrix is deposited in thin layers called **lamellae**, which are arranged in concentric patterns around tiny tubes called **haversian canals**. One or two small blood vessels occupy the canal along with a nerve and possibly a lymphatic vessel.

Lying between or within the lamellae are cavities known as **lacunae** (the same as are found in cartilage). Each lacuna provides enough space for an individual bone cell to reside. The osteocyte inside the lacuna is responsible for secreting the bone salts surrounding it.

Osteocytes within their cavelike lacunae communicate with each other via cytoplasmic extensions through unique passages called **canaliculi**. These passages provide an avenue for diffusion of nutrients and wastes. Canaliculi of bone are essential for osteocytes because diffusion cannot occur across crystalline solids.

Blood and Hematopoietic Tissues

Blood is a unique connective tissue because its intercellular matrix is composed of a liquid (plasma) in which cells (white blood cells, red blood cells, and platelets) is suspended. Hematopoietic tissues form red blood cells and white blood cells. Red blood cells

are formed within red bone marrow of certain bones, and white blood cells are formed by lymphoid organs. Because red bone marrow and lymphoid organs form these types of cells, they are known as hematopoietic tissues (see Chapter 10 for details about blood).

Reticuloendothelial tissue

Another specialized connective tissue is reticuloendothelial tissue, composed of various cells that are phagocytic, meaning that they attack foreign invaders of the body and ingest them. The most common type of these phagocytic cells is the **macrophage**, these cells remain fixed in place until they sense an invasion by a foreign particle. Once stimulated, they become motile and pursue the invader until they catch it and ingest it. Because they function to protect the body from infection, phagocytic cells are an instrumental aspect of the front line of the immunity system.

MUSCLE TISSUE

Muscle tissue, through its ability to relax and contract, causes movement that brings about locomotion and other types of internal movement necessary for survival (such as the cardiac movement and movement of the alimentary canal for the expulsion of waste). Muscles can be divided into three main groups according to their structure:

- Smooth muscle tissue
- Skeletal muscle tissue
- Cardiac muscle tissue

Smooth Muscle Tissue

Smooth muscle tissue is made up of thin, elongated muscle fibers. Each fiber has a large, oval nucleus, and each cell is filled with a specialized cytoplasm (called the **sarcoplasm**) that is surrounded by a thin cell membrane (called the **sarcolemma**).

The myofibrils of the muscle cell run parallel to each other, interlacing to form flattened sheets. Because they do not form bundles, the sheets of muscle appear smooth (unlike skeletal muscle, smooth muscle fibers do not form a striped, striated pattern). This type of muscle tissue makes up the walls of hollow organs, such as those of the alimentary canal, bladder, uterus, and blood vessels, and is therefore outside the voluntary control of the brain.

Smooth muscle controls slow contractions of the walls of the stomach and intestines, and also controls the artery wall contractions for the regulation of blood pressure and flow of blood. Uterine wall and bladder wall contractions are also controlled by smooth muscle.

Skeletal Muscle Tissue

Skeletal muscle, the most abundant tissue in the body, is attached to various bones of the skeleton (hence the name), and is under the conscious control of the brain. These muscles are used for locomotion: as they contract, the bones move and a motion is carried through. Skeletal muscles function in pairs to bring about the coordinated movements of limbs, eyes, trunk, jaws, and so on. Skeletal muscle makes up approximately 40% of our total weight.

The skeletal muscle is enclosed in a sheath of connective tissue, called the epimysium. This sheath folds inward into the substance of the muscle to surround a large number of smaller bundles, the **fasciculi**. These fasciculi consist of still smaller bundles of elongated, cylindrical muscle cells, called fibers. Each fiber contains many nuclei found at the periphery of the cell, just beneath the sarcolemma. Alternating thin protein filaments of actin and dark bands of the thicker protein filaments of myosin give skeletal muscle a striated (striped) appearance.

Cardiac (Heart) Muscle Tissue

Cardiac tissue is found only in the walls of the heart, and exhibits some of the characteristics of smooth muscle and some of skeletal muscle tissue. Like skeletal muscle, it has fibers with cross-striations that contain numerous nuclei; but, like smooth muscle, it is involuntary (not under the conscious control of the brain). Cardiac muscle fibers are shorter than striated muscle fibers, and the striations are not as striking in appearance. There is only one nucleus present in the center of each cardiac fiber, and adjacent fibers branch but are linked to each other by so-called muscle bridges. The spaces between different fibers are filled with areolar connective tissue, which contains blood capillaries to supply the tissue with oxygen and nutrients. This branching effect by muscle bridges ensures that the muscles contract in coordinated movements.

Cardiac muscle tissue plays the most important role in the contraction of the atria and ventricles of the heart. By causing the rhythmical beating of the heart and expelling blood, it circulates the blood and its contents throughout the body.

NERVOUS TISSUE

Nerve tissue, made up of specialized cells called **neurons**, is found in the brain and spinal cord (central nervous system) and peripheral nerves (peripheral nervous system). Nervous tissue is specialized to react to stimuli and to conduct impulses to various organs in the body that bring about a response to the stimulus, thereby coordinating and regulating many body functions.

A nerve is made up of many neurons bound together by connective tissue, with a sheath of dense connective tissue (called the **epineurium**) surrounding the entire nerve. This sheath penetrates the nerve to form the perineurium, which surrounds bundles of nerve fibers. Blood vessels of various sizes can be seen in the epineurium. The endoneurium, which consists of a thin layer of loose connective tissue, surrounds the individual nerve fibers.

MEMBRANES

Membranes are thin, sheetlike structures composed of connective and epithelial tissues. They line body cavities and cover body surfaces. There are four major types: serous, mucous, cutaneous, and synovial. Serous, mucous, and cutaneous membranes are composed of epithelial tissue (with some underlying connective tissue), and synovial membranes are composed of connective tissues.

Serous membranes line body cavities that do not open to the outside of the body. They cover the organs within the abdomen and thorax (called the **visceral layer**), and form the inner linings of those cavities (called the **parietal layer**). Serous membranes are composed of two different layers of tissue: a thin layer of simple squamous epithelium, covering a layer of loose connective tissue that acts as a basement membrane for support of epithelial cells. Serous membranes secrete a thin, watery fluid (called serous fluid) that lubricates the surface of the membrane and reduces friction between adjacent organs.

In the thoracic cavity, serous membranes are referred to as **pleura**. In the abdominal cavity, they are referred to as **peritoneum**. Therefore, we refer to the layer of serous membrane that lines the thoracic cavity as the parietal pleura, and the one covering the abdominal cavity as the parietal peritoneum. The serous membrane that lines the organs of the thoracic cavity is called the visceral pleura, and the one lining the abdominal organs is called the visceral peritoneum. Figure 3-1 illustrates the mucous and serous membranes.

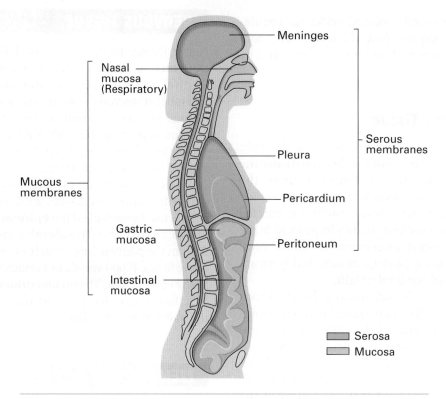

FIGURE 3-1 **Mucous and serous membranes**

Mucous membranes are epithelial membranes that line cavities and tubes that open to the outside of the body, such as the oral and nasal cavities, and the tubes of the reproductive, digestive, urinary, and respiratory systems. The epithelial component of the membrane varies according to its location. The oral cavity is lined with stratified squamous epithelium (as is the esophagus), and the lower intestinal tract is lined with simple columnar epithelium. Specialized epithelial cells of mucous membranes secrete a thick fluid called **mucus**, which keeps the membranes lubricated.

The cutaneous membrane is commonly referred to as skin, and is an organ of the integumentary system, which is described in detail in a later chapter.

Synovial membranes line the inner linings of freely moveable joints between the ends of bones. They secrete a thick, slippery fluid called synovial fluid, which lubricates the ends of the bones within the joint cavities.

POSTOPERATIVE TISSUE REPAIR

The surgical technologist must be knowledgeable of the types of tissues, the way that they heal, and the techniques and methods used for tissue approximation in order to prevent postoperative wound infection and enhance healing. An understanding of surgical-wound classification, the types of wound healing, and the complications that can arise from the creation of a surgical-wound or the treatment of a traumatic wound is essential to the proper practice of surgical technology.

Classification of Surgical Wounds

Surgical wounds are either incisional or excisional: An **incision** is an intentional cut through intact tissue for the purpose of exposing underlying structures. **Excision** is the removal of tissue. They are also classified according to their degree of microbial intrusion. The categories are as follows:

1. Class I (clean): occurs when an incision is made under ideal conditions, and aseptic technique is not broken. The wound is closed primarily, and the aerodigestive or genitourinary tract is not entered. No wound drain is necessary, and the infection rate for Class I wounds is 1%–5%.
2. Class II (clean-contaminated): occurs after a primary closure, but the wound is drained and either a minor break in aseptic technique occurred, or the aerodigestive, biliary, or genitourinary tract was entered. Infection rate is 8%–11%.

3. Class III (contaminated): occurs when an open traumatic wound is encountered, the aerodigestive, biliary, or genitourinary tract was entered (often with fluid spillage), or a major break in aseptic technique occurred. Usually acute inflammation is present, and the infection rate is 15%–20%.
4. Class IV (dirty-infected): occurs in open traumatic wounds in which microbial contamination had previously occurred. Perforated viscus with fluid spillage is common, and the infection rate is 27%–40%.

Types of Wound Healing

There are three types of wound healing: (a) first intention or primary union, (b) second intention or granulation healing, and (c) third intention or delayed primary closure.

First Intention Healing

First intention healing (primary union) is considered the optimal type of healing because tissues heal from side to side without infection. Dead space (space between tissue layers that can accumulate fluids and lead to infection) is not present and the wound heals without complications.

First intention healing occurs in three phases:

1. Lag (inflammatory response) phase: begins within minutes of injury and lasts approximately three to five days. It is defined by the physiologic changes associated with inflammation: heat, redness, swelling, and pain. Bleeding is controlled at this stage through platelet aggregation, and epithelial cells are formed for repair. A scab forms to seal the wound and protect it from microbial invasion. Protein-rich fluid leaks into the extravascular fluid compartment, resulting in swelling (edema) and pain.

    Neutrophils and macrophages begin to phagocytize foreign particles, and basal cells migrate across skin edges to close the wound surface. Fibroblasts begin reconstructing nonepithelial tissue.
2. Proliferation phase: begins on the third postoperative day and continues for up to 20 days. Fibroblasts bind the wound edges and secrete collagen, which gives the wound a quarter of its original strength. New capillary networks are established and lymphatic networks are reformed by the 10th day.
3. Maturation or differentiation phase: begins on the 14th postoperative day and continues until

the wound is completely healed. Tensile strength is slowly established to normal, and wound contraction resulting from dermal and subcutaneous myofibroblasts is finished by the 21st day. Collagen density increases and angiogenesis (creation of new blood vessels) stops. A small, white surface scar, called a cicatrix, appears during this phase. Figure 3-2 illustrates the tissue response to injury.

Second Intention Healing

Second intention healing (granulation) is characterized by healing that takes place from the bottom upward in which the wound fills in with granulation tissue. It occurs when a wound fails to heal by primary union, and generally occurs in large wounds that cannot be directly reapproximated by primary union. It also occurs in wounds in which infection has caused a breakdown of tissues and suture; wounds in which it is highly likely an infection will occur, such as a wound heavily contaminated with soil and dirt; and wounds that required extensive excision of necrotic tissue.

After debridement (excision) of necrotic tissue, second intention healing may occur from the inner layer to the outside surface in a complicated and prolonged process. Granulation tissue that contains myofibroblasts forms in the wound, causing closure by contraction. Large gaps are filled from the bottom up with granulation tissue, resulting in a wide irregular scar.

Third Intention Healing

Third intention healing (delayed primary closure) occurs when two granulated surfaces are approximated, and is employed when the wound is infected, dirty, or contaminated. The traumatic surgical wound is thoroughly irrigated and debrided, and left open to heal by second intention for approximately one week. During that period the patient is kept on antibiotic treatment. When the wound is infection free, it is closed and allowed to heal by first intention. Therefore, the wound heals by contraction, granulation, and connective tissue closure.

Complications of Wound Healing

Complications of a healing wound can arise even if strict sterile technique is maintained by the surgical technologist. **Dehiscence** is a partial or total separation of a layer or layers of tissue after closure, and it occurs most frequently between the fifth and 10th postoperative day. It can be caused by a variety of -

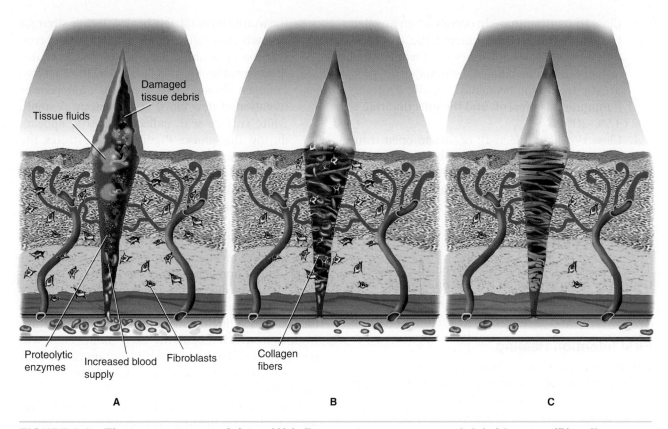

FIGURE 3-2 Tissue response to injury: (A) inflammatory response and debridement, (B) collagen formation (scar tissue), and (C) sufficient collagen laid down (Reproduced with permission from Ethicon, Inc., Somerville, NJ, 2002)

conditions, including abdominal distension, increased tension on the wound (from coughing or vomiting), or improper suturing techniques or suture types. Figure 3-3 shows dead space within a wound.

Complications from the use of suture for wound approximation occur when the suture is not absorbed properly or the suture irritates the wound. The result of either is usually an inflammatory state. Silk and cotton suture materials (seldom used today) are most often implicated. Suture "spits" from the wound when this condition occurs. Table 3-2 describes postoperative wound complications.

TISSUE TYPING

Human have genetic markers on the surface of most of their white blood cells. One of those markers is called **human leukocyte antigen** or HLA (antigen refers to a genetic marker). The test that identifies an individual's HLA is called tissue typing, and the performance of this test is essential for any patient receiving a donor organ.

Laboratory personnel mix the white blood cells from the donor (or the donor tissue) and the recipient and look for an immune response. If leukocytes proliferate, this signals the triggering of an immune response, and that the tissue is likely to be rejected by the recipient.

Another newer technique involves the analysis of the donor's and recipient's DNA for tissue typing. This technique diminishes the likelihood of rejection in the case of tissue transplantation. DNA testing is done for bone marrow transplants to determine whether the leukocytes and their precursors repopulating a recipient's bone marrow are the recipient's or those of the donor.

DNA tissue typing targets a specific set of genes where the **major histocompatibility complex** (MHC) resides. These particular genes are unique to each individual, and they code for the production of specific glycoprotein antigens that recognizes each individual's tissues and targets as foreign those different from that individual's tissue. These are the antigens that trigger an immune response that leads to rejection of an organ in a transplantation procedure.

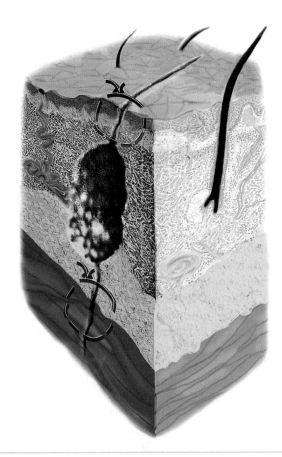

FIGURE 3-3 **Dead space in a wound (Reproduced with permission from Ethicon, Inc., Somerville, NJ, 2002)**

BOX 3-1

Infection of Tissue

For the surgical technologist, infection of tissue presents a significant challenge that can permanently affect the patient's quality of life. It is estimated that the patient with a postoperative surgical-wound infection stays in the hospital on average an additional 7–10 days, contributing to the higher cost of health care. The surgical technologist receives extensive training in aseptic technique that is designed to prevent postoperative wound infections, but an infection can arise even if there are no breaks in sterile technique. There are two categories of postoperative wound infections:

1. Incisional infection is one that penetrates the skin, subcutaneous tissue, and muscle. It occurs at the incisional site usually within 30 days of the surgical procedure. The wound may be reopened for extensive irrigation and drainage, with placement of a drain. The wound may also be left open to heal by third intention. Packing with or without impregnated antibiotic may be necessary if the wound is to heal by third intention.

2. Deep-tissue infection also occurs at the surgical site within 30 days of the surgical procedure. The infection is established in the deep tissues of the body below the fascia or peritoneal layer, thereby increasing the risk of dehiscence. The surgeon will often have to perform a procedure to irrigate the wound with antibiotic saline, with placement of a wound drain. If the infection occurs around an implant, such as screws or a plate, the implant will most likely have to be removed.

TABLE 3-2 Postoperative Complications of Wound Healing

COMPLICATION	DEFINITION
Evisceration	The protrusion of viscera through the edges of a totally separated wound. This situation requires immediate attention to prevent peritonitis.
Hemorrhage	Uncontrolled bleeding that can occur immediately following a procedure, and can lead to hypovolemic shock. The patient must be returned to the operating room, reopened, and hemostasis must be achieved.
Adhesions	Abnormal attachments of two surfaces or structures that are normally separate. Fibrous tissue may develop within the abdominal or pelvic cavity from previous procedures, infections, or the presence of a foreign body. These attachments can cause organs to stick together, thereby disrupting function and causing pain.
Herniation	The result of wound dehiscence that could cause incarceration of the bowel. Surgery is required for repair.
Fistula	A tract between two epithelium-lined surfaces; it is open at both ends. It typically occurs after bladder, bowel, and pelvic procedures. Surgery is required to correct this condition.
Keloid scarring	A hypertrophic scar formation that occurs mainly in dark-skinned individuals. Surgery is often required for plastic repair of these wounds.
Sinus tract	A tract between two epithelium-lined surfaces that is open at only one end. It typically occurs after bladder, bowel, and pelvic procedures. Surgery is required for repair.

The HLA within the MHC is the region used for DNA analysis for tissue typing for transplantation. This region, called HLA-D, is further subdivided into regions HLA-DR, HLA-DQ, and HLA-DP, depending on the type of glycoprotein antigen for which they code. These regions of the genes of the recipient and donor are carefully compared and contrasted to determine the transplant's chances for rejection.

SURGICAL SPECIMENS

The surgical technologist must also understand how surgical pathology personnel prepare the tissue for study once the specimen leaves the operating room. Tissues are submitted to the pathology department to diagnose benign and malignant neoplasms and inflammatory or infectious diseases.

Tissue for specimen is removed from the body intraoperatively by knife, biopsy forceps, or Tru-cut needle biopsy devices. The type of tissue (and its origin), and the decision to make it a frozen or permanent specimen, are ascertained during the procedure (permanent specimens are routinely fixed in 10% neutral buffered formalin, although some special studies require fresh tissue, frozen tissue, or tissue submitted in other fixatives). Once the tissue is identified, labeled, and properly "fixed" in the operating room, it is transferred to the pathology department with a tissue specimen request form. This form is typically filled out by the circulator in the operating room (OR) and should include the following:

Patient's first and last name
Medical record number
Date
Physician
Date of birth
Billing information
Social Security Number (optional)
Identity of tissue specimen
Procedure done to obtain the tissue
Clinical history

The container should be legibly and properly labeled on adhesive tape or addressograph label adhered to the container with the name of the patient and the medical record number.

For permanent sections, the circulator should add 10% formalin to the container before the specimen is placed into it. Prefilled formalin containers are supplied by the pathology department upon request. Specimens must be placed in formalin as soon as possible to avoid compromising histopathologic evaluation.

Once the tissue is received in pathology, it is routinely processed through a tissue processor, and then embedded in paraffin wax. A thin section is then cut, placed on a slide, stained with dyes, and then examined under the microscope.

For the surgical technologist in the intraoperative role, it is important to understand the identity and origin of the specimen when receiving it from the surgeon. This information should be properly communicated to the circulator when it is passed from the sterile field. If specimen edges are marked by suture for tumor margins, the significance of the markers must be explained as well.

When the specimen is to be removed from the sterile field, it should be done in a sterile fashion. The specimen should be placed in a sterile specimen container, Telfa pad, towel, or basin. A counted surgical sponge should never be used for specimen transport. If the specimen is to remain on the back table (for permanent section), then precautions should be taken to prevent drying. A specimen obtained for frozen section should be immediately handed to the circulator (usually in a folded sterile towel) after receiving it from the surgeon so that it can be taken to the lab for immediate diagnosis. Once received by the pathologist, the tissue is frozen, sliced into thin sections, and then stained for viewing under the microscope. The preliminary results are phoned into the surgeon in the OR, and a decision is made about the removal of the affected organ.

BOX 3-2
Special Circumstances for Specimen Preparation in the OR

- Breast Biopsy: The circulator should place the biopsy in formalin, and indicate on the requisition whether the surgeon desires DNA ploidy analysis or estrogen/progesterone receptor analysis or both (these can be done on the formalin-fixed tissue).
- Lymph Nodes: The pathologist should be contacted one to two days prior to the biopsy if malignant lymphoma is suspected. The pathologist may need to order special processing (e.g., flow cytometry, gene rearrangement studies). The node should be sectioned into 3 to 4 mm slices if it is large, and the specimen should be placed in fixative as soon as possible.

IMPLICATIONS FOR THE SURGICAL TECHNOLOGIST

The surgical technologist spends a good deal of time dealing with human tissues, so an understanding of how they are classified, how they heal, and the complications that can accompany their incision or excision, handling, and closure is imperative for proper patient care. Different types of tissues heal in different ways, and the surgical technologist must understand the techniques and suture materials that best fit the tissue to be handled. In addition, an understanding of the specific instrumentation needed to grasp, excise, or retract different types of tissue must be understood. Because the excision and handling of specimens for pathologic study is routine practice for the surgical technologist, an understanding of the proper procedure for procurement and transfer is important. In addition, the surgical technologist assists with transplantation procedures on a regular basis, and must know the importance of proper tissue typing for successful outcomes.

Case Study 2

Dr. Morgan is performing an emergency procedure on a gunshot wound (GSW) to the abdomen that has perforated the bowel, spilling the contents into the abdominal cavity. The surgical technologist is using a specific bowel technique to isolate and minimize the contamination.

1. How would this wound be classified? What is the infection rate for these types of wounds?

2. What is the bowel technique utilized by the surgical technologist in this procedure?

3. What are the possible complications for this type of wound?

CHAPTER SUMMARY

- When groups of cells that have similar function and structure are grouped together, they form tissues.

- There are four major types of tissue in the human body: epithelial, connective, muscle, and nervous.

- Epithelial tissues are found throughout the body, and cover all body surfaces.

- A single layer of cells within epithelial tissue is said to be simple, and those with multiple layers are called stratified.

- Cells that are thin, flattened, and slightly irregular in shape are called squamous, whereas cells with a cubelike appearance are called cuboidal. Cells with an elongated, rectangular appearance are referred to as columnar.

- The cells of simple squamous epithelium have the appearance of thin, flat plates and form the lining of cavities (mouth, blood vessels, heart, and lungs), and make up the outer layers of the skin.

- The cells of simple cuboidal epithelium are shaped like cubes, and are found in glands, gland ducts, and in the lining of the kidney tubules.

- The cells of simple columnar epithelium are elongated and column-shaped, with nuclei that are elongated and located at the base of the cells near the basement membrane. These cells form the lining of the uterus, stomach, and intestines.

- Columnar and cuboidal epithelial cells often become specialized as gland cells that synthesize and secrete enzymes, hormones, milk, sweat, wax, and saliva.

- Glands that secrete their substances into ducts are called exocrine glands, and those that secrete their products into tissue fluid or blood are called endocrine glands.

- Where the body is exposed to conditions that cause wear and tear, the epithelia located there are composed of several layers of cells, and are called stratified squamous epithelia.

- Transitional epithelium is designed to handle tension in tissues, and lines the walls of the urinary bladder, urethra, and ureters.

- Connective tissue, the most varied and abundant tissue of the body, functions to support the body and to bind together all types of tissue. It can be classified according to three subgroups: loose, dense, and specialized.

- The fibers of loose connective tissue are delicate and loosely woven together, and serve to fill spaces between organs. There are three main types: areolar, adipose, and reticular.

- Collagenous fibers are thick, tough fibers that are composed of the protein collagen. They are important in keeping separate structures together due to their tensile strength.

- Elastic fibers are made of the protein elastin. Their elasticity makes them ideal for body structures that require a good amount of stretching for proper function.

- Areolar tissue surrounds various organs, and lies beneath the layers of the epithelium. Its fibers are constructed of these cells: fibroblasts, histiocytes, and mast cells.

- Adipose tissue cells (adipocytes) store fat droplets.

- Reticular tissue consists of a network of delicate collagenous fibers that mechanically support the liver, bone marrow, spleen, and lymphoid organs.

- Dense connective tissue forms tendons, ligaments, and aponeuroses.

- Fibrous connective tissue is made of dense collagenous fibers and a network of delicate elastic fibers. It is strong and elastic, and binds separate structures together (tendons and ligaments).

- Elastic connective tissue is made up of yellow, elastic fibers that make up the ligamenta flava that binds adjacent vertebra together. It also occurs in the walls of hollow organs, arteries, and airways.

- Specialized connective tissue consists of cartilage, bone, blood and hematopoietic tissues, and reticuloendothelial tissue.

- There are three types of cartilage found in the body: hyaline, fibrous, and elastic.

- Hyaline cartilage has a matrix of delicate collagenous fibers.

- Elastic cartilage has a matrix of dense elastic fibers.

- Fibrocartilage is a dense, tough tissue with many collagenous fibers embedded within its matrix.

- Bone is the hardest of the connective tissues because it contains mineral salts such as calcium phosphate and calcium carbonate.

- The skeleton anchors muscles and tendons, and enables support and movement. Bones are protective structures for critical organs and contain red marrow for the formation of red blood cells.

- Blood is composed of a liquid (plasma) in which white blood cells, red blood cells, and platelets are suspended.

- Hematopoietic tissues form red blood cells and white blood cells.

- Reticuloendothelial tissue is composed of various phagocytic cells.

- Muscle tissue causes movement that brings about locomotion and other types of internal movement necessary for survival. Muscles can be divided into three main groups according to their structure: smooth, skeletal, and cardiac.

- Nerve tissue, made up of specialized cells called neurons, is found in the brain and spinal cord (central nervous system) and peripheral nerves (peripheral nervous system).

- Membranes are thin, sheetlike structures composed of connective and epithelial tissues. They line body cavities and cover body surfaces. There are four major types: serous, mucous, cutaneous, and synovial.

- Serous membranes line body cavities that do not open to the outside of the body. They cover the organs within the abdomen and thorax (visceral layer), and form the inner linings of those cavities (parietal layer).

- Mucous membranes are epithelial membranes that line cavities and tubes that open to the outside of the body, such as the oral and nasal cavities, and the tubes of the reproductive, digestive, urinary, and respiratory systems.

- The cutaneous membrane is commonly referred to as skin.

- Synovial membranes line the inner linings of freely moveable joints between the ends of bones.

- Surgical wounds are either incisional or excisional. They are also classified according to their degree of microbial intrusion: Class I (clean), Class II (clean-contaminated), Class III (contaminated), Class IV (dirty-infected).

- There are three types of wound healing: (a) first intention or primary union, (b) second intention or granulation healing, and (c) third intention or delayed primary closure.

- First intention healing occurs in three phases: lag (inflammatory response) phase, proliferation phase, and maturation (differentiation) phase.

- Complications of a healing wound include dehiscence, evisceration, hemorrhage, adhesions, herniation, fistula, keloid scarring, and sinus tract.

- There are two categories of postoperative wound infections: Incisional infection is one that penetrates the skin, subcutaneous tissue, and muscle. Deep-tissue infection is established in the deep tissues of the body below the fascia or peritoneal layer.

- The test that identifies an individual's HLA is called tissue typing, and the performance of this test is essential for any patient receiving a donor organ.

- DNA tissue typing targets a specific set of genes where the MHC resides.

- The HLA within the MHC is the region used for DNA analysis for tissue typing for transplantation.

- Tissue for specimen is removed from the body intraoperatively by knife, biopsy forceps, or Tru-cut needle biopsy devices.

- Once the tissue is received in the pathology department, it is processed through a tissue processor and then embedded in paraffin wax. A thin section is then cut, placed on a slide, stained with dyes, and examined under the microscope.

CRITICAL THINKING QUESTIONS

1. How should the surgical technologist handle certain projectile specimens such as bullets?
2. Should an incision into the trachea be treated the same as an incision into the bowel?
3. Would you consider a fistula and an adhesion to be the same thing? If not, why?
4. What is the difference between dehiscence and evisceration?
5. Why should a counted sponge never be used for specimen transfer?

BIBLIOGRAPHY

Adorno, D., Maccarone, D., & Papola, F. (2000). Tissue-typing laboratories for organ transplantation. *Annali dell'Istituto Superiore di Sanita, 36*(2), 179–183.

Association of Surgical Technologists. (2003). *Surgical technology for the surgical technologist: A positive care approach* (2nd ed.). Clifton Park, NY: Thomson Delmar Learning.

Blystone, R., & Cooper, R. (2004). *Synergistic learning in biology and statistics.* Retrieved May 4, 2005, from http://www.trinity.edu/rblyston/bone/intro2.htm

Hole, J.W. Jr. (1987). *Human anatomy and physiology* (4th ed.). Dubuque, IA: Brown.

Moore, F. D. (1995). Clinical transplants 1993. *New England Journal Medicine, 332*, 65–67.

Scott, A. S., & Fong, E. (1998). *Body structures and functions* (9th ed.). Clifton Park, NY: Thomson Delmar Learning.

Tortora, G. J., & Grabowski, S. R. (1996). *Principles of anatomy and physiology* (8th ed.). New York: Harper-Collins.

Unknown. *Surgical specimens.* Retrieved, June 25, 2004, from http://www.lcpath.com/pathology.html

Unknown. (2003). *Tissue typing for transplantation.* Retrieved May 4, 2005, from http://www.lcpath.com/manual.asp

Wisniewska-Roszkowska, K. (1973). *Aging of tissues and organs. Pieleg Polozna, 5*, 8–10.

4

ORGAN SYSTEMS

CHAPTER OUTLINE

Introduction
Homeostasis and Organ Systems
Feedback Systems in Homeostasis
Organ Replacement

CHAPTER OBJECTIVES

After completing the study of this chapter, you should be able to:

1. Compare and contrast the various organ systems of the body.
2. Describe the function of homeostasis and its importance to health.
3. Compare and contrast negative and positive feedback.
4. Describe the problems associated with organ replacement and the methods that will solve them.

Case Study 1

Margaret is a surgical technologist employed by a medical center that specializes in all forms of organ transplantation. She has been performing kidney and liver transplantations for years, but only this year has begun to perform heart transplantations. She is preparing to transplant a heart into a 44-year-old man with advanced congestive cardiomyopathy. The heart is being flown in by jet from a donor in a nearby state.

1. What is cardiomyopathy?

2. Heart transplantations are the third most common transplantation procedures in the United States. What are the two most common?

3. What is the biggest lifelong struggle for the postoperative transplantation patient?

INTRODUCTION

An **organ** is a structure that is made up of two or more different types of tissue that are organized for the performance of a specialized function. Organs are arranged within systems that allow for more complex functions that cannot be performed by one organ alone. The organ systems of the body are as follows:

Integumentary system
Skeletal system
Muscular system
Nervous system
Endocrine system
Circulatory system (including lymphatics)
Immune system
Respiratory system
Digestive system
Excretory (urinary) system
Reproductive system

ORGAN SYSTEMS

The integumentary system (Chapter 5) is the outermost protective layer. It prevents water loss and invasion of foreign microorganisms into the body. It also helps regulate body temperature and houses a variety of sensory receptors. The components of the integumentary system are the *skin, hair, nails, sweat glands,* and *sebaceous glands.*

The skeletal system (Chapter 6) provides support and protection, attachment points for muscles, and a rigid framework for movement. It supports and protects the body and body parts, produces blood cells, and stores inorganic salts. It is composed of *bones, joints, ligaments,* and *cartilage.*

The muscular system (Chapter 7) allows movement and locomotion. It produces body movements and body heat, maintains posture, and supports the body. Action of this system is closely tied to that of the skeletal system. See Figure 4-1, which illustrates the integumentary, skeletal, and muscular systems. The muscular system consists of *muscles* and *tendons.*

The nervous system (Chapter 8) coordinates and controls actions of internal organs and body systems. Memory, learning, and conscious thought are a few aspects of the functions of the nervous system. Maintaining autonomic functions such as heartbeat, breathing, and control of involuntary muscle actions are performed by some of the parts of this system. Its components are the *brain, spinal cord,* and *associated nerves.*

The endocrine system (Chapter 18) works with the nervous system to control the activity of internal organs as well as coordinate long-range response to external stimuli. The endocrine system secretes hormones that regulate body metabolism, growth, and reproduction, and consists of the *pituitary gland, pineal gland, ovaries, testes,* and *thyroid gland.*

The circulatory system (Chapters 11, 12, and 13) transports oxygen, carbon dioxide, nutrients, waste products, immune components, and hormones. The lymphatic system is considered part of the circulatory system because it transports excess fluids to and from the circulatory system and carries lipids away from the digestive organs. It helps to defend the body against infection by removing microorganisms from tissue fluid and by supporting the activities of immune cells (lymphocytes). Figure 4-2 illustrates the nervous, endocrine, and cardiovascular or circulatory systems. The components of the cardiovascular system are the *heart, arteries, veins, capillaries,* and

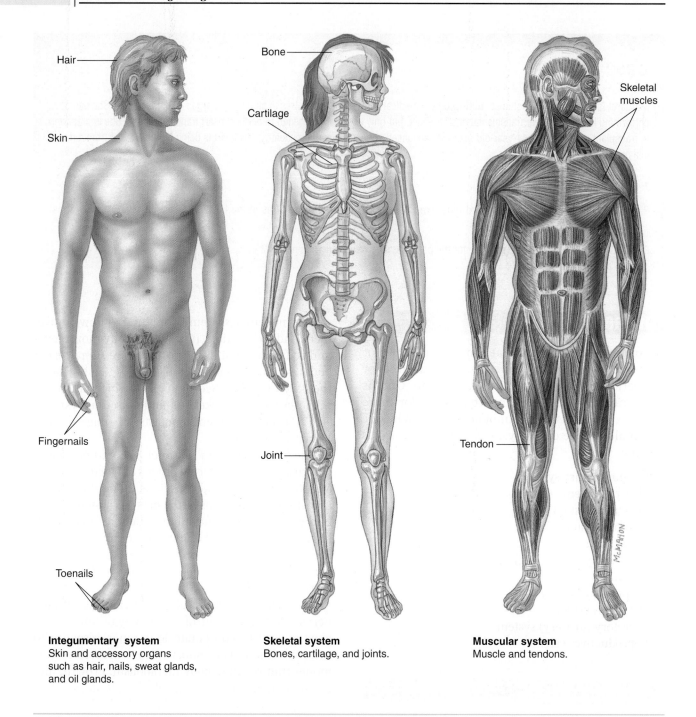

Integumentary system
Skin and accessory organs
such as hair, nails, sweat glands,
and oil glands.

Skeletal system
Bones, cartilage, and joints.

Muscular system
Muscle and tendons.

FIGURE 4-1 The integumentary, skeletal, and muscular systems of the body

blood. The lymphatic system consists of the *lymph nodes* and *vessels, thymus,* and *spleen.*

The **immune system** defends the internal environment from invading microorganisms and viruses, as well as cancerous cell growth. The immune system provides cells that aid in protection of the body from disease via the antigen–antibody response. A variety of general responses are also part of this system.

The respiratory system (Chapter 14) moves oxygen from the external environment into the internal environment; it also removes carbon dioxide and maintains pH of the blood. It consists of the *nasal cavity, pharynx, larynx, trachea, bronchi,* and *lungs.*

The digestive system (Chapter 15) digests and absorbs food into nutrient molecules by chemical and mechanical breakdown, breaking food into particles small

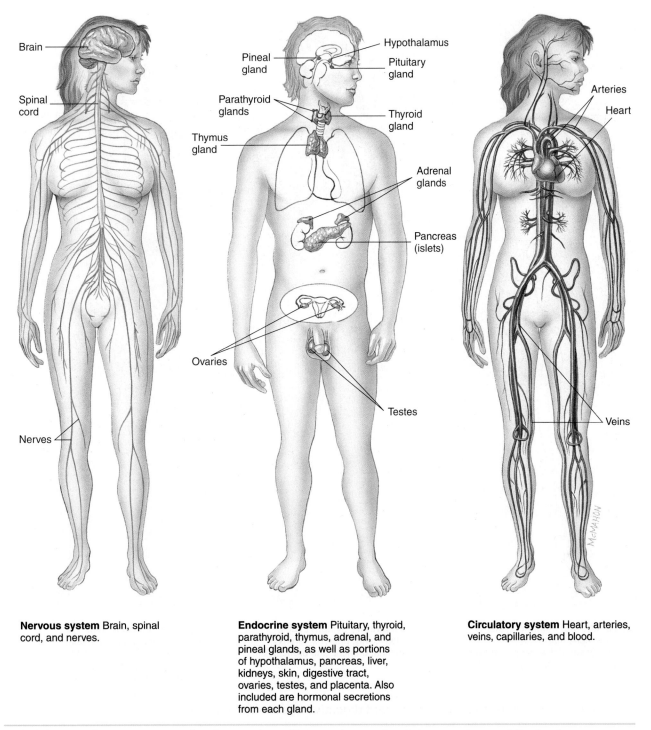

Nervous system Brain, spinal cord, and nerves.

Endocrine system Pituitary, thyroid, parathyroid, thymus, adrenal, and pineal glands, as well as portions of hypothalamus, pancreas, liver, kidneys, skin, digestive tract, ovaries, testes, and placenta. Also included are hormonal secretions from each gland.

Circulatory system Heart, arteries, veins, capillaries, and blood.

FIGURE 4-2   The nervous, endocrine, and cardiovascular or circulatory systems of the body

enough to pass into the bloodstream; it eliminates solid wastes from the body into the environment. The digestive system also recycles water and reclaims vitamins from food in the large intestine. Figure 4-3 illustrates the lymphatic, respiratory, and digestive systems. The components of the digestive system are the *mouth, tongue, teeth, salivary glands, pharynx, esophagus, stomach, liver, gallbladder, pancreas, small intestine,* and *large intestine.*

The **excretory (urinary) system** (Chapter 16) regulates the fluid volume and electrolyte balance of the body. It removes organic wastes from the blood,

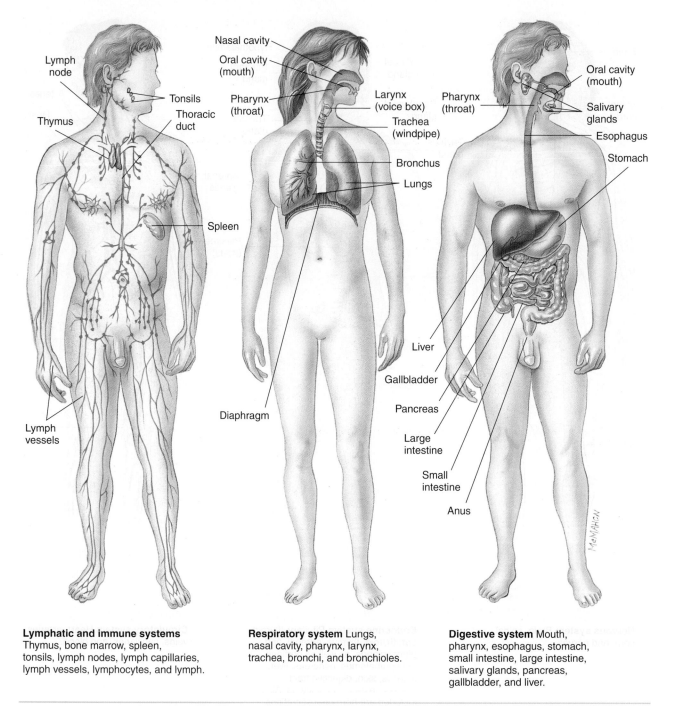

Lymphatic and immune systems
Thymus, bone marrow, spleen, tonsils, lymph nodes, lymph capillaries, lymph vessels, lymphocytes, and lymph.

Respiratory system Lungs, nasal cavity, pharynx, larynx, trachea, bronchi, and bronchioles.

Digestive system Mouth, pharynx, esophagus, stomach, small intestine, large intestine, salivary glands, pancreas, gallbladder, and liver.

FIGURE 4-3   The lymphatic, respiratory, and digestive systems of the body

and sends them out of the body as urine. It consists of the *kidneys, urinary bladder, urethra,* and *ureters.*

The reproductive system (Chapter 17) is mostly controlled by the endocrine system, and is responsible for survival and perpetuation of the species. Elements of the reproductive system produce hormones (from endocrine control) that control and aid in sexual development. Organs of this system produce gametes that combine in the female system to produce the next generation (embryo). See Figure 4-4, which illustrates the urinary and reproductive systems. The male reproductive system consists of the *scrotum, testes, penis, epididymides, vas deferentia, seminal vesicles, prostate, bulbourethral glands,* and *urethra.* The female reproductive system comprises the *ovaries, uterine tubes, uterus, vagina, vulva,* and *mammary glands.*

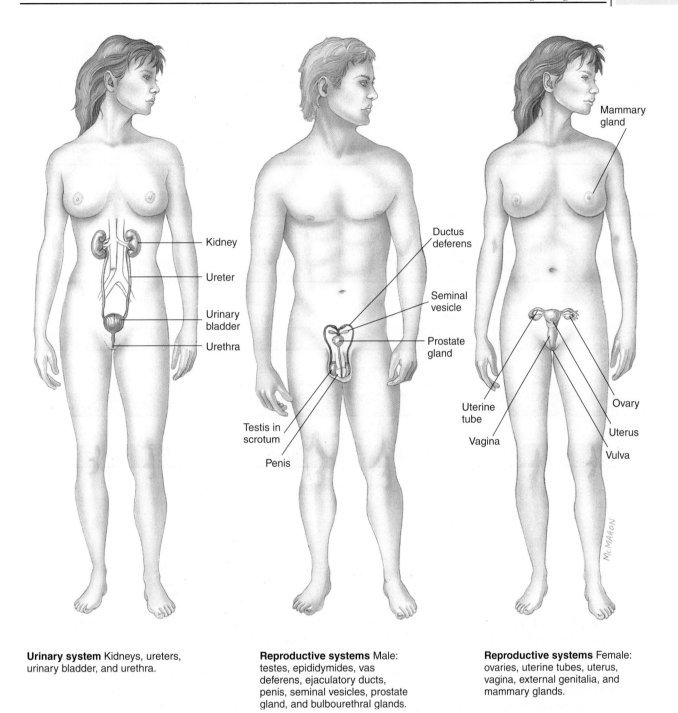

Urinary system Kidneys, ureters, urinary bladder, and urethra.

Reproductive systems Male: testes, epididymides, vas deferens, ejaculatory ducts, penis, seminal vesicles, prostate gland, and bulbourethral glands.

Reproductive systems Female: ovaries, uterine tubes, uterus, vagina, external genitalia, and mammary glands.

FIGURE 4-4 The urinary and reproductive systems of the body

Table 4-1 describes abnormalities related to cell growth and organ development.

HOMEOSTASIS AND ORGAN SYSTEMS

The cells that make up organs need a stable environment (free from wild fluctuations in activity) to effec-tively contribute to survival. **Homeostasis** (*homeo* = same; *stasis* = standing still) is the ability to maintain a relatively constant internal environment. It de-scribes the physical and chemical parameters that an organism must maintain to allow proper functioning of its component cells, tissues, organs, and organ systems.

Single-celled organisms are surrounded by their external environment, whereas the cells of most

TABLE 4-1 Common Terms Related to Organs

ANAPLASIA	
	When cells divide (mitosis) rapidly and bear little or no resemblance to normal cells in appearance or function. A loss of differentiation of cells and of their orientation to one another and to their axial framework and blood vessels, a characteristic of tumor tissue.
APLASIA	
	Lack of development of an organ or tissue.
ATROPHY	
	A wasting or decrease in size of a body organ, tissue, or part owing to disease, injury, or lack of use (if something develops, but then wastes away, it is said to have atrophied).
DYSPLASIA	
	Abnormal development (of organs or cells) or an abnormal structure resulting from such growth (cells that look abnormal under a microscope but are not cancer).
HYPERPLASIA	
	An increase in the number of cells in a tissue or organ, not due to tumor formation. It differs from hypertrophy, which is an increase in bulk without an increase in the number of cells.
HYPERTROPHY	
	An increase in bulk of tissue without an increase in the number of cells.
HYPOPLASIA	
	Incomplete development or underdevelopment of an organ or tissue.

multicellular organisms consist of an intercellular matrix (an aqueous internal environment) separated from the external environment by a semipermeable membrane. This internal environment must be maintained in such a state as to allow maximum efficiency.

Humans possess a series of organs and organ systems that function in homeostasis. Changes in the external environment can trigger changes in the internal environment as a response. The ultimate control of homeostasis is done by the nervous system in the form of negative feedback loops. Heat control, as a major function of homeostatic conditions, involves the integration of integumentary, muscular, nervous, and circulatory systems.

The primary internal components of homeostasis are concentration of oxygen and carbon dioxide, pH of the internal environment, concentration of nutrients and waste products, concentration of salt and other electrolytes, and volume and pressure of extracellular fluid.

FEEDBACK SYSTEMS IN HOMEOSTASIS

Negative feedback mechanisms (used by most of the body's systems) are called negative because the information caused by the feedback causes a reverse of the response. **Positive feedback** control is used in some cases, meaning that input increases or accelerates the response. During uterine contractions, oxytocin is produced, which causes an increase in frequency and strength of uterine contractions. This in turn causes further production of oxytocin.

The control mechanisms for the maintenance of homeostasis are either open or closed. Open systems are linear and have no feedback (similar to a light switch that is switched on). Closed systems have two components: a **sensor** and an **effector**, such as a thermostat (sensor) and furnace (effector). If room temperature is to remain at 72°F, and the thermostat is set at this point, the thermostat (which is sensitive to temperature changes) will signal the furnace to fire up when the temperature drops below the set point, thereby bringing the temperature back to the set point. Once the temperature is restored, the furnace will shut down, allowing for a relatively stable constant temperature to be maintained.

A homeostatic mechanism achieves similar effects. The brain (specifically, the hypothalamus of the brain) acts as the thermostat, and the set point for humans is approximately 98.6°F. If a person goes outside into the cold, the hypothalamus senses the drop in internal temperature and begins a series of mechanisms to raise the temperature to the set point: the muscles shiver, producing extra heat as a by-product, and surface vessels constrict, forcing warm blood deeper into tissues. These mechanisms continue until the set point is reached.

If a person becomes overheated, the hypothalamus will signal mechanisms to release heat from the body. Sweat glands open up, releasing fluids that cool the skin. The heart rate increases, causing a greater volume of blood to move to the surface vessels and release heat to the outside. Breathing rate increases as well, forcing more heated air to be released.

The maintenance of blood pressure at preset levels is also an important homeostatic mechanism. Pressure-sensitive centers located in the walls of the peripheral vessels are stimulated if the pressure rises. The signal they release tells the brain to slow the contractions of the heart so that less blood is released. The pressure of blood against the arterial walls is decreased, and the centers signal the brain that pressure is normal again. Below-normal pressure levels signal the brain to cause the heart to contract with more force, so that blood is released at higher volumes. Pressure then rises, as signaled by the arterial pressure points.

The endocrine system has a homeostatic mechanism that involves a chemical component to the reflex. Sensors detect a change within the body and send a message to an endocrine effector (parathyroid), which makes parathyroid hormone (PTH). PTH is released into the blood when blood calcium levels are low. PTH causes bone to release calcium into the bloodstream, thereby raising the blood calcium levels and shutting down the production of PTH (See Figure 4-5 for an illustration of this homeostatic effect).

Some reflexes have a combination of nervous and endocrine response. The thyroid gland secretes thyroxin (which controls the metabolic rate) into the bloodstream. Falling levels of thyroxin stimulate receptors in the brain to signal the hypothalamus to release a hormone that acts on the pituitary gland to release thyroid-stimulating hormone (TSH) into the blood. TSH acts on the thyroid, causing it to increase production of thyroxin.

Local, or intrinsic, controls usually involve only one organ or tissue. When muscles use more oxygen,

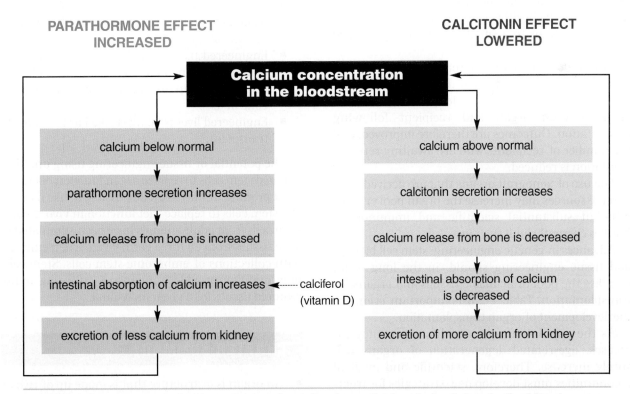

FIGURE 4-5   Effects of parathormone and calcitonin on the level of calcium in the blood

and also produce more carbon dioxide, intrinsic controls cause dilation of the blood vessels, allowing more blood into those active areas of the muscles. Eventually the vessels will return to "normal."

ORGAN REPLACEMENT

Damage to or loss of an organ is common, as any surgical professional can attest. A large fraction of the nation's health care costs are attributable to tissue loss or organ failure, and approximately 8 million surgical procedures are performed annually in the United States to treat these disorders. Currently, transplantation of organs is limited by the lack of available and viable organs (tens of thousands await viable organs, but expansion of the donor pool is unlikely). Advances in mechanical artificial organs have improved the treatment of organ failure, but this is limited by the technology. Artificial organs often act as temporary life support until an actual organ can be found (ventricular-assist devices, intra-aortic balloon pumps, intravenous oxygenators, and dialysis machines, among others).

The number of available organs has increased slightly with the expansion of acceptable donor criteria. The recent development of procedures that implant portions of organs, such as the liver, from healthy individuals has helped as well. However, the risks incurred by healthy donors will likely limit living-related donations to a small number of specialized situations.

Although it does not increase the donor pool, improved organ preservation during transport between donor and recipient is lengthening the survival of both organ and recipient following implantation. Outcomes are therefore improved, and the number of recipients who are awaiting retransplantation is reduced.

The use of xenograft organs that are derived from porcine sources may increase the organ pool eventually, but substantial scientific and immunologic hurdles currently limit their use.

Advances in genetic engineering, stem cell biology, and tissue engineering should, in the long term, increase the pool of available tissues and organs for transplantation. Table 4-2 lists important events in the development of organ transplantation.

As the population ages and life expectancy increases, age-related degeneration of organs will surely increase. Therefore, scientific and medical communities must develop new strategies for treatment of organ and tissue failure. Tissue will soon be created in laboratories for the formation of viable

TABLE 4-2 Historical Milestones in Transplantation
1944: Kolff and Berk report the successful dialysis of a uremic patient for 26 days.
1950s: The development of life-sustaining devices such as extracorporeal membrane oxygenators, ventricular-assist devices, and automatic–implantable cardiac defibrillators.
1954: Murray and colleagues begin the era of solid organ transplantation by performing the first successful kidney transplantation between identical twins.
1959: Murray implants the first renal allograft.
1967: First human heart transplantation (see Figure 4-6).
1970–1975: Artificial heart devices developed.
1982: The first successful implantation of an artificial heart in a patient, who survived for 112 days.

organs that are not rejected because they were formed from the cells of the afflicted patient. However, to reach this stage, an improved understanding of tissue development and cellular differentiation must be accomplished. In addition, enhancement of immune tolerance of transplanted tissues will be necessary.

Research is currently under way with the following accomplishments:

- Engineering of replacement tissues from autologous cells cultured on biocompatible synthetic or natural substrates.
- Engineered tissues (such as blood vessels and bladder) are functional in preclinical studies.
- Engineered skin and cartilage are currently in clinical use.
- Engineered liver is being studied as a "bridge to transplant."

The potential of tissue engineering using undifferentiated stem cells to replace organ function offers the most promise. It may soon be possible to use pancreatic stem cells to replace islet function in vivo. Neural stem cells from adult animals have been stimulated to form tissues from all three germ layers when cultured with collections of embryonic stem cells. Stem cells may one day provide a means of culturing many required tissues for a given individual.

CHAPTER SUMMARY

- An organ is a structure that is made up of two or more different types of tissue that are organized for the performance of a specialized function.

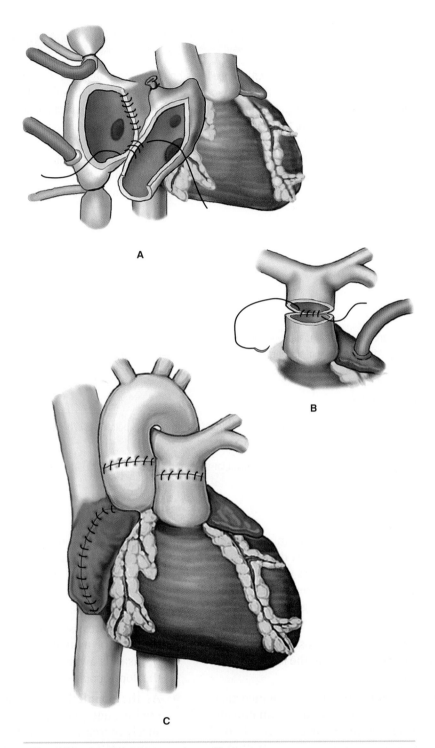

FIGURE 4-6   Heart transplantation

- The organ systems of the body are:

Integumentary system	Respiratory system
Skeletal system	Digestive system
Muscular system	Excretory (urinary) system
Circulatory system (including lymphatics)	Reproductive system
Nervous system	Endocrine system
	Immune system

IMPLICATIONS FOR THE SURGICAL TECHNOLOGIST

Surgical technologists assist with procedures on all organs of the body. An understanding of those organ systems and their functions will help provide better intraoperative patient care. In addition, each organ requires specific instruments for handling, and each also requires specific sutures and needles that are best suited for the type of tissue that makes up the organ. For example, suture for replacement of a heart valve must be strong; therefore, a multifilament, nonabsorbable heavy-gauge suture is required.

Organ replacement procedures (transplantation) are becoming routine as better techniques that prevent rejection are perfected. The surgical technologist assists with all transplantation procedures, and must have an intimate knowledge of the affected organ's anatomy. In addition, an understanding of homeostasis systems is an essential part of the administration of general anesthesia for surgical procedures.

Case Study 2

Chris is a surgical technologist who is privately employed by a cardiovascular surgeon. Today she is assisting the physician with a carotid endarterectomy. After exposure of the common, external, and internal arterial branches, the surgeon asks Chris to inject lidocaine 1% without epinephrine into the carotid body.

1. What is the carotid body?

2. What is lidocaine, and why is it injected into the carotid body during this procedure? Why is epinephrine not included with the lidocaine?

3. Can you name other chemoreceptors of the cardiovascular system that are involved in negative feedback?

- Homeostasis is the ability to maintain a relatively constant internal environment. It describes the physical and chemical parameters that an organism must maintain to allow proper functioning of its component cells, tissues, organs, and organ systems.

- The ultimate control of homeostasis is accomplished by the nervous system in the form of negative feedback loops.

- The primary internal components of homeostasis are concentration of oxygen and carbon dioxide, pH of the internal environment, concentration of nutrients and waste products, concentration of salt and other electrolytes, and volume and pressure of extracellular fluid.

- Negative feedback mechanisms are called negative because the information caused by the feedback causes a reverse of the response.

- Positive feedback control is used in some cases, meaning that input increases or accelerates the response.

- A large fraction of the nation's health care costs are attributable to tissue loss or organ failure, and approximately 8 million surgical procedures are performed annually in the United States to treat these disorders.

- Currently, transplantation of organs is limited by the lack of available and viable organs (tens of thousands await viable organs, but expansion of the donor pool is unlikely).

- As the population ages and life expectancy increases, age-related degeneration of organs will surely increase. Therefore, scientific and medical communities must develop new strategies for treatment of organ and tissue failure.

CRITICAL THINKING QUESTIONS

1. What function does the pancreas serve in a negative feedback system?

2. What role does diabetes play in this negative feedback system?

3. What diseases or conditions make liver transplantation necessary?
4. Can the spleen be safely removed, or would it require transplantation?
5. Are their moral and ethical dilemmas associated with organ transplantation and procurement?

BIBLIOGRAPHY

Association of Surgical Technologists. (2003). *Surgical technology for the surgical technologist: A positive care approach* (2nd ed.). Clifton Park, NY: Thomson Delmar Learning.

Clancy, B., & McVicar, A. (1998). Homeostasis—the key concept to physiological control. Surgery, stress and metabolic homeostasis. *British Journal of Theatre Nursing, 8*(3), 12–18.

Farabee, M. J. (2000). *Animal organ systems and homeostasis.* Retrieved May 4, 2005, from http://www.emc.maricopa.edu/faculty/farabee/BIOBK/BioBookANI MORGS YS.html

Hole, J. W. (1987). *Human anatomy and physiology* (4th ed.). Dubuque, IA: Brown.

Horton, R. L. & Horton, P. J. (1993). Improving the current system for supplying organs for transplantation. *Journal of Health Politics, Policy and Law, 18*(1), 175–188.

Langer, R., & Vacanti, J. P. (1993). Tissue engineering. *Science, 260,* 920–926.

Niklason, L. E., & Langer, R. L. (2001). Prospects for organ and tissue replacement. *Journal of the American Medical Association, 285,* 573–576.

Scott, A. S., & Fong, E. (1998). *Body structures and functions* (9th ed.). Clifton Park, NY: Thomson Delmar Learning.

Strukov, A. I., & Strukova, S. M. (1980). Structural and functional bases of hemostasis and its pathology. *Arkhiv Patologii, 42*(9), 3–16.

Tortora, G. J., & Grabowski, S. R. (1996). *Principles of anatomy and physiology* (8th ed.). New York: HarperCollins.

Urbaszek, W. (1986). Therapeutic principle of organ replacement—artificial organs. *Zeitschrift für die Gesamte Innere Medizin, 41*(10), 281–283.

Vacanti, J. P., & Langer, R. (1999). Tissue engineering: The design and fabrication of living replacement devices for surgical reconstruction and transplantation. *Lancet, 354*(Suppl. 1), SI32–SI34.

5

INTEGUMENTARY SYSTEM

CHAPTER OUTLINE

Introduction
Structure of the Skin and Subcutaneous
Layer
    Epidermis
    Thick and Thin Skin Layers
    Dermis
    Subcutaneous Tissue Layer
    Blood and Lymph Vessels and Nerve Supply
    Skin Pigmentation
    Immune Response of the Skin
Appendages
    Hair
    Ceruminous Glands
    Nails
    Sweat Glands
Burns
Healing of the Skin
    First Intention Healing
    Second Intention Healing
    Third Intention Healing
    Suturing of Skin and Subcutaneous Layers
Functions of the Skin
    Cutaneous Sensation
    Protection
    Body Temperature Regulation
    Vitamin D Production
    Secretion
Aging

CHAPTER OBJECTIVES

After completing the study of this chapter, you should be able to:

1. Describe the importance of skin lines in surgery.
2. Name the layers of the skin.
3. Describe the functions of the skin.
4. Describe the growth process of skin.
5. Describe the blood, lymph, and nerve supply of the skin.
6. Describe the functions of the subcutaneous layer.
7. Describe the anatomy of hair and nails.
8. Describe the functions of melanocytes.
9. Describe the two types of glands located in the skin and their functions.
10. Explain the differences between eccrine and apocrine sweat glands.
11. Describe how sweat aids in regulating body temperature.
12. Describe the ceruminous glands.
13. Name and describe the three types of burns.
14. Explain the difference between an autograft, allograft, and xenograft.
15. Describe the Rule of Nines.
16. Explain the various effects of aging on the skin.
17. Describe the three types of wound healing.
18. Describe the stages of primary wound healing.
19. Describe the suture that is best used on the skin and subcutaneous layers.

KEY TERMS

allograft (homograft)
apocrine sweat glands
autologous graft (autograft)
cerumen
ceruminous glands
dead space
eccrine sweat glands
encapsulated nerve endings

epithelialization
eschar
free nerve endings
keratinocytes
Langerhans cells
matrix
Meibomian glands
reactive hyperemia

Rule of Nines
stratum basale
stratum corneum
stratum germinativum
stratum granulosum
stratum lucidum
stratum spinosum

subcutaneous layer
  (hypodermis)
sweat glands (sudoriferous
  glands)
ultraviolet rays
urocanic acid
xenograft

Case Study 1

A patient is brought to the Emergency Department after sustaining burns over the body from a house fire. The patient is burned on the anterior head and neck and the entire surface of the anterior trunk. The burns are observed as being red with blisters in some body areas to charred in appearance. Answer the following questions based on this case study:

1. Based on the information provided and using the Rule of Nines, estimate the total body surface that has been burned.

2. What type of burns has the patient sustained?

3. Describe the usual course of treating blisters.

4. Will the patient be able to receive autologous grafts or will some other type of graft have to be used?

INTRODUCTION

The integumentary system consists of the first line of defense, the skin and its accessory structures. The skin is actually a more complicated anatomic structure than what it seems and carries out many important physiologic functions, such as aiding in the control of the body temperature. It is, obviously, also a highly visible structure of the body, which many individuals go to great lengths to preserve in an attempt to stay "younger looking"; the cosmetics industry and plastic surgery industry generate a huge amount of revenue for companies and plastic surgeons. This chapter will discuss all aspects of the anatomic structures of the body and physiologic functions.

STRUCTURE OF THE SKIN AND SUBCUTANEOUS LAYER

The skin and accessory structures that cover and protect the external surface and internal structures of the body are together called the integumentary system. The skin is the largest organ of the body. The accessory structures are the nails, glands, and hair. The skin has the unique characteristic of self-repair and regeneration, is waterproof, aids in regulating body temperature, serves as a barrier to the **ultraviolet rays** of the sun, and is the principal organ for sensing touch.

The skin consists of two layers—an ectoderm-derived layer composed of stratified squamous keratinizing epithelium called the epidermis and a second mesoderm-derived layer composed of connective tissue called the dermis. The ectoderm is the outer layer of three primary layers of a developing embryo and the mesoderm is the middle layer. Beneath the dermis

is the **subcutaneous layer (hypodermis)**. Figure 5-1 illustrates the structure of the skin.

Epidermis

The epidermal layer is composed of stratified squamous keratinized epithelial cells called **keratinocytes**. Keratinized refers to the fact that the cells have no nuclei. The epidermis does not contain any blood vessels, and only the deeper layers of the epidermis receive nourishment, which is delivered by diffusion from the capillaries located in the dermal layer.

The surface of the epidermis is indented with a number of skin lines, some deeper than others such as those near joints. The lines vary in arrangement; for instance, those on the back of the hand are very fine and intersect at different angles, whereas the lines of the palm are deeper and curvilinear in arrangement. The surgeon pays attention to the arrangement of these skin lines when performing certain types of procedures. For example, when performing surgery that requires an incision on the palm, the surgeon will attempt to follow the skin lines to promote healing, prevent contracture, preserve the ability to fully open the hand, and hide the scar as much as possible. Or, for lower abdominal procedures, the surgeon will use the Pfannenstiel incision (bikini incision) to follow the skin line to aid in reducing the visibility of the scar.

The keratinocytes are located at the base of the epidermis and divide by mitosis. As new cells are produced, they push the older cells to the surface of the skin. As the older cells move upward, they lose their water content, become flattened in shape, and soon die. This transformation into keratin scales is referred to as keratinization, because the cells become filled

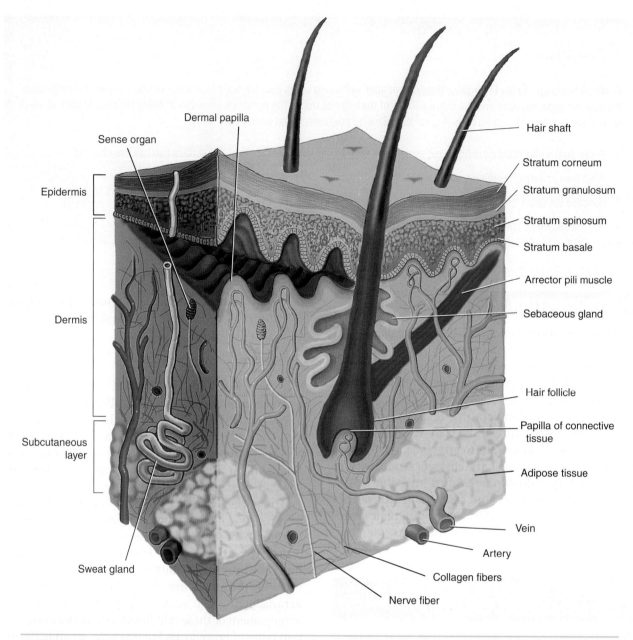

FIGURE 5-1 Structure of the skin

with keratin, a protein substance. Keratinization ensures that the upper layer of the skin that is worn off is replaced at the same rate as production. It takes approximately four weeks for the keratinocytes to make their way to the skin surface. Due to the cellular changes that occur during the journey to the surface, the skin has five distinct layers called stratum (singular) or strata (plural). Figure 5-2 shows the layers of the epidermis and dermis.

The **stratum germinativum** is the deepest layer of the epidermis. The cells of this layer are columnar and arranged perpendicular to the surface of the

dermis, in a single, double, or triple layer. It is the only layer to contain keratinocytes, which divide by mitosis; mitosis does not occur in any of the other four epidermal layers. A basale layer, which is a subdivision of the stratum germinativum, is called the **stratum basale** and it connects the epidermis to the basement membrane. The keratinocytes in the stratum basale are anchored to the basement membrane by a series of interlocking adhesive bridges called hemidesmosomes (Cormack, 2001). The cells of the stratum germinativum itself are attached to each other and to the cells in the stratum spinosum by

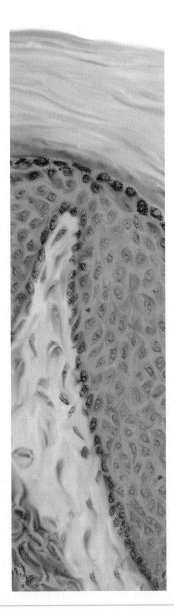

FIGURE 5-2 The epidermal and dermal layers of the skin

The next layer is the **stratum granulosum**, which is only a few cells thick and consists of two to three layers of flattened cells. The cells contain easily recognized basophilic granules called keratohyalin granules, which produce the protein component called soft keratin (Cormack, 2001). Within this layer the keratinocytes lose their nuclei.

The most difficult layer to identify, due to its thin, transparent nature, is the **stratum lucidum**. It is usually only one cell layer thick. The cells are flat, tightly packed, and transparent with no nuclei. In other words, they are essentially a cell membrane and contained within the cell membrane are keratin filaments.

The outermost layer of the epidermis is the **stratum corneum**. It is composed of dead cells that contain no nuclei or organelles and have transformed into flat keratin scales, but remain tightly attached by desmosomes. The intercellular lipid prevents the passage of fluid through this layer, rendering it waterproof. The keratin cells are also waterproof to aid in preventing the evaporation of water. This layer also protects the body from light, heat, microorganisms, and chemicals.

Thick and Thin Skin Layers

Two types of skin are distinguishable by the thickness of the epidermis—thick skin and thin skin. The thickness of the epidermis is influenced by the amount of stimulation on the skin's surface and weight bearing. Hence, thick skin is found primarily on the palms of the hands and soles of the feet. On the thick skin a pattern of friction ridges, called primary epidermal ridges, is easily visible. These dermatoglyphic patterns, are unique to each person, which is why fingerprinting is so important in determining an individual's identity (Cormack, 2001). These ridges are discussed in further detail in the dermis section.

The areas of the body surface that are not exposed to as much abrasion and weight bearing have a decreased layer of epidermis and thin layer of keratin, hence the name thin skin. But this is actually something of a misnomer. In fact, thin skin has a thicker dermal layer than thick skin; therefore, the total thickness of thin skin is more than that of thick skin. This thicker layer of dermis in thin skin makes it easier to suture. Furthermore, thin skin does not have friction ridges, the distribution of eccrine and apocrine sweat glands in thin skin is limited, and the epidermal layers of thin skin are more difficult to distinguish as compared to thick skin. The stratum spinosum is much thinner, the stratum granulosum is indistinguishable, and the stratum lucidum is not present. The stratum corneum is also thin.

another set of interlocking adhesive sites called desmosomes (macula adherens). The stratum germinativum also contains the melanocytes, which are responsible for producing skin color, which is discussed in detail later in this chapter.

The next layer above the stratum germinativum is the **stratum spinosum**. It is several cells thick. The cells are polyhedral in shape and under the microscope appear to be connected by spinelike processes, hence the alternative name prickle cells. Desmosomes are abundant in this layer and play a key role in distributing the tensile stress from cell to cell, thereby allowing the epidermal layer to survive rough treatment.

Dermis

The dermis, also called the corium, is directly inferior to the epidermis. It is composed of loose, fibrous connective tissue. The dermis is divided into two sections: the papillary layer and reticular layer. The papillary layer is the uneven junction of the dermis to the epidermis and is the more vascular of the two layers. The boundary is uneven due to the dermal papillae. The papillae arise from the dermis and push into the stratum germinativum, raising the skin into the uniquely individual primary epidermal ridges discussed previously. The underlying fibrous layer of the dermis, called the reticular layer, is located between the papillary layer and subcutaneous tissue layer and contains tough white collagenous fibers that form a woven network of tissue. In addition to the collagenous fibers, the dermis contains numerous yellow elastin fibers. Recall that fibroblasts produce collagen and elastin fibers. The collagen fibers are strong and tough, and elastic fibers are just that—elastic, meaning they can resume their original postion after being stretched. Elasticity and strength are the two main physiologic characteristics of dermis. With age, however, the elastin fibers deteriorate to some degree, causing the skin to lose some of its elasticity. The dermis contains the capillary vessels, lymph vessels, nerves, hair follicles, sweat glands, and sebaceous glands.

Subcutaneous Tissue Layer

The subcutaneous layer or hypodermis consists of loose areolar connective tissue interspersed with a substantial proportion of adipose tissue. The subcutaneous layer (often abbreviated as *subq* in surgery) connects the dermis to the underlying structures, provides insulation from the cold, and protects and cushions internal body organs and bony prominences. The adipose tissue contained in the layer is formed by adipocytes, specialized cells that store fat, making the subcutaneous layer a storehouse for fat. The excess nutrients contained therein are seen as a source of energy.

Blood and Lymph Vessels and Nerve Supply

The arteries that supply blood to the skin divide into numerous branches in the subcutaneous tissue, forming a network called the rete cutaneum between the dermis and subcutaneous layer. These arteries travel into the dermis and further divide into a complex capillary network that supplies the sudoriferous and sebaceous glands and the hair follicles terminating in the superior layers of the dermis. The larger vessels, which divide into capillaries and play an important physiologic role within the skin, are the arterioles. The middle smooth muscle layer of the arteriole, called the tunica media, can dilate or constrict. For example, during hot weather the arterioles vasodilate to increase the blood flow through the dermis, transferring heat to the skin surface so it can escape from the body. During cold weather the arterioles vasoconstrict to decrease the flow of blood through the dermis and conserve heat within the body. Vasoconstriction may also occur during times of stress, but this is actually a physical response to a "fight or flight" situation, such as having a weapon pointed at one. The vasoconstriction in that situation redirects the blood to more vital organs such as the muscles and heart that require additional blood flow. The body senses that the skin is able to temporarily function with a less then normal blood supply. The vasoconstriction and vasodilation of the arterioles is controlled by the nervous system.

The lymphatic vessels form a minute network of small branches in the superior layers of the dermis. The vessels are interwoven with the capillary vessels and nervous plexuses. They are particularly dense in the scrotum and around the nipple (Gray, 1991).

The nerves that innervate the skin travel upward through the deep layer of the dermis to the superior layers to form minute mesh networks. Obviously, these networks of nerve meshes are most numerous where the body is most sensitive.

Reactive hyperemia, an increase in the amount of blood in an area of the body in which circulation has been reestablished after a short period of occlusion (Ganong, 1993), is a reaction of the blood vessels that not only can be seen in the skin but also occurs within body organs. For instance, in surgery, after a tourniquet is deflated that has been in place while a procedure is being performed on an extremity, the skin "pinks" up with the reestablishment of the blood flow. When the blood supply is blocked, the cutaneous arterioles inferior to the tourniquet dilate due to local hypoxia (Ganong, 1993). When circulation is reestablished the blood flows into the arterioles, making the skin pink in color. Oxygen, transported by the blood, diffuses through the skin and the tissue is reoxygenated.

Skin Pigmentation

The stratum germinativum contains cells called melanocytes. The variations in skin color of individuals and races, and suntans and freckles after exposure to the sunlight are attributed to the distribution and concentration of melanin in the epidermis. Melanocytes are the melanin-synthesizing cells that develop from neural crest cells and travel to the stratum germinativum layer (Cormack, 2001). Melanocytes put forth cytoplasmic extensions, which travel between the keratinocytes in the stratum germinativum. The melanocytes produce melanin granules, which are transferred to the keratinocytes by phagocytosis. In light-skinned individuals, the melanin is concentrated in the stratum germinativum. The melanin protects the keratinocytes from the carcinogenic ultraviolet rays of the sun.

Regardless of racial or ethnic background, all people have approximately the same number of melanocytes in the skin. What accounts for the differences in skin color is the amount of melanin the cells produce, which is controlled by the genes. The more melanin that is produced, the darker the skin. The size of the melanin granules as well as distribution within the melanocytes also affects the skin color. The granules in lighter-skinned individuals are formed in clusters of two or more granules and are small; in individuals with darker skin, the granules are single and large-sized.

Occasionally, a recessive gene, or a mutation, can prevent the production of melanin, resulting in an individual with no skin color, a condition called albinism. A person with albinism is called an albino. Albinos have no skin pigment; therefore, the skin is very white, the hair is white, and the eyes are pink. Albinos have to be very careful to avoid overexposure to the sun to prevent skin cancer from developing and, due to the lack of pigment in their eye's condition, exposure to bright lights can be painful.

Immune Response of the Skin

Located in the epidermis are specialized cells called **Langerhans cells**, which are irregularly shaped dendritic cells that are formed in the bone marrow. The cells are located throughout the layers of the epidermis, in particular the stratum germinativum between the other cells of the skin tissue. The cytoplasm contains granules called Langerhans cell granules or Birbeck granules. Currently, the origin and function of the granules is not understood.

The Langerhans cells are mobile phagocytic cells that phagocytize bacteria that enter through breaks in the skin. Langerhan cells, as part of the immune system, also attack cancerous cells.

Langerhans cells are also the skin's primary antigen-presenting cells for helper T cells, which are important in cutaneous-contact hypersensitivity reactions, such as allergic contact dermatitis that occurs when an individual is allergic to latex (Cormack, 2001). Scientific research has been focused on the role of the skin in the immune system, and preliminary indications are that the skin is much more active in aiding immunity than previously thought.

APPENDAGES

The appendages of the skin include hair, nails, sebaceous glands, arrector pili muscles, sweat glands, and ceruminous glands.

Hair

Hair is a unique feature of mammals. Animals tend to have hair on all parts of the body, but humans do not have hair on the soles of the feet or palms of the hands. Genetics plays a large role in determining the amount of hair a person develops and, as individuals become older, if baldness will or will not occur. Human hair functions much differently from that of animals. Whereas most animals depend on their large amount of hair for warmth, human hair does not serve this function. Eyebrows and eyelashes aid in keeping dust, debris, and perspiration out of eyes. The hairs that line the nares (nostrils) catch dust and debris to prevent their entrance into the respiratory tract. The hair on the scalp does help in preventing the escape of heat and insulates the head during cold weather.

Hair follicles are an invagination of the epidermis that lie in the subcutaneous layer, the growth region of hair. Two types of keratin are present in hair follicles: Soft keratin, the type found in the epidermis, forms the inner root and is found in the soft center of the strands of hair. Hard keratin forms the main substance of hair. The wall of the hair follicle is composed of three sheaths—connective tissue sheath, external root sheath, and internal root sheath. The outer layer that surrounds the hair follicle is the connective tissue sheath. Next is the tubular-shaped invagination of the epidermis called the external root sheath. The third layer, the internal root sheath, is made of soft keratin. At the base of the hair follicle is the hair matrix, a group of epidermal cells that lie over the connective tissue papilla. These epidermal cells are responsible for producing hair and the internal root sheath. The cells mature and divide by mitosis and, as more cells form, the older cells are pushed upward. As these cells are displaced, they begin forming keratin and eventually form the layers of the hair shaft. The area at the base of the hair follicle where hair growth begins is called the hair bulb. Capillary vessels in the hair bulb provide the nourishment needed for the production of hair (Figure 5-3).

The growth of hair alternates between a growing and resting phase. The growing phase signifies the division of the epidermal cells and production of keratin. The resting phase is when mitosis eventually discontinues; the hair stops growing and falls out of the follicle to allow a new hair to form in the same follicle. The growing phase for hair in most parts of the body is shorter than the resting phase (Cormack, 2001). But this is not true for the scalp, where hair can grow for three years and the resting phase is fairly short.

Men tend to experience permanent hair loss more frequently than women. Many men inherit an autosomal-dominant tendency that causes male pattern alopecia; that is, they are genetically predisposed to hair loss. The hair follicles of these men are affected by the male hormone androgen. Not only does the hair fall out, but the hair follicle comes with it and so the hair will not grow back.

Each hair has three parts: the inner medulla, cortex, and cuticle. The inner portion of the hair is the medulla, which is made of soft keratin. The next layer is the cortex, which forms the majority of the hair and is made of hard keratin. The cells of the cortex are flattened and elongated. The outer layer is the cuticle, also made of hard keratin. It consists of overlapping scales that interlock with similar scales located in the internal root sheath to lock the hair in the follicle (Cormack, 2001). The soft, small hairs of the body are called vellus; the coarser hairs found on the scalp, beard, axillae, eyebrows, and pubic regions are called terminal hairs.

Hair color is determined by the type of melanin, such as yellow pheomelanin, which causes the hair to be blond, or red pheomelanin, which makes it red (Cormack, 2001). The melanocytes are interspersed within the hard keratin of the hair. Eventually, in old age, the melanocytes stop producing melanin and the hair turns white.

The sebaceous gland is a kind of small alveolar gland that develops along the side of the hair follicles.

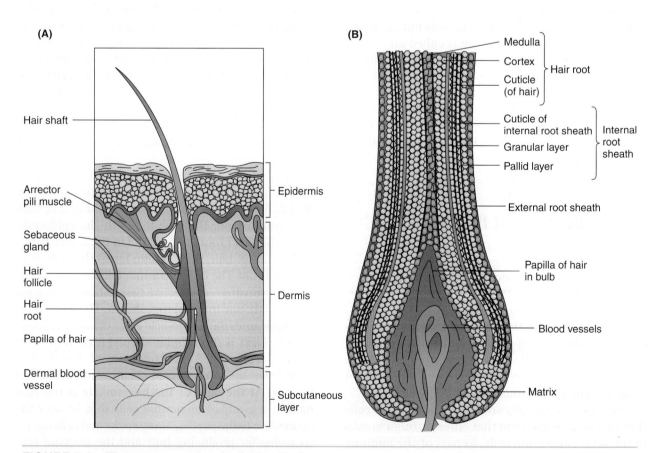

(A)

Hair shaft

Arrector pili muscle

Sebaceous gland

Hair follicle

Hair root

Papilla of hair

Dermal blood vessel

Epidermis

Dermis

Subcutaneous layer

(B)

Medulla

Cortex

Cuticle (of hair)

Hair root

Cuticle of internal root sheath

Granular layer

Pallid layer

Internal root sheath

External root sheath

Papilla of hair in bulb

Blood vessels

Matrix

FIGURE 5-3 **The anatomy of an individual hair**

Sebaceous glands are a type of holocrine gland in which the cells of the gland disintegrate in order to release their secretory product. Several sebaceous glands can be found on each side of hair follicles and are located in all parts of the body, but the largest number of glands are located in the face. On the nose and face, the glands are of a large size as compared to the glands in other parts of the body. The largest sebaceous glands, called the **Meibomian glands**, are located in the eyelids.

Each sebaceous gland consists of a single duct that terminates in a pouchlike shape, or sac, in the dermis. The membrane that forms the wall of the sac and duct is lined by epithelium filled with small particles of sebaceous material called the sebum, the oily substance produced by the sebaceous glands. The purpose of sebum include lubricating the surface of the skin to keep it from drying and keeping hair soft, supple, and lubricated. All the cells of the sebaceous glands contain sebum. Within the gland the cells disintegrate, becoming the sebum that travels along the hair shaft to the surface of the skin.

The secretion of the sebaceous glands is influenced by the endocrine system. As an individual ages a gradual decrease in glandular activity occurs. During puberty, however, the size and activity of the glands increase due to stimulation by androgen (Cormack, 2001). The glands become hyperactive and overproduce secretory cells, resulting in an excess of sebum within the glands. The opening of the gland can become plugged with the excess sebum so that the oily substance cannot travel through the hair follicle to its opening on the skin surface, consequently rupturing into the dermis. The oily substance oxidizes in the presence of normal air and produces what is known as a blackhead. The sebum also serves as an excellent medium for the growth of bacteria. If the blockage of the gland is near the skin surface, the result is a pimple. The pimple eventually assumes a white color caused by the fluid within it, which is a mixture of dead bacterial cells and white blood cells. If the blockage is deep in the gland, the result is a boil. Due to their severity, some boils must be lanced by a physician to release the infectious fluid, and the area irrigated to aid in preventing reinfection.

In the thin skin, each hair follicle has a bundle of smooth muscle attached to it called the arrector pili muscle. The contraction of the muscle causes the hair to "stand on end." The muscle extends in an oblique direction from its attachment at the base of the connective tissue sheath to the papillary layer of the dermis (Cormack, 2001). When the muscle contracts, not only does the hair straighten, but the sebaceous gland is slightly squeezed, causing it to release sebum onto the skin surface.

Ceruminous Glands

Ceruminous glands are a modified type of sebaceous gland located in the dermis in the auditory canal of the ear. They secrete a yellowish substance called **cerumen**, more commonly referred to as ear wax. Cerumen prevents the auditory canal and tympanic membrane from drying out. However, if there is a buildup of cerumen, it can become impacted against the tympanic membrane, preventing the sound waves from vibrating the membrane and impairing the hearing of the person.

Nails

The ends of the fingers and toes have nails. The nail is composed of hard keratin. The structure of the nails consists of cells that are laminated in arrangement and are similar to the cells that compose the epidermis. The cells of the deepest layer are elongated, arranged perpendicular to the surface, and have nuclei. The cells near the surface become thin, flattened, and broad in shape, and are formed closely together.

The visible portion of the nail is called the body. The portion of the cutis beneath the body is called the nail matrix. The nail matrix is thick and covered with vascular papillae, which is evident by the color that can be seen through the transparent tissue. Behind the nail matrix near the root of the nail, the papillae are smaller and less vascular, and air is mixed with the keratin matrix to from the white crescent at the proximal end of each nail, which is called the lunula. Figures 5-4 and 5-5 show the fingernail and its anatomy.

The nail grows outward from a transverse curved area called the nail groove. The floor of this groove is the area where the cells are located, the aforementioned nail matrix. As the cells come closer to the dorsal surface of the nail, they change into the hard keratin, causing the nail to grow outward and strengthen. The thin layer of epidermis that is attached to the undersurface of the nail plate is referred to as the nail bed. Due to this thinness, the vascularity of the dermis shows through, giving the nail, except for the lunula, its characteristic light pink color. The continual growth of new cells at the root and under the surface of the body, combined with the cells moving forward, maintains the uniform thickness of the nail and ensures that it grows in the correct direction. As old cells are replaced by new cells, they lose their

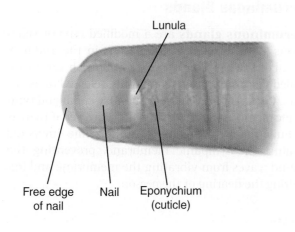

FIGURE 5-4   Fingernail

nuclei and become the hard keratin. The function of nails is to aid the individual in picking up small items and protect the ends of fingers and toes from injury.

Sweat Glands

Sweat glands, called **sudoriferous glands**, are tubular with a base that is coiled and a duct that that transports the sweat to the skin surface. The coiled portion is located just below the dermis in the subcutaneous tissue layer. There are thousands of sweat glands located throughout the body, but they are most numerous in the palms of the hands and soles of the feet. These are the only skin appendages present in thick skin. When a person experiences stress, anxiety, or fear, the characteristic sweaty palms are evident. Sweat is a clear fluid that contains the same inorganic materials as blood but in much lower concentration. Its chief salt is sodium chloride, which is why sweat tastes salty. Its organic constituents include urea, amino acids, potassium, ammonia, sugar, lactic acid, and ascorbic acid. Sodium chloride that has been secreted can be resorbed by the duct cells (Cormack, 2001). The hormone aldosterone, produced in the outer portion of the adrenal gland, increases the amount of sodium chloride that is resorbed.

There are two types of sweat glands: **eccrine** and **apocrine**. Eccrine sweat glands, also called merocrine sweat glands, are located all over the body. Eccrine glands release their fluid products by exocytosis. They are most numerous in the regions just above the upper lip, palms, soles, and forehead. The duct of the eccrine gland opens onto the skin's surface through a pore. The sweat produced by the glands plays an important role in the maintenance of normal body temperature.

The apocrine sweat glands are located primarily in the axillary and genital regions. The apocrine glands are larger than the eccrine glands (Caruthers & Price, 2001), and are activated during times of stress, exercise, and emotional events. The sweat is odorless. What produces the characteristic odor evident in a locker room or after exercise is the interaction of sweat with bacteria. If the sweat from apocrine glands accumulates on the skin, bacteria metabolize the chemicals in the sweat, producing waste products that give off a somewhat foul odor. Personal hygiene and the use of antiperspirants will keep the odors under control. Table 5-1 compares apocrine and eccrine sweat glands.

Sweat is important in helping to cool the surface of the body. When an individual has been sweating,

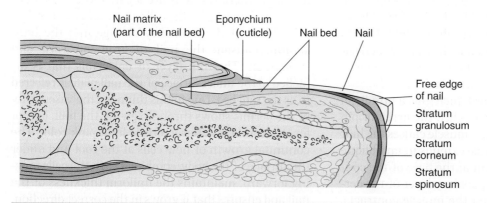

FIGURE 5-5   Fingernail and underlying structures

TABLE 5-1 Differences Between Apocrine and Eccrine Sweat Glands

APOCRINE SWEAT GLANDS	ECCRINE SWEAT GLANDS
Ducts open into upper part of hair follicles	Ducts open through pore in skin
Only secrete sweat with the onset of puberty	Secrete sweat through all stages of life
Secretion is cloudy	Secretion is clear

such as during exercise, they often feel a chill or coolness on the skin surface. Heat is required to evaporate the water in sweat; therefore, the loss of body heat aids in cooling the body, which lowers the body temperature, and the internal organs, tissues, and cells of the body do not overheat. The regulation of body temperature is discussed in detail later in the chapter.

BURNS

Burns can result from thermal effects (heat or cold), chemicals, gases, electricity, and radiation. A burn is classified according to degree, which indicates the depth of the burn (Figures 5-6 and 5-7). First-degree burns affect only the epidermis. Signs and symptoms include some slight swelling due to the vasodilation of the blood vessels in the dermis, erythema, and pain, but no blistering is evident. Healing usually occurs in approximately one week and leaves no scarring. Sunburns are a common form of first-degree burn.

Second-degree burns involve the dermis to varying degrees. Signs and symptoms include extreme pain, blisters, and swelling. Superficial second-degree burns heal in about two weeks and usually do not leave a scar. Deep second-degree burns take much longer to heal and often leave a scar. Deep burns often require debridement of dead skin and skin grafting. Infection is the primary complication in second-degree burns. The source of the infection can be the patient, but is most often due to breakdowns in aseptic technique by health care providers caring for the patient. Emphasis must be placed on strict aseptic technique in the care of a burn patient to prevent a possible life-threatening infection.

Large blisters often occur with second-degree burns due to the escape of fluid from damaged dermal capillaries, and the management of blisters presents an interesting dilemma. The physician must decide whether to protect the blisters or rupture them by excising epithelium (Peacock, 1984). However, the fluid does not aid in epitheliazation and it is not normal for the dermis to be in constant contact with fluid (Peacock, 1984). The usual course of treatment is to protect the blisters for 24 to 36 hours to prevent rupture; then the physician will excise partially detached epithelium. The wound can then be treated with a dressing or allowed to dry and epitheliazation can begin.

Third-degree burns involve all layers of the skin and the upper portion of the subcutaneous tissue layer. Signs and symptoms include shock, possibly pain, and dehydration. Destruction of all layers of the skin leaves what is called **eschar**, which is black in color and composed primarily of collagen. Interestingly, patients with third-degree burns often have no pain, since the nerves in the skin layers have been destroyed, whereas with second-degree burns the patient experiences severe pain due to the exposure and damage done to the superficial nerves. Patients who sustain a third-degree burn to a large portion of the body are placed in a life-threatening situation. The patient may require immediate intubation for respiratory support, and the administration of fluids and antibiotics will also be immediately begun. Intubation is necessary because even the tissues of the throat may have been damaged by the burn and may be swollen, thereby cutting off the airway. Fluid loss will be dramatic due to the loss of the protective skin layer, and the fluids must be quickly replaced; in addition, fluid will continue to be lost, since it has an easy route by which to escape. As stated previously, the loss of the skin layer leaves the patient open to acquiring an infection. With extensive third-degree burns, this potential is even more exaggerated because all layers of the skin have been destroyed. Even if the affected area of the body is small, the risk for infection any time a third-degree burn occurs is great. Because the epithelial cells in the area will be destroyed, healing can occur only by inward growth of the epithelial cells on the borders of the burn. If the burn covers too much of the body, skin grafting will be necessary.

Fourth-degree burns are called char burns (Caruthers & Price, 2001). The depth of these burns involves the muscles, tendons, and possibly down to and affecting the bone. Surgery will be immediately performed to remove the necrotic tissue, irrigate the area, and protect with dressings. The patient will undergo extensive reconstructive surgery.

The method of determining how much of the surface of the body has been burned is referred to as the **Rule of Nines**. The areas of the body are subdivided into 9% or multiples of 9% of the body surface area (BSA). Estimating the BSA helps to determine fluid

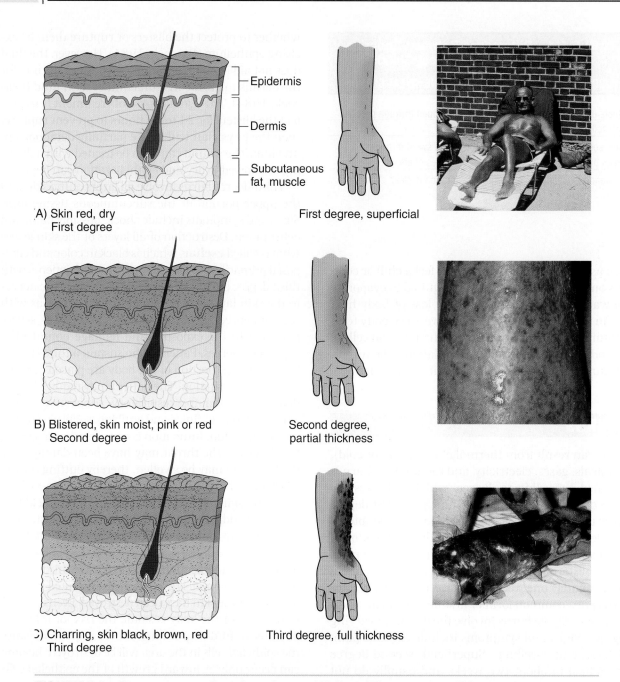

- Epidermis
- Dermis
- Subcutaneous fat, muscle

A) Skin red, dry
First degree

First degree, superficial

B) Blistered, skin moist, pink or red
Second degree

Second degree, partial thickness

C) Charring, skin black, brown, red
Third degree

Third degree, full thickness

FIGURE 5-6   Burns are usually referred to as (A) first, (B) second, or (C) third degree. (Photos courtesy of The Phoenix Society for Burn Survivors, Inc.)

and electrolyte replacement therapy and the amount of skin or skin substitutes that will be required to cover the burned area. The following is a breakdown of the BSA percentages:

1. Anterior and posterior head and neck—9% ($4\frac{1}{2}$% anterior and posterior)
2. Anterior and posterior trunk—36% (18% anterior and posterior)
3. Anterior and posterior upper extremities—18% ($4\frac{1}{2}$% anterior and posterior of each arm)
4. Perineum—1%
5. Anterior and posterior lower extremities—36% (9% anterior and posterior of each leg)

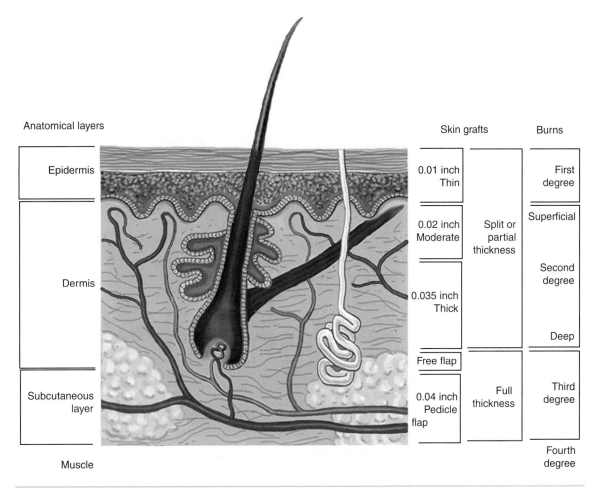

FIGURE 5-7 Burn depth

HEALING OF THE SKIN

The three types of wound healing, which were discussed in Chapter 3, are first intention (primary union), second intention (granulation), and third intention (delayed primary closure).

First Intention Healing

First intention healing is considered the ideal type of healing because the wound heals side to side without infection. There is usually minimal scarring and 70%–80% of the original tensile strength, the amount of tension that a suture strand will withstand before breaking, is obtained by the third month. First intention healing occurs in three phases:

1. Lag or inflammatory response phase: begins immediately after injury, lasts three to five days, and is characterized by the signs of inflammation: swelling, pain, redness, heat, and loss of function. Bleeding is controlled by the clumping of platelets and formation of epithelial cells. A scab forms on the surface of the skin to aid in closing the wound to prevent microbes from entering. Neutrophils and macrophages migrate to the area to remove foreign particles by phagocytosis. The surface of the wound is further closed by migrating basal cells. Fibroblasts begin the job of reforming nonepithelial tissue. No tensile strength is gained by the wound during this phase (Caruthers & Price, 2001).

2. Proliferation phase: begins on the 3rd or 4th day after surgery and continues for approximately 20 days. The fibroblasts continue to multiply and close the wound edges. They also secrete collagen, which forms into fibers to provide the wound about 30% of its original tensile strength. A new capillary network is established from the capillaries that were not damaged; the network is established by the fifth or sixth postoperative day.

BOX 5-1

Skin Grafting

Skin grafting is necessary when a patient has lost an extensive amount of skin that will require a long time to heal and could form a disfiguring scar in the process. Patients who sustain third-degree burns and occasionally second-degree burns will undergo one or possibly several skin-grafting procedures, depending on the amount of BSA involved. The skin grafts will replace the area of lost tissue, thus preventing further complications such as infection, and aid in healing.

Skin that is taken from the patient to be transferred to the recipient site is called autologous graft or autograft. The skin is usually obtained from the buttocks, or the lateral or posterior portion of the thigh. If too much of the body is burned or autograft donor sites require healing, a temporary solution for covering the burned areas is the use of allografts (also called homografts), skin or tissue from the same species, in this case, humans but not twins, or xenografts, skin or tissue from another species. The allograft most often used is cadaveric skin obtained from a skin bank and a popular xenograft is pig skin. Another substitute that has been used is the amniotic membrane. These substitutes are temporary solutions used to cover the wound, preserve the deeper tissues, prevent the escape of body fluid, and prevent infection. When healing has begun the allograft or xenograft will be removed and replaced with autograft from areas of the body where the skin has healed. The use

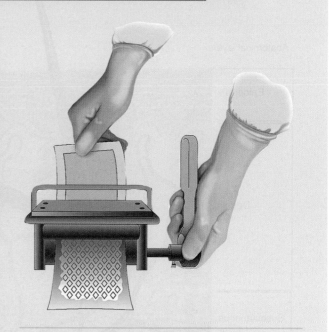

FIGURE 5-9   Mesh graft device

of allografts and xenografts has decreased since the development of effective topical agents that prevent bacterial infection of the eschar (Peacock, 1984). Advances are being made in the development of various skin substitutes, a focus of biomedical tissue engineering. In the laboratory, small pieces of skin that were not burned are taken from the patient and grown to a very large size on artificial dermis (Swerdlow, 2002). The new skin is then grafted onto the patient. Research is also focused on the development of artificial membranes.

Skin grafts are either full-thickness skin graft (FTSG) or split-thickness skin graft (STSG). An FTSG is composed of the epidermis and dermis, and possibly some of the subcutaneous tissue layer. Due to its depth, FTSG is limited in use to small areas. STSG involves the epidermis and approximately half of the dermis, and is most frequently used to cover large areas of the body. A powered dermatome, which has a very sharp cutting blade that moves back and forth, is used to procure the STSG. Also a hand-turned mesh graft device is used to expand the size of the skin graft, allowing it to cover a larger area of the body (Figures 5-8 and 5-9).

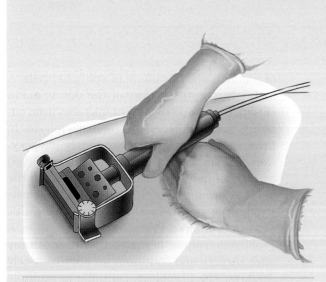

FIGURE 5-8   Oscillating blade type dermatome

3. Maturation or differentiation phase: begins approximately on the 14th postoperative day and ends when the wound is healed. The tensile strength of the wound increases aided by the network of collagen fibers. Wound contraction due to the action of myofibroblasts is completed around 21 days postoperative. The collagen reaches maximum density and the formation of capillaries decreases, leaving a mature scar called a cicatrix.

Second Intention Healing

Second intention healing occurs when a wound fails to heal by first intention healing. It is appropriate for large wounds in which the wound edges cannot be reapproximated with suture, large wounds on which undue tension will be placed, or infected wounds. The wound is left open to heal from the bottom to the surface. As the wound heals, the space is filled in with granulation tissue that contains myofibroblasts, and wound closure occurs by contraction. Wounds that heal by granulation tend to be weak and form a wide, irregular-shaped scar. Herniation is common.

Third Intention Healing

Third intention healing occurs when the edges of the granulated surface are approximated. Surgeons use this method for the management of contaminated wounds including dirty traumatic wounds. The surgeon treats the injury by debridement of the dead tissue and leaves the wound open to heal by second intention for four to six days. Once the wound is infection free, it is closed with suture or staples to finish healing by first intention.

Suturing of Skin and Subcutaneous Layers

Because skin wounds heal slowly, so too do they slowly regain tensile strength, indicating that the choice of suture should be nonabsorbable rather than absorbable to provide a longer period of support to the wound. Typically, skin suture is removed between 3 and 10 days postoperatively, even when the skin wound has regained only approximately 5%–10% of its tensile strength, because most of the stress to the healing wound is placed on the fascia, the tissue layer that holds the wound closed (Ethicon, 2002). Because the minute spaces in multifilament suture can be a breeding ground for microorganisms, a monofilament nonabsorbable suture is the suture of choice to prevent wound infection. Furthermore, monofilament suture usually causes less tissue reaction. The most popular suture materials are nylon and polypropylene. Skin is a tough tissue requiring a type of surgical needle that can pass smoothly through the skin and cause minimal tear, so the conventional cutting and reverse cutting surgical needles are optimal.

Because the composition of subcutaneous fat is primarily water and therefore has little tensile strength, it does not tolerate suturing well. However, many surgeons will place sutures in the layer to prevent dead space, the accumulation of fluid and/or air within the tissue causing pockets, which delay wound healing, and, because bacteria can grow in the space, contribute to the development of infection. In this case, an absorbable suture is the suture of choice, often polyglactin 910.

A surgeon, using either absorbable or nonabsorbable suture according to his or her preference, will often perform a closure of the subcuticular tissue to minimize the skin scar. A subcuticular closure holds the edges of the skin in very close approximation.

FUNCTIONS OF THE SKIN

The skin functions include cutaneous sensation, protection, body temperature regulation, manufacturing of vitamin D, secretion, and drug absorption.

Cutaneous Sensation

The four cutaneous senses are touch-pressure, pain, warmth, and cold. The skin contains thousands of cutaneous receptors, which are made of afferent nerve endings. The receptors respond to several environmental stimuli, such as temperature, pressure, and pain, and then send messages to the cerebral cortex to interpret the messages. The interpretation can be sufficiently specific to indicate to the person exactly what area of the body is being affected by the stimulus. There are three categories of cutaneous receptors: (a) thermoreceptors, which respond to temperature; (b) nociceptors, which respond to painful irritants; and (c) mechanoreceptors, which respond to pressure or stretching (Cormack, 2001). From a morphological standpoint, there are two primary categories of afferent nerves: (a) free nerve endings and (b) encapsulated nerve endings.

The deep layers of the epidermis and the dermal papillary layer contain afferent nerve endings that have no Schwann cells, hence the term free nerve endings. The endings in these layers are both nociceptors and thermoreceptors. The free nerve endings next to hair follicles are mechanoreceptors, which allow an individual to be receptive to the movement of hair. Located in the palms of the hands and soles of the feet are disk-shaped afferent nerve endings attached to the epidermal cells called Merkel cells. These cells are mechanoreceptors.

By contrast, encapsulated nerve endings contain Schwann cells. There are several types of encapsulated nerve endings. The largest is the mechanoreceptor called the pacinian corpuscles. Pacinian corpuscles are located in the dermis, subcutaneous tissue layer, and joint capsules—areas of pressure. Their purpose is to sense heavy pressure and relay the information to the hypothalamus (Shier, Butler, & Lewis, 2002). Located in the areas of highest tactile sensation, the palmar surface of the fingers and plantar surface of the toes, are Meissner's corpuscles. They lie in the papillary layer of the dermis and are very sensitive mechanoreceptors for the sensation of touch. Ruffini corpuscles are small spindle-shaped encapsulated nerve endings located in the deep dermis and subcutaneous tissue layer (Cormack, 2001). Finally, Krause end bulbs, also called mucocutaneous corpuscles, are not as abundant as the other nerve endings, but are scattered through the dermis and are mechanoreceptors.

Interestingly, studies reveal that being able to perceive touch is a highly important social-psychological factor. Studies of different cultures have shown that a high rate of touching and physical affection corresponds with a low rate of adult physical violence (Swerdlow, 2002).

Protection

The unbroken skin is the first line of defense against microbes, substances such as chemicals, and the ultraviolet rays of the sun. The melanin produced by the melanocytes protects us to a limited degree from the sun's ultraviolet rays. However, if an individual does not take the right precautions and exposes himself or herself to the sun's rays for a length of time, damage to the skin can occur. And if the person does this often, this damage could lead to skin cancer. Most chemicals cannot gain entrance to the body through the skin; however, there are a few, such as DDT and the chemicals that make up Agent Orange, that can penetrate the skin layer and poison the person.

Skin also has a certain acidity level, which either aids in preventing the growth of bacteria or kills the bacteria. However, some diseases can alter the pH level of the skin, allowing the bacteria to grow and cause infections.

Body Temperature Regulation

Normal body temperature stays at or close to 98.6°F (37°C). When the external temperature increases, the capillaries in the dermis dilate, allowing the blood to flow to the surface of the body to release heat. As previously mentioned, when a person sweats, the water in the sweat evaporates, which requires energy thus releasing more heat to maintain the body tempera-

ture. When the external temperature decreases, the dermal capillaries dilate to bring heat to the body surface and warm the body. However, if the person remains exposed to the cold, the brain sets in motion another set of responses. The muscles in walls of the capillaries contract, thereby decreasing the flow of blood to the skin and conserving the heat for the vital organs. Sweat glands are inactive, decreasing heat loss by evaporation. The muscle fibers in the skeletal muscles may begin to contract, causing the person to shiver, which generates additional heat.

These are three processes by which body heat is lost: radiation, conduction, and convection. During radiation, the heat rays leave the warmer surface for a cooler environment, radiating every which way. During conduction, heat travels into the molecules of cooler objects that are in contact with the body. For example, heat is lost through conduction when a person sits on cold metal outdoor bleachers. During convection, as air becomes heated, it tends to move away from the body, taking the heat with it. This is then replaced by cooler air that travels toward the body.

Hyperthermia and hypothermia are two abnormal conditions that can occur with body temperature. Hyperthermia means the body temperature is elevated above the normal range, and may be caused by many things, including heatstroke. For instance, on a hot, humid day the air can hold only so much water vapor and eventually becomes saturated. Due to the heat, the sweat glands are active, but the water from the sweat cannot evaporate quickly enough and so the body temperature remains elevated. The condition can be complicated by not taking in enough fluids, resulting in dehydration. (Shier, Butler, & Lewis, 2002).

Prolonged exposure to cold temperatures can lead to hypothermia. Hypothermia begins with excessive shivering and coldness, which leads to frostbite, mental confusion, lethargy, loss of consciousness, and eventually the vital organs stop functioning. In the operating room (OR) the temperature is kept low to help keep the growth of microbes to a minimum, and the patient can quickly lose body heat due to exposure of body parts; so the patient must be protected from hypothermia. A warming blanket is placed on the OR bed that the patient lays upon and, because the majority of heat is lost through the scalp, the anesthetist often covers the patient's head with a towel.

Vitamin D Production

When exposed to the ultraviolet rays of the sun the skin is stimulated to produce a progenitor molecule of vitamin D. The molecules travel to the liver and kidneys where they mature to vitamin D molecules. Vitamin D is essential in the metabolism of calcium, which is necessary for bone development and the contraction of the muscles, and of phosphate, used by the intestines to manufacture adenosine triphosphate (ATP).

Secretion

As previously discussed, sweat and sebum are produced by accessory structures of the skin. In addition to the other properties mentioned concerning sebum, it also has limited antifungal and antibacterial properties. Besides aiding in thermoregulation of the body, sweat contains waste products such as uric acid, urea, and ammonia. These waste products are rid from the body when the sweat is excreted and evaporated.

AGING

Aging skin changes in both appearance and physiology. Age spots, which are the result of oxidation of fats in the secretory cells of the apocrine and eccrine sweat glands, appear in various regions of the body. The thickness of the dermis decreases and is less elastic, plus fat is lost from the subcutaneous tissue layer, leading to sagging and wrinkling of the skin and causing the elderly to be more sensitive to cold weather. The number of lymphocytes decreases, which causes wounds to heal slower. The oil secretion from sebaceous glands decreases and the skin becomes drier and more brittle. This also can cause a delay in wound healing.

Melanin production slows, causing the hair to become gray or white. The activity of the hair follicles lessens, resulting in hair loss on the scalp and body. Blood flow to the skin decreases, and the skin becomes thinner and looks more translucent as mitosis in the stratum basale decreases and the fibroblasts that die in the dermis are not replaced. The blood supply to the nail beds also decreases, impairing their growth and hardening them. The number of receptors in the skin diminishes with age, resulting in a decreased sensitivity to pain and pressure.

Aging also affects the bones of the skeleton. Skin in the elderly has a decreased ability to activate vitamin D, which, as discussed earlier, is required for the absorption of calcium to take place in the bone tissue and keep bones sturdy. Additionally, many older people do not go outdoors as much or, because of health reasons, can't get outside at all. But the skin, as the site of activation of vitamin D, requires sunlight.

BOX 5-2

Skin Cancer

Excessive exposure to sunlight not only accelerates the body's aging process but serious side effects can also occur. The epidermis thickens in response to exposure to sunlight and the elastin is damaged. The damaged elastin predisposes the individual to the development of premalignant and malignant cells (Caruthers & Price, 2001). Individuals with fair skin are more prone to skin damage from sun exposure as compared to darker-skinned individuals. The ultraviolet (UV) rays of the sun are responsible for damaging the skin. There are three types of ultraviolet radiation, which is measured in nanometers (nm) (Caruthers & Price, 2001):

1. Type A (UVA 320–400 nm): It is potentially as harmful as type B.
2. Type B (UVB 290–320 nm): It is associated with sunburn and skin cancer.
3. Type C (UVC 200–290 nm): The danger increases as the ozone layer diminishes.

There are three types of skin cancer: basal cell carcinoma, squamous cell carcinoma, and malignant melanoma. Basal cell carcinoma, the most common, is easily treated with surgery and/or radiation therapy. Squamous cell carcinoma is much more dangerous. A keratinized nodular tumor forms in the epidermis. If left untreated, it can easily spread to the dermis and metastasize. Malignant melanoma is life-threatening. It is linked to moles, which are a group of melanocytes that become cancerous and easily metastasize to the lungs, liver, or other vital organs. In the last two decades, cases of melanoma have almost doubled in the United States, making it one of the most rapidly increasing types of cancer (Swerdlow, 2002). Each year more than 50,000 new cases are reported by the American Cancer Society (Swerdlow, 2002). Researchers are currently studying a vaccine that would prompt the immune system to prevent a recurrence in individuals who had melanoma (Scanlon & Sanders, 1999). Researchers have also discovered the role of **urocanic acid** in the skin. The cells of the immune system normally attack cells damaged and altered by the sun's UV rays. But when the molecules of urocanic acid are exposed to UV rays, they bend into a form that suppresses the immune response to the damaged cells (Swerdlow, 2002). Researchers believe this reaction evolved over time to give the damaged cells of the skin an opportunity to repair themselves.

IMPLICATIONS FOR THE SURGICAL TECHNOLOGIST

Because the skin is the first organ that is penetrated during a surgical procedure or when injured by trauma, the surgical technologist must be aware of its anatomy and physiology. Once the skin is broken, the body's first line of defense has been compromised, requiring the surgical team to practice strict aseptic technique, in particular when treating a burn patient, to prevent the patient from acquiring an infection. Hand washing has long been known to be the number one method to prevent the spread of disease. The surgical technologist must perform a hand wash prior to contact with a patient, if contact with blood or body fluids occurs, and after removing the surgical gloves. When wearing surgical gloves the hands sweat (remember the large number of sweat glands that are found in the palms of the hands) and this provides ready environment for the growth of bacteria. As soon as the sterile gloves are removed, the surgical technologist should perform a 30- to 60-second hand wash to remove as much of the bacterial growth as possible.

A second important consideration for the surgical technologist is the healing of skin. For patients who are young and undergo surgery, whether routine or traumatic, the skin usually heals with few or no complications. However, as previously mentioned, in the elderly the skin heals much slower. This does not affect the choice of using nonabsorbable sutures or staples to close the skin, but it may affect how long the sutures or staples are left in place. As with both examples of patient types, the key to successful healing of the skin is removal of the suture as soon as possible before **epithelialization** of the suture tract occurs and infection sets in (Ethicon, 2002).

Case Study 2

A patient is brought to the operating room for excision of a keloid above the right eyebrow that continues to enlarge and is painful. The keloid formed as a result of a traumatic wound sustained during a motor vehicle accident. Answer the following questions based on this information:

1. Define a keloid.

2. How can surgeons avoid causing the formation of a keloid?

3. Why is the removal of keloids by surgical excision alone usually not successful?

4. What other methods of treatment have been successful in the removal of keloids?

5. Which type of lasers are most commonly used in the removal of keloids?

Therefore, Vitamin D supplements are recommended for many older individuals to maintain the bone structure and density of the skeleton.

CHAPTER SUMMARY

- The integumentary system comprises the skin, hair, glands, and nails.

- The skin is the largest organ of the body.

- The skin consists of two layers—epidermis and dermis. Beneath the dermis is the subcutaneous tissue layer.

- The epidermis receives its nourishment from capillaries located in the dermal layer.

- The surface of the epidermis is indented with a number of skin lines.

- Keratinization is the process by which older cells move upward, become flat, and die, thereby transforming, into keratin scales.

- There are two types of skin characterized by the thickness of the epidermis—thick skin, found on the palms of the hands and soles of the feet, and thin skin.

- The dermis is located posterior to the epidermis and is composed of loose, fibrous connective tissue. It is divided into two sections—papillary layer and reticular layer.

- The subcutaneous (subq) tissue layer consists of loose areolar connective tissue interspersed with adipose tissue. The purpose of the subq layer is to connect the dermis to the body's underlying structures, provide insulation from the cold, protect and cushion internal body organs and bony prominences, and store fat.

■ The arteries in the skin divide into a network of branches called the rete cutaneum. The branches travel into the dermis, further divide, and terminate in the superior layers of the dermis.

■ The lymphatic vessels form a network of small branches in the upper layers of the dermis.

■ The nerves of the skin travel from the deep layer of the dermis to the upper layers to form a mesh network.

■ The melanocytes are located in the stratum germinativum. Melanocytes secrete melanin, which is responsible for skin color, suntans, and freckles. Melanin protects the skin from the UV rays of the sun.

■ Albinism is a mutation that causes the nonproduction of melanin.

■ Langerhans cells are dendritic cells that are formed in the bone marrow and are located throughout the epidermis. The cells are mobile phagocytic cells that phagocytize bacteria that enter through breaks in the skin and attack cancerous cells.

■ The purpose of hair includes keeping dust and debris out of the eyes, catching dust and debris in the nose, preventing the escape of heat from the head, and insulating the head during cold weather.

■ Hair follicles are invaginations of the epidermis, and the follicles lie in the subq layer. Soft and hard keratins form the hair shaft. The wall of the hair follicle is composed of three sheaths—connective tissue, external root, and internal root.

■ Sebaceous glands secrete sebum. The largest sebaceous glands are the Meibomian glands.

■ Sebum lubricates the surface of the skin to keep it from drying, and keeps hair soft and prevents it from drying.

■ The secretion of sebum is influenced by the endocrine system. Hyperactivity of the glands leads to the secretion of excess sebum and the formation of blackheads, acne, and boils.

■ Ceruminous glands are located in the auditory canal and secrete cerumen.

■ Nails are composed of hard keratin. The visible portion of the nail is called the body. The portion beneath the body is called the nail matrix and the white crescent at the proximal end of each nail is called the lunula.

■ Sudoriferous glands are a tubular gland with a coiled base and a duct for the transport of sweat to the skin's surface. The coiled base is located just below the dermis in the subq layer.

■ There are two types of sweat glands—eccrine and apocrine. Eccrine sweat glands are located all over the body and the ducts open onto the skin's surface through the pores. Apocrine sweat glands are primarily located in the axillary and genital regions and are larger than the eccrine glands. They are activated during times of stress, exercise, and emotional stress. Sweat plays an important role in cooling the surface of the body.

■ Burns are classified according to the depth of the burn. First-degree burns involve only the epidermis; second-degree burns involve the dermis to varying degrees and blisters form; third-degree burns involve the epidermis, dermis, and upper portion of the subq layer; fourth-degree burns go as deep as involving the muscles, tendons, and possibly bone—referred to as a char burn.

■ The Rule of Nines is a method of determining the extent of burn of the body surface area. The method helps to determine fluid and electrolyte fluid replacement therapy and the amount of skin or skin substitutes that will be needed to cover the burned area.

■ First intention healing is primary healing in which the wound heals from side to side with no infection present. It occurs in three phases: lag or inflammatory response, proliferation, and maturation or differentiation.

■ Second intention healing occurs by granulation. The wound is left open to heal from the bottom to the surface, the space is filled in with granulation tissue, and the wound closes by contraction.

■ Third intention healing, also called delayed primary closure, refers to initial healing by second intention and then primary closure. Infected wounds are allowed to heal in this manner.

■ Skin heals slowly, and thus slowly regains tensile strength. The choice of suture is nonabsorbable due to the slow healing time. The needle of choice is conventional cutting and reverse cutting, since the tissue of the skin is tough.

■ The subcutaneous tissue layer does not tolerate suturing well due to weak tensile strength. Surgeons will place sutures in the subq layer to prevent the formation of dead space.

■ The cutaneous senses are touch-pressure, pain, warmth, and cold. There are three categories of cutaneous receptors: thermoreceptors, nociceptors, and mechanoreceptors. The cutaneous nerves are afferent nerves, which are categorized as free nerve endings and encapsulated nerve endings.

- A type of free nerve ending attached to epidermal cells are Merkel cells, which are mechanoreceptors.

- The types of encapsulated nerve endings are pacinian corpuscles, Meissner's corpuscles, Ruffini corpuscles, and Krause end bulbs.

- The unbroken skin is the first line of defense against microbes, chemicals, and other substances, and UV rays of the sun.

- Dilation and constriction of the blood vessels in the skin layer play an important role in maintaining the homeostasis of the body by aiding thermoregulation.

- Heat is lost from the body through three methods—radiation, conduction, and convection.

- The UV rays of the sun stimulate the skin to begin the production of vitamin D.

- In addition to other properties, sebum has limited antifungal and antibacterial properties. Sweat contains waste products that are eliminated from the body when the sweat is excreted and evaporated.

- Age spots appear due to the oxidation of fats in the secretory cells of the apocrine and eccrine sweat glands.

- The thickness of the dermis decreases and is less elastic, plus the fat in the subq layer decreases, leading to sagging and wrinkling of the skin.

- The decreased fat in the subq tissue causes the elderly to be more sensitive to cold weather.

- Lymphocytes decrease in number causing wounds to heal slower.

- The secretion of sebum decreases and the skin becomes drier and more brittle.

- Hair turns gray or white due to the decrease in melanin production.

- Blood flow to the skin decreases; mitosis in the stratum basale decreases and the fibroblasts that die in the dermis are not replaced, leaving the skin thinner.

- The blood supply to the nail beds decreases, impairing their growth and hardening them.

- The number of cutaneous receptors diminishes, resulting in decreased sensitivity to pain and pressure.

- Due to decreased time in the sun, the level of vitamin D can be diminished in the elderly, requiring the intake of supplements.

- Strict emphasis must be placed on aseptic technique, especially when treating burn patients, since the skin is the first organ penetrated during all surgical procedures or when injured by trauma.

- Hand washing is the number one method of preventing the spread of infection. The surgical technologist should perform a hand wash as soon as possible after the sterile gloves are removed.

- The surgical technologist must understand the anatomy and physiology of the skin in order to understand the healing of the skin. The skin of elderly patients will most likely heal slower than that of patients of a younger age.

CRITICAL THINKING QUESTIONS

1. Describe the difference between eccrine and apocrine sweat glands.
2. How should a wound that has been debrided due to infection be allowed to heal?
3. What medical term is used to refer to a deficiency in vitamin D and what is the result of the deficiency?
4. Why is the subcutaneous tissue layer conducive to the formation of dead spaces during healing after a surgical procedure?
5. Where are the merocrine glands located in the body?

BIBLIOGRAPHY

Caruthers, B. L., & Price, P. (Eds.). (2001). *Surgical technology for the surgical technologist: A positive care approach.* Clifton Park, NY: Thomson Delmar Learning.

Cormack, D. H. (2001). *Essential histology* (2nd ed.). Philadelphia: Lippincott, Williams, & Wilkins.

Ethicon Products Worldwide. (2002). *Wound closure manual.* Somerville, NJ: Ethicon.

Ganong, W. F. (1993). *Review of medical physiology* (16th ed.). Norwalk, CT: Appleton & Lange.

Gray, H. (1991). *Anatomy: descriptive and surgical.* St. Louis, MO: Mosby-Year Book.

Peacock, E. E., Jr. (1984). *Wound repair* (3rd ed.). Philadelphia: W. B. Saunders.

Scanlon, V. C., & Sanders, T. (1999). *Essentials of anatomy and physiology* (3rd ed.). Philadelphia: F. A. Davis.

Shier, D., Butler, J., & Lewis, R. (2002). *Hole's human anatomy & physiology* (9th ed.). Boston: McGraw-Hill.

Swerdlow, J. L. (2002). Unmasking the skin. *National Geographic, 202* (5), 38–63.

6

SKELETAL SYSTEM

CHAPTER OBJECTIVES

After completing the study of this chapter, you should be able to:

1. Describe the anatomic structure of bone.
2. Describe the embryonic development of bone.
3. Describe the two types of bone by discussing their anatomic and functional differences.
4. List and describe the different types of bones.
5. List and describe the different types of joints.
6. List the clinical reference points of bones and their location.
7. Discuss the functions of bone.
8. Describe pathologies of bone.
9. List and describe the bones of the axial skeleton.
10. List and describe the bones of the appendicular skeleton.
11. Discuss the importance of understanding the anatomy and physiology of the skeletal system by surgical technologists and how that affects their role on the surgical team.

acetabulum
acromioclavicular (AC) joint
acromion process
amphiarthrosis
anterior cruciate ligament
    (ACL)
anterior superior iliac spine
appendicular skeleton
articulation
atlas
axis
ball-and-socket joint
bursae
cancellous bone (spongy
    bone)
capitulum
carpals
clavicle
coccyx
condyloid joint
coronoid process
cortical bone (compact bone)
costal cartilages
deltoid tuberosity
diaphysis
diarthrosis joint
endochondral ossification
endosteum
epicondyle
epiphyseal disk (epiphyseal
    plate)
epiphysis
ethmoid bone
external auditory meatus

fibula
flat bones
fontanel
foramen magnum
frontal bone
glenoid cavity
glenoid fossae
gliding joint
greater trochanter
greater tubercle
haversian system
hematopoiesis (hemopoiesis)
hinge joint
humerus
hyoid bone
iliac crest
ilium
inferior nasal conchae
intervertebral disks
intramembranous ossification
irregular bones
ischial spine
ischial tuberosity
ischium
lacrimal bones
lamellae
lateral malleolus
lesser trochanter
lesser tubercle
long bones
mandible
mandibular condyle
mandibular foramen
mandibular fossa

mastoid process
maxillary bones
medial malleolus
medullary canal
menisci
metacarpals
metatarsals
middle nasal concha
nasal bones
occipital bone
occipital condyles
olecranon process
origin
ossification (osteogenesis)
osteoblasts
osteoclasts
osteocytes
osteon
osteoprogenitor cells
palatine bones
paranasal sinuses
parietal bone
patella
patellar ligament
pelvis
phalanges
pivot joint
posterior cruciate ligament
    (PCL)
pubis
radial tuberosity
radius
ramus
red bone marrow

rotator cuff
sacroiliac joint
saddle joint
scapula
sesamoid bones
short bones
sphenoid bone
sphenoidal sinuses
sternum
styloid process
superior nasal concha
surgical neck
suture lines
symphysis pubis
synarthrosis
synovial joint
synovial membrane
tarsal bones
temporal bones
tibia
tibial tuberosity
trabeculae
transverse process
trochlea
ulna
vertebrae
vertebral canal (vertebral
    foramen)
vertebral column
vomer bone
zygomatic bones

Case Study 1

A 15-year-old patient is brought into the operating room to undergo repair of a broken radius. The surgeon is going to perform an open-reduction internal fixation, the placement of a plate over the fracture site that is held in place with screws. The surgical technologist makes sure she has enough cortical screws for the operation.

1. Why is the surgical technologist confirming that sterile cortical screws are available for the surgeon to use?

2. Describe the location of the radius.

3. When moving the forearm, what is the movement of the radius?

4. Just proximal to the head of the radius is a process called the radial tuberosity. What is the function of the tuberosity?

5. The distal end of the radius articulates with the carpal bones. Define the term *articulate*.

INTRODUCTION

When viewing bone it appears to be a nonliving material, but that is far from the truth. Bones are a specialized type of tissue that are the beginning structure of the body. They also support the body and perform many functions that maintain homeostasis. The skeletal system is composed of the 206 bones of the body and includes the ligaments, tendons, aponeuroses, and cartilage.

STRUCTURE OF BONE TISSUE

Bone is a specialized type of connective tissue. The bone cells are called **osteocytes**. Osteocytes function to transport nutrients and wastes to and from nearby cells through small channels that are further discussed in subsequent text. The inactive matrix that surrounds the osteocytes is composed of collagen and calcium salts. The calcium salts give the bone its hardness so it can support the body. Collagen provides strength and resistance to the bone and a limited degree of flexibility in order to withstand pressure. There are two types of bone tissue: compact or cortical bone and cancellous or spongy bone.

Cortical bone, also called **compact bone**, is the hard, dense tissue that surrounds the bone marrow cavity and comprises the majority of bone. Approximately 75% of the bone in the body is compact bone. The basic structural unit of compact bone is the **osteon**. When viewed under the microscope the osteon consists of concentric rings of **lamellae** and the haversian canal; together these structures comprise what is called a **haversian system**. There are hundreds of haversian systems within the compact bone. The haversian canal travels in a longitudinal direction, and traversing each canal is a single venule, nerve, and arteriole. Radiating from the lacuna, a space within the matrix of each haversian unit, are tiny passages called haversian canaliculus, which connect to the larger haversian canals that are interconnected within the bone matrix. In addition, another type of canal, called Volkmann's canal, connects with the haversian canals; this is a vascular canal that contains small blood vessels. An osteocyte is situated in the lacuna. The osteocyte transversely extends protoplasmic projections, which contact adjacent osteocyte projections (Figure 6-1).

Cancellous bone, also called **spongy bone**, is located at the ends of bone and lines the medullary marrow cavity. The name spongy bone is derived from the appearance of the bone; when viewed it gives the impression of a sponge due to its porous matrix. Approximately 25% of the bone in the body is cancellous bone (Ganong, 1993). Cancellous bone is composed of interspersed columns of bony substance called **trabeculae** with spaces between the columns. It would seem upon first look that this type of bone would be weak, but actually, because of their formation along stress lines, the columns are well adapted for load bearing and spreading out the load. Cancellous bone is composed of bone matrix and osteocytes.

With the exception of the ends of long bones, a thin, outer layer of fibrous tissue called the periosteum surrounds the bone. The following are the functions of the periosteum:

1. It provides a layer of defense to protect the bone from infection.
2. The inner elastic cambium layer is the area where new bone cells are formed.
3. It is permeated with nerves and blood vessels, which aid in nourishing the underlying bone.
4. The outer collagenous layer serves as an area of attachment that merges with those of the tendons and ligaments that are attached to bone.

Due to these various functions, in particular providing protection and containing blood vessels, the orthopedic surgeon will approximate the periosteal layer with suture when it has been incised.

In the middle of bones is a canal that runs the length of the bone called the **medullary canal** or cavity. Within the canal the semisolid tissue called **red bone marrow** is located. In infants, adolescents, and young adults, the red bone marrow is located in the spaces of cancellous bone found in the ends of the long bones, sternum, vertebrae, and ribs. The red bone marrow functions in the production of erythrocytes, leukocytes, and platelets. In long bones a fibrous layer of tissue that is similar to the periosteal layer lines the cavity and is called the **endosteum**. In adults, the red bone marrow is converted to yellow bone marrow, which does not produce red blood cells (RBCs). However, yellow bone marrow is highly vascular and supplies the cortex of the bone. It is interesting to note that the yellow bone marrow will convert back to red bone marrow in reaction to hemorrhagic trauma in order to produce needed RBCs. The conversion is not a quick process, but does signal the body's attempt to compensate for the loss of the RBCs. When homeostasis is returned, the marrow reconverts back to yellow bone marrow.

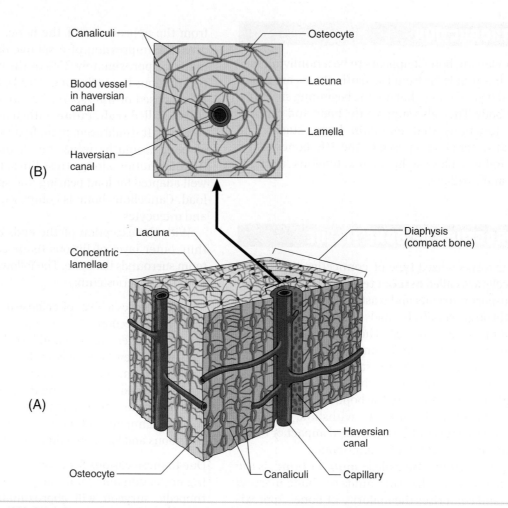

(B)

(A)

FIGURE 6-1   (A) Structure of a typical long bone; (B) cross section of bone body (B is from *Atlas of Microscopic Anatomy: A Functional Approach: Companion to Histology and Neuroanatomy,* by R. Bergman, A. Afifi, P. Heidger, 1999. www.vh.org/Providers/Textbooks/Microscopic Anatomy.html. Reprinted with permission.)

Bone Cells

There are four types of bone tissue cells including the stem cells: osteoprogenitor cells, osteoblasts, osteocytes, and osteoclasts.

Osteoprogenitor cells (formerly called osteogenic cells) are the stem cells of skeletal tissue. As previously mentioned, the inner layer of the periosteum is the cambium layer, which is composed of osteoprogenitor cells. In addition, the endosteum is made up of a single layer of osteoprogenitor cells; the cells from the cambium layer and endosteum can participate in both the formation of fetal bone and the repair of bone fractures. The osteoprogenitor cells differentiate into osteoblasts in regions with a good blood supply and into chondroblasts in regions that do not have a blood supply.

Osteoblasts are specialized basophilic cells that cannot divide. They are responsible for synthesizing the collagen and glycoprotein to form the bone matrix. They are a large polygonal cell, much larger than osteoprogenitor cells. The also have a role in bone resorption, which is discussed later in the chapter. The osteoblasts eventually develop into osteocytes, which makes sense because the osteoblasts are originally responsible for creating the cytoplasmic processes that connect the cells and canaliculi.

Osteocytes are smaller basophilic cells than osteoblasts. The lacunae, cytoplasmic processes, and canaliculi, which were discussed in detail earlier in this book, are responsible for maintaining the bone matrix and, in the fetus, represent the last stage of bone maturation.

Osteoclasts are large cells that are easily distinguished from the other bone cells because they are multinucleated. Under the microscope, osteoclasts will be seen residing in recesses of the bone called Howship's lacunae. The osteoclast functions in the development, growth, and repair of bone, including breakdown and resorption. Osteoclasts are activated by parathyroid hormone, and the area of the bone undergoing resorption has a ruffled border, which is the edge of the osteoclast cell and indicates a bone resorption site. The ruffles are actually fingerlike processes of the osteoclast cell that are penetrating the bone matrix. Osteoclasts are differentiated from blood monocytes. The monocytes are attracted to the bone surface where they form osteoclasts by joining together. Therefore, osteoclasts do not necessarily belong to the family of osteoprogenitor cells, but represent a line of differentiation of the monocyte and are derived from hematopoietic stem cells via monocytes (Cormack, 2001; Ganong, 1993).

EMBRYONIC DEVELOPMENT OF BONE

During the embryonic development of bone the skeleton is initially composed of cartilage and connective tissue. This is gradually replaced by bone through one of two methods: intramembranous ossification and endochondral ossification. However, it must be emphasized that although the two methods of bone development occur separately, the end product is still the same kind of bone tissue (Figure 6-2).

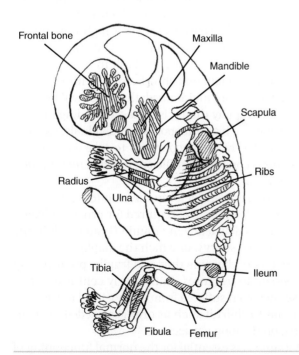

Frontal bone
Maxilla
Mandible
Scapula
Radius
Ulna
Ribs
Tibia
Ileum
Fibula
Femur

FIGURE 6-2   Embryonic skeleton

Intramembranous Bone

The terms **ossification** and **osteogenesis** both refer to the development of bone. The flat bones of the cranium, facial bones, mandible, and clavicle develop by the process of **intramembranous ossification**. Let's take the mandible as an example. A site amply supplied by capillaries is where osteogenesis begins. Mesenchymal cells in this center differentiate into osteoprogenitor cells, which are the stem cells of skeletal tissue. The osteoprogenitor cells differentiate into round basophilic osteoblast cells that synthesize the collagen and glycoproteins to form the bone matrix and with the growth of bone develop into osteocytes.

As previously mentioned, the osteoblasts form many cytoplasmic processes to interconnect the cells and they secrete the organic matrix that forms around the cell bodies and processes. At the same time the lacunae and canaliculi are formed. After calcification, the canaliculi are responsible for the transport of nutrients to the lacunae and bone tissue from the capillaries.

Endochondral Bone

The rest of the bones, in particular the long bones of the embryonic skeleton, develop by **endochondral ossification**. The growth of a long bone begins in the area located in the center of the developing bone called the primary ossification center, and the bone tissue develops from the center toward the ends. Mesenchymal cells collect and differentiate into chondroblasts, marking the site of where a bone will soon form. The chondroblasts synthesize matrix, and the long bone is now formed of hyaline cartilage and a perichondrium has begun to develop. The growth of the cartilage continues as the chondrocytes further divide and more matrix is produced. In the midsection, or what will become the diaphysis of the bone, the perichondrium becomes the periosteum, which produces osteoblasts that begin the process of forming bone matrix in the shaft. Eventually subperiosteal bone is formed under the periosteum and the medullary cavity is formed. The medullary cavity is formed when osteoclasts resorb the cancellous bone that formed in the center of the diaphysis and is surrounded by cortical bone. The canal later fills with red bone marrow (Figure 6-3).

The bone now grows in length, but the ends, called the epiphyses, are still composed of cartilage. A transverse disk of hyaline cartilage known as the **epiphyseal disk** or **epiphyseal plate** forms between the junction of the diaphysis with each epiphysis. The epiphyseal plate is the area of growth that allows the bone to keep lengthening until the diaphysis and

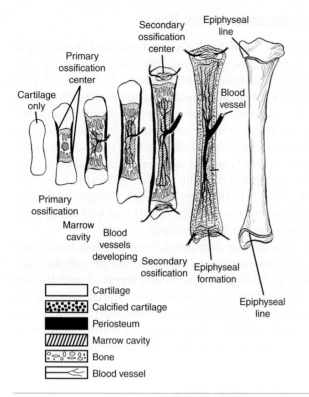

FIGURE 6-3 Long bone development

Labels in figure: Secondary ossification center; Epiphyseal line; Primary ossification center; Cartilage only; Blood vessel; Primary ossification; Marrow cavity; Blood vessels developing; Secondary ossification; Epiphyseal formation; Epiphyseal line

Legend:
Cartilage
Calcified cartilage
Periosteum
Marrow cavity
Bone
Blood vessel

epiphysis join together, marking that the bone has reached full length and maturity, usually occurring between the ages of 16 and 25 years.

BONE REMODELING

Once the bones have reached maturity and full growth, it appears that they become inactive, but this is hardly the situation. Bones undergo a lifetime of remodeling and adapting to stresses. For example, the trabecula found in the cancellous bone at the end of long bones forms according to the unique stresses that each person places upon the bone. Athletes who run long distances, such as marathons, will have trabeculae that become aligned to adjust to the stress of the locomotion of the feet constantly hitting hard ground or pavement. Conversely, if a limb is not used for a long period and the bone is not subjected to some amount of stress, the bone may atrophy due to disuse.

Compact bone is constantly undergoing remodeling to maintain its structure and strength, as well as to ensure a constant supply of calcium to the body. Osteoclasts absorb bone that is then replaced by new compact bone. The action of the osteoclasts is hormonally regulated. Approximately 90% of the calcium in the body is stored by the bones of the skeleton. Calcium is essential for many processes of the body, including transmission of nerve impulses, muscle contraction, blood coagulation, cardiac function, and many other metabolic functions. Maintaining a normal blood level of calcium is a constant, ongoing process, accounting for the high level of activity of bone tissue. When the body detects that a low level of calcium is present in the blood, parathyroid hormone is released and it affects the osteoclasts, which break down the bone tissue, thereby releasing calcium for absorption into the blood and returning the level of calcium to normal. When the normal level has been attained, the thyroid gland secretes the hormone calcitonin, which acts on the osteoclasts to inhibit their activity and decrease the resorption of bone and subsequent release of calcium. Osteoblasts are then stimulated to form new bone tissue. This counteraction of osteoblasts and osteoclasts keeps the bone matrix strong because the calcium in bone is replaced at a rate equal to its removal (Caruthers & Price, 2001).

The calcium in bone is replaced at a rate of 100% per year for infants and approximately 18% per year in adults (Ganong, 1993). The renewal rate for compact bone is about 4% per year in adults and 20% per year for cancellous bone (Ganong, 1993).

Factors That Affect Bone Maintenance

Two other important factors affect bone maintenance in conjunction with hormonal influence: exercise and nutrition. Weight-bearing exercise is highly important in maintaining the strength of bone and preventing an abnormal bone loss. Bones are built to support a person's normal weight and absorb stress. Without stress, homeostasis is not maintained; the bones will lose calcium more rapidly than it is replaced, leading to bone pathologies such as osteoporosis. Individuals, particularly the elderly, are encouraged to take daily walks, since this is considered sufficient to aid in maintaining the density of bone.

Nutrition is a key factor in the maintenance of normal bones. Vitamin C is required for proper collagen formation; a deficiency in vitamin C can result in the disease called scurvy, in which the diaphysis and epiphyseal plates become thin and fragile, predisposing the person to fractures. In the early centuries, navy personnel often suffered from scurvy until it was realized that fresh fruit such as oranges needed to be ingested on the long voyages.

Vitamin A is essential for the normal functioning of osteoblasts and osteoclasts during normal bone growth and development. A deficiency of vitamin A causes other pathologies, such as night blindness, but also can contribute to poor bone development.

Vitamin D is necessary to promote the absorption of calcium and phosphate from the small intestine. Approximately one third of the calcium ingested by a person is absorbed from the small intestine. Vitamin D itself also forms a substance called dehydrocholesterol, which is produced in the digestive tract or obtained from the diet. Dehydrocholesterol is transported via the circulatory system to the skin and upon exposure to the ultraviolet rays of the sun is converted to vitamin D (Shier, Butler, & Lewis, 2002). Individuals deprived of vitamin D by poor diet and minimum exposure to the sun are predisposed to developing the bone disorder called rickets, wherein the bones are poorly calcified and semirigid, causing the weight-bearing bones to bend under the stress of the body's weight. Common physical signs of rickets are bowed legs or knock-knees.

Heredity is a factor that must be taken into consideration. Individuals inherit from parents a genetic potential for determining height. If a person has parents and other relatives who are tall, there is a good chance the bones of the body will grow in a manner so as to indicate that the person has inherited this propensity for being tall.

BLOOD SUPPLY TO LONG BONES

Bone has an excellent blood supply and has a total blood flow of 200–400 mL/min in the adult (Ganong, 1993). The blood supply of the diaphysis, bone marrow cavity, and metaphyses of a long bone is supplied by the nutrient artery. The metaphyseal arteries also provide blood to the metaphyses. The epiphyses receive their blood supply primarily from the epiphyseal arteries. The outer layers of compact bone also receive nutrients and oxygen delivered by blood via the canaliculi, which receive the supply from the periosteal arteries. The blood supply to long bones is advantageous in that if the blood supply from the nutrient artery is interrupted due to trauma or disease, the rest of the bone will remain viable due to the other arterial supply.

The arteries develop during bone development as follows. The nutrient artery develops from the capillaries called the periosteal bud, which were initially formed in the primary ossification center. The epiphyseal arteries soon develop from the same periosteal bud. Metaphyseal arteries develop from periosteal arteries, which became part of the bone

tissue when the metaphyses widened (Cormack, 2001). When the epiphyseal plates disappear upon maturity of the bone the terminal branches of the nutrient, metaphyseal, and epiphyseal arteries anastomose.

TYPES OF BONES

There are four types of bones: long, short, flat, and sesamoid. Examples of **long bones** include the humerus, femur, and phalanges. The shaft or middle portion of the bone is called the **diaphysis** and the end is called the **epiphysis** (plural, epiphyses). The diaphysis is composed of compact bone and the epiphyses are made of cancellous bone (Figure 6-4).

The joints of the body are composed of the epiphyses. The ends of the epiphyses are covered by a type of cartilage called articular cartilage. Articular cartilage protects the ends of the bones by providing a smooth surface for the movement of the joints and tendons and preventing the bone from rubbing against bone. Articular cartilage is composed of vertical columns of chondrocytes. Articular cartilage is avascular and depends on nourishment by diffusion from the capillaries outside of the cartilage. The joint is lined by a **synovial membrane**, which does not cover the articular cartilage. The combination of the ligaments of a joint and the synovial membrane is referred to as the joint capsule (Caruthers & Price, 2001). The synovial membrane is discussed in further detail in text in which the joints are described.

As previously mentioned, the area of active bone growth in the long bone is called the epiphyseal plate. When the growth of a long bone is complete, the epiphyseal plate disappears and the area is then referred to as a closed epiphysis.

The **short bones** of the body are the carpal bones located in the wrist joint and tarsal bones located in the ankle joint. The carpals and tarsals are a group of bones that aid in the movement of the wrist and ankle joints.

Examples of **flat bones** include cranial bones, scapula, sternum, and ribs. The bones of the cranium and face are also referred to as **irregular bones**. In adults, the majority of erythrocytes are developed and supplied to the body by the sternum and ribs.

Sesamoid bones, or round bones, are usually stabilized by tendons. The two most commonly known sesamoid bones are the patella, or kneecap, and the two bones located on the head of the metatarsal in the foot that form the "ball" of the foot (Figure 6-5).

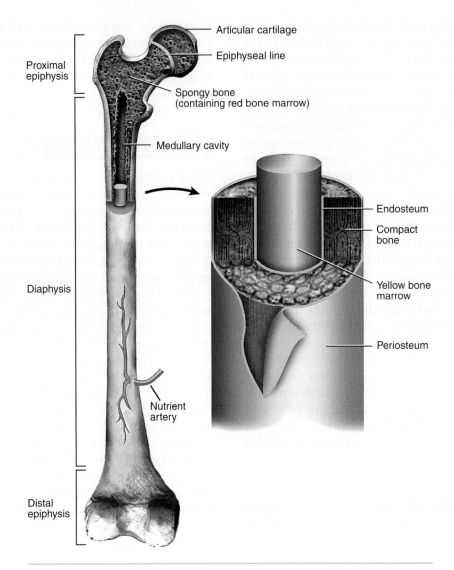

FIGURE 6-4 **Structure of long bones**

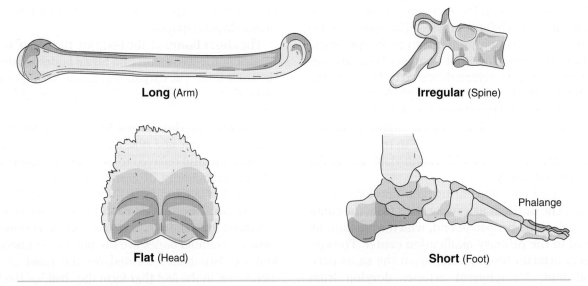

FIGURE 6-5 **Bone shapes**

Anatomic Reference Points of Bones

The surgical technologist should be familiar with the many anatomic terms used in reference to bones so as to be able to identify a particular area of the bone on which the surgeon may be focussing. Refer to Table 6-1.

Functions of Bones

Bones have five functions:

1. Support the body and aid in protecting the internal organs.
2. Serve as points of attachment for the tendons of the muscles.
3. Aid in body movement.
4. Serve as a source of erythrocytes.
5. Serve as a storage site of minerals.

The bones support the body and give shape to the individual's structure. The pelvis, lower leg bones, and vertebral column are the weight-bearing bones of the body and provide the needed support. Certain bones also aid in protecting internal organs from injury: for instance, the cranial and facial bones protect the brain, eyes, and ears; the ribs and sternum protect the lungs and heart; and the pelvic bones protect the lower abdominal organs and internal reproductive organs of the female.

The bones serve as points of attachment of the tendons of the muscles. As will be discussed in the following chapter, the muscles are not directly attached to bones, but are attached by tendons. An example listed in Table 6-1 is the anatomical landmark referred to as a trochanter, which serves as a point of attachment for various muscles.

Bones interact with muscles to create the various body movements. The bones and muscles form a mechanical device referred to as a lever. A lever has four components: (a) rigid bar, (b) pivot on which the bar turns, (c) object that moves against resistance, and (d) force the supplies the energy for the bar to move (Shier, Butler, & Lewis, 2002). The bending of the forearm at the elbow is a good example of a lever of the body. When an individual bends the upper limb, the radius and ulna of the forearm are the rigid bars, the elbow joint is the pivot, the hand is moved against the resistance of its own weight, and the force is supplied by the biceps brachii while the triceps brachii is relaxed. When the upper limb is straightened, all the structures of the lever have the same action with exception of the two muscles—the triceps brachii now supplies the force and the biceps brachii relax.

There are many levers throughout the body, which provide a range of movements. In addition, some levers are arranged to give a person the ability to produce a rapid motion, whereas others, such as those that aid in head movements, are designed to maintain posture.

TABLE 6-1	**Anatomic Landmarks and Terms for Bone**
Appendicular skeleton	The 126 bones comprising the upper and lower extremities of the body.
Axial skeleton	The 80 bones comprising the cranium, vertebral column, sternum, and ribs.
Condyle	Rounded projection/process at the epiphysis of a bone that articulates with another bone and serves as the point of attachment for ligaments.
Crest	Narrow elongated ridge/elevation of bone, such as the iliac crest.
Distal	Away from the origin of the extremity.
Epicondyle	Projection on the surface of a bone located above a condyle.
Foramen	Opening in the bone for the passage of structures such as blood vessels, nerves, or ligaments. An example is the foramen magnum, a passage in the occipital bone through which the spinal cord passes into the spinal column.
Fossa	Hollow or depression on the surface end of a bone, such as the olecranon fossa.
Fovea	Another name for a depression on the bone but smaller than a fossa. An example is the fovea on the head of the femur, which serves as the point of attachment for the ligamentum teres.
Head	The enlarged, rounded, proximal portion of a bone, usually a long bone.
Process	Natural growth that projects from a bone. Condyles are an example of a process.
Proximal	Near the origin of the limb.
Trochanter	Large process on a bone. Examples are the lesser and greater trochanters of the femur that serve as points of attachment for various muscles.
Tubercle	Small knoblike nodule or eminence on a bone.
Tuberosity	Nodule or eminence on a bone that is larger than a tubercle.

As previously mentioned, bone is the source of blood cell formation called **hematopoiesis** or **hemopoiesis**. In infants and adolescents, the red marrow within the medullary cavity of long bones functions in the formation of erythrocytes, leukocytes, and platelets. As the person ages, the red marrow is slowly replaced by yellow marrow, which stores fat and does not function in hematopoiesis. In adults, red bone marrow is located primarily in the skull, clavicles, sternum, ribs, vertebrae, and pelvis.

Recall that the matrix of the bone tissue is composed of collagen and inorganic mineral salts. The mineral salts, which make up approximately 70% of the matrix, are a type of calcium phosphate called hydroxyapatite (Shier, Butler, & Lewis, 2002). The functions of calcium have already been discussed. In addition to storing calcium and phosphorus, small amounts of sodium, potassium, and magnesium are stored. Bone also has an affinity for storing harmful metallic elements that are unintentionally ingested by a person, such as lead, radium, plutonium, and strontium. The last three elements are by-products of atomic bomb explosions or nuclear accidents, such as what occurred at Chernobyl in the former Soviet Union. The radiation from these elements almost always leads to pathologic changes to the bone cells, causing the formation of osteogenic sarcomas. Fluoride is another element, but it aids in the formation of new bone and is present in the enamel of the teeth to help increase the resistance to the formation of cavities.

TYPES OF JOINTS

An **articulation** refers to an area where the ends of two bones meet to form a joint or the bones articulate to form a joint. There are three classifications of joints: immovable, slightly movable, and freely movable.

Synarthrosis is a type of immovable joint. Synarthroses joints are close together and separated by a thin layer of cartilage. The most well known example of synarthroses is the **suture lines** of the cranial bones.

Amphiarthrosis is a joint that is slightly movable. Between the joint is a layer of fibrous cartilage that serves as a connection between the bones. This type of joint has very little movement due to the slight flexibility of the cartilage. Examples include the symphysis pubis, which is a disk of cartilage that connects the pubic bones of the pelvis and the cartilage that connects the vertebrae.

Diarthrosis joints are freely movable joints. They allow the most movement of any type of joint.

The articular ends of a diarthrosis joint are covered with a thin layer of hyaline cartilage called the articular cartilage. It protects the ends of the bone from wear and tear and reduces friction during body movement. The joint capsule is composed of two layers: an outer layer of dense connective tissue that attaches to the periosteum around each bone of the joint near the articulation thus enclosing the joint; and the synovial membrane, which lines the capsule but does not cover the articular cartilage, produces synovial fluid, and is the reason why diarthroses are also called **synovial joints**. The synovial membrane, also called synovium, is a highly vascularized connective tissue membrane. The function of the synovial fluid is to lubricate the joint, reducing friction between the articular cartilages and aiding joint movement, and provide nourishment to the articular cartilages (Figure 6-6).

Some synovial joints contain flat disks of tough fibrocartilage called **menisci** (singular, meniscus). The menisci are located between the two articulating ends of the bones. For example, in the knee joint two crescent-shaped (half-moon–shaped) menisci are located laterally and medially within the joint to aid in joint movement, protect the ends of the bones, and serve as cushions, since the bones of the leg are weight-bearing bones.

Many of the synovial joints also contain small fluid-filled sacs called **bursae** (singular, bursa). Each bursa has an inner lining of synovial membrane that may be continuous with the synovial membrane of the joint cavity. The sacs contain synovial fluid and are commonly located between the tendons and bony prominences of the joint, such as the bursa located in the shoulder and knee joints. Bursae cushion and aid the movement of tendons to slide easily as the bones are moved. Occasionally, if a joint undergoes excessive use such as in weight lifting, or jarring activities such as running on hard surfaces, the bursae will become inflamed, a condition referred to as bursitis.

Joints

There are six types of joints: ball-and-socket, gliding, hinge, pivot, condyloid, and saddle (Figure 6-7). The **ball-and-socket joint** allows for the widest range of motion. It is made up of a bone with a ball-shaped head at one end that fits into or articulates with a bone that has a cup-shaped socket. Movement in all planes is possible, including rotation (Caruthers & Price, 2001). Two examples are the hip and shoulder joints.

Gliding joints allow twisting and side-to-side movements. The articulating surfaces of both bones are slightly curved or flat. The carpals in the wrist

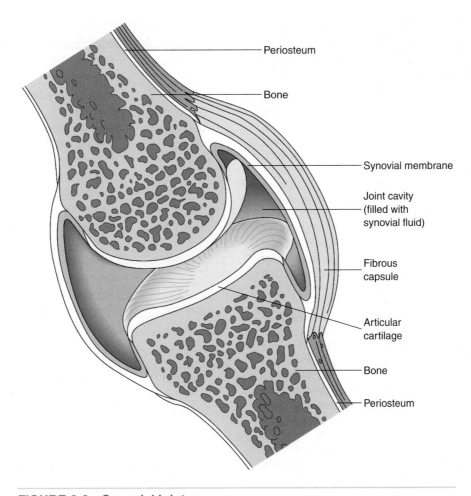

FIGURE 6-6 Synovial joint

Labels: Periosteum; Bone; Synovial membrane; Joint cavity (filled with synovial fluid); Fibrous capsule; Articular cartilage; Bone; Periosteum

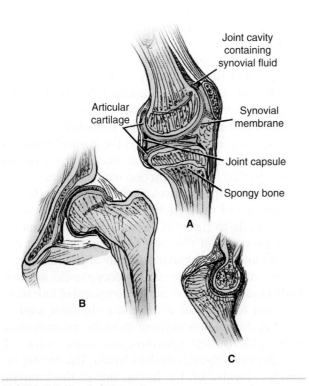

Labels: Joint cavity containing synovial fluid; Articular cartilage; Synovial membrane; Joint capsule; Spongy bone; A; B; C

FIGURE 6-7 Joint types

joint and the tarsals in the ankle joint are each examples of a gliding joint.

Hinge joints allow only extension and contraction. The joint is formed by the convex surface of one bone end articulating with the concave surface of the other bone. The elbow is an example of a hinge joint.

Pivot joints allow movement in only one plane, a rotational movement around a central axis. The proximal ends of the ulna and radius form a pivot joint. When moved the radius rotates around the ulna.

Condyloid joints also allow movement in only one plane with limited lateral movement. The joint is formed by the end of one bone articulating with the fossa of another bone. The most popular example is the temporomandibular joint (TMJ) in which the condyle of the mandible articulates with the fossa of the temporal bone.

Saddle joints allow movement in many planes. The articulating ends of both bones have concave and convex surfaces. The surface of one bone fits into the same surface of the other bone. The trapezium of the wrist and the metacarpal of the thumb form a saddle joint.

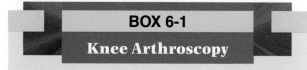

BOX 6-1

Knee Arthroscopy

An arthroscopy is a surgical procedure in which a rigid scope is inserted within a joint to view the interior. It is performed both for diagnostic reasons and for procedures such as repair of a torn meniscus, removal of joint mice, arthroscopic repair of the anterior cruciate ligament (ACL), or removing tissue from the joint with the use of a shaver, a special piece of power equipment that utilizes various types of rotating cutting heads. Arthroscopy can be performed on almost every joint of the body. The size of the scope and instrumentation will vary according to the joint that will be worked on. For example, the scope used for viewing the knee joint will be much larger in diameter than a scope used to view the ankle joint. The following is a brief description of a diagnostic knee arthroscopy.

Small, stab incisions are made in the knee to accommodate the scope and instrumentation. The first stab incision is made just lateral to the patellar tendon and superior to the tibia and fibula. A cannula called the irrigation/inflow cannula is placed into the knee joint through the incision. Tubing leading from the cannula to a bag of fluid called lactated Ringer's allows the fluid to flow into the joint to distend it. This helps the surgeon view the internal structures of the knee joint. A second stab incision is made on the anterolateral area of the knee, and a sheath larger in diameter than the irrigation cannula is inserted into the knee joint. The scope is inserted through this sheath. The surgeon will visualize the underside of the patella, menisci, and ACL. Another incision is made on the anteromedial area of the knee and the scope is inserted through this portal. This allows the surgeon to view the medial femoral condyle, medial meniscus, and posterior cruciate ligament. At the end of the procedure, the cannula and sheaths are removed, the fluid in the knee is allowed to escape through the incisions, and the incisions are closed with suture.

Joint Movement Terms

The muscles attached to diarthroses are called the skeletal muscles and, along with the bone, produce the movements of the body. The **origin** of the muscle is the end attached to the immovable end of one bone. The other end of the muscle, called the **insertion**, is attached to the movable end of the bone. When the muscle contracts the muscle fibers draw the insertion toward the origin, causing joint movement. The clinical terms used most frequently to describe joint movement are given in Table 6-2.

TABLE 6-2   Joint Movement Terminology

Abduction	Moving a body part away from the midline of the body
Adduction	Moving a body part toward the midline of the body
Circumduction	Moving a particular body part in a circular path without moving the entire body part (e.g., moving a finger in a circular motion without moving the hand)
Rotation	Moving a body part around a central axis
Dorsiflexion	Bending the foot upward at the ankle joint
Plantar flexion	Bending the foot downward at the ankle joint
Eversion	Turning the foot outward or inside out at the ankle joint so the sole of the foot is shown outward
Inversion	Turning the foot outward at the ankle joint so the sole of the foot is pointing inward
Flexion	Bending a joint
Extension	Straightening a joint
Pronation	Pointing a body part downward (e.g., facing the palm of the hand downward)
Supination	Pointing a body part upward

Examples: Shoulder Joint and Knee Joint

The following is a description of two joints of the body to serve as examples of how joints have both common and unique structures. Because of their complexity, the shoulder and, in particular, the knee were chosen.

The shoulder joint is a type of ball-and-socket joint composed of the head of the humerus that fits into the glenoid cavity of the scapula. It is capable of the following movements: extension, flexion, rotation, circumduction, adduction, and abduction. Two projections of the scapula, called the coracoid process and acromion process, aid in protecting the joint and strengthening it in conjunction with ligaments.

The joint capsule envelops the joint along the circumference of the glenoid cavity and humeral neck. The capsule along with the muscles and ligaments hold the bones of the joint together to prevent displacement. The muscular anatomy of the shoulder is composed of the rotator cuff, biceps muscle, and deltoid muscle. The rotator cuff is composed of four muscles that form a cuff around the shoulder joint to stabilize and allow a range of motions: infraspinatus, subscapularis, supraspinatus, and teres minor. All four muscles originate in the scapula. The greater tubercle is located on the lateral side of the humeral head. The tendons of the infraspinatus, supraspinatus, and teres minor all insert on the greater tubercle. The lesser tubercle is located on the anterior side of the head at the insertion of the subscapularis tendon. Between the two tuberosities is a groove in the bone called the bicipital groove, and the tendon of the biceps muscle inserts in the groove. In the middle of the humeral shaft is the deltoid tuberosity, and this serves as the point of attachment for the tendon of the deltoid muscle. The deltoid muscle aids in raising the arm horizontally and laterally.

The ligaments of the joint are as follows:

1. Glenohumeral ligaments: Three bands of fiber located in the ventral wall of the capsule, extending from the edge of the glenoid cavity to the lesser tubercle and humeral neck.
2. Glenoid labrum: Composed of fibrocartilage, it is attached along the edge of the glenoid cavity forming a rim around the cavity.
3. Transverse humeral ligament: A narrow band of connective tissue that is situated in a transverse direction between the lesser and greater tubercles of the humerus. In conjunction with the intertubercular groove, it forms the retinaculum (canal) through which the head of the biceps brachii muscle travels (Shier, Butler, & Lewis, 2002).
4. Coracohumeral ligament: A broad band of connective tissue that connects the coracoid process to the greater tubercle. It aids in strengthening the superior region of the joint capsule.

The shoulder joint contains four bursae:

1. Subcoracoid bursa: located between the joint capsule and coracoid process
2. Subdeltoid bursa: located between the deltoid muscle and joint capsule
3. Subscapular bursa: located between the tendon of the subscapularis muscle and joint capsule
4. Subacromial bursa: located between the acromion process and the joint capsule

The knee joint is the most complex of the synovial joints. It is composed of the lateral and medial condyles located at the distal end of the femur and the lateral and medial condyles located at the proximal end of the tibia. Also, the anterior portion of the femur articulates with the posterior portion of the patella. The knee joint is actually three types of joints: primarily a hinge joint for extension and flexion; a condyloid joint for articulation between the femur and tibia, allowing limited rotation upon flexing the knee; and a gliding point for articulation between the femur and patella.

The joint capsule is a thin layer but is reinforced by the muscles and ligaments of the knee. For example, the tendons of the quadriceps muscle connect the femur to the patellar tendon, which passes anteriorly over the knee covering the joint capsule and attaches to the patella. The tendon then continues as the patellar ligament and attaches to the tibia.

The primary ligaments that hold the knee joint in place include:

1. Oblique popliteal ligament: connects the lateral condyle of the femur to the edge of the tibial head.
2. Arcuate popliteal ligament: extends from the lateral condyle of the femur to the head of the fibula.
3. Fibular collateral ligament: a band located between the lateral condyle of the femur and head of the fibula.
4. Tibial collateral ligament: a flattened band of tissue located between the medial condyle of the femur and the medial condyle of the tibia.
5. Patellar ligament: a strong, thick ligament that is a continuation of the patellar tendon of the quadriceps muscle that extends from the inferior border to the patella to the tibial tuberosity. A portion of the patellar ligament is often removed to serve as a replacement of the anterior cruciate ligament when it has been injured.
6. **Anterior cruciate ligament (ACL):** one of two cruciate ligaments. Its origin is from the anterior intercondylar area of the tibia and it inserts on the lateral condyle of the femur. The ACL prevents the femur from sliding posteriorly on the tibia, limits the medial rotation of the femur when the leg is in a fixed position with foot planted, and prevents hyperextension of the knee. A common injury of the knee, particularly with athletes, is a torn ACL, in which the ligament is either repaired or replaced.
7. **Posterior cruciate ligament (PCL):** the other of the two cruciate ligaments, its orgin is from the posterior intercondylar area of the tibia and inserts on the medial condyle of the femur. The PCL prevents the femur from sliding anteriorly on the tibia (Figures 6-8 and 6-9).

As stated earlier, two crescent-shaped fibrocartilages are located in the knee joint, which are called the menisci (singular, meniscus). They separate the ends of the femoral and tibial bones and are a tough, thick tissue. The tibial head has slight depressions for attachment of the medial and lateral menisci, and the superior portion of the menisci have depressions to fit the

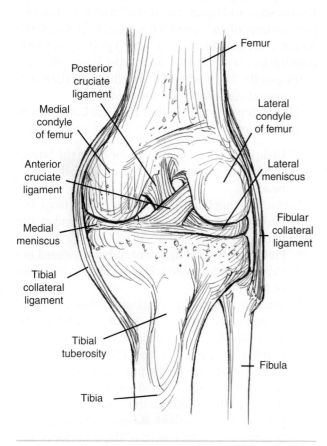

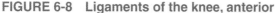

FIGURE 6-8 **Ligaments of the knee, anterior**

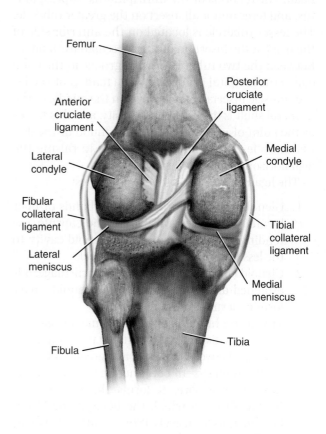

FIGURE 6-9 **Ligaments of the knee, posterior**

condyles of the femur. They serve to keep the bones from rubbing against each other, and thereby avoid friction and breaking down of the bone, and as cushions, especially for active individuals such as basketball players, who are constantly jumping and landing on hard surfaces.

The three bursae of the knee joint include:

1. Prepatellar bursa: located between the patella and skin
2. Infrapatellar bursa: located between the proximal end of the tibia and patellar ligament
3. Suprapatellar bursa: located between the anterior surface, distal end of the femur and quadriceps located superiorly

PATHOLOGIES OF BONE

There are numerous pathologies of the skeletal system. Table 6-3 lists and describes some of the more common ones encountered in the surgical setting.

BONE HEALING

A fracture is the discontinuity of the normal alignment of bone. Most fractures are caused by accidents, although some are pathological (fractures caused by diseased bones). Table 6-4 explains how fractures are classified and Table 6-5 lists the types of fractures and their causes. The healing of bone fractures occurs in a series of stages to reach the final result of the bone returning to its original contour and strength. The normal process of bone healing takes place in five stages: (a) inflammation, (b) cellular proliferation, (c) callus formation, (d) ossification, and (e) remodeling.

Normal Bone Healing

A fracture completely heals in approximately 8–12 weeks. For proper healing and complete union of the two ends of the fractured bone to take place, the site of the injury must be completely immobilized by

BOX 6-2

Total Joint Arthroplasty

Total joint arthroplasty refers to replacing a joint in the body with prosthetic joint implants. The procedure is performed to replace a joint that has irreversible damage due to trauma or arthritis. Because of osteoarthritis, osteomalacia, or other types of degenerative joint diseases, a large population of the elderly undergo hip joint and knee joint replacement surgery. Athletes such as football players undergo joint replacement due to repeated injuries or wear and tear. An injury to the hip joint wherein the blood supply to the femoral head is damaged or interrupted leads to necrosis of the head and requires joint replacement surgery.

Almost all joints of the body can be replaced including finger, toe, wrist, elbow, shoulder, hip, knee, and ankle. The prostheses for the larger joints of the body are composed of metal alloys that the body does not reject. Over the years much improvement has been made in both the alloys and the design of the prostheses, surgical instrumentation, and surgical technique. Research is ongoing to find materials that better resemble the chemistry of the body. For example, in the future implants may be developed that have a coating that would allow the bone tissue to grow into the prostheses to better stabilize the joint and provide a longer life to the prostheses.

The following is a short description of a total hip arthroplasty with the use of bone cement; cement is not always used and the type of prostheses determines whether it will be.

The patient is placed on the nonoperative side, called the lateral position, to expose the hip joint. A long incision is made and carried down to the hip joint. The joint is manually dislocated in order to deliver the femoral head into the surgical wound. The head of the femur is removed with a power saw approximately 1 cm proximal to the lesser trochanter. Next, powered acetabular cutting heads, referred to as acetabular reamers, are used to remove the articular cartilage and osteophytes. The acetabulum is reamed until osteochondral bone is exposed. A trial acetabular prosthesis is placed to determine the correct size. Once the correct size is determined, bone cement is placed into the acetabulum and the permanent acetabular prosthesis is placed.

Next, rasps are inserted down the femoral canal to create an opening for the femoral prosthesis. The final size of rasp also serves as the femoral trial component. The trial femoral head and neck are placed on the rasp to confirm the correct sizes. The rasp/trial are removed and cement is injected down the femoral canal. The femoral component that has a long stem is placed down the femoral shaft. Next, the femoral head is positioned onto the stem. An insert made of polyethylene is inserted into the acetabular prosthesis so the metal head is not rubbing against the metal acetabulum, but moves freely on the smooth surface of the polyethylene insert. The hip is put back into place and moved through a range of motions. If all looks good, the wound is closed with sutures.

---

either external fixation such as with a cast, an external fixation device, or internal fixation such as with plates and screws. In addition, the bone ends must be as perfectly aligned as possible.

The first stage, called the inflammatory stage, begins when the fracture occurs and lasts approximately two days. The fracture hematoma or blood clot forms at this time and serves as the basis for the cellular proliferation stage.

The cellular proliferation stage begins on about the third day after the injury. Macrophages have migrated to the site of the injury for purposes of debridement and a fibrin mesh forms, which seals the approximated edges of the fractured ends of the bone. The fibrin mesh allows for the ingrowth of capillaries and fibroblasts. The soft-tissue periosteal callus is formed on the surface or cortex of the fractured bone by collagen-producing fibroblasts and osteoblasts.

The next stage, callus formation, lasts about three to four weeks. The ingrowth of soft tissue continues to bring the bone fragments toward each other to close the gap. Osteoblasts synthesize collagen, which penetrates the periosteal callus to further close the gap and aid in uniting the two fractured ends. Together cartilage, immature bone, and fibrous tissue provide stabilization to the fracture site.

The ossification stage is the longest of the five stages, lasting three to four months. The collection of osteoblasts (called the osteoid) calcifies, thereby completing the unification of the bone ends. The bone can now store mineral deposits.

The last stage is the remodeling stage and signifies the return of homeostasis to the bone. Any devitalized tissue left over from the fracture is removed and the new bone is mature and resumes all normal functions.

Sutures Used in Repair of Bone

The two most common areas of the skeleton in which suture is used for repair are the sternum and

TABLE 6-3   Common Pathologies of the Skeletal System

CLINICAL TERMS	DESCRIPTION
Ankylosis	Abnormal stiffness or fixation of a joint usually resulting from the destruction of articular cartilage as occurs in rheumatoid arthritis.
Arthralgia	Pain in a joint.
Bunion	A bony protuberance on the medial aspect of the first metatarsal. The condition is associated with hallux valgus deformity. A bony prominence projecting from a bone is called an exostosis.
Chondroma	Benign tumor of cartilage.
Dislocations	A dislocation is the displacement of a bone from its socket, usually caused by trauma. The types of dislocations include compound, or open, which is the complete displacement of the bone from its socket along with a break in the skin; complete, which is the complete displacement of the bone from its socket with no break in the skin; and incomplete, subluxation, or partial, which is the slight displacement of the bone from its socket and does not involve a break in the skin.
Genu valgum	Knock-kneed; the knees are in close position and the space between the ankles is increased.
Genu varum	Bow-legged; the space between the knees is abnormally increased and the lower leg bows inward.
Hallux valgus	The outward turning of the great toe away from the midline.
Hallux varus	The inward turning of the great toe toward the midline.
Hammer toe, claw toe, mallet toe	Acquired or congenital deformity of the toe as a result of abnormal positioning of the interphalangeal joints.
Joint mice	Joint mice, so called because of loose particles within the joint, are caused by repeated trauma to the knee. Joint mice often create a constant irritation within the joint cavity. When a particle becomes lodged between articulating surfaces, pain or a locking of the joint may occur.
Kyphosis	Commonly referred to as hunchback; it is an abnormal humped curvature in the thoracic region of the spine. Adolescent kyphosis is the most common form of the disorder. Two other abnormal curvatures of the spine are lordosis and scoliosis. Lordosis is referred to as swayback and involves an inward curvature of the lumbar spine just superior to the sacrum. Scoliosis is a lateral curvature of the spine, most often in the lumbar region. Scoliosis may be functional or structural. Functional scoliosis is most often due to poor posture. Structural scoliosis is either congenital, paralytic due to paralysis of the muscles resulting from disease such as polio or muscular dystrophy, or idiopathic, the most common reason for the appearance of scoliosis in a previously straight spine (Figure 6-10).
Osgood–Schlatter disease	A painful, incomplete separation of the epiphysis of the tibial tubercle from the bone shaft. Most commonly occurs in active adolescent males. It is most likely the result of some type of trauma to the epiphyseal region before it has completely fused to the main bone, which usually occurs between the ages of 10 and 15.
Osteoarthritis (OA)	OA is a degenerative disease of the joint and is a normal part of aging. The degeneration results from the breakdown of chondrocytes and the articular cartilage wears away, often because of overuse, thereby exposing underlying bone. Pain is caused by the friction between the two bones as they glide across each other without the protection of the articular cartilage. Primary osteoarthritis is associated with aging; secondary osteoarthritis is associated with a predisposing factor such as trauma or obesity.
Osteochondritis	Inflammation of bone and cartilage.
Osteogenesis imperfecta (OI)	Genetic and congenital condition that involves the defective development of connective tissue resulting in deformed and abnormally brittle bones that are easily fractured.
Osteogenic sarcoma; osteosarcoma	Malignant tumor of the long bones, particularly the femur, commonly metastasizing to the lungs.
Osteoma	Tumor of the bone.
Osteomalacia	Abnormal condition characterized by softening of the bone due to a loss of calcification of the bone matrix. The condition is a result of an inadequate amount of phosphorus and calcium in the blood for the mineralization of bone, caused by a deficiency of vitamin D or malabsorption of calcium, and is called rickets in children.

(continues)

TABLE 6-3 Common Pathologies of the Skeletal System *(continued)*

CLINICAL TERMS	DESCRIPTION
Osteomyelitis	Inflammation and infection of bone and bone marrow usually caused by bacteria. Staphylococci are the most common causative bacteria. The infection can spread to the bone through the blood from a previously injured site, or the microorganisms can infiltrate the bone directly following open fractures, surgical reductions, or other exposure to the air. Osteomyelitis occurs more often in male children than adults. As the microbe population grows and forms pus within the bone, tension increases within the medullary cavity and the pus is forced out through the haversian canals. This forms a subperiosteal abscess that inhibits the blood supply to the bone and necrosis eventually occurs.
Osteonecrosis	Destruction and death of bone tissue. Occurs frequently in the head of the femur due to a disease process or trauma that obstructs or destroys the blood supply to the femoral head.
Osteoporosis	Disorder characterized by the excessive loss of calcium from bone without replacement, causing a loss in bone density. The bone becomes porous and fragile, and fractures are common.
Rheumatoid arthritis (RA)	Rheumatoid arthritis involves connective tissue throughout the entire body, but mainly involves the synovium in the joint. RA is considered an autoimmune disease. In the disease process, the body does not recognize its own natural antibodies as "self." Because the body thinks its own natural antibodies are foreign, it produces antibodies called rheumatoid factors (RFs) that fight against its own natural antibodies. The disease starts with a simple synovitis and can progress through several stages, the last being joint immobility. Because of the role of the RF antibodies, an RF test confirms RA.

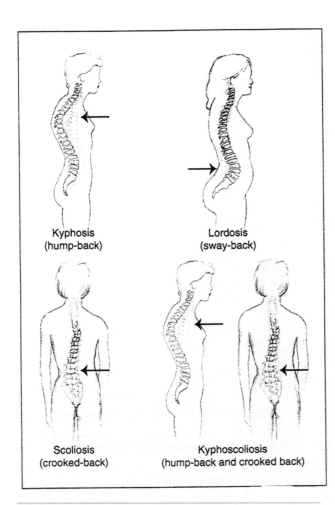

FIGURE 6-10 **Abnormal scoliosis**

facial bones. Surgeons most often use steel suture to close a sternotomy; occasionally a type of suture called Vicryl will be used, in which case a very thick or heavy-stranded size of Vicryl suture must be chosen in order to hold the sternum in place. Sternum closure can be difficult and the two sides must be properly approximated to ensure normal healing. If motion occurs, the healing will be delayed and the patient will experience postoperative pain.

Steel suture is also ideal for the repair of facial fractures. It is the most inert suture material available and lacks elasticity. Facial bones do not heal by the process previously discussed, but rather by fibrous union (Ethicon, 2002). Healing by fibrous union can take a long time—in some instances months. Therefore, the suture material must remain in place for a long time until the fibrous tissue has formed and remodeling taken place. Steel suture is not absorbed and does not lose its tensile strength, and thus provides long-term support to the facial fracture.

Pathologic Bone Healing

A number of abnormal conditions can disrupt the normal healing process of a fracture and the end results can be severe for the individual. Examples of pathologic bone healing include movement of the fracture bones,

TABLE 6-4   Classification of Fractures

FRACTURES CAN BE GROUPED ACCORDING TO THE FOLLOWING

■ *Whether the bone pierces the skin*	If the fractured bone pierces the skin, it is called a compound or open fracture. If the fracture does not pierce the skin, it is called a simple or closed fracture.
■ *Type of fracture line through the bone*	If the fracture line is continuous through the bone, it is called complete. If the fracture line is not continuous through the bone, it is called incomplete or partial. A type of partial fracture is a greenstick fracture, which, like a green stick or twig from a tree, will bend on one side and break on the other.
■ *Direction of the fracture line*	In a linear fracture, the line of the fracture runs parallel to the axis of the bone. A spiral fracture is where the fracture line curves around the bone. A transverse fracture is where the fracture line is across the bone. In an intra-articular fracture, the fracture line is on the joint surfaces of bone.
■ *Miscellaneous fractures*	Pott's fracture, a break of the lower fibula, is an outdated term. Colles' fracture is a break of the distal radius.

TABLE 6-5   Types of Fractures and Causes

TYPE	DESCRIPTION	CAUSE
Avulsion	Bone and other tissues are pulled from normal attachments.	Direct force, most often extremity is bent in abnormal manner.
Bucket handle	Dual vertical fractures on the same side of the pelvis.	Direct force or anterior compression of the pelvis.
Butterfly	Associated with comminuted type of fracture; butterfly-shaped piece of fractured bone.	Direct or rotational force.
Comminuted (segmental)	Fracture with more than two pieces of bone fragment; may have notable amount of associated soft-tissue trauma.	Direct crushing force.
Compound (open)	Broken end of bone has penetrated skin exposing the bone. Significant damage may be present to surrounding blood vessels, nerves, and muscles.	Moderate to severe energy that is continuous until bone reaches level of tolerance. Usually produced by direct force.
Depressed	Fracture occurs when bone is driven inward; frequently seen with cranial fracture.	Moderate to severe direct force.
Displaced	Fracture in which bone ends are out of alignment.	Direct force to area.
Greenstick	The fracture occurs in only one cortex of the bone. The bone splits longitudinally and is not a complete break; sometimes referred to as an incomplete or stress fracture.	Minor direct energy. Repetitive direct force such as jogging on a hard surface every day or jumping (basketball).
Impacted	The broken ends of each bone are forced into each other, usually creating many bone fragments.	Compressive force.
Intra-articular	Bones inside a joint are fractured.	Direct force to the joint area.
Oblique (type of linear structure)	Fracture occurs at an oblique angle across both cortices.	Direct force possibly with some compression.
Simple (closed)	Fracture is in normal anatomic position and the skin is not broken.	Moderate energy that continues until bone reaches level of tolerance. Usually direct force.
Spiral	Fracture that curves around bone.	Direct twisting force or distal part of bone unable to move.
Spontaneous (pathologic)	Fracture occurs without trauma; usually associated with bone weakened by a tumor or other disease process.	Minor force can cause fracture, such as leaning on the arm for support.
Stellate	Fracture occurs at central point in which additional breaks in bone radiate from the central point.	Direct force of moderate energy.
Transverse	Horizontal fracture through the bone.	Direct force toward the bone.

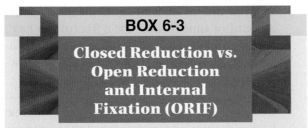

BOX 6-3

Closed Reduction vs. Open Reduction and Internal Fixation (ORIF)

Surgeons will treat fractures in one of two ways: closed reduction where an incision is not made or ORIF. If the fracture is uncomplicated such as a greenstick or transverse and the skin has not been penetrated, the surgeon will set the bone back into place by closed reduction with the aid of fluoroscopic x-ray. The patient will be taken into the operating room and anesthetized. A type of x-ray machine called a C-arm, so called due to the C shape of the x-ray machine arm, will be used to view the fracture while it is being set. The surgeon will manually manipulate the fractured bones into place, aligning the fracture so proper healing can take place, and will apply a cast to immobilize the site.

An ORIF involves the surgeon making an incision down to the fracture site. The two ends of the fractured bone are aligned and temporarily held in place with bone-holding forceps or wire that has been drilled into place. The surgeon will choose the correct size plate that will hold the fracture together; it is held in place over the fracture site. The surgical technologist places the correct size drill bit on the power drill and the surgeon drills the first hole through the opening in the plate and into the bone. Next, the surgeon uses a depth gauge to determine the depth of the hole and that will be the size of the screw. A tap is used to prepare the drill hole for the threads of the screw. The surgical technologist will choose the correct size screw, place it on the screwdriver, and hand it to the surgeon for placement. These steps are repeated for all the holes in the plate and the wound is closed with suture.

distraction and interposition of soft tissues, disruption of the blood supply, infection, and compartmental syndrome.

As previously discussed, it is imperative that the fracture site be immobilized in order for the fractured ends of the bone to be held in place and a normal union occur. If the bones are not properly immobilized, movement can occur at the fracture site, causing disruption of the hematoma and leading to additional bleeding and a lengthier healing process.

The term *distraction* is used to describe the situation in which the fractured bone ends are abnormally separated and contact is not occurring. Surgeons will use distraction to help align the bone ends in surgery by using either weights or a special type of operating room table called a fracture table. The fracture table has devices that help to slightly stretch the leg to aid in aligning the bone, and then the surgeon can apply either a cast and/or external fixator to immobilize the bone ends. However, postoperatively after the bone ends are aligned and immobilized, the surgeon must be careful not to apply too much weight to the skeletal traction, creating a gap between the fractured bone ends. The abnormal gap will fill in with granulation tissue, which delays healing. In addition, the excessive distraction places too much tension on the blood vessels, thereby decreasing the blood supply to the fracture site and increasing the healing time.

Interposition of soft tissues is another complication of distraction. The gap can allow soft tissue to grow over either one or both ends of the fractured bone. This prevents the formation of the hematoma and callus, resulting in a poor union of the fracture.

Vascular necrosis refers to the blood supply not being reestablished after a fracture occurs. If the capillary network cannot re-form, the bone will necrose due to lack of nourishment and oxygen, and the necrosis is most likely irreversible. For example, the femoral head receives three sets of arteries that anastomose in the femoral neck region with a main artery that enters the femoral head. When a femoral neck fracture occurs the blood supply can be easily disrupted and the femoral head is in danger of necrosis due to the disruption of the blood supply. Often individuals will require surgical replacement of the femoral head with a metal prosthesis.

Compound or open fractures in which the bone penetrates the skin, creating an opening and exposing the fractured bone ends, can allow for the easy entry of microorganisms leading to an infection. Infections of bone tissue are extremely serious and can have devastating results. Once exposed to microorganisms, bone tissue is easily infected and the infections are difficult to control and resolve. The infection can quickly lead to a generalized infection of the whole bone, including the bone marrow where microbial growth is rapid. Osteomyelitis is a type of serious bone and bone marrow infection that rapidly expands from a local infection to an infection of the entire bone. Osteomyelitis can become chronic, resulting in the person possibly losing the limb through surgical amputation.

Compartment syndrome is an increase in pressure within the compartments of a limb formed by the skin and fascia. The syndrome most commonly occurs with fractures of the forearm bones and tibia. The radius, ulna, and tibia are divided into compartments composed of the muscles, nerves, and bone; surrounding these structures are the skin and fascia, which actually form the compartments. When a fracture occurs, the swelling of the surrounding tissues and bleeding cause pressure within the compartment. The fascia has limited flexibility and can expand only so far in response to the swelling; upon reaching maximum expansion the pressure is directed inward. This pressure compresses the internal blood vessels and nerves, inhibiting the blood flow of the capillaries. Due to the compromise of the circulation, the muscles and bone become ischemic; necrosis begins in 2 to 4 hours and becomes irreversible if allowed to continue for 12 hours (Caruthers & Price, 2001). Nerve damage begins in 30 minutes and, if the swelling is not resolved within 12 hours, the muscles will sustain irreversible loss of function (Caruthers & Price, 2001).

Other terms associated with bone-healing pathology include the following:

1. Nonunion: fractured bone ends do not unite; infection and movement of the fracture site are the two primary reasons for nonunion.

2. Delayed union: an abnormal increase in the amount of time it takes for a fracture to heal; reasons include pathologies such as osteomalacia or osteoporosis, poor immobilization allowing bone movement, and distraction.

3. Malunion: fracture heals in an abnormal position that does not represent the original anatomic form, structure, and contouring of the bone prior to the fracture; this can alter the mechanics and weight-bearing ability of the bone.

BONES OF THE AXIAL SKELETON

The skeleton has two divisions: the axial skeleton, which consists of the cranial bones, ribs or thoracic cage including sternum, hyoid bone, and vertebrae; and the appendicular skeleton, which consists of the extremities, pectoral girdle, and pelvic girdle (Figure 6-11).

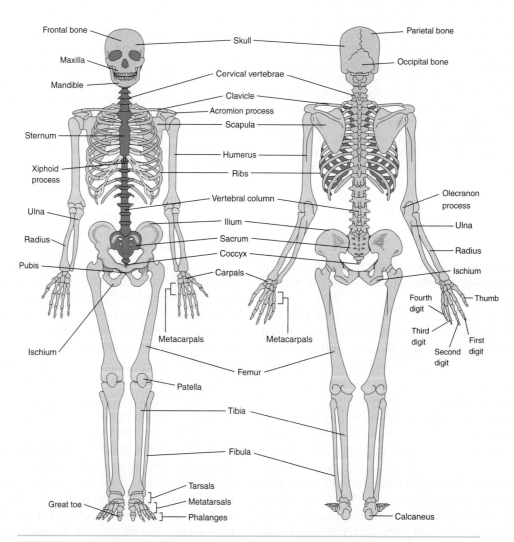

FIGURE 6-11   The axial skeleton (blue) and the appendicular skeleton

Cranium

The cranium consists of 8 immovable cranial bones and 14 facial bones, 13 that are immovable and 1 movable (Figure 6-12). The purpose of the cranium is to enclose and protect the brain, serve for attachments of muscles that aid in head movement and chewing, and contain the **paranasal sinuses**, air-filled cavities that are lined by mucous membrane and have openings that connect to the nasal cavity. The sinuses affect the tone of the voice by serving as resonant sound chambers. In addition, the sinuses reduce the weight of the skull due to the air within the cavities, allowing the individual to hold the head up without fatigue.

There are eight cranial bones (Figure 6-13):

1. **Frontal bone**: Forms the anterior portion of the skull superior to the eyes and includes the forehead, roof of the nasal cavity, and roofs of the bony socket of the eyes. Just superior to each bony eye socket, in the eyebrow region, the supraorbital foramen is located through which blood vessels and nerves travel to supply the tissue of the forehead. Also within the frontal bone are the

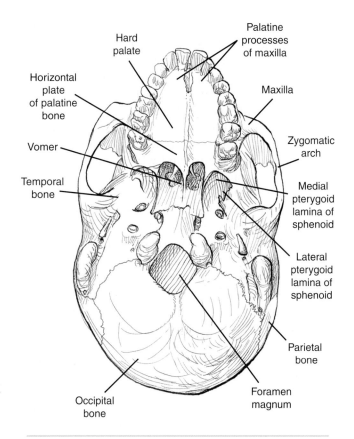

FIGURE 6-13   External view of inferior skull

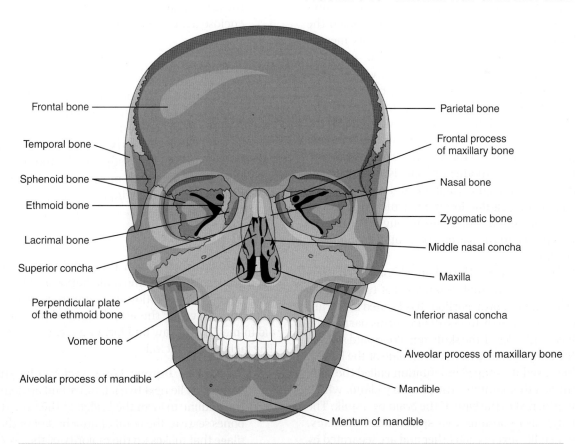

FIGURE 6-12   External frontal view of facial bones

two frontal sinuses, located superior to the bony eye sockets in the midline of the forehead.

2. **Parietal bone**: There are two parietal bones, one forming each side of the skull inferior to the frontal bone. The parietal bone has a curved shape with four sides or sutures. Parietal bones form part of the sides of the skull and roof of the cranium. They are joined at the midline by the sagittal suture and with the frontal bone at the coronal suture.

3. **Occipital bone**: Forms the back and base of the skull. It has a large opening called the **foramen magnum** through which the nerve fibers of the brain pass to become the spinal cord. On each side of the foramen magnum are two rounded processes called the **occipital condyles**, which articulate with the first vertebra of the vertebral column. The bone is joined to the parietal bone at the lambdoidal suture.

4. **Temporal bones**: There are two temporal bones, which form a portion of the sides and base of the skull. The **external auditory meatus** is an opening located in each of the temporal bones for the ear canal and the bones also contain the internal ear structures, thus providing protection. The temporal bones have a slight depression called the **mandibular fossa**, which articulates with the condyles of the mandible to form the TMJ. Just inferior to the external auditory meatus are two projections, the rounded **mastoid process**, which serves for attachment of neck muscles, and the pointed **styloid process**, which serves for attachment of the muscles of the tongue and pharynx. An opening called the carotid canal is located next to the mastoid process and allows the internal carotid artery to pass through. Another opening is located on the border of the temporal bone and occipital bone called the jugular foramen, which allows the internal jugular vein to pass through. The temporal bones join the parietal bone at the squamosal suture.

5. **Sphenoid bone**: The sphenoid bone is a butterfly-shaped bone that is composed of two winglike sides and a central portion. It is located in the anterior portion of the skull and forms part of the base and sides of the skull, and floors and sides of the bony eye sockets. In the midline of the bone it has a saddle-shaped indentation called the sella turcica that contains the pituitary gland, which is attached to the base of the brain by a stalk. The bone also contains two **sphenoidal sinuses**, which lie next to each other and are separated by a thin septum made of bone that travels downward into the nasal cavity.

6. **Ethmoid bone**: The ethmoid bone is located anterior to the sphenoid bone. It is complex in structure in that laterally it consists of two masses of bone that are joined in the midline by a long, thin piece of bone called the cribriform plates and perpendicular plate. The cribriform plates form a portion of the roof of the nasal cavity. Located in the plates are tiny openings called olfactory foramina through which the olfactory nerves pass. The perpendicular plate projects downward to form the majority of the nasal septum. The lateral portions of the ethmoid bone are delicate and scroll-shaped, projecting toward the perpendicular plate; they are called the **superior nasal concha** and **middle nasal concha**. They aid in supporting the mucous membranes that line the nasal cavity. The purpose of the mucous membranes is to humidify, warm, and filter the air an individual breathes in. Also located on the lateral portions of the bone are small air spaces called the ethmoidal sinuses. Projecting superiorly from the bone into the cranial cavity between the cribriform plates is a triangular-shaped process called the crista galli. The meningeal membranes that enclose the brain tissue attach to this process.

Hyoid Bone

The **hyoid bone** is the only bone in the body that does not articulate or connect to another bone. It is located in the neck between the mandible and larynx. It is held in position by muscles and ligaments. The function of the hyoid is to support the tongue and to serves as an attachment of muscles that aid in tongue movement during swallowing.

Facial Bones

As previously mentioned, the facial portion of the skull consists of 13 immovable bones and the movable mandible. In addition to giving shape to the face, the bones serve for the attachment of muscles that aid in moving the jaw and forming facial expressions. The facial bones include:

1. Two **nasal bones**: Long, rectangular-shaped bones that lie next to each other and are joined at the midline to form the bridge of the nose. These bones serve as the point of attachment of the cartilage that makes up the majority of the nose.

2. **Vomer**: A thin, flat bone located in the midline of the nasal cavity. Posteriorly it connects to the perpendicular plate of the ethmoid bone to form the nasal septum.

3. Two **inferior nasal conchae**: Scroll-shaped bones that are thin and fragile, attached to the lateral walls of the nasal cavity. They are located inferior to the superior and middle nasal conchae of the ethmoid bone and are much larger. They also support the mucous membranes of the nasal cavity.

4. Two **lacrimal bones**: Each lacrimal bone is located in the medial wall of each bony socket between the ethmoid bone and the maxilla. It is a very thin bone. A groove on its anterior surface travels from the bony eye socket to the nasal cavity and serves to hold in place the lacrimal duct that transports tears to the nasal cavity.

5. Two **palatine bones**: The palatine bones are shaped like the letter *L* and are located inferior to the maxillae. The horizontal sections form the posterior portion of the hard palate of the mouth and the floor of the nasal cavity. The perpendicular sections form the lateral walls of the nasal cavity.

6. Two **zygomatic bones**: The zygomatic bones form the lateral walls and floors of the bony eye socket. They also form the cheek prominences that are inferior and slightly lateral to each eye. Each bone has a process, called the temporal process, which travels posteriorly to join the zygomatic process and together form the zygomatic arch.

7. Two **maxillary bones**: The maxillae are the bones of the upper jaw. They form a portion of the anterior hard palate, floors of the bony eye sockets, floor of the nasal cavity, and contain the openings or sockets for the upper teeth. The inferior border of the maxillae projects downward to form the alveolar process. The processes form the alveolar arch and the teeth are situated in the cavity of the arches. Connective tissue binds the teeth to the arches in the maxillae. The maxillae contain the largest of the sinuses, called the maxillary sinuses, which are located lateral to the nasal cavity.

8. **Mandible**: The mandible is the lower bone of the jaw shaped like a horseshoe, and on each side the bone flattens and projects upward to form the **ramus** (plural, rami). The rami are divided into the **mandibular condyle** and coronoid process, which is situated anteriorly to the condyle. The condyles articulate with the mandibular fossae, also called **glenoid fossae**, of the temporal bones to form the TMJ. The coronoid processes serve as points of attachment for muscles used when chewing. The superior border of the mandible contains the sockets for the lower teeth. A condition called TMJ syndrome is marked by mandibular dysfunction that causes pain due to a defective or dislocated TMJ. Indications of the syndrome include a clicking sound of the joint when the jaws are moved, limitation in range of motion of the jaw, and subluxation. Surgery is often indicated to repair the joint.

On the medial side of the mandible, inferior to each rami, is the opening called the **mandibular foramen**. The opening allows blood vessels and a nerve to travel through to supply the roots of the lower teeth. This is the area into which dentists inject local anesthetic drugs, in order to block the nerve impulses so the patient will feel no pain when the teeth of the lower jaw are being worked upon. Two other foramen, called the mental foramen, are located on the front of the mandible and slightly lateral. Blood vessels and a nerve travel through this opening to supply the tissues of the chin and lower lip.

Development of the Infantile Skull

The bones of the skull at birth have not matured and completed their growth. Fibrous connective tissue is located between the bones and these areas are called **fontanels**, commonly referred to as soft spots. This is advantageous, allowing the bones to be slightly compressed and shaped, called molding, to allow the infant's skull to pass through the narrow birth canal. The fontanels must be protected from trauma, but eventually by the age of 2 all the fontanels will have become ossified and closed. In addition, the bones of the infant's skull are connected by suture lines, serrated connections between the bones that also become more stable with time. Examples of suture lines include the coronal suture, frontal suture, and sagittal suture. There are four fontanels: posterior fontanel, anterior fontanel, mastoid fontanel, and sphenoid fontanel.

Other characteristics of the infant skull include the following:

1. Frontal bone is in two parts that eventually fuse.
2. Cranial bones are thinner than that of adults.
3. The forehead is prominent.
4. Paranasal sinuses are not completely formed.
5. Nasal cavity is small, as is the jaw.

Thoracic Cage

The thoracic cage, also called the rib cage, consists of the ribs and the sternum (Figure 6-14). The function of the rib cage is to enclose and protect the lungs and heart. The ribs are also flexible so as to allow the lungs to expand during respiration. When a person inhales air the ribs are pulled upward and outward by the intercostal muscles. This expands the chest cavity, the lungs expand, and the person takes in air. There are 12 pairs of ribs, each attached to the 12 thoracic vertebrae. The first seven pairs are referred to as the true ribs and they join the sternum via the **costal cartilages**. The next three pairs are called the false ribs, since they are not attached to the sternum but are attached to the seventh rib by costal cartilage. The last two pairs are called floating ribs, since they are not attached to the sternum or other ribs.

The **sternum**, also called the breastbone, is located along the midline in the anterior portion of the rib cage. It is a flat, elongated bone that has three parts: upper manubrium, middle body, and lower xiphoid process, which is the delicate structure of the sternum that projects downward. The manubrium connects to the clavicles by facets located on its superior border. The true ribs attach to the body. The ster-

num is the bone that is pushed upon to compress the heart during cardiopulmonary resuscitation (CPR). The xiphoid process is easily found by running the fingers upward along the edge of the lower ribs until the edge stops—the process is in the middle. Two finger breadths above the xiphoid process is where the palm of the hand is placed to apply pressure to the sternum in order to provide compressions to the heart.

Vertebral Column

The **vertebral column** begins close to the foramen magnum of the skull and extends posteriorly to the pelvis (Figure 6-15). The functions of the column include

1. Supporting the head and trunk
2. Being flexible to allow the person to bend forward, backward, and to the side, and turn at the waist
3. Forming the passageway called the **vertebral canal** or **vertebral foramen** to allow the spinal cord to pass through

The column consists of bone called the **vertebrae**, which are separated by a fibrocartilage called

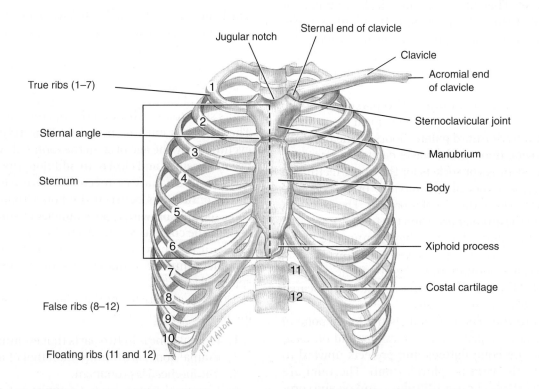

FIGURE 6-14   Anterior external view of thoracic skeletal structures

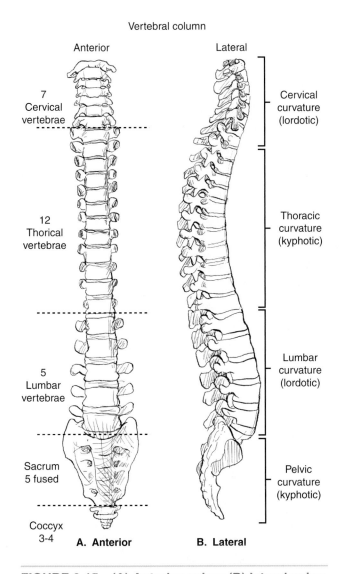

Vertebral column

Anterior — Lateral

7 Cervical vertebrae

12 Thorical vertebrae

5 Lumbar vertebrae

Sacrum 5 fused

Coccyx 3-4

A. Anterior — **B. Lateral**

Cervical curvature (lordotic)

Thoracic curvature (kyphotic)

Lumbar curvature (lordotic)

Pelvic curvature (kyphotic)

FIGURE 6-15 (A) Anterior spine; (B) lateral spine

the anterior portion of the vertebra (Figure 6-16A). The vertebrae are arranged in a longitudinal fashion the length of the vertebral column and provide the support for the head and trunk. As previously mentioned, between each vertebra is the fibrocartilage structure called the intervertebral disk (Figure 6-16B). The disks cushion the column, especially in athletic individuals whose activity involves a lot of jumping and running such as basketball players and gymnasts. The vertebrae are also kept in place by the anterior longitudinal ligaments that attach to the anterior surface of the body and the posterior longitudinal ligaments that attach to the posterior surface.

Posteriorly the pedicles project from the body. They form the sides of the vertebral foramen. Continuous with the pedicles are the laminae, which join to form the posterior spinous process. Together the pedicles, laminae, and spinous process form the vertebral foramen.

Between both pedicles and lamina is the **transverse process**, which projects at a slight angle laterally and posteriorly. The spinous process and transverse process serve as points of attachment of

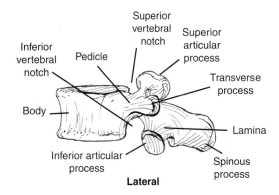

Inferior vertebral notch — Pedicle — Superior vertebral notch — Superior articular process — Transverse process

Body — Lamina

Inferior articular process — Spinous process

Lateral

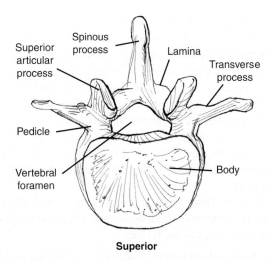

Superior articular process — Spinous process — Lamina — Transverse process

Pedicle

Vertebral foramen — Body

Superior

FIGURE 6-16A Lateral and superior views of typical vertebra

intervertebral disks and are connected to each other by ligaments. The vertebral column has four natural curvatures:

1. Cervical curvature: located in the neck and curves in a convex anterior direction
2. Thoracic curvature: located in the thoracic region; concave anterior curvature
3. Lumbar curvature: located in the lower back; convex anterior curvature
4. Pelvic curvature: located in the pelvic region; concave anterior curvature

The vertebrae in each region vary somewhat but have common features. The following is a general description of a vertebra. The body makes up the majority of the bone and is an irregular-shaped circle; it forms

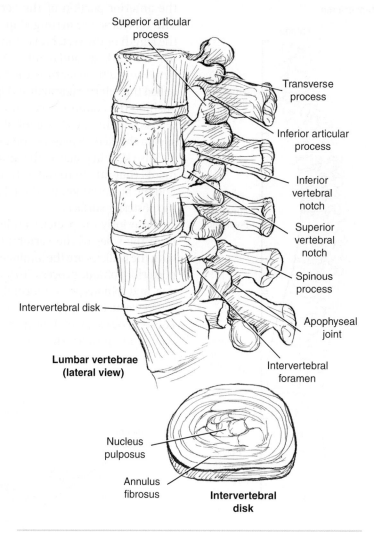

Superior articular process

Transverse process

Inferior articular process

Inferior vertebral notch

Superior vertebral notch

Spinous process

Apophyseal joint

Intervertebral disk

Lumbar vertebrae (lateral view)

Intervertebral foramen

Nucleus pulposus

Annulus fibrosus

Intervertebral disk

FIGURE 6-16B **Lateral view of articulating vertebrae and superior view of intervertebral disk**

the ligaments and muscles of the vertebral column. The articulating area of each vertebra is marked by the superior and inferior articulating processes. These are cartilage-covered facets by which each vertebra contacts the other vertebra superiorly and inferiorly.

On the undersurface of the pedicles are small openings called intervertebral foramina, which are aligned. The openings are the passageways for the spinal nerves that connect to the spinal cord and are responsible for transmitting information to and from the brain.

There are three types of vertebrae and each slightly varies in structure. The following is a brief description of the variances of each type:

1. Cervical vertebrae: There are seven that are located in the neck. They are smallest of the vertebrae. The transverse processes contain transverse foramina, which are openings for arteries to pass

through to the brain. The spinous processes of the second through sixth cervical vertebrae are slightly split at the end, called a bifid spinous process, and they serve as attachments for muscles. The spinous process of the seventh vertebra is unusually long, projecting beyond the spinous process of the other vertebra, and is called the vertebra prominens. It is a useful anatomic landmark in the neck. The first cervical vertebra is called the **atlas** and it supports the head. It has no distinguishable body and no spinous process. It is seen as an oval circle with two transverse processes. On the superior surface, located on each side of the vertebral foramen are two facets that articulate with the occipital condyles of the occipital bone. The second cervical vertebra is called the **axis**. On its superior surface, a process called the odontoid process projects upward. It lies within the ring of the atlas and when the head is turned from side to side the atlas pivots around the odontoid process.

2. Thoracic vertebrae: There are 12 thoracic vertebrae. The vertebrae have a long spinous process that ends in a point, slightly curving downward. Facets are located laterally on the body and articulate with a rib. Starting with the third thoracic vertebra and traveling downward, each of the vertebrae increases in size in order to aid in weight bearing of the body.

3. Lumbar vertebrae: There are five lumbar vertebrae. They perform the majority of the weight-bearing function as compared to the other vertebrae of the body; thus they have large bodies, thicker, shorter spinous processes, and the transverse processes project posteriorly at an increased angle.

The last two portions of the vertebral column are the sacrum and coccyx. The sacrum is shaped like a triangle and is located at the base of the vertebral column connected to the fifth lumbar vertebra. It consists of five vertebrae that have fused. The spinous processes form a ridge called the median sacral crest. Located laterally to the processes are openings called the dorsal sacral foramina, which serve as a passageway for nerves and blood vessels.

The sacrum is located between the ilia of the pelvic girdle and is joined to each ilium by fibrocartilage at the **sacroiliac joints**. The sacrum forms the posterior portion of the pelvic cavity. The anterior edge is the first sacral vertebra and is called the sacral promontory, an important anatomic landmark in females. During physical examination of a pregnant woman the physician can palpate the sacral promontory and use it to aid in determining the size of the pelvis. This is helpful to determine if the pelvic cavity is large enough for the fetus to be vaginally delivered or whether a cesarean section will have to be performed. On the surface of the sacrum, located laterally, are four pairs of openings called the pelvic sacral foramina, which provide passageways for blood vessels and nerves.

The **coccyx**, better known as the tailbone, is the most inferior portion of the vertebral column. It is composed of four fused vertebrae. It is held in place by ligaments that attach it to the sacral hiatus. A person notices the coccyx when they fall to the ground landing on their buttocks, which puts extreme pressure on the coccyx causing pain, or after riding a horse for a long period. The coccyx is often dislocated or fractured and if chronically fractured, it may require surgery such as placing steel sutures to hold it in place or a coccygectomy.

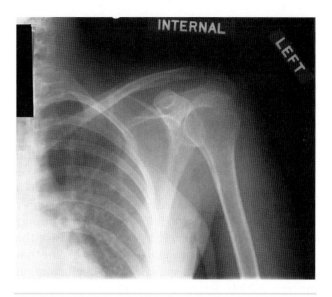

FIGURE 6-17   AP shoulder, internal rotation

BONES OF THE APPENDICULAR SKELETON

The bones of the **appendicular skeleton** include the pectoral girdle, upper extremities, pelvic girdle, and lower extremities.

Pectoral Girdle

The pectoral girdle consists of the two clavicles and two scapula and two shoulder joints (Figures 6-17 and 6-18). It serves as support for the humerus and attachment for muscles that move the shoulder joint and upper extremity bones.

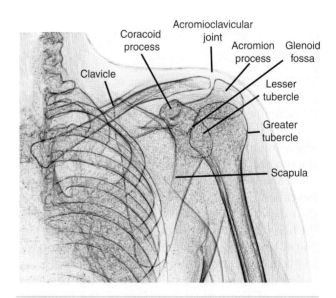

FIGURE 6-18   AP shoulder, internal rotation

The **clavicle**, commonly referred to as the collarbone, is a long, slender, doubly curved bone that aids in keeping the shoulder joint in place and braces the movable scapula. It is situated in a horizontal fashion between the sternum and shoulder joint. The medial end of the clavicle articulates with the manubrium and the lateral end articulates with the **acromion process** of the scapula. The clavicles also serve as attachments of the muscles of the chest, back, and upper extremities.

The **scapula**, referred to as the shoulder blade, is a flat, broad triangular-shaped bone located in the upper lateral region of the back. It forms the posterior portion of the pectoral girdle. The posterior surface of the scapula is divided into unequal portions by a spine that is a ridge of bone. The spine leads to the acromion process, which serves as an important anatomic landmark of the shoulder, since the process forms the tip of the shoulder and the coracoid process. Both processes are points of attachment of muscles for the humerus and chest. Located at the head of the scapula between the two processes is a fossa called the **glenoid cavity**, which serves as the socket for the head of the humerus.

The pectoral girdle also consists of three joints: glenohumeral, sternoclavicular, and **acromioclavicular (AC)**. The glenohumeral has the widest range of motion. The AC joint, another important anatomic landmark, is an articulation between the lateral head of the clavicle and the acromion process. The **rotator cuff** surrounds the shoulder joint to strengthen and provide stability to the joint, and provide for a wide range of joint movements. The rotator cuff consists of four muscles the tendons of which insert onto the capsule of the humeral head: supraspinatus, subscapularis, infraspinatus, and teres minor.

Humerus

The **humerus** is the largest bone of the upper trunk of the body (Figures 6-19 and 6-20). It extends from the scapula to the elbow and aids in forming the shoulder joint at its proximal end, and forming the elbow joint at its distal end. The proximal end is a smooth, rounded ball that fits into the glenoid fossa of the scapula. Just distal to the head are two tuberosities called the greater and lesser tuberosities. Between the tuberosities is a narrow, lengthwise depression in the bone called the bicipital groove in which the tendon of the biceps brachii muscle travels along to the shoulder joint. A narrow circumferential depression, called the anatomic neck, travels along the lower margin of the articular surface of the humerus,

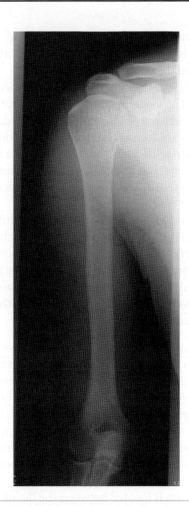

FIGURE 6-19   AP humerous

separating the head from the tubercles. Just inferior to the anatomic neck is a region called the **surgical neck**, which receives its name due to the common occurrence of fractures in this region of the humerus.

The **greater tubercle** is located on the lateral side of the humeral head. This tubercle serves as the insertion point for the tendons of the supraspinatus, infraspinatus, and teres minor muscles. The **lesser tubercle** is located on the anterior side and serves as the site of insertion of the subscapular tendon. In the midshaft of the humeral bone on the lateral side is a tubercle called the **deltoid tuberosity**. The deltoid muscle, which raises the arm horizontally and laterally, attaches at the tuberosity.

At the distal end of the humerus are two condyles. The lateral condyle is called the **capitulum**, and it articulates with the radius at the elbow joint. The medial condyle, called the **trochlea**, articulates with the ulna. Just proximal to the two condyles are **epicondyles**, which provide attachments for the

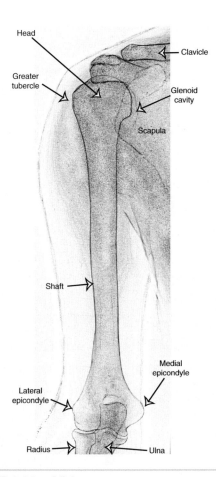

FIGURE 6-20   AP humerus

ligaments and muscles of the elbow. A small depression in the bone, called the coronoid fossa, is located between the epicondyles. When the elbow is bent the coronoid process of the ulna fits into the coronoid fossa. On the posterior surface of the bone is another depression, called the olecranon fossa. When the elbow is extended, straightening out the upper limb, the olecranon process fits into the olecranon fossa.

Radius and Ulna

The **radius** extends from the elbow to the wrist and rotates around the **ulna** upon movement of the upper limbs (Figures 6-21 and 6-22). A way to remember the side of the forearm in which the radius lies is to place the hand in anatomic position (palm of the hand forward); the radius lies on the thumb side of the hand. The proximal head of the radius articulates with the capitulum of the humerus and the radial notch of the ulna. This provides the ability of the radius to rotate around the ulna during movement. Just inferior to the head is the **radial tuberosity**, which

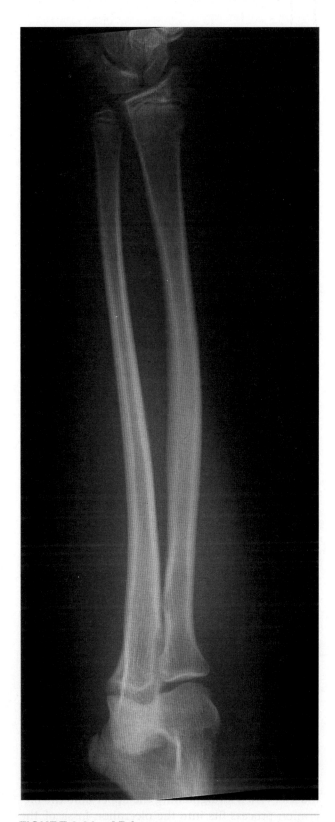

FIGURE 6-21   AP forearm

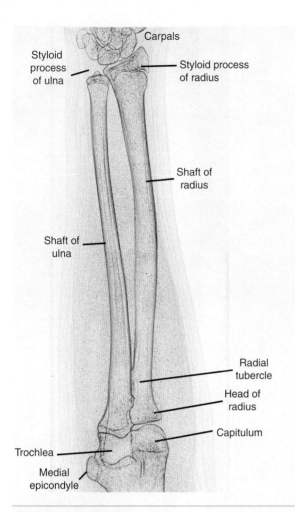

FIGURE 6-22   AP forearm

serves at the point of attachment for the tendon of the biceps brachii muscle. The distal end of the radius articulates with the carpal bones of the wrist. Located on the lateral side of the distal end is the styloid process, which provides attachments for the ligaments of the wrist.

The ulna is longer than the radius (Shier, Butler, & Lewis, 2002). The proximal end of the ulna has a depression, called the trochlear notch, that articulates with the humerus. On each side of this articulation are two processes called the **olecranon process** and the **coronoid process**. The olecranon process provides attachment for the tendon of the triceps brachii muscle. When straightening the upper limb the olecranon process fits into the olecranon fossa of the humerus. When bending the elbow the coronoid process fits into the coronoid fossa of the humerus (Figures 6-23 and 6-24).

The rounded head at the distal end of the ulna articulates with a notch in the radius called the ulnar

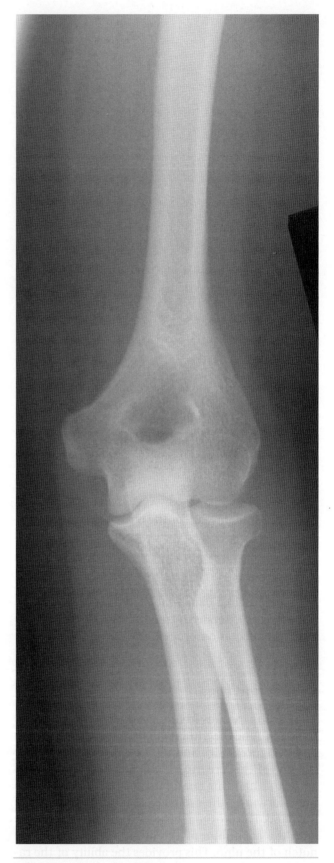

FIGURE 6-23   AP elbow

notch. Also located at the distal end is the styloid process, which provides attachment for ligaments of the wrist.

Wrist and Hand

The bones of the wrist joint are called **carpals** (Figures 6-25 and 6-26). There are eight carpal bones arranged in two rows of four. Each carpal bone has a smooth, rounded, articular surface that contacts the other carpal bones, reducing friction during movement and providing a smooth surface for the attachment of ligaments. The distal row of carpal bones from the radial to the ulnar side is as follows: trapezium, trapezoid, capitate, and hamate. The proximal row is as follows: scaphoid (also called navicular), lunate, triquetrum, and pisiform. The scaphoid is the primary bone of the carpals, since it stabilizes and coordinates the movements of the other carpals.

The hand and fingers consist of **metacarpals** and **phalanges**. The five metacarpal bones are located in the palm and are cylindrical in shape.

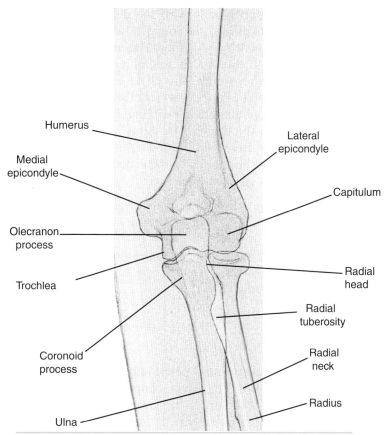

FIGURE 6-24   AP elbow

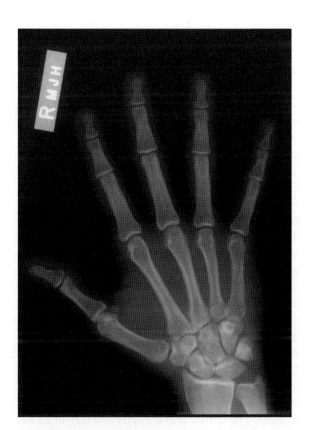

FIGURE 6-25   PA hand

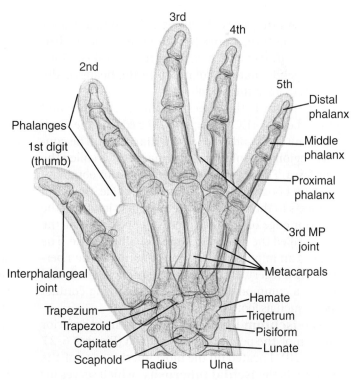

FIGURE 6-26   PA hand

They articulate proximally with the distal row of carpal bones and distally the rounded head of each bone articulates with a phalange. The metacarpals are numbered 1 through 5 beginning with the metacarpal of the thumb. The distal ends of the metacarpals form the knuckles when a fist is made.

There are 14 phalanges in each hand, 3 in each finger, and 2 in the thumb. The joints of the phalanges are often sites of dislocations. Abbreviations are used to describe the site of the dislocation; two common areas of dislocation include:

1. PIP joint: proximal interphalangeal joint; this is the joint between the distal and middle phalanx.
2. MCP joint; metacarpophalangeal joint; this is the joint between the metacarpal bone and the proximal phalanx.

Pelvis

The sacrum, coccyx, and pelvic girdle form the bowl-shaped **pelvis**. The pelvis is important in providing support for the upper and lower trunk of the body, serves for attachments of muscles of the femur, and aids in protecting the internal organs such as the urinary bladder, female reproductive organs, and distal end of the colon. The pelvis is formed by the fusion of the ilium, ischium, and pubis, and they are collectively referred to as the ox coxae. The three bones fuse to form the **acetabulum**, a round cavity located on the lateral portions of the pelvis that articulates with the heads of the femora to form the hip joint.

The **ilium** is the largest of the three bones and forms the majority of the pelvis. The edge of the ilium flares outward and is called the **iliac crest**. The concave region just inferior to the iliac crest is called the iliac fossa. The crest is an important site for obtaining bone for bone grafts. On the posterior side, the ilium connects to the sacrum at the sacroiliac joint. On the anterior edge of the iliac crest is a projection of the ilium called the **anterior superior iliac spine**. The spine is an important anatomic landmark when performing surgery, since it can be easily palpated, and also is a common site for injuries involving contact sports such as football.

The **ischium** forms the lowest or most inferior portion of the pelvis and is L-shaped (Figures 6-27 and 6-28). Located on the most inferior edge of the ischium is the **ischial tuberosity**, which serves for

---

BOX 6-4

Bone Grafting

The iliac crest is the best source for obtaining autogenous cancellous and cortical bone for bone grafting. Bone grafting may have to be performed for the following reasons: filling in a cavity after the removal of a large amount of bone, filling in a large area in which bone was lost due to trauma or disease, and promoting the fusion of a joint such as the ankle. The most abundant source of cancellous bone is located in the posterior portion of the iliac spine, just inferior to the iliac crest (Caruthers & Price, 2001).

The following is a brief description of the procedure. The incision is made from the highest point of the iliac crest traveling downward and medially. Once the iliac crest is exposed, the gluteal muscles are separated and retracted for exposure. With use of a curved surgical instrument that has a sharp end called an osteotome, small cuts are made around the periphery of the ilium to outline the area of bone to be taken as graft material. Next, using another sharp instrument called a gouge and hammer, the surgeon begins to take strips of cancellous bone. Once removed, the gluteal muscle, fascia, and periosteum are sutured to the iliac crest.

---

the attachment of ligaments and leg muscles, and aids in supporting the weight of the body while sitting. Superior to the ischial tuberosity is a pointed projection called the **ischial spine**. Along with the sacral promontory, the spine can be felt during a diagnostic digital vaginal examination and is used by the physician as a guide in determining the pelvic size. The distance between the ischial spines is the smallest diameter of the pelvic outlet (Shier, Butler, & Lewis, 2002).

The **pubis** forms the anteromedial portion of the pelvis. The two pubic bones join at the midline to form the **symphysis pubis**, which is a disk of fibrocartilage that connects the two pubic bones and serves as a cushion between them. The ischium and pubis join to form the large opening called the obturator foramen, the largest foramen in the skeleton. A thin tissue called the obturator membrane covers the foramen.

The female and male pelvis have key differences, all relating to the female pelvis functioning as part of the birth canal. The female pelvic cavity is wider in all as-

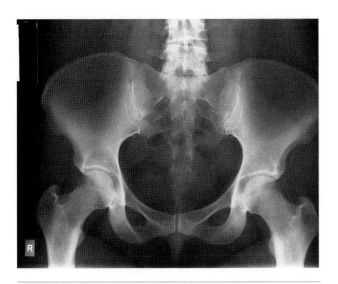

FIGURE 6-27   AP pelvis

Hip, Femur, Patella, and Knee Joint

The hip is a ball-and-socket joint formed by the head of the femur fitting into the acetabulum of the pelvis (Figures 6-29 and 6-30). The hip joint capsule, ligaments, and muscles stabilize the joint. The iliofemoral ligament connects the ilium with the femur anteriorly and superiorly, and the ischiofemoral and pubofemoral ligaments connect the ischium and pubis to the femur (Caruthers & Price, 2001).

The femur is the largest and longest bone of the body, extending from the hip to the knee joint (Figure 6-31). The proximal end of the femur consists of the rounded head, femoral neck, and **greater** and **lesser trochanters**. The femoral head has a small depression located approximately in the center, which serves

pects as compared to the male pelvis. The differences are as follows:

1. Female iliac crests are more dramatically flared causing the hips to be much broader.
2. The female pubic arch is at a greater angle.
3. There is more distance between the female ischial spines and tuberosities.
4. The female sacral curvature is decreased and flatter.
5. The bones of the female pelvis tend to be more delicate, thus lighter in weight.

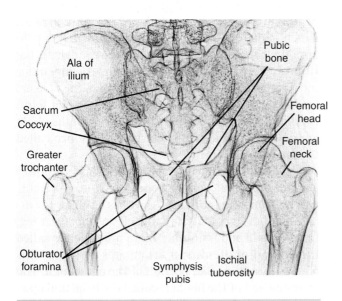

FIGURE 6-28   AP pelvis

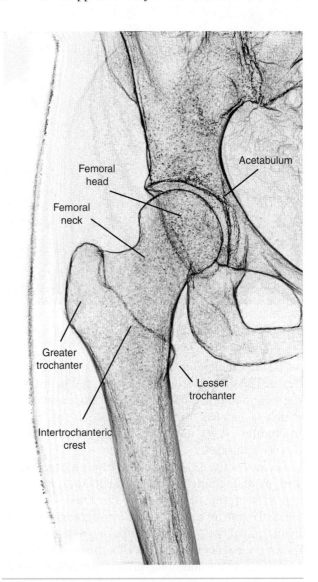

FIGURE 6-29   Anatomy of the hip

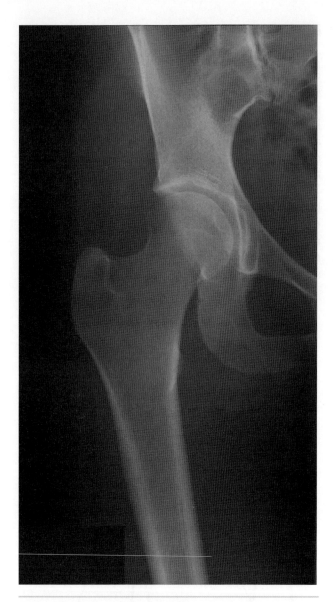

FIGURE 6-30   AP of the hip

as the attachment for the ligament of the head of the femur. The greater trochanter is located laterally on the femur and is superior to the lesser trochanter, which is located on the medial side. The greater trochanter serves as the point of insertion for the iliopsoas muscle.

Located at the distal end of the femur are the lateral and medial condyles, which articulate with the condyles of the tibia to form the knee joint. The femoral condyles are separated by a depression in the femur called the patellar surface or groove, forming the anterior articulating surface for the patella. Next to each condyle are additional projections called the lateral and medial epicondyles, which provide attachments for ligaments and muscles.

The **patella**, more commonly known as the kneecap, is a flat, irregularly shaped circle that is contained within the quadriceps tendon. The patellar tendon passes over the anterior surface of the patella, originating superior to the patella and inserting inferior to it.

The capsule of the knee joint is attached as follows (Caruthers & Price, 2001):

1. Proximally to the lateral and medial condyles of the femur
2. Distally to the lateral and medial condyles of the tibia
3. Superior end of the fibula

The capsule is kept in position as follows (Caruthers & Price, 2001):

1. Anteriorly by the patellar and quadriceps tendons
2. Laterally and medially by the medial and lateral collateral ligaments
3. Posteriorly by the popliteus and gastrocnemius muscles

As previously discussed, the two thick ligaments known as the anterior cruciate ligament and posterior cruciate ligament help stabilize the movement of the joint.

Tibia and Fibula

The **tibia**, or shinbone, is the larger and stronger of the two bones of the lower portion of the leg (Figures 6-32 and 6-33). It is located on the medial side. At the proximal end are the medial and lateral condyles, which articulate with the condyles of the femur to form the knee joint. Just inferior to the condyles is the **tibial tuberosity**, which provides an attachment for the **patellar ligament**. At the distal end, the tibia articulates with the talus to form part of the ankle joint. On the lateral side, the tibia articulates with the fibula and on the medial side is a large prominence called the **medial malleolus**.

The **fibula** is located on the lateral side of the lower leg and is a long, slender bone. It is a non–weight-bearing bone that primarily serves as a site for the attachment of ligaments and muscles of the lower leg. On the distal end is another large prominence called the **lateral malleolus**; it articulates with the talus bone to form the other portion of the ankle joint. The proximal end of the fibula is called the head and it articulates with the tibia slightly inferior to the tibial lateral condyle.

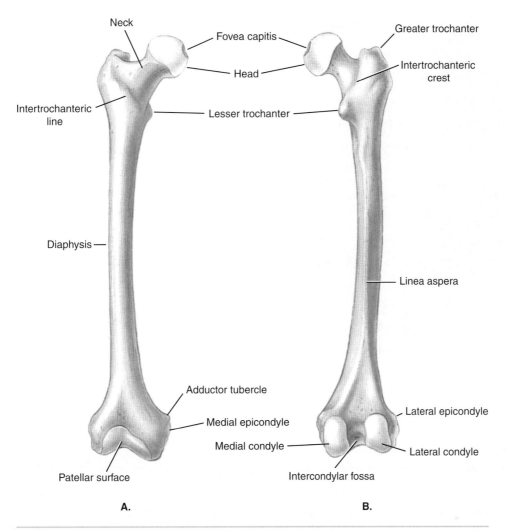

Neck
Fovea capitis
Greater trochanter
Head
Intertrochanteric crest
Intertrochanteric line
Lesser trochanter
Diaphysis
Linea aspera
Adductor tubercle
Medial epicondyle
Lateral epicondyle
Medial condyle
Intercondylar fossa
Lateral condyle
Patellar surface

A.

B.

FIGURE 6-31   Femur, (A) anterior view (B) posterior view

Frequently, both bones of the lower leg will be fractured during a traumatic event and this will be referred to as a tib-fib fracture. The surgeon can often set the fracture of the fibula by closed reduction with the aid of a C-arm x-ray machine due to the slender structure of the bone. However, since the tibia is a thick, strong bone, fixation of the fracture is usually required with either a plate held in place with screws or an external fixation device.

Ankle and Foot

The ankle joint consists of seven **tarsal bones**, which are equivalent to the carpal bones of the wrist. The names of the seven bones are as follows: talus, calcaneus, navicular, cuboid, medial cuneiform, middle cuneiform, and lateral cuneiform. The talus articulates with the tibia and fibula and is freely movable in order to form the ankle joint. The other tarsal bones are held firmly together by tendons and ligaments (Figure 6-34).

The largest tarsal is the calcaneus, more commonly known as the heel. The calcaneus aids in supporting the weight of the body and provides an attachment for the muscles of the foot.

There are five **metatarsals**, which are equivalent to the metacarpals of the hand, and they articulate with the tarsals. They are numbered 1 to 5 from the medial to the lateral side. The heads form the ball of the foot. The distal ends articulate with the proximal phalanx of each toe. There are three phalanges per toe except for the great toe, which has only two.

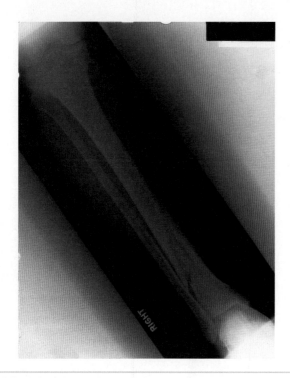

FIGURE 6-32   AP lower leg

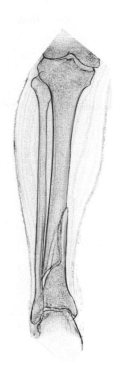

FIGURE 6-33   AP lower leg

IMPLICATIONS FOR THE SURGICAL TECHNOLOGIST

Orthopedic surgery is one of the more complicated specialties due to the vast number and types of orthopedic instruments, equipment, and supplies. In addition, surgical instruments have been developed—and are constantly improved upon—that are for specific surgical procedures. For example, when a patient undergoes a total hip arthroplasty, the surgical technologist has to deal with five to seven trays of surgical hip instruments, including power equipment, such as a reciprocating and oscillating saw, and drill and reamer. Another example is when an open reduction internal fixation (ORIF) will be performed to repair a fracture and the set of instruments to be used is unique for the placement of the plate and screws.

The surgical technologist must know and understand all of the joint movement terminology and anatomic landmarks. For example, when a surgeon is performing a knee arthroscopy, she or he will often ask the surgical technologist to put the leg through various ranges of motion in order to view the entire inside of the joint. Knowing terms such as abduction and adduction are key to being able to assist the surgeon. If the surgeon asks the surgical technologist to move a retractor distally when working on an extremity, he or she must know which direction to move the retractor without having to ask.

Having a basic understanding of the common pathologies of bone aids a surgical technologist in determining the types of instruments, equipment, and supplies that may be needed, and the position in which the patient will be placed. If a surgeon indicates that a patient has a bucket handle tear, the surgical technologist should immediately realize that the surgeon is referring to a tear of either the lateral or medial meniscus. Next, the surgical technologist should know without having to ask that the surgeon will be performing a knee arthroscopy and will need instrumentation available to either remove the meniscus that is torn or repair it.

These are just a few examples that illustrate how important it is for the surgical technologist to have a thorough understanding of the anatomic structure of the skeleton, including important physiological aspects such as the normal healing of bone. This information serves as a basis for learning the many types of orthopedic surgical procedures and performing the role of first scrub, incorporating all factors such as terminology, patient positioning that is unique to orthopedics, instrumentation and power equipment, and postoperative care of the patient.

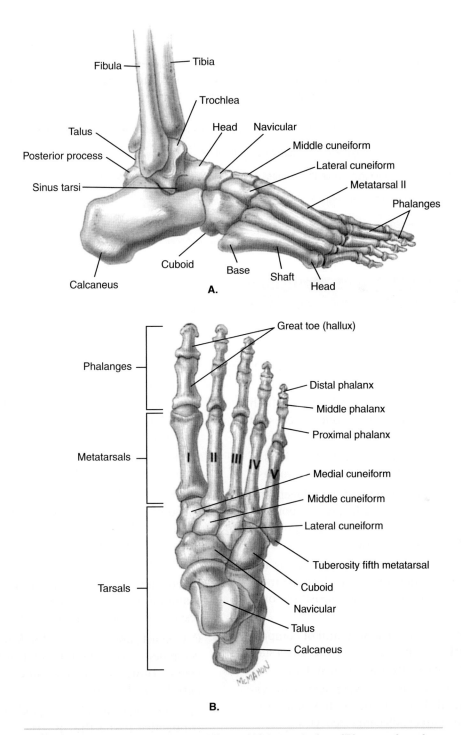

FIGURE 6-34   Right ankle and foot, (A) lateral view (B) superior view

Case Study 2

A 10-year-old female patient is admitted to the Emergency Room with the following clinical signs and symptoms of the tibia in the left leg: pain especially upon movement or weight bearing, tenderness, swelling, redness, and heat. The patient recently recovered from furunculosis. The physician diagnosed the patient with osteomyelitis.

1. How does knowing the patient recently recovered from furunculosis aid the physician in making a diagnosis?

2. What is the most common microorganism that causes osteomyelitis?

3. Osteomyelitis occurs more often in children than adults. What are the most common sites of infection in children?

4. Describe the clinical course of the infection.

5. How is osteomyelitis treated?

CHAPTER SUMMARY

- Bones are a living, specialized type of tissue that form the structure of the body.

- The bones support the body and aid in maintaining homeostasis.

- The skeletal system consists of 206 bones, which includes ligaments, tendons, aponeuroses, and cartilage.

- Bone cells are called osteocytes, the functions of which include transporting nutrients and wastes.

- The inactive matrix is composed of collagen and calcium salts. The calcium salts provide bone its hardness to support the body. Collagen provides strength and resistance to bone.

- Cortical bone, also called compact bone, is the hard, dense tissue that surrounds the bone marrow cavity. The majority of bone consists of cortical bone.

- The osteon is the basic structural unit of compact bone. It consists of lamallae and the haversian canal, which make up the haversian system.

- Osteocytes rest in lacunae of each haversian system and extend filaments through Volkmann's canals, which contact adjacent osteocytes.

- Cancellous bone, also called spongy bone, is located at the ends of bones and lines the medullary marrow cavity. Cancellous bone is composed of trabeculae, which consist of bone matrix and osteocytes.

- Periosteum is a thin fibrous layer of tissue that surrounds the surface of bone and functions to protect bone, form new bone cells, nourish the underlying bone, and serve as attachment for tendons and ligaments. It is often reanastomosed with suture after the bone repair surgery is completed.

- The medullary canal travels the length of bone and contains the red bone marrow.

- Red bone marrow produces erythrocytes, leukocytes, and platelets. The endosteum lines the cavity. In adults the red bone marrow is converted to yellow marrow.

- Osteoprogenitor cells are the stem cells of the skeletal tissue. They differentiate into osteoblasts and chondroblasts.

- Osteoblasts are basophilic cells that are responsible for synthesizing collagen and glycoprotein to form the bone matrix. They eventually develop into osteocytes.

- Osteocytes are basophilic cells, responsible for maintaining the bone matrix, and in the fetus represent the last stage of bone maturation.

- Osteoclasts are large cells that function in the development, growth, and repair of bone. They reside in Howship's lacunae and are activated by parathyroid hormone.

- The skeleton is initially composed of cartilage and connective tissue that is gradually replaced by bone.

- The cranial bones, facial bones, mandible, and clavicle develop by intramembranous ossification. Mesenchymal cells differentiate into osteoprogenitor cells, which differentiate into osteoblasts that synthesize the collagen and glycoproteins to form the bone matrix; the osteoblasts develop into osteocytes.

- Long bones and all other bones of the skeleton develop by endochondral ossification. Bone begins growth in the primary ossification center and develops from the center toward the ends. Mesenchymal cells differentiate into chondroblasts that synthesize matrix, and the bone is formed of hyaline cartilage and perichondrium. More cartilage is formed and the perichondrium in the diaphysis develops into periosteum, which produces osteoblasts to form the bone matrix of the shaft. The medullary canal is formed and filled with red bone marrow. The bone continues to grow at the epiphyseal plate until maturity.

- Bones constantly undergo remodeling and adaptation to stresses.

- Compact bone is particularly important in the remodeling process, since it affects the calcium level in the circulation of the body. Osteoclasts resorb bone, which is then replaced with new bone. The action of osteoclasts is hormonally regulated by parathyroid hormone and calcitonin. Osteoblasts are responsible for the formation of new bone tissue.

- Calcium is important for the transmission of nerve impulses, muscle contraction, blood coagulation, cardiac function, and many other metabolic functions.

- Other factors that affect bone maintenance include exercise and nutrition. Vitamins A, C, and D are important for maintaining healthy bones.

- The nutrient artery supplies the diaphysis, bone marrow cavity, and metaphyses of long bones. During fetal development the artery develops from the periosteal bud.

- Metaphyseal arteries supply the metaphyses. The artery develops from periosteal arteries that had become part of the bone tissue.

- Epiphyseal arteries supply the epiphyses. The artery develops from the periosteal bud.

- Periosteal arteries supply the outer layers of the compact bone.

- Long bones include the humerus and femur. They consist of a diaphysis and epiphyses. The ends of epiphyses are covered by articular cartilage.

- Short bones are the carpal and tarsal bones.

- Flat bones include the cranial bones, scapula, sternum, and ribs. The cranial and facial bones are also referred to as irregular bones. The ribs and sternum in adults are the sites for the development of erythrocytes.

- Sesamoid bones include the patella and the two bones located at the head of the metatarsal in the foot that form the ball of the foot.

- The surgical technologist should be highly familiar with the anatomic terms used in reference to bones.

- Bones have five functions: support the body and protect internal organs; serve for attachment of tendons of the muscles; aid in body movement; provide a source of erythrocytes; store minerals.

- Bones and muscles form levers to provide the body the ability to have a wide range of movements.

- Bone is the source of hematopoiesis.

- Besides calcium, the elements sodium, potassium, and magnesium are also stored by bone.

- An articulation refers to the ends of two bones that meet to form a joint.

- Synarthrosis is a type of immovable joint.

- Amphiarthrosis is a slightly movable joint.

- Diarthrosis joints, also called synovial joints, are freely movable joints.

- The joint capsule is composed of an outer connective tissue layer and a synovial membrane, which produces synovial fluid.

- Menisci are fibrocartilages located between the two articulating ends of some synovial joints.

- The synovial joints contain small sacs called bursae, which contain synovial fluid. The sacs are located between the tendons and bony prominences of joints to cushion and aid in movement. Bursitis is an inflammation of the bursa.

- There are six types of joints: ball-and-socket, gliding, hinge, pivot, condyloid, and saddle.

- The origin of a muscle is the end attached to the immovable end of a bone. The insertion is the end of the muscle that is attached to the movable end of the bone.

- Normal bone healing takes place in five stages: (a) inflammatory stage, (b) cellular proliferation stage, (c) callus formation, (d) ossification stage, (e) remodeling stage.

- The most common areas of the skeleton that require suturing are the sternum after a sternotomy and facial bones that have been fractured. Steel suture is the suture of choice, but occasionally Vicryl will be used.

- Examples of pathologic bone healing include movement of the fractured bones, distraction, interposition of soft tissues, disruption of the blood supply leading to vascular necrosis, infection especially in conjunction with open fractures, which can lead to osteomyelitis, and compartment syndrome.

- Terms associated with poor union of fractured bone ends include nonunion, delayed union, and malunion.

- Cranium: 8 immovable bones and 14 facial bones. Encloses and protects the brain, serves for attachment of muscles, and contains the paranasal sinuses. Cranial bones: (a) frontal; (b) parietal; (c) occipital, which has the large opening called the foramen magnum; (d) temporal, which has the following openings: external auditory meatus, carotid canal, and jugular foramen, and a slight depression called the mandibular fossa that forms part of the TMJ; (e) sphenoid, which has the indentation called the sella turcica that contains the pituitary gland; and (f) ethmoid, which is partially formed by the superior and middle nasal concha.

- The hyoid bone is the only bone of the body that does not articulate with or connect to another bone. It supports the tongue and serves for attachment of the muscles that aid in tongue movement during swallowing.

- The facial bones are as follows: nasal bones, vomer, inferior nasal conchae, lacrimal bones, palatine bones, zygomatic bones, maxillary bones, and mandible, the only movable facial bone.

- The mandibular condyles articulate with the glenoid fossae of the temporal bones to form the TMJ.

- The mandibular foramen is located on the medial side of the mandible and allows blood vessels and a nerve to supply the roots of the lower teeth.

- The mental foramen is an opening located on the front of the mandible and allows blood vessels and a nerve to travel through to supply the tissues of the chin and lower lip.

- At birth the infant has four fontanels: posterior fontanel, anterior fontanel, mastoid fontanel, and sphenoid fontanel. These are known as soft spots and by the age of 2 they will all have become ossified and closed.

- The thoracic cage consists of the ribs and sternum. The functions of the rib cage include enclosing and protecting the lungs and heart, and allows for expansion of the lungs during respiration.

- There are 12 pairs of ribs: 7 pairs called the true ribs, which join the sternum via the costal carti-

lages; 3 pairs called the false ribs, which attach to the seventh rib by costal cartilage; and 2 pairs called the floating ribs.

- The sternum is divided into three parts: manubrium, body, and xiphoid process.

- The functions of the vertebral column include: supporting the head and trunk, allowing flexibility, and forming the vertebral canal for passage of the spinal cord.

- The column consists of vertebrae that are separated by intervertebral disks. The column has four curves: cervical curvature, thoracic curvature, lumbar curvature, and pelvic curvature.

- The common parts of a vertebra are: body, intervertebral disk, anterior and posterior longitudinal ligaments, pedicles, laminae, spinous process, transverse processes, superior and inferior articulating processes, facets, and intervertebral foramina.

- There are three types of vertebrae and each varies slightly in structure: cervical vertebrae of which the first is called the atlas and the second is called the axis, thoracic vertebrae, and lumbar vertebrae.

- The sacrum consists of five vertebrae that are fused into a triangular shape. It forms the posterior portion of the pelvic cavity. The sacroiliac joints mark where the sacrum joins the ilium. The anterior edge of the first sacral vertebra is called the sacral promontory, which is an important anatomic landmark used in determining the size of the pelvis in a female.

- The coccyx consists of four fused vertebrae and is better known as the tailbone.

- The pectoral girdle consists of the clavicles, scapulae, and shoulder joints.

- The clavicle is a long, slender bone situated horizontally that serves for attachment of muscles of the chest, back, and upper extremities. It articulates with the manubrium and acromion process of the scapulae.

- The scapulae are large, triangular-shaped bones located in the upper lateral region of the back. Each scapula has two important anatomic landmarks, the acromion process and the coracoid process. The head of the scapula is a fossa called the glenoid cavity, which serves as the socket for the head of the humerus.

- The pectoral girdle consists of three joints: glenohumeral, sternoclavicular, and acromioclavicular (AC).

- The rotator cuff surrounds the shoulder joint to provide strength and stability. It consists of four muscles: supraspinatus, subscapularis, infraspinatus, and teres minor.

- The humerus extends from the scapula to the elbow and forms part of the shoulder and elbow joints. It has a rounded head that fits into the glenoid fossa; greater, lesser, and deltoid tuberosities; and bicipital groove for the tendon of the biceps brachii muscle. In addition are the capitulum and trochlea, which form part of the elbow joint. A region called the surgical neck is a common area of fractures.

- The radius rotates around the ulna upon movement of the upper limbs and is on the thumb side of the hand. The proximal head forms part of the elbow joint. Other important structures include the radial tuberosity and styloid process. The distal end articulates with the carpal bones.

- The proximal end of the ulna forms part of the elbow joint at the trochlear notch, which articulates with the humerus. Two important processes are the olecranon process and coronoid process. The distal end of the ulna articulates with the radius at the ulnar notch.

- There are eight carpal bones of the wrist arranged in two rows of four. The distal row includes the trapezium, trapezoid, capitate, hamate; the proximal row includes the scaphoid or navicular, lunate, triquetrum, and pisiform.

- The hand and fingers consist of the 5 metacarpals and 14 phalanges.

- Common areas of dislocations in the finger are the PIP joint and MCP joint.

- The functions of the pelvis are to support the trunk of the body, provide attachment for muscles of the femur, and protect internal organs. It is formed by the fusion of the ilium, ischium, and pubis, collectively referred to as the ox coxae. The three bones also fuse to form the acetabulum.

- The ilium forms the majority of the pelvis. The edge of the ilium is called the iliac crest, which serves as an important site for retrieving bone graft material. On the anterior edge of the iliac crest is the anterior superior iliac spine, which is a common site of injuries from contact sports.

- The L-shaped ischium forms the inferior portion of the pelvis. The ischial spine is another anatomic landmark used to determine the size of the pelvis.

- The pubis forms the anteromedial portion of the pelvis. The two pubic bones are joined by the symphysis pubis. The ischium joins the pubis to form the obturator foramen.

- The female and male pelvis have key differences due to the female pelvis functioning as part of the birth canal.

- The hip is a ball-and-socket joint formed by the head of the femur and the acetabulum of the pelvis. The ligaments that stabilize the hip joint include the iliofemoral ligament, ischiofemoral ligament, and pubofemoral ligament.

- The femur is the largest bone of the body. The important structures of the femur include head, femoral neck, greater and lesser trochanters, lateral and medial condyles, patellar groove, and lateral and medial epicondyles.

- The patella is contained in the quadriceps tendon. The patellar tendon passes over the anterior surface of the patella and inserts inferior to it.

- Several tendons and ligaments keep the knee capsule in position.

- The tibia is the larger and stronger of the two bones of the lower leg, located on the medial side. The medial and lateral condyles on the proximal end articulate with the condyles of the femur to form the knee joint. The distal end articulates with the talus bone to form part of the ankle joint. On the medial side is the medial malleolus.

- The fibula is located on the lateral side of the lower leg. It is a non–weight-bearing bone. On the distal end on the lateral side is the lateral malleolus, which articulates with the talus bone to form part of the ankle joint. The proximal head articulates with the tibia.

- A common fracture is a tib-fib fracture, meaning both bones have broken.

- The ankle joint consists of seven tarsal bones: talus, calcaneus, navicular, cuboid, medial cuneiform, middle cuneiform, and lateral cuneiform. The talus is the freely movable bone of the joint that articulates with the tibia and fibula. The heel of the foot is made up of the calcaneus, the largest tarsal bone.

- There are five metacarpals that articulate with the tarsals. They are numbered 1–5 from medial to lateral side. The distal ends articulate with the proximal phalanx of each toe. There are three phalanges per toe except for the big toe for which there are two.

- Orthopedic surgery is one of the more complicated surgical specialties due to the number of procedures that are performed and the large number and many types of orthopedic instruments, equipment, and supplies.

- The surgical technologist must be familiar with joint movement terminology and anatomic landmarks of bone in order to adequately assist the surgeon.

- Understanding the pathologies of bone will aid the surgical technologist in preparing for a surgical procedure.

CRITICAL THINKING QUESTIONS

1. A surgeon will be performing a total hip arthroplasty. Answer the following: (a) What ligament of the femur will be incised? (b) What part of the femur is removed in preparation for the insertion of the prosthesis?

2. A child is brought into the Emergency Room for a fracture of the radius. The child has a history of fractures in various bones throughout the body and the surgeon is now starting to suspect that the child has a particular type of bone pathology. What bone pathology is most likely contributing to the occurrence of the fractures?

3. Why is bone marrow the most ideal tissue for the treatment of certain diseases, such as leukemia, through a bone marrow transplantation?

4. A football player is running and has his left foot and leg planted in the turf when he is hit from the side. He feels a popping sensation in the knee joint and when the team physician examines the knee he tells the player that a ligament has been injured. What ligament has been injured and how did it occur?

5. A surgeon has completed a physical examination of a patient's shoulder. When writing in the patient's chart she notes that the patient does not have full range of motion on abduction and adduction. What does the surgeon mean?

REFERENCES

Caruthers, B. L., & Price, P. (Eds.). (2001). *Surgical technology for the surgical technologist: A positive care approach.* Clifton Park, NY: Thomson Delmar Learning.

Cormack, D. H. (2001). *Essential histology* (2nd ed.). Philadelphia: Lippincott Williams & Wilkins.

Ethicon Products Worldwide. (2002). *Wound closure manual.* Somerville, NJ: Ethicon, Inc.

Ganong, W. F. (1993). *Review of medical physiology* (16th ed.). Norwalk, CT: Appleton & Lange.

Shier, D., Butler, J., & Lewis, R. (2002). *Hole's human anatomy & physiology* (9th ed.). Boston: McGraw-Hill.

7

MUSCULAR SYSTEM

CHAPTER OUTLINE

CHAPTER OBJECTIVES

After completing the study of this chapter, you should be able to:

1. Describe the various types of muscle tissue.
2. List the categories of types of muscle tissue.
3. Describe the purpose and functions of muscles.
4. List and describe the different movements that muscles can produce.
5. Explain the microscopic structure of a muscle fiber.
6. Describe the whole structure of a muscle.
7. Explain the chemical and physiologic processes of producing muscle movement and contraction.
8. Name the skeletal muscle groups.
9. Name and describe the various major muscles of the body.
10. Describe the factors that affect the healing of muscle tissue.
11. List and describe the sutures that are best used for muscle tissue.
12. List and describe the factors that are important to the surgical technologist's understanding of muscle anatomy and physiology.

KEY TERMS

acetylcholine (ACh)
actin
agonist
anaerobic threshold
antagonists
aponeurosis
cardiac muscle tissue
cisternae
compartment syndrome
cross-bridge
electromyography (EMG)

endomysium
epimysium
facial compartments
fascia
fascicle
fasciotomy
fast-twitch fibers
ligaments
motor end plate
motor neuron
motor unit

multiunit smooth muscle
muscle sense
muscle tone
myofibril
myofilament
myogenic
myoglobin
myogram
myoneural junction
myosin
neuromuscular junction

neurotransmitter
oxygen debt
pericytes
perimysium
peristalsis
prime mover
sarcolemma
sarcomere
sarcoplasm
sarcoplasmic reticulum (SR)
skeletal muscles

Case Study 1

For several months, a patient has been receiving nonsurgical treatment for torticollis. The treatment has included stretching exercises and proper positioning during sleep. However, the therapy has not improved the patient's condition and surgery will be performed to correct the condition.

1. What muscle is affected by torticollis?

2. What are the origin and insertion of the muscle affected by torticollis?

3. What are the actions of the muscle?

4. What nerves innervate the muscle?

5. The anterior edge of the muscle is used as an anatomic landmark for locating an artery of the neck. What artery is located adjacent to the anterior edge?

INTRODUCTION

As previously mentioned in Chapter 6, functions of the skeletal system include providing the basic shape and structure to the human body and aiding in body movement. The muscles work with the bones to give the body shape—as evidenced by body builders, athletes, and how individuals vary in their muscular build—and aide in body movement. The physiology of body movement involving the muscles is a complex interaction of nerve impulses and chemicals that coordinate every move. Muscular movement is either voluntary or involuntary, which contributes to the homeostasis of the body.

There are three types of muscular tissue: skeletal, smooth, and cardiac. **Skeletal muscles**, also called voluntary muscles, are the muscles that attach to bones that we consciously move. The cells of skeletal muscles are long and narrow. Skeletal muscle tissue is easily recognized due to the **striations**. The cells have alternating light and dark bands that make up the striations. In addition, the cells are distinguished by the multiple number of nuclei, referred to as multinucleated. The muscle fibers are stimulated to contract by nerve cells, causing protein filaments to slide past each other. Then the muscle fibers relax. The skeletal muscles are responsible for movements of the head and neck, jaw, eyes, and limbs, and the actions of chewing, swallowing, breathing, and facial expressions.

Smooth muscle is so called because it does not have striations. Smooth muscle is also called involuntary muscle, since its movements are not under the control of the person. Smooth muscle cells are shorter and narrower than skeletal muscle cells. They are spindle-shaped with one nucleus located in the center of each cell. Smooth muscle is located in the wall of the stomach, intestines, urinary bladder, blood vessels, and uterus. Therefore, it functions to aid in churning food in the stomach, moving food through the small intestine and colon, emptying the urinary bladder, constricting the arteries, and contracting during childbirth.

Cardiac muscle tissue is located only in the heart. It is the only muscle tissue in the body that has striations but is also composed of smooth muscle. The cells form an interconnecting complex network of branches in which the muscle fibers are joined end to end. The junction at which one cell joins another is marked by a slightly raised band called the intercalated disk, which is seen only in cardiac muscle tissue. Each cell has one nucleus. The muscle is responsible for contracting and relaxing to pump the blood through the four chambers of the heart and into the blood vessels.

MOVEMENT AND THE NERVOUS SYSTEM

The contraction and relaxation of the skeletal muscles rely on the impulses from the central nervous system. The nerve impulses for movement generate from the frontal lobes of the cerebrum. The cerebrum is the largest portion of the brain and the frontal lobes are located underneath the frontal bone of the cranium. The frontal lobes contain the motor areas that generate electrochemical impulses that travel along motor nerves to the muscle fibers, stimulating them to contract.

When movements are made, such as walking, eating, jumping, and running, most of us are not attentive to the movement. The movements are taken for granted and do not require our constant focus. This is referred to as **muscle sense**. Muscle sense is the brain's ability to sense where the muscles are and what they are performing during a movement, thus not requiring us to consciously look at them during the movement. For example, the basketball player who leaps through the air to slam dunk the ball does not have to watch his or her feet to make sure they land on the ground right; muscle sense takes care of that.

Within muscles are receptors called **stretch receptors**, also referred to as proprioceptors. They work in conjunction with the sensory receptors. The stretch receptors sense the changes in the length of a muscle as it stretches. These signals or sensory impulses generated by the stretch receptors travel to the brain. The brain can now interpret the impulses to create a mental picture of where the muscles are, thus providing the person an unconscious sense of the body.

The impulses related to muscle sense are coordinated by the parietal lobes of the cerebrum, which integrate conscious muscle sense with the unconscious muscle sense coordinated by the cerebellum. The cerebellum is located inferior to the occipital lobes of the cerebrum.

SKELETAL MUSCLE

Skeletal muscles aid in a large variety of body movements (Figure 7-1). The action of a muscle depends on the joint to which it is connected and the type of movement(s) the joint can make. It must also be understood that when a muscle is stimulated, it is an all-or-nothing response; the muscle does not partially contract.

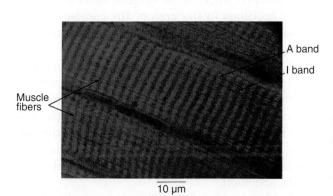
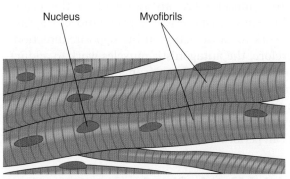

FIGURE 7-1 Voluntary or striated (skeletal) muscle cells (Photo is from *Atlas of Microscopic Anatomy: A Functional Approach: Companion to Histology and Neuroanatomy,* by R. Bergman, A. Afifi, and P. Heidger. 1999. www.vh.org/Providers/Textbooks/MicroscopicAnatomy.html. Reprinted with permission.)

Movement of Skeletal Muscles

Recall from Chapter 6 the terms origin and insertion. One end of a skeletal muscle will be attached to the immovable part of a bone and this is called the origin. The other end of the muscle is attached to the movable part of a bone and this is called the insertion. A few muscles in the body have more than one origin or insertion. A classic example is the biceps brachii muscle, which has two origins, reflected by the name biceps, bi- meaning two. The origin of the tendon of the short head of the muscle is the coracoid process of the scapula and the origin of the tendon of the long head of the muscle is the tubercle of the scapula just superior to the glenoid cavity. The muscle is situated along the anterior length of the humerus and inserts by one tendon on the radial tuberosity of the radius. When a person bends the elbow, the biceps brachii contracts and the insertion is pulled toward the origin. This is the action of every muscle when a joint is bent—the insertion is pulled toward the origin.

When a person moves a body part, it involves a group of muscles and not just a single one. Therefore, groups of muscles can be identified for each particular movement of the body. There are three important terms that must be defined in order to understand body movements. Abduction of the arm will be used as an example. When the arm is abducted it requires the deltoid muscle to contract; therefore, the muscle is the **prime mover**, since it does most of the work of flexing. Also referred to as **agonist** in the motion, it is the muscle primarily responsible for producing the action. But this is not the only muscle involved. When the deltoid muscle has contracted other muscles are needed to keep the shoulder and arm steady to remain in an abducted position, thereby assisting the prime mover. Muscles that contract and assist the prime mover are called **synergists**.

Other muscles are **antagonists** to the prime mover. Antagonists resist the prime mover's action and work to cause action in the opposite direction. Therefore, the antagonistic muscles work to adduct the arm. However, the person's ability to execute smooth body movements depends on the nervous system to communicate to the antagonist to relax and allow the prime mover to contract, and then the agonist can perform its role.

Skeletal Muscle Structure

The composition of a skeletal muscle is complex and involves ancillary structures such as fascia, tendons, and ligaments. **Fascia** is a type of fibrous connective tissue that is off-white to gray in color. It varies in thickness and density, and in the amounts of fat, collagenous fiber, and elastic fiber it contains. There are three types of fascia: deep, subcutaneous, and subserous. The most extensive of the three is deep fascia, which consists of a series of sheets and bands of tissue that surround muscles to hold them together and provide support. The deep fascia is a complex continuous system of tissue that is attached to the skeleton and consists of three layers: outer layer, internal layer, and intermediate membranes. The subcutaneous fascia, also called the subcutaneous layer, is a continuous layer of connective tissue over the entire body that is located between the skin layer and deep fascia. It is composed of an outer fatty layer and an inner elastic layer. The subserous fascia lies between the internal layer of the deep fascia and the serous membranes that line the body cavities and cover the organs of the body.

The deep fascia of the body will form **fascial compartments**, an example of which is an individual muscle or group of muscles that also contains nerves and blood vessels that are tightly surrounded by fascia, walling the tissue off from the body. The majority of compartments are found in the extremities. A complication that can occur due to hemorrhage, edema, or malfunction of the arthroscopic pump machine during an arthroscopy of a joint is **compartment syndrome**. If fluid accumulates within a compartment, the pressure inside increases. The increased pressure inhibits the blood flow to the tissues, thereby causing ischemia and pressure on the nerves. If not treated, the muscle tissue will necrose and permanent nerve damage can occur, impairing the function of the body part. The condition is treated by performing the surgical procedure called **fasciotomy**, wherein the surgeon makes a series of small incisions in the area of the compartment to allow the fluid to escape, reducing the pressure in the compartment.

A special type of fascia, which serves to bind muscle to muscle, is called **aponeurosis**. It is a strong sheet of fibrous connective tissue. An example is the aponeurosis of the external abdominal oblique muscle. The muscle is located on each side of the body with fibers that slant downward, and is connected by the aponeurosis that covers the entire ventral surface of the abdomen.

Tendons are a dense fibrous connective tissue, which is easily recognized by its glistening white appearance. Tendons vary in length and thickness, and are composed of parallel fibers kept together by a connective tissue sheath called the **tenosynovium** to form the tough, inelastic, cordlike structure. The fibers in the tendon merge with the periosteum of a bone at certain points such as a tubercle or process, serving to attach muscle to bone. Tendons also merge with the fascia. Atheletes often experience **tendinitis**, inflammation of a tendon, or **tenosynovitis**, inflammation of the tendon sheath. The injuries are often a result of overuse and stress due to repeated activity. The inflammation is treated by RICE: rest, ice, compression, and elevation. Surgery is rarely indicated except in cases of chronic tenosynovitis.

Ligaments are also white; they are slightly elastic and more flexible than tendons. Ligaments are a fibrous tissue composed of parallel collagenous bundles that bind bone to bone to form joints. Refer to Chapter 6 for detailed information concerning major ligaments such as the anterior and posterior cruciate ligaments.

For the purpose of easily remembering the function of the ancillary structures, the following review is provided:

1. Fascia: covering of the muscles to bind them together
2. Tendon: connects muscle to bone or in the case of aponeurosis, binds muscle to muscle
3. Ligament: connects bone to bone

Another layer of connective tissue that more intimately surrounds a skeletal muscle is called the **epimysium**. It can be thicker in some areas and more delicate in others, and may fuse with the fascia as it merges with the tendon. Inward extensions of the epimysium, called the **perimysium**, continue between the bundles of muscle fibers, dividing the muscle tissue into sections. The sections or bundles of skeletal muscle fibers that are surrounded by the perimysium are referred to as **fascicles**. The blood vessels, nerves, and lymphatic vessels are conveyed by the fascicles inward from the epimysium. Muscles with more fasciculi have greater strength and power but less range of motion as compared to muscles with fewer fasciculi. In addition, each muscle fiber in the fascicle is surrounded by a thin layer of connective tissue called the **endomysium**. Therefore, each portion of a skeletal muscle is surrounded and separated by connective tissue.

Structure of a Skeletal Muscle Fiber

A skeletal muscle fiber is actually a single muscle cell (Figure 7-2). Each fiber during development joins together to form a muscle. The fibers are thin, long, and cylinder-shaped with a rounded end, and attach to the connective tissue layers previously described.

Each fiber is covered by a membrane called the **sarcolemma**, which is electrically polarized, and underlying the sarcolemma is the **sarcoplasm**, the semifluid cytoplasm of muscle cells that contains the nuclei and mitochondria. On examination, the muscle fiber can be further broken down and is composed of parallel slender threadlike strands called **myofibrils**, which are composed of **myofilaments**.

The myofibrils are the major component of muscle contraction and relaxation. There are two kinds of protein myofilaments: **myosin**, which is a thick filament that makes up approximately one half of the proteins that occur in muscle tissue, and the thin fibrils called **actin**, which are pulled on by the myosin crossbridges to cause muscle contraction and relaxation. The two myofilaments are responsible for producing the alternating dark and light bands or striations that identify a muscle as either skeletal or cardiac. The myofibrils are further broken down into **sarcomeres**, the functioning unit of a myofibril. Sarcomeres occur as repeating sections along the length of a myofibril; therefore, a myofibril can actually be considered as a line of sarcomeres that are joined end to end.

The striation pattern of skeletal muscle is broken down into several minute sections. The first part is referred to as the I band (for isotropic), which is the light band. It is composed of actin myofilaments that are attached to the Z lines, which are situated in the center of the I band. Sarcomeres occupy the region between the Z lines. The second portion of the striation is the A band (for anisotropic), which is the dark band that consists of myosin myofilaments. In the region of the A band, the actin and myosin myofilaments overlap. Also within the A band is a zone called the H zone, located in the center of the A band and slightly lighter in color, which consists of myosin myofilaments. In the center of the H zone is a thickening called the M line, which is made up of proteins that hold the thick myosin myofilaments in place. The myosin myofilaments are held in place not only by the Z lines, but also by a protein called connectin.

On microscopic examination of a myosin myofilament, it can be seen that the myosin molecule consists of twisted proteins strands with globular extensions called **cross-bridges** that project outward toward the nearby actin myofilaments. An actin myofilament consists of two strands of actin twisted to form a helix. The actin molecule is also globular and contains a binding site for the cross-bridges of the myosin filament to attach (Figure 7-3).

Two other proteins that are part of the actin myofilaments are **tropomyosin** and **troponin**. Tropomyosin molecules are thin, rod-shaped strands

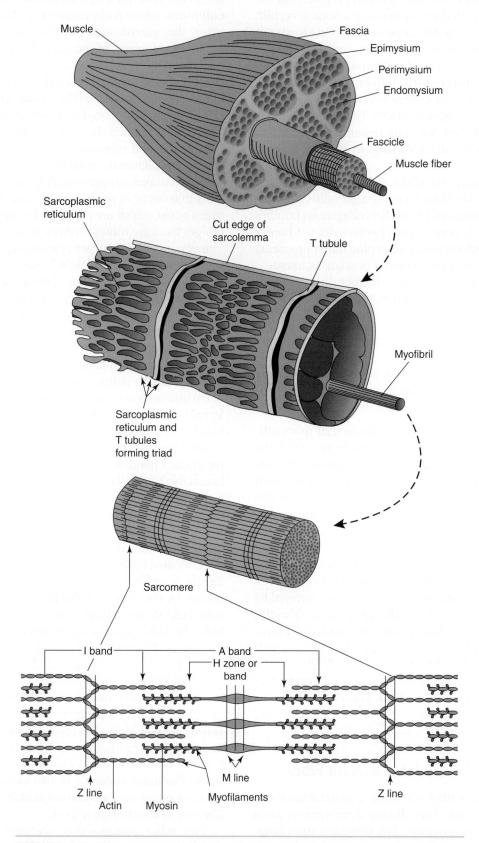

FIGURE 7-2 **The anatomy of skeletal muscle at the microscopic, cellular, and molecular levels**

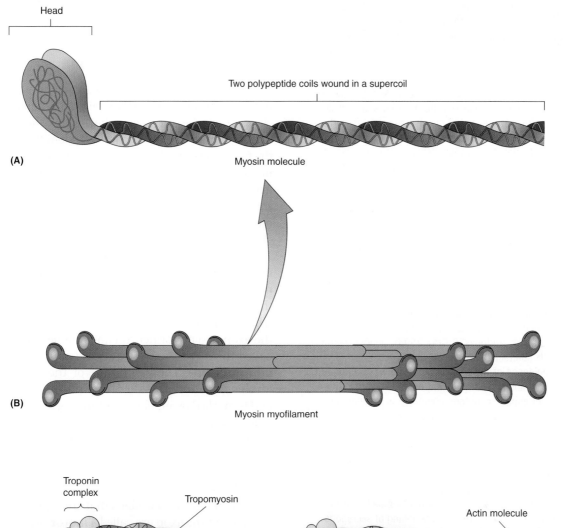

Head

Two polypeptide coils wound in a supercoil

(A)   Myosin molecule

(B)   Myosin myofilament

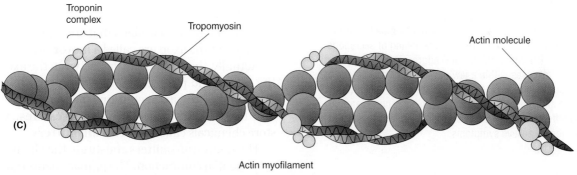

Troponin complex

Tropomyosin

Actin molecule

(C)

Actin myofilament

FIGURE 7-3   The structure of the actin and myosin myofilaments of a muscle cell. (A) Myosin molecule, (B) Myosin myofilament, (C) Actin myofilament

that are located within the longitudinal grooves of the helix formed by the actin. Each tropomyosin molecule is held in position by a troponin molecule. Together these two molecules regulate the interactions of myosin and actin in muscle contractions.

Surrounding each myofibril is a complex network of tubules and sacs called the **sarcoplasmic reticulum (SR)**. This network is analogous, but not identical in structure, to the endoplasmic reticulum of other body cells. Sarcoplasmic reticulum plays an important role in muscle contraction and relaxation by storing and releasing calcium ions; therefore, its primary role is to regulate calcium ion concentration within the myofibrils. Attached to the surface of the reticulum are open channels called the transverse tubules or T-tubules, and they contain extracellular fluid. The T-tubules have openings onto the surface of the skeletal muscle fiber. Each T-tubule is located

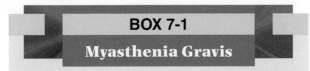

BOX 7-1

Myasthenia Gravis

Myasthenia gravis results in progressive weakness of skeletal muscles. Due to the weakness, the muscles fatigue easily, especially with exercise, and as the disease progresses, the fatigue occurs with normal movements such as walking. The majority of the time the disease affects muscles innervated by the cranial nerves such as the lips, tongue, face, throat, and neck (Weinstock, Andrews, & Cray, 1998). The disease follows a course of recurring activity and remissions.

The exact cause of myasthenia gravis is not known. It causes a failure in the transmission of nerve impulses at the neuromuscular junction. During a muscle contraction acetylcholine (ACh) diffuses across the synaptic junction. Normally, it will bind with the receptor sites on the motor end plates, thereby depolarizing the muscle fiber and causing the muscle to contract. With myasthenia gravis, the receptor sites are weakened or destroyed by antibodies that have attached to the sites and block the ability of ACh to bind (Weinstock, Andrews, & Cray, 1998). Depolarization and muscle contraction are not allowed to occur.

The incidence of the disease peaks between ages 20 and 40 years and occurs much more often in women than men. The dominant symptom, obviously, is skeletal muscle weakness and fatigue. The muscle weakness is progressive and as the disease progresses additional muscles are involved.

The most serious complication is respiratory difficulties. Respiratory muscle weakness can lead to a life-threatening myasthenic crisis. The patient will most likely require an emergency tracheostomy combined with mechanical ventilation and frequent suctioning of secretions. However, if treated quickly and aggressively, the patient usually improves within a few days. In the early stages of the disease, anticholinergic drugs are taken to counteract fatigue and muscle weakness. But these drugs eventually are ineffective as the disease progresses. Corticosteroids occasionally relieve symptoms.

between two transverse **cisternae** (singular, cisterna), which serve as a reservoir for extracellular fluid. The two cisternae and a T-tubule together are referred to as a **triad**, and the triad marks the region where myosin and actin myofilaments overlap.

PHYSIOLOGY OF MUSCLE MOVEMENT

The contraction of a muscle is a complex interaction involving the structures of the muscle fiber, the nervous system, and chemicals. The contraction and

relaxation of a muscle occurs according to what is referred to as the **sliding filament theory**.

Contraction and Relaxation

As previously mentioned, the sarcomere is the functioning portion of the skeletal muscle. When the muscle contracts the sarcomeres shorten, but the actin and myosin filaments do not change in length. However, the filaments slide past one another with the actin filaments moving toward the center of the sarcomere from each end. During this action, the I bands and H zones narrow, the region where the actin and myosin filaments overlap is widened, and the Z lines move closer together, thereby shortening the sarcomere.

The nervous system is involved in the following manner. Skeletal muscle fibers are innervated by **motor neurons**, which are neurons extending from the spinal cord. The skeletal muscle fibers contract when stimulated by motor neurons. The region where the axon of a motor neuron and muscle fiber touch is called the **myoneural junction** (or **neuromuscular junction**). The membrane of the muscle fiber at this junction is called the **motor end plate** and is marked by an abundant number of nuclei and mitochondria.

The muscle fiber will have only one motor end plate, but the axon of a motor neuron will have many branches. This allows the motor neuron to connect to several muscle fibers at the motor end plate. The motor neuron and the muscle fibers that are connected to the branches of the axon are called a **motor unit**.

Actually, there is a small gap between the axon and the motor end plate called the **synaptic cleft**. The distal end of the axon contains many mitochondria and tiny vesicles called **synaptic vesicles**, which store chemicals called **neurotransmitters**.

The neurotransmitters constitute the chemical involvement in contraction. The primary neurotransmitter of motor neurons when interacting with skeletal muscles is **acetylcholine (ACh)**. ACh is synthesized in the cytoplasm of the motor neuron and transported to the distal end of the axons to be stored in the synaptic vesicles. When a nerve impulse, or what is called an action potential, travels to the end of an axon, the vesicles are stimulated to release ACh into the synaptic cleft. The motor end plate has receptor sites for the ACh, which travels across the cleft to combine with the sites and stimulate the muscle fiber. The ensuing muscle impulse is an electrical stimulus that causes the muscle cell membrane to transmit the impulse in all directions along the length of the muscle cell, into the sarcoplasm, and farther into the SR and cisternae.

The membrane of the SR contains a high level of calcium ions. Responding to the muscle impulse, the cisternae are more impermeable to the calcium ions, and the ions diffuse from the cisternae into the cytosol of the muscle fiber (remember cytosol is the clear liquid within the cytoplasm of a cell in which the organelles are suspended).

When a muscle fiber is at rest, the tropomyosin–troponin complex prevents the formation of cross-bridge linkages between the actin and myosin filaments by blocking the binding sites on the actin filaments. However, as the level of calcium ions in the cytosol increases, the ions bind to the troponin, change their conformation, and change the position of the tropomyosin. With the change in position, the binding sites on the actin filaments are exposed and the cross-bridge linkages are formed between the myosin cross-bridges and actin filaments (Figure 7-4).

Relaxation of the muscle begins when the nerve impulses stop. The remaining ACh in the synaptic cleft is broken down by the enzyme called acetylcholinesterase (AChE). The enzyme is always present in the synapse and located within the membrane of the motor end plates. The action of AChE hydrolyzes ACh to choline and acetate and prevents the continuous firing of neurons at the neuromuscular junction.

Additionally, the breakdown of ACh in the sarcolemma and muscle fiber membranes is no longer stimulated. The calcium pump causes the quick transfer of calcium ions back into the SR, thereby decreasing the level of calcium ions in the cytosol. The cross-bridge linkages break and tropomyosin reoccupies the longitudinal grooves of the actin helix, which prevents any cross-bridge attachments to form. The end result is the relaxation of the muscle fibers.

Chemical Sources for Contraction

ATP supplies the energy that is needed for the action of the myosin and actin filaments during muscle fiber contraction. However, ATP is not available in unlimited quantity within the muscle fiber to sustain a muscle contraction and, when a muscle is active, the ATP must somehow be regenerated.

The initial enzyme that is available to regenerate ATP from adenosine diphosphate (ADP) and phosphate is creatine phosphate. Creatine phosphate does not directly supply energy to the cells. Rather, it stores the excess energy that is released from mitochondria. When ATP is present at a sufficient level, the enzyme creatine phosphokinase, located in the mitochondria, stimulates the synthesis of creatine phosphate.

When ATP is broken down to ADP, the energy from creatine phosphate molecules transfers to the ADP molecules in order to convert them back to ATP. However, as previously mentioned, the level of ATP and creatine phosphate in the skeletal muscle fibers is not sufficient to sustain a high level of muscle activity for more than 15 seconds. Therefore, the next step is for the muscle fibers to depend on the cellular respiration of glucose as the source of ATP. Muscles store glucose in the form of the polysaccharide called glycogen. Glycogen is the primary carbohydrate stored in animal cells.

The Role of Oxygen

The following is a short review of cellular respiration, oxygen debt, and muscle fatigue. Recall that glycolysis is one of the early stages of cellular respiration and it takes place in the cytoplasm; therefore, it does not require oxygen (anaerobic). But glycolysis does not completely break down glucose; therefore, only a few ATP molecules are released. Glucose is completely broken down in the mitochondria, a process that requires oxygen (aerobic). The aerobic process in conjunction with the whole complex citric acid cycle produces a large number of ATP molecules.

The erythrocytes in the circulatory system transport the oxygen from the lungs to the cells of the body to support aerobic respiration. Oxygen molecules bind to the hemoglobin molecules that are located in the erythrocyte. Hemoglobin is the pigment responsible for giving the erythrocytes their red color. The oxygen molecules are released from hemoglobin and are then available for aerobic respiration.

Myoglobin is another pigment that aids in providing oxygen to muscles. Myoglobin is synthesized in the muscle cells and is responsible for giving skeletal muscle its reddish-brown color. Myoglobin, like hemoglobin, can bind to oxygen molecules and temporarily store oxygen in the muscle tissue. This aids in reducing the muscles' requirement of circulating hemoglobin.

When the skeletal muscles are at rest or not involved in performing a strenuous activity, the supply of oxygen is usually sufficient to adequately support aerobic respiration. However, in situations in which the muscles are heavily tasked, the respiratory and circulatory systems may not be able to supply the level of oxygen required to sustain aerobic respiration. The muscle fibers will then switch to the anaerobic phase of cellular respiration to create energy. The outcome of this phase is an increase in the level of lactic acid in the circulatory system called the anaerobic threshold (or lactic acid threshold).

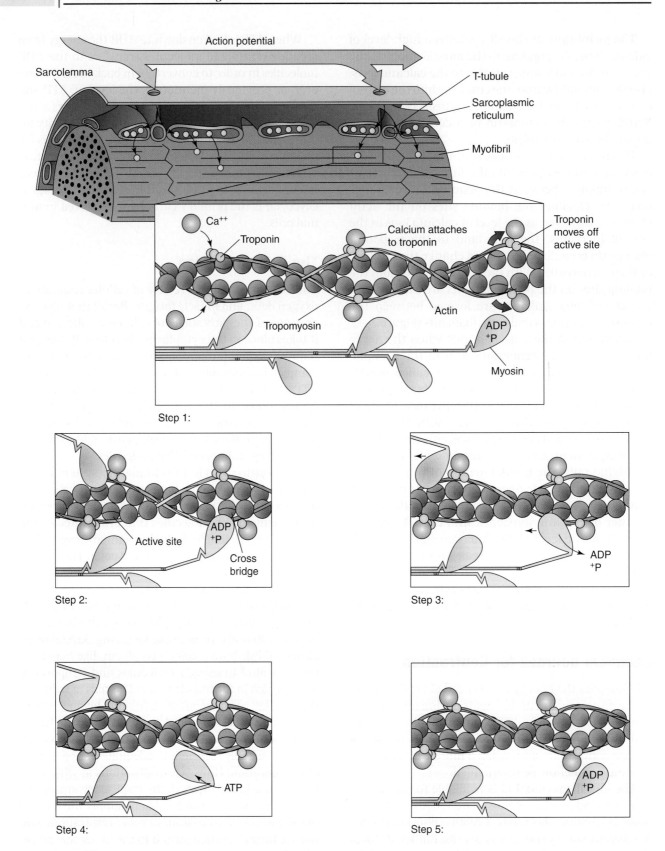

FIGURE 7-4 **The interaction of the activated myosin cross-bridges with the actin filaments pulling the actin in among the myosin, resulting in contraction**

When anaerobic conditions exist, glycolysis breaks down glucose into pyruvic acid, which is further broken down into lactic acid, and then transported through the circulatory system to the liver. The hepatocytes form glucose from the lactic acid, but this requires ATP. However, during active exercise, the priority of oxygen is to aid in synthesizing the ATP needed for muscle contraction; the oxygen is not being diverted for synthesizing ATP for use in converting lactic acid to glucose. The consequence is the buildup of lactic acid, resulting in **oxygen debt**. The level of oxygen debt approximately equals the amount of oxygen the hepatocytes require to convert the lactic acid to glucose and represents the amount of oxygen needed to return the blood and tissue oxygen levels to their preexercise levels. In other words, oxygen debt is the quantity of oxygen that the lungs take up during recovery from exercise that is in excess of the quantity that is normally needed during rest or preexercise. It represents payback of oxygen and energy stores that were depleted during the time that oxygen uptake was inadequate during exercise to sustain aerobic metabolism.

A sustained strenuous level of activity can lead to muscle fatigue, in which the muscle temporarily loses the ability to fully contract. Muscle fatigue is most often due to the buildup of lactic acid in the muscle. As the lactic acid accumulates in the muscle, it also is transferred into the circulatory system; this allows lactic acid to be transferred throughout the muscles of the body and leads to muscle fatigue. Muscle fatigue occurs at varying rates in individuals. High-caliber athletes tend to produce less lactic acid and do not produce it as soon as individuals who are less active. Individuals who exercise regularly stimulate the development of new capillaries within muscles, allowing for an increased level of oxygen delivery. Also, exercise stimulates the muscle fibers to form more mitochondria, which increases the body's ability to sustain aerobic respiration for a longer period.

SLOW- AND FAST-TWITCH MUSCLE FIBERS

The contraction of muscle fibers can be recorded and the fibers are placed in one of two categories based on how they synthesize ATP and the speed of their contractions.

Muscle Twitch

Many individuals are familiar with dissecting a frog and applying a small amount of electrical current to

---

BOX 7-2
Muscular Dystrophy

Muscular dystrophy (MD) is a genetic, congenital disorder characterized by a progressive wasting of the skeletal muscles. An individual with MD physiologically presents an appearance of healthy muscles because they tend to enlarge, but that is due to the abnormal deposit of connective tissue and fat. There are four types of MD: Duchenne's, Becker's, facioscapulohumeral, and limb-girdle.

Duchenne's accounts for about 50% of all cases (Weinstock, Andrews, & Cray, 1998). It usually begins during childhood, between the ages of 3 and 5 and the individual does not survive past the age of 20. Males are primarily affected. Muscle deterioration rapidly occurs and contractures develop. By age 9–12 the patient is confined to a wheelchair. In the late stages of the disease, the cardiac muscle weakens combined with pulmonary complications.

Diagnosis is based on clinical findings, family history, and diagnostic tests. Electromyography and muscle biopsy are the two diagnostic tests often used. Muscle biopsy will reveal the absence of dystrophin, a protein located in the sarcolemma. Its absence results in abnormal cell permeability and cell death. There is no cure for MD. Palliative measures are taken such as exercise, physical therapy, orthopedic braces, and surgery to correct contractures.

---

the leg to see it move. In a more advanced laboratory setting, a skeletal muscle will be removed from the frog then mounted on a special device that can electrically stimulate the muscle and cause it to contract. The stimulation of the muscle is then recorded and a recording of the contraction, called a **myogram**, is obtained.

When a single stimulus is transmitted to the frog muscle, some of the motor units are activated, causing the muscle to contract and relax. This instantaneous single contraction is called a **twitch**. Figure 7-5 is a representation of a myogram showing a twitch. Note the delay between the application of the stimulus to the muscle and the time the muscle contracted. This period of time is called the latent period; in humans the latent period is less than 0.01 second. After the latent period is a period of contraction when the muscle pulls at its attachments and then a period of relaxation when the muscle assumes its former length. If two rapid stimuli are transmitted to the muscle, it will twitch in response to the first stimulus, but not the second. The reason is that it takes less than a second following a muscle contraction for the muscle fibers to recover and to be responsive to the

BOX 7-3

Muscle Biopsy

A muscle biopsy is a minor surgical procedure that involves the excision and examination of a piece of muscle tissue. Specific reasons for performing a muscle biopsy include:

1. Identify specific muscular disorders, in particular muscular dystrophy.
2. Identify metabolic defects of the muscle.
3. Identify diseases of the connective tissue and blood vessels, in particular polyarteritis nodosa, a widespread inflammation and necrosis of arterioles and ischemia of the tissues they supply.
4. Identify infections that are specific to muscles such as trichinosis.
5. Check the progress of an existing diagnosed condition.

The majority of the time the biopsy is obtained with the patient awake and the biopsy site numbed with local anesthesia. A needle biopsy is the most common method of obtaining a sample of the muscle tissue. The procedure is as follows:

1. Local anesthetic is injected.
2. Hollow-bored needle is inserted.
3. A small piece of tissue containing a large number of muscle fibers remains in the needle as it is withdrawn.
4. The tissue is sent to the pathologist for examination and diagnosis.
5. If necessary, to obtain a large enough specimen for testing and examination, the procedure may require repeating more than once.

The advantages of a needle biopsy include:

1. It can be performed on children and adults.
2. Repeat biopsies can easily be performed.
3. There is little scarring or cosmetic effects.
4. It is cost-effective.
5. There is very little chance of infection occurring.
6. There is little to no bleeding.

Occasionally, an open muscle biopsy must be performed, in which case the patient will most likely receive general anesthesia. The surgeon makes an incision approximately 2 inches in length over the muscle that has been selected for the biopsy. Once the incision has been made, the muscle identified, and area of biopsy chosen, the doctor uses scissors and forceps to remove the muscle tissue. The wound is then closed with absorbable suture and skin staples. An advantage of open biopsy is that a sizable piece of tissue can be removed, therefore eliminating the need to repeat the procedure.

The most common sites for excising muscle include:

1. Quadriceps femoris on the lateral aspect of the thigh
2. Deltoid muscle
3. Biceps brachii muscle

A muscle that has recently sustained trauma such as from a previous biopsy or being bruised or cut by accident, or that is affected by a preexisting condition such as nerve compression, should not be used as the muscle biopsy site.

The pathologist will examine the tissue with and without staining under a light microscope and electron microscope. He or she will also perform a frozen biopsy procedure, which is effective in viewing thin slices of the tissue.

second or further stimuli. During this brief moment the muscle is not capable of response; this time lapse is called the refractory period.

When muscles appear to be at rest, there is always a certain level of sustained contraction within the muscle fibers. This is referred to as **tonus** or **muscle tone** and occurs in response to the repeating nerve impulses traveling from the spinal cord. Therefore, a continuous state of partial contraction is present.

Tonus is important in the body's ability to maintain posture without fatigue. The tonus of the muscles of the neck, back, trunk, and extremities allows an individual to hold the head and body upright, stand, or sit

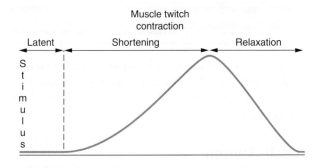

FIGURE 7-5   A laboratory analysis of a muscle twitch

and for long periods if necessary. An example of when tonus is lost is when a person loses consciousness, falling to the ground due to the complete collapse of the body. Tonus is also lost if trauma or disease interferes with the continual transmission of the nerve impulses to the muscles.

Categories and Types of Muscle Fibers

Muscle fibers vary in the speed of contraction and are thus categorized as **slow-twitch fibers** or **fast-twitch fibers**. These two categories are further broken down into types. The category to which a muscle fiber belongs is also determined by whether the fiber produces ATP glycolytically or oxidatively.

Slow-twitch fibers are type I and are always oxidative; therefore, they do not fatigue quickly. Fast-twitch fibers are type II and are either glycolytic, susceptible to fatigue, or oxidative. The slow-twitch fibers are also referred to as red fibers because they contain myoglobin, the red-colored pigment that stores oxygen. The blood supply to the type I fibers is rich with oxygen and the fibers contain multiple mitochondria, organelles that are important in sustaining aerobic respiration. Therefore, the red fibers can synthesize ATP quickly enough to equal the ATP breakdown that occurs during contraction and sustain contractions for a long period without fatigue setting in.

Fast-twitch fibers that are glycolytic are type IIa and are referred to as white fibers, since they contain less myoglobin and the blood supply is not as abundant. The white fibers also have fewer mitochondria, thus reducing the respiratory level. However, in comparison to red fibers, the SR in white fibers is much more comprehensive, allowing calcium ions to be stored and reabsorbed, and ATP is synthesized faster. These qualities allow white fibers to rapidly contract, but they fatigue much sooner with the accompanying accumulation of lactic acid and as the biochemicals needed to synthesize ATP are depleted.

The third kind of fibers are fast-twitch oxidative, which are a type IIb and referred to as intermediate fibers. These fibers combine the fast-twitch contraction speed of white fibers with the oxidative level of red fibers.

Most of the muscles of the body are a combination of the fiber types. However, the fibers are adapted to meet the need of the particular area of the body they are servicing. For example, the extraocular muscles, which aid in moving the eye, contract quickly, compared to the slower contracting muscles of the neck and back, which are responsible for maintaining the posture of the body.

SMOOTH MUSCLES

The mechanism of smooth and cardiac muscle contraction is basically the same as that of skeletal muscles. The difference lies in the structure and functions of the cells of the smooth and cardiac muscle (Figure 7-6).

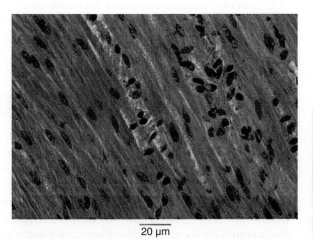

20 μm

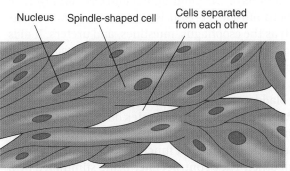

Nucleus   Spindle-shaped cell   Cells separated from each other

FIGURE 7-6   Involuntary or smooth muscle cells (Photo is from *Atlas of Microscopic Anatomy: A Functional Approach: Companion to Histology and Neuroanatomy,* by R. Bergman, A. Afifi, and P. Heidger. 1999. www.vh.org/Providers/Textbooks/MicroscopicAnatomy.html. Reprinted with permission.)

Muscle Fiber Structure

As compared to skeletal muscle fibers, smooth muscle cells are shorter and have a single central nucleus. When viewed under the microscope the cells are elongated and taper at both ends. The myofibrils contain actin and myosin, but they are not neatly arranged like skeletal muscle fibers, but rather are randomly arranged, which is why smooth muscle is not striated. Smooth muscle fibers also differ from skeletal muscle fibers in that they do not have transverse tubules and the SR is less developed.

There are two types of smooth muscles: multiunit and visceral. **Visceral smooth muscle** is the most common type of smooth muscle and is located in the walls of hollow organs including the stomach, intestines, urinary bladder, and uterus. Most often there will be at least two layers of smooth muscle. The fibers of the outer layer of smooth muscle travel in a longitudinal fashion and those of the inner layer are arranged in a circular pattern. The two-layer arrangement of the fibers allows the organ to change in shape and size, such as the action of the stomach after a meal.

Visceral smooth muscle consists of spindle-shaped cells that are in close contact. The thick portion of the cell lies next to and is in contact with the thin portion of the adjacent cells in order to form the tight bond. When one fiber is stimulated by a nerve impulse, the impulse travels over the surface of the fiber to stimulate the adjacent fibers and the domino effect continues. This causes the visceral smooth muscle to respond as a single element. Some visceral muscles experience spontaneous repeated contractions called rhythmicity.

The domino effect of the nerve impulses and rhythmicity is responsible for causing the wavelike motion called **peristalsis**, the coordinated contractions and relaxations of the longitudinal and circular layers of smooth muscle. Peristalsis occurs in tubular organs such as the esophagus, intestines, and ureters. It aids in forcing the contents within the tube forward, such as pushing digested food forward in the colon or moving urine forward through the ureters to empty into the bladder.

Multiunit smooth muscles do not function as a unit like visceral smooth muscle. They are separate, independent units that function independently from each other. They contract after being stimulated by a motor nerve impulse or particular kinds of hormones. The walls of blood vessels and the irises of the eyes are examples of where multiunit smooth muscles are located.

Physiology of Contraction

The contraction of smooth muscle is the same as skeletal muscle contraction in the following ways:

1. Actin and myosin are necessary for contraction to occur.
2. Contractions are stimulated by membrane impulses.
3. Both types of muscle release calcium ions.
4. Both types of muscle acquire energy from ATP molecules.
5. Acetylcholine affects both muscles.

But there are several differences:

1. Smooth muscle fibers do not contain troponin, but rather use the protein called calmodulin, which binds to the calcium ions that are released when the smooth muscle fibers are stimulated. This activates the contraction of actin–myosin.
2. As mentioned in the preceding text, acetylcholine affects smooth muscle, but norepinephrine is also required for smooth muscle function. The two neurotransmitters have two different effects—they either stimulate contractions in some smooth muscles or inhibit contractions in other muscles.
3. Certain types of hormones affect smooth muscles by stimulating or inhibiting contractions.
4. When smooth muscle fibers are stretched contractions can be stimulated. This is especially important in visceral smooth muscle that is located in the wall of a hollow or tubular organ. For example, when digested food stretches the wall of the colon, peristalsis is stimulated to begin.
5. Smooth muscle contracts and relaxes slower than skeletal muscle. However, smooth muscle can sustain contractions much longer using the same amount of ATP as the skeletal muscle.

CARDIAC MUSCLE

Cardiac muscle is the only smooth muscle that contains striations, but it is a specialized type of smooth muscle in that it works involuntarily. The cardiac muscle cells are arranged end-to-end to form fibers that are interconnected in a complex branching network (Figure 7-7). Each muscle cell has a single nucleus centrally located in the fibers, and actin and myosin filaments. Under the microscope, the endomysium appears as thin regions between the muscle fibers and is a loose connective tissue that is well supplied with capillaries and lymphatics.

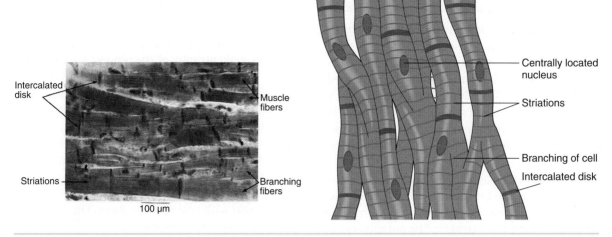

FIGURE 7-7 Cardiac muscle cells (Photo is from *Atlas of Microscopic Anatomy: A Functional Approach: Companion to Histology and Neuroanatomy,* by R. Bergman, A. Afifi, and P. Heidger. 1999. www.vh.org/Providers/Textbooks/MicroscopicAnatomy.html. Reprinted with permission.)

The transverse tubules are well developed and the cells contain many mitochondria. In addition, the transverse tubules are wider in comparison to skeletal muscle and release a large amount of calcium ions into the SR when stimulated by a single nerve impulse. But the cardiac muscle contains fewer transverse tubules as compared to skeletal muscle. The tubules lie at the Z line, not at the junction of the A and I bands (Cormack, 2001). Consequently, there is only one level of transverse tubules per sarcomere.

The SR is also well developed, but has a smaller compartment. Additionally, the cisternae are not present, but rather the SR compartment consists of connected longitudinal sarcotubules; therefore, this muscle has storage capacity for calcium as compared to skeletal muscle fiber.

Because the SR can store only a small amount of calcium and does not meet the level needed for contractions to occur, the cardiac muscle cells are dependent on a supply of extracellular calcium ions. The ions enter through the sarcolemma and transverse tubules. The entrance of the extracellular calcium ions stimulates the release of calcium ions stored in the SR, and together the ions enter the myofibrils and stimulate contractions. Just as with skeletal muscles, relaxation occurs when the ions are pumped back into the SR. Therefore, the contraction of the cardiac muscle relies on both extracellular and intracellular calcium ions. The calcium is responsible for helping to control the strength of heart contractions and allows the cardiac muscle fibers to contract for a longer period than skeletal muscle fibers. Because the force of

contractions is dependent on the calcium ions, during exercise the force of the cardiac muscle contractions increases (Cormack, 2001).

Cells are joined together at each end by traversing cross-bands called intercalated disks, structures that are unique to cardiac muscle fibers. The cross-bands not only connect cells, but also are a membrane junction that allows ions to travel between the cells. This cellular connection provides for the rapid transfer of impulses from cell to cell. When a portion of the cardiac muscle is stimulated, the impulse travels throughout the other muscle fibers, causing the whole cardiac muscle to respond to the stimulation in an all-or-nothing manner.

The cardiac muscle contracts and relaxes in a rhythmic pattern and the pattern repeats itself over and over. The refractory period of cardiac muscle is longer than that of skeletal muscle and does not end until the contraction has ended. Involuntary contraction of the cardiac muscle occurs through filament sliding (Cormack, 2001). The contraction is referred to as **myogenic**, meaning it is a spontaneous, involuntary rhythmic activity. The rate of contractions is controlled by the nerve impulses of the autonomic nervous system.

The rhythmic pattern of a person's heartbeat can be recorded with the use of an electrocardiogram (ECG). The device is used for recording the electrical activity of the cardiac muscle to detect the transmission of the impulse through the muscle. Electrocardiography aids in detecting and diagnosing abnormalities of the heart beat and rate by producing a graph.

ELECTROMYOGRAPHY

Previously, obtaining a myogram through myography by stimulating the muscle of a frog was discussed. In this section, recording the electrical activity in human skeletal muscle will be described. A record of the electric activity in a skeletal muscle is called an electromyogram and is obtained by performing **electromyography (EMG)**. The data obtained from EMG aids in diagnosing neuromuscular pathologies.

EMG is performed by applying skin electrodes or inserting a needle electrode intramuscularly. An oscilloscope is used to display the electric variations on a screen along with a loudspeaker. The patient will be asked to flex and extend the particular muscle in which the electrodes are placed and a graphic recording can be printed. Besides recording the electric activity of the muscle, EMG also measures the electric or muscle action potentials induced by voluntary muscle contraction.

EMG has proved that there is very little spontaneous activity in skeletal muscles that are at rest. It has also shown that with minimal voluntary activity on the part of the individual a few motor units discharge and, as voluntary activity is increased, more motor units are involved (Ganong, 1993). This is referred to as recruitment of motor units (Ganong, 1993).

HEALING OF TENDON AND MUSCLE TISSUE

Muscle tissue and tendon do not tolerate suturing well and tend to heal slower as compared to other body tissues. In addition, skeletal and cardiac muscle cells do not have the capability to divide but healing obviously takes place. This section will discuss the growth, regeneration, and healing of the three types of muscle tissue.

Healing of Tendon

Tendon surgery is generally scheduled due to a traumatic injury. This complicates the surgery for three reasons:

1. The wound is most likely dirty and therefore contaminated.
2. If the tendon is partially or totally ruptured, the ends will be frayed, making suturing difficult.
3. A tendon does not have much flexibility as far as stretching and, when injured, it is comparable to snapping a rubber band apart—both ends recoil.

Therefore, surgery must be performed as soon as possible to avoid atrophy of the tendon. But if the wound is contaminated, it will need to be thoroughly irrigated to avoid infection. Tendons heal slowly as it is, and an infection would further slow the healing process.

When a tendon is injured, the fibroblasts that are responsible for beginning the process of repair are derived from the peritendinous tissue and migrate to the injury site (Ethicon, 2002). The two ends initially heal by the development of scar tissue, and eventually that is replaced with new tendon fibers. The surgeon must achieve close approximation of the two ruptured ends of the tendon for good healing results.

The suture material chosen for repair must have the following characteristics:

1. It must be inert.
2. It must be strong to hold the tendon in place.
3. It must have little or no elasticity, because the tendon ends can separate due to the contraction and relaxation of a muscle.

The most popular type of suture material is stainless steel. It is the most inert of all suture materials so it is best used in the presence of infection, and it is strong and without elasticity so it will hold the tendon tissue in place. Other suture materials that can be used are polyester, polypropylene, and nylon.

The suture technique performed by the surgeon is just as important as the choice of suture material. The suture should be placed so as to cause the least interference possible with the surface of the tendon, since this is where the gliding mechanism is located (Ethicon, 2002). The tendon fibers are arranged in a longitudinal, parallel fashion, which challenges the secure placement of sutures and achieving good approximation. The figure-of-eight suturing technique is popular to keep sutures from slipping and cutting through the tendon, which would create additional trauma to the tissue.

Another suturing technique used for the repair of tendons, especially in the digits of the hand and foot, is the Bunnell technique. This involves placing sutures in a figure-of-eight fashion to approximate the ruptured ends. Next, the suture ends both above and below the incision site are brought out through the skin and tied over two polyethylene buttons that are placed on each end of the surgery site; this is referred to as pull-out suture. This maintains excellent tension on the tendon and once healing has occurred, the sutures can be withdrawn.

Healing of Muscle

As previously mentioned, muscle does not tolerate suturing. To avoid disrupting the blood supply and innervation by nerves, the goal of the surgeon is to open the muscle in the direction of its fibers. The surgeon avoids disrupting the nerve supply because if the muscle must be incised across the direction of its fibers, the patient will most likely experience increased pain. To achieve this goal, the surgeon will open the muscle either with the use of a knife and scissors, by splitting or separating the fibers of the muscle using their fingers (called blunt dissection), or by using retractors to separate the fibers (another method of blunt dissection). When muscle is opened in this manner it does not need to be sutured, since the fibers will naturally approximate. Instead, the fascia will be sutured (Ethicon, 2002).

If muscle must be sutured, the best types of suture are stainless steel and polypropylene. Both cause little to no tissue reaction, have excellent strength, have little to no elasticity, and can be used in the presence of infection. When either type is used the sutures may be palpable under the surface of the skin and cause irritation. To avoid this complication, the surgeon buries the knots in the fascia instead of the subcutaneous tissue.

Skeletal Muscle Regeneration

An important fact to remember in relation to the healing of muscles is that muscle cells do not regenerate. Muscle does not develop through mitosis or development of new cells, but myofibrils have the capability of regenerating. The development of new skeletal muscle fibers is derived from myosatellite cells that lie close to the skeletal muscle fibers (Cormack, 2001). The myosatellite cells are a source of new myoblasts, which fuse to form new skeletal muscle fibers when needed.

Smooth Muscle Regeneration

Smooth muscle, as compared to skeletal and cardiac muscle, has a much better ability to regenerate. Smooth muscle cells have the ability to regenerate through mitosis and subsequently increase in number. Additionally, new smooth muscle cells can be generated from **pericytes**. Pericytes are located in the endothelial layer of capillaries and venules; they lie wrapped around the endothelium (Cormack, 2001). These cells are incompletely differentiated and can divide by mitosis. An important role is the ability to produce smooth muscle cells when the blood vessels or connective tissue are injured due to trauma or surgical incision.

Cardiac Muscle Replacement

It should be mentioned that a response of all three types of muscle tissue to increased functional demands is enlargement or hypertrophy of the existing fibers. This is a normal reaction of the muscle to compensate for the additional load placed on the muscle. For example, many long-distance runners who train in high altitudes have cardiac hypertrophy, which allows the heart muscle to adapt to the intense training regimen of the athlete.

Cardiac muscle cells that die, such as during a cardiac arrest, are not replaced. Cardiac muscle cells do not have the ability to divide by mitosis and they are not associated with any type of cells that are comparable to myosatellite cells located in skeletal muscle or pericytes located in smooth muscle. If a portion of the myocardium is injured and dies, it is replaced by ineffective fibrous scar tissue that does not have the ability to contract. Therefore, if a person sustains a severe cardiac arrest and they survive, it is likely that a large portion of the myocardium has been destroyed and that they will experience complications and disability for the rest of their life.

SKELETAL MUSCLE GROUPS

This section contains a series of tables that address the locations, actions, origins and insertions, and nerve innervation of the major skeletal muscles of the body. A hint for remembering the names of muscles is that the name often describes the muscle. The name may describe the shape, location, action, number of attachments, or direction of the muscle fibers. For example, the deltoid muscle is named after the Greek *delta*, meaning triangle, since the muscle has that shape. Another example is the sternocleidomastoid muscle. When the name is broken down it indicates the three attachments of the muscle:

1. Sterno: sternum
2. Cleido: clavicle
3. Mastoid: mastoid process

A last example is the external oblique muscle. The name oblique indicates that the fibers of the muscle travel at an angle or in a slanting fashion, and external refers to the fact that it is an outer layer of muscle.

IMPLICATIONS FOR THE SURGICAL TECHNOLOGIST

Orthopedic surgery involves not only the bones of the body, but also the various muscles. Obviously, to repair a fractured bone or perform a total hip arthroplasty, the muscle must be incised to reach the bone(s). In addition to tendons, muscles do become injured, so the surgeon must have knowledge of each muscle in order to properly repair the injury. However, orthopedic surgeons are not the only individuals who must intimately know the muscles of the body. Every surgical specialty involves muscles: for instance, general surgery procedures involve muscles of the abdomen, neck, and chest; maxillofacial procedures involve muscles of the face; and gynecological procedures involve muscles of the lower abdomen and pelvis.

Consequently, in order to assist the surgeon, the surgical technologist should also be knowledgeable about the major muscles of the body, which will aid him or her with regard to the following:

1. What surgical instruments will be required
2. Position of patient
3. Draping of patient
4. Type of sutures to be used
5. Positioning of retractors during the surgical procedure
6. Identification of the nerve(s) that innervate a muscle(s)
7. Understanding the pathology affecting muscles

BOX 7-4

Torticollis

Torticollis is a neck deformity that involves the sternocleido-mastoid muscle of the neck. The muscle is shortened, causing the head to be tilted to one side and the chin rotated to the opposite side. Commonly referred to as wryneck, it is congenital or acquired.

Causes of congenital torticollis include malposition of the fetal head in utero, fibroma, prenatal injury, or interruption of the blood supply to the muscle. Treatment of the congenital type includes stretching, thereby lengthening the shortened muscle. Nonsurgical treatments include passive neck stretching and positioning the infant properly while sleeping, and active stretching exercises for the older child. Surgical correc-tion involves sectioning the muscle in order to lengthen it and is performed during the preschool years.

There are three types of acquired torticollis: acute, spasmodic, and hysterical. The acute form is caused by muscular damage, which is a result of an inflammatory disease such as tuberculosis or myositis, or trauma due to cervical spine injury that produces scar tissue causing a contracture. The spasmodic type is the result of rhythmic muscle spasms that are caused by an organic central nervous system disorder such as irritation of the nerve root by arthritis (Weinstock, Andrews, & Cray, 1998). Hysterical torticollis originates from a psychogenic origin when an individual does not want to control the neck muscles.

Case Study 2

A 6-year-old patient has been diagnosed with Becker's muscular dystrophy (MD). The parents have been told that patients with this type of MD live well into their 40s and 50s, since it is a progressively slow disease process.

1. Why do the muscles in a person with MD enlarge?

2. What are the three other types of MD and which one has the worst prognosis?

3. What surgical procedure is performed to examine the variations in the size of muscle and determine if fat and connective tissue deposits are occurring?

4. What is the cause of Becker's MD?

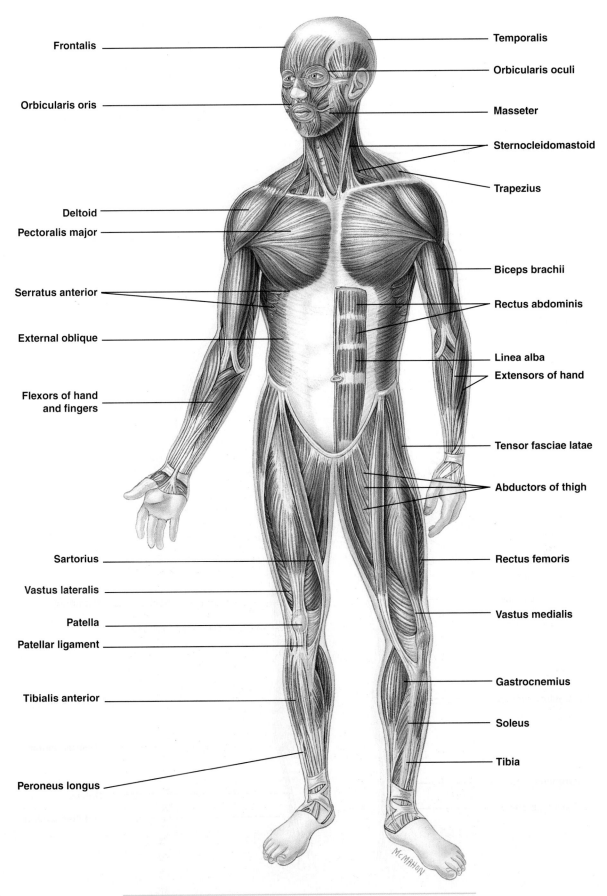

Frontalis

Orbicularis oris

Deltoid

Pectoralis major

Serratus anterior

External oblique

Flexors of hand
and fingers

Sartorius

Vastus lateralis

Patella

Patellar ligament

Tibialis anterior

Peroneus longus

Temporalis

Orbicularis oculi

Masseter

Sternocleidomastoid

Trapezius

Biceps brachii

Rectus abdominis

Linea alba

Extensors of hand

Tensor fasciae latae

Abductors of thigh

Rectus femoris

Vastus medialis

Gastrocnemius

Soleus

Tibia

**FIGURE 7-8 The superficial muscles of the body
(anterior view)**

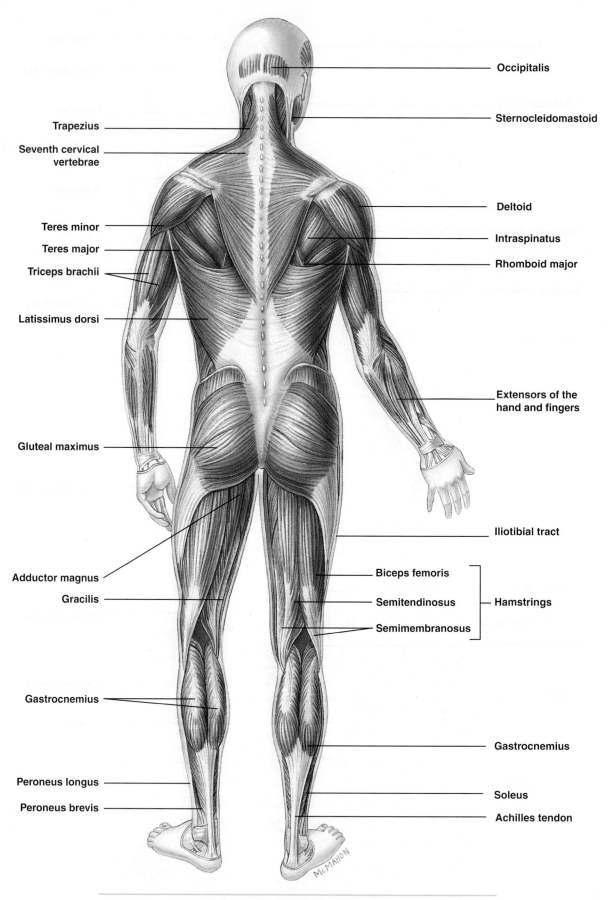

Occipitalis

Sternocleidomastoid

Trapezius

Seventh cervical
vertebrae

Deltoid

Teres minor

Intraspinatus

Teres major

Rhomboid major

Triceps brachii

Latissimus dorsi

Extensors of the
hand and fingers

Gluteal maximus

Iliotibial tract

Biceps femoris

Adductor magnus

Semitendinosus

Hamstrings

Gracilis

Semimembranosus

Gastrocnemius

Gastrocnemius

Peroneus longus

Soleus

Peroneus brevis

Achilles tendon

FIGURE 7-9   The superficial muscles of the body (posterior view)

TABLE 7-1 Muscles of Facial Expression

MUSCLE	ORIGIN	INSERTION	ACTIONS	INNERVATION
Buccinator (trumpet muscle)	Maxillae and mandible	Orbicularis oris	Smiling; blowing air out of the mouth as in playing a trumpet	Facial nerve
Corrugator supercilii	Frontal bone	Skin of eyebrow	Vertical wrinkles of the forehead	Facial nerve
Epicranius: consists of frontalis and occipital muscles (occipitofrontalis); muscles united by epicranial aponeurosis	Occipital bone	Tissues of eyebrows	Horizontal wrinkles of the forehead; raises eyebrows	Facial nerve
Orbicularis oculi (sphincter muscle that surrounds the eye)	Maxillary and frontal bones	Skin around eye	Closes or blinks the eye; compresses lacrimal gland to aid in flow of tears; contraction causes "crow's feet" to develop at lateral corners of eyes	Facial nerve
Orbicularis oris (kissing muscle and type of sphincter muscle that surrounds the mouth)	Muscles near the mouth	Skin of the lips	Closes and puckers lips	Facial nerve
Zygomaticus major	Zygomatic bone	Orbicularis oris	Raises angle of mouth as in laughing or smiling	Facial nerve
Platysma	Fascia of upper chest	Lower border of mandible	Draws angle of mouth downward as when pouting; aids in movement of mandible	Facial nerve

TABLE 7-2 Muscles of Mastication

MUSCLE	ORIGIN	INSERTION	ACTIONS	INNERVATION
Lateral pterygoid	Sphenoid bone	Anterior of mandibular condyle	Opens the mouth; pulls on mandible to make it protrude; moves mandible from side to side	Trigeminal nerve
Masseter	Zygomatic arch	Lateral external surface of mandible	Closes jaw	Trigeminal nerve
Medial pterygoid	Maxillary, sphenoid, and palatine bones	Medial external surface of mandible	Closes jaw; moves mandible from side to side	Trigeminal nerve
Temporalis	Temporal bone	Mandible	Closes jaw	Trigeminal nerve

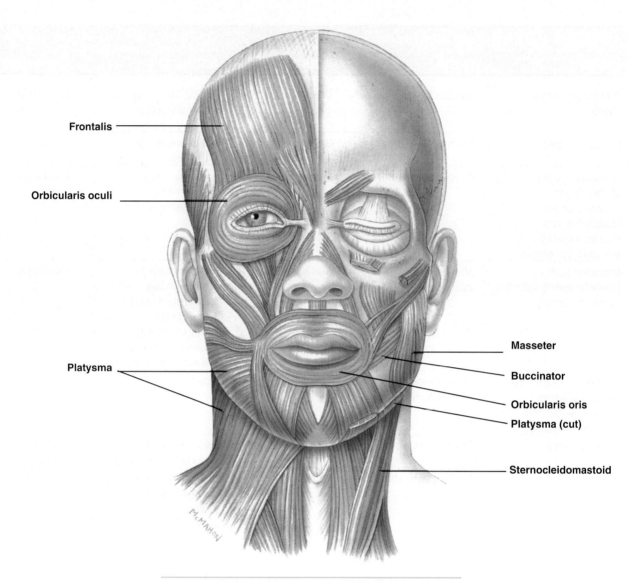

Frontalis

Orbicularis oculi

Platysma

Masseter

Buccinator

Orbicularis oris

Platysma (cut)

Sternocleidomastoid

McMAHON

FIGURE 7-10 Some muscles of the head and neck (anterior view)

TABLE 7-3 Muscles of the Head, Neck, and Vertebral Column

MUSCLE	ORIGIN	INSERTION	ACTIONS	INNERVATION
Sternocleidomastoid (prayer muscle)	Sternum and clavicle	Mastoid process of temporal bone	Flexes head; one muscle alone rotates head to one side	Accessory nerve
Semispinalis capitis	Processes of upper thoracic and lower cervical vertebrae	Occipital bone	Bends head to one side; extends neck and head; rotates head	First five cervical nerves
Splenius capitis	Spinous processes of lower cervical and upper thoracic vertebrae	Mastoid process of temporal bone and occipital bone	Connects base of skull to vertebrae in neck and upper thorax; extends head and neck; bends to same side as contracting muscle; rotates head	2nd–4th cervical nerves

(continues)

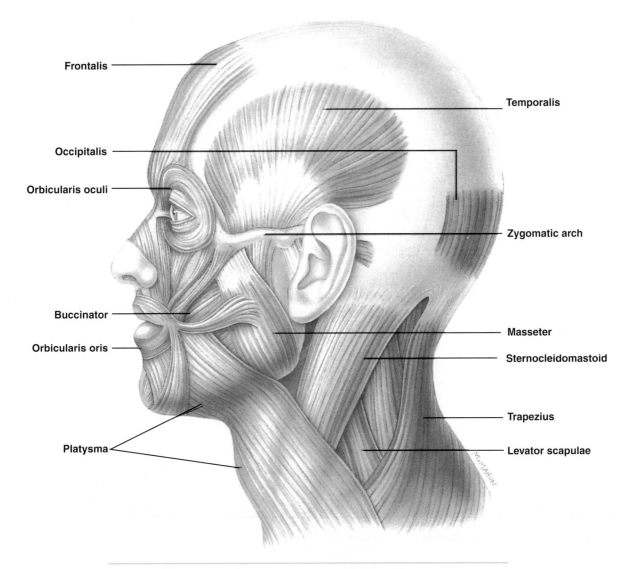

Frontalis

Temporalis

Occipitalis

Orbicularis oculi

Zygomatic arch

Buccinator

Masseter

Orbicularis oris

Sternocleidomastoid

Trapezius

Levator scapulae

Platysma

FIGURE 7-11   Some muscles of the head and neck (lateral view)

TABLE 7-3 Muscles of the Head, Neck, and Vertebral Column *(Continued)*				
MUSCLE	**ORIGIN**	**INSERTION**	**ACTIONS**	**INNERVATION**
ERECTOR SPINAE GROUPS				
Lateral group: *Iliocostalis group:*				
Iliocostalis lumborum	Iliac crest, spinous processes of lumbar vertebrae, posterior surface sacrum	Lower six ribs	Extends lumbar regions of vertebral column and spine	Lumbar spinal nerves
Iliocostalis dorsi	Lower six ribs	Upper six ribs	Maintains erect spine to aid in an erect posture of the trunk	Thoracic spinal nerves
Iliocostalis cervicis	Upper six ribs	4th–6th cervical vertebrae	Extends cervical region of vertebral column	Cervical spinal nerves

(continues)

TABLE 7-3 Muscles of the Head, Neck, and Vertebral Column *(Continued)*

MUSCLE	ORIGIN	INSERTION	ACTIONS	INNERVATION
Medial group: *Longissimus group:*				
Longissimus dorsi	Iliac crest, spinous processes of lumbar vertebrae, posterior surface sacrum	Thoracic and lumbar vertebrae; thoracic ribs	Extends thoracic portion of vertebral column	Spinal nerves
Longissimus cervicis	First thoracic vertebrae	2nd–6th cervical vertebrae	Extends cervical portion of vertebral column	Spinal nerves
Longissimus capitis	First six thoracic vertebrae and last four cervical vertebrae	Mastoid process of temporal bone	Rotates head toward contracting side of muscle; extends head	Cervical spinal nerves
Second medial group: *Spinalis group:*				
Spinalis dorsi	Upper lumbar and lower thoracic vertebrae	Upper thoracic vertebrae	Extends vertebral column and spine	Spinal nerves
Spinalis cervicis	Ligamentum nuchae, 5th and 6th cervical vertebrae	Spinous processes of the axis	Extends vertebral column and spine	Spinal nerves
Quadratus lumborum	Iliac crest and last three lumbar vertebrae	12th ribs and first four lumbar vertebrae	Extends spine; abducts trunk toward side of contracting muscle	First three lumbar nerves

TABLE 7-4 Muscles of the Shoulder Girdle

MUSCLE	ORIGIN	INSERTION	ACTIONS	INNERVATION
Trapezius	Occipital bone	Clavicle and acromion process of scapula	Raises and lower shoulders by raising the scapula, pulls scapula medially, moves scapula downward	Accessory nerve
Pectoralis minor	2nd–5th ribs	Coracoid process of scapula	Pulls shoulder down and forward by pulling on scapula; raises ribs to aid in forceful inhalation	Pectoral nerve
Levator scapulae	Transverse processes of C1–C4	Superior angle (medial margin) of scapula	Connects cervical vertebrae to scapula; elevates scapula and abducts neck	Dorsal scapular nerve
Serratus anterior	First eight or nine ribs	Anterior surface of scapula	Pulls shoulder down and forward by pulling scapula anteriorly and downward; abducts and rotates scapula upward	Long thoracic nerve
Rhomboideus major	T1–T4	Medial border of scapula	Connects upper thoracic vertebrae to scapula; adducts, rotates, raises, and fixes scapula	Dorsal scapular nerve
Rhomboideus minor	C6–C7	Medial border of scapula	Adducts, rotates, raises, and fixes scapula	Dorsal scapular nerve

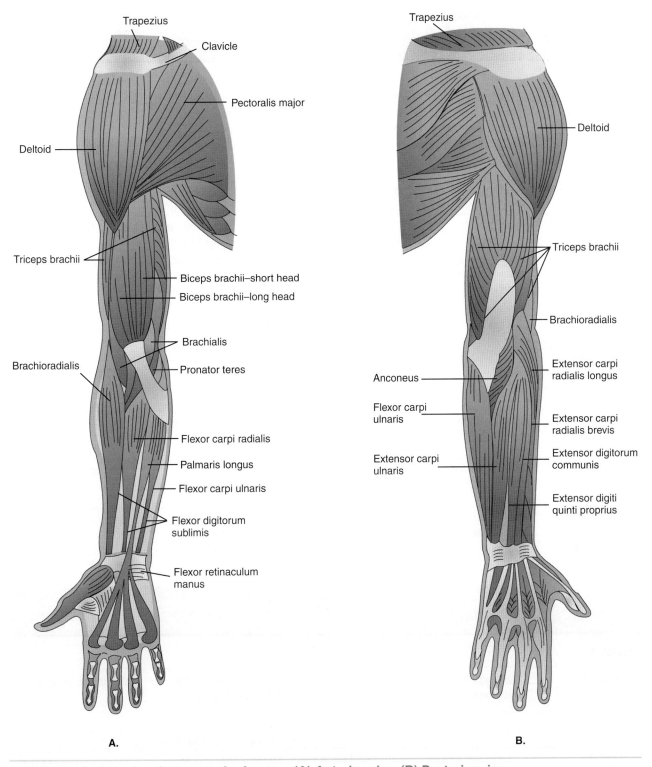

FIGURE 7-12   Muscles that move the forearm (A) Anterior view (B) Posterior view

TABLE 7-5 Muscles of the Upper Arm

MUSCLE	ORIGIN	INSERTION	ACTION	INNERVATION
Pectoral major	Clavicle, sternum, costal cartilages of true ribs	Greater tubercle of humerus	Flexes and adducts arm; draws arm across chest	Pectoral nerve
Latissimus dorsi	Spines of lower thoracic, lumbar, and sacral vertebrae; iliac crest	Intertubercular groove of humerus	Extends the arm; adducts the arm posteriorly; rotates arm medially. Used to pull arm back in climbing, rowing, swimming	Thoracodorsal nerve
Coracobrachialis	Coracoid process of scapula	Middle of humeral shaft, medial surface	Flexes and adducts arm; medial rotation of arm	Musculocutaneous nerve
Teres major	Axillary border of scapula	Proximal portion of humerus, anterior surface	Extends and adducts arm; medial rotation of arm	Lower subscapular nerve
Deltoid	Clavicle; spine and acromion process of scapula	Deltoid tubercle of humerus	Connects clavicle and scapula to lateral side of humerus; abducts arm; assists flexing and extending the arm	Axillary nerve
ROTATOR CUFF GROUP				
Teres minor	Axillary border of scapula	Greater tubercle of humerus	Connects scapula to humerus; rotates arm laterally	Axillary nerve
Supraspinatus	Supraspinous fossa on posterior surface of scapula	Greater tubercle of humerus	Connects scapula to greater tubercle of humerus; abducts the arm	Suprascapular nerve
Subscapularis	Subscapular fossa on anterior surface of scapula	Lesser tubercle of humerus	Connects scapula to humerus; medial rotation of arm	Subscapular nerve
Infraspinatus	Posterior surface of scapula below the spine	Greater tubercle of humerus	Connects scapula to humerus; lateral rotation of arm	Suprascapular nerve

TABLE 7-6 Muscles of the Forearm

MUSCLE	ORIGIN	INSERTION	ACTIONS	INNERVATION
FLEXORS				
Biceps brachii	Supraglenoid tuberosity of scapula	Radial tuberosity	Connects scapula to the radius. Flexes forearm at elbow; rotates hand as in opening a doorknob; supinates forearm and hand	Musculocutaneous nerve
Brachialis	Distal half, anterior surface of humerus	Coronoid process of ulna	Connects shaft of humerus to ulna. Strongest flexor of elbow; flexes forearm at elbow	Musculocutaneous nerve
Brachioradialis	Superior to lateral epicondyle of humerus	Styloid process of radius	Connects humerus to radius. Flexes forearm at elbow; supinates forearm and hand	Radial nerve

(continues)

TABLE 7-6   Muscles of the Forearm *(Continued)*

MUSCLE	ORIGIN	INSERTION	ACTIONS	INNERVATION
EXTENSOR				
Triceps brachii	Tubercle inferior to glenoid cavity; medial and lateral surfaces of humerus	Olecranon process	Has three heads. Only muscle located on back of arm. Connects humerus and scapula to ulna; extends forearm at elbow; primary extensor of elbow	Radial nerve
SUPINATOR				
Supinator	Lateral epicondyle of humerus and upper portion of ulna	Lateral surface of proximal portion of radius	Supinates forearm	Radial nerve
PRONATORS				
Pronator teres	Medial epicondyle of humerus; ulnar coronoid process	Lateral surface of radius	Connects ends of humerus and ulna to the radius; pronates and flexes forearm	Median nerve
Pronator quadratus	Ulnar anterior surface, distal end	Radial anterior surface, distal end	Pronates forearm	Median nerve

TABLE 7-7   Muscles of the Wrist, Hand, and Fingers

MUSCLE	ORIGIN	INSERTION	ACTIONS	INNERVATION
FLEXORS				
Flexor carpi radialis	Medial epicondyle of humerus	Base of second metacarpal	Flexes and abducts hand at wrist; flexes forearm	Median nerve
Flexor carpi ulnaris	Medial epicondyle of humerus	Pisiform bone; metacarpals	Connects distal end of humerus and proximal end of ulna to carpal and metacarpal bones; flexes and adducts hand at wrist	Ulnar nerve
Palmaris longus	Medial epicondyle of humerus	Fascia of palm	Connects distal end of humerus to fascia of palm; flexes hand at wrist	Median nerve
Flexor digitorum profundus	Ulnar anterior surface	Bases of distal phalanges of fingers 2–5	Connects the ulna to the distal phalanges; flexes interphalangeal joints of fingers	Median and ulnar nerves
Flexor digitorum superficialis	Medial epicondyle of humerus, radius, coronoid process of ulna	Tendons of fingers	Flexes fingers	Median nerve
Flexor pollicis brevis	Flexor retinaculum	Proximal phalanx of thumb	Flexes thumb	Median and ulnar nerves
Lumbricales	Tendons of flexor digitorum profundus	2–5 phalanges	Flexes 2–5 proximal phalanges	Median and ulnar nerves

(continues)

TABLE 7-7 Muscles of the Wrist, Hand, and Fingers *(Continued)*

MUSCLE	ORIGIN	INSERTION	ACTIONS	INNERVATION
EXTENSORS				
Extensor carpi radialis longus	Distal end of humerus	Base of second metacarpal	Connects humerus to hand; extends and abducts hand at wrist	Radial nerve
Extensor carpi radialis brevis	Lateral epicondyle of humerus	Bases of 2nd and 3rd metacarpals	Extends and abducts hand at wrist	Radial nerve
Extensor carpi ulnaris	Lateral epicondyle of humerus; upper portion of ulna	Base of 5th metacarpal	Connects humerus to hand; extends and adducts hand at wrist	Radial nerve
Extensor digitorum	Lateral epicondyle of humerus	2–5 phalanges	Extends fingers	Radial nerve
Opponents pollicis	Trapezium	Metacarpal of thumb	Opposes thumb to fingers	Median nerve
Abductor pollicis brevis	Trapezium	Proximal phalanx of thumb	Abducts thumb	Median nerve
Adductor pollicis	Trapezoid, capitate, 2nd and 3rd metacarpals	Proximal phalanx of thumb	Adducts thumb	Ulnar nerve

TABLE 7-8 Muscles of the Abdomen

MUSCLE	ORIGIN	INSERTION	ACTIONS	INNERVATION
External oblique	Last eight ribs	Linea alba via aponeurosis; iliac crest and pubis via inguinal ligament	Compresses abdomen; rotates trunk laterally. Abdominal muscles are important in maintaining normal posture by pulling front of pelvis upward, thereby flattening the lumbar curve of the spine. The muscles also compress the abdominal cavity and aid in defecation, forced expiration, urination, vomiting, and childbirth. They are antagonists of diaphragm, relaxing when it contracts and vice versa.	7–12 intercostal nerves
Internal oblique	Iliac crest and inguinal ligament	Last three ribs, linea alba, crest of pubic bone	Same as external oblique	Last three intercostal nerves; iliohypogastric and ilioinguinal nerves
Transversus abdominis	Last six ribs, processes of lumbar vertebrae, iliac crest, inguinal ligament	Linea alba; crest of pubic bone	Same as external and internal obliques	Last five intercostal nerves; iliohypogastric and ilioinguinal nerves
Rectus abdominis	Symphysis pubis and crest of pubic bone	Costal cartilage of 5–7 ribs, xiphoid process	Same as other muscles; flexes vertebral column	Last six intercostal nerves

TABLE 7-9 Muscles of the Pelvic Floor

MUSCLE	ORIGIN	INSERTION	ACTIONS	INNERVATION
PELVIC DIAPHRAGM				
Levator ani	Spine of ischium and pubic bone	Coccyx	Sheet of muscles across the pelvic outlet. Connected at midline by ligament. Male: anteriorly separated by the urethra and anal canal; female: urethra, vagina, and anal canal. Forms floor of pelvic cavity to support pelvic organs	Pudendal nerve
External and internal anal sphincters (circular muscles)	Coccyx	Central tendon of median raphe	External anal sphincter consists of voluntary muscle and internal anal sphincter consists of involuntary muscle. Both work to close the anal canal	Pudendal and S4 nerves
Coccygeus	Ischial spine	Sacrum and coccyx	Aids levator ani in its actions	S4–S5 nerves
UROGENITAL DIAPHRAGM				
Ischiocavernosus	Ischium	Pubic arch	Compresses base of penis or clitoris	Pudendal nerve
Superficial Transversus perinei	Ischium	Central tendon	Supports pelvic floor	Pudendal nerve
Sphincter urethrae	Pubic ramus and ischium	Central tendon	Constricts and opens urethra	Pudendal nerve
Bulbospongiosus:				
Male	Bulb of penis	Perineum	Constricts urethra; erects penis	Pudendal nerve
Female	Perineum	Base of clitoris	Erects clitoris	

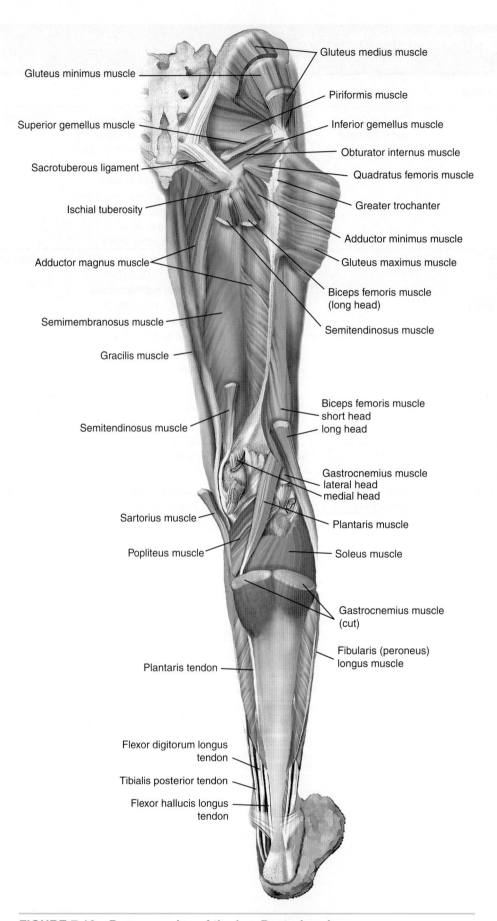

Gluteus medius muscle

Gluteus minimus muscle

Piriformis muscle

Superior gemellus muscle

Inferior gemellus muscle

Sacrotuberous ligament

Obturator internus muscle

Quadratus femoris muscle

Ischial tuberosity

Greater trochanter

Adductor minimus muscle

Adductor magnus muscle

Gluteus maximus muscle

Biceps femoris muscle
(long head)

Semimembranosus muscle

Semitendinosus muscle

Gracilis muscle

Biceps femoris muscle
short head
long head

Semitendinosus muscle

Gastrocnemius muscle
lateral head
medial head

Sartorius muscle

Plantaris muscle

Popliteus muscle

Soleus muscle

Gastrocnemius muscle
(cut)

Plantaris tendon

Fibularis (peroneus)
longus muscle

Flexor digitorum longus
tendon

Tibialis posterior tendon

Flexor hallucis longus
tendon

FIGURE 7-13 **Deep muscles of the leg, Posterior view**

TABLE 7-10   Muscles of the Leg

MUSCLE	ORIGIN	INSERTION	ACTIONS	INNERVATION
Iliopsoas (iliacus and psoas major)	Ilium; bodies of 12th thoracic to 5th lumbar	Lesser trochanter of femur	Flexes thigh	Femoral nerve; 2nd–4th lumbar nerves
ADDUCTOR GROUP				
Adductor brevis	Pubic bone	Femur	Adducts, flexes, and rotates thigh laterally	Obturator nerve
Adductor longus	Pubic bone	Femur	Adducts, flexes, and rotates thigh laterally	Obturator nerve
Adductor magnus	Ischial tuberosity	Femur	Adducts, extends, and rotates thigh laterally	Obturator nerve
Gracilis	Just inferior to symphysis pubis	Medial surface of tibia deep to sartorius	Adducts thigh and flexes leg	Obturator nerve
Pectineus	Spine of pubic bone	Femur, distal end to lesser trochanter	Adducts and flexes thigh	Obturator and femoral nerves
GLUTEAL GROUP				
Gluteus maximus	Crest and posterior surface of ilium; posterior surface of sacrum and coccyx	Femoral gluteal tuberosity; fascia of thigh (iliotibial tract)	Extends thigh at hip; rotates thigh laterally	Inferior gluteal nerve
Gluteus minimus	Lateral surface of ilium	Femoral greater trochanter	Abducts and rotates thigh medially; stabilizes pelvis on femur	Superior gluteal nerve
Gluteus medius	Lateral surface of ilium	Femoral greater trochanter	Abducts and rotates thigh medially; stabilizes pelvis on femur	Superior gluteal nerve
Piriformis	Sacrum	Medial aspect of femoral greater trochanter	Abducts, extends, and rotates thigh laterally	Second sacral nerve
Tensor fasciae latae	Anterior iliac crest	Iliotibial band	Abducts thigh	Superior gluteal nerve
QUADRICEPS FEMORIS GROUP				
Rectus femoris	Anterior and inferior iliac spine	Tibial tuberosity via patellar tendon	Flexes thigh	Femoral nerve
Vastus lateralis	Femoral greater trochanter	Tibial tuberosity via patellar tendon	Extends leg	Femoral nerve
Vastus medialis	Medial surface of femur	Tibial tuberosity via patellar tendon	Extends leg	Femoral nerve
Vastus intermedius	Anterior surface of femur	Tibial tuberosity via patellar tendon	Extends leg	Femoral nerve
Sartorius	Anterior and superior iliac spine	Medial surface of upper portion of tibia	Abducts and adducts leg; flexes leg; rotates thigh laterally; permits crossing of legs	Femoral nerve

(continues)

TABLE 7-10   Muscles of the Leg *(Continued)*

MUSCLE	ORIGIN	INSERTION	ACTIONS	INNERVATION
HAMSTRING GROUP				
Biceps femoris	Ischial tuberosity; linea aspera of femur	Head of fibula and lateral condyle of tibia	Flexes and rotates leg laterally; extends thigh	Hamstring nerve (branch of sciatic nerve)
Semitendinosus	Ischial tuberosity	Proximal end of tibia, medial surface	Flexes and rotates leg medially; extends thigh	Hamstring nerve
Semimembranosus	Ischial tuberosity	Tibial medial condyle	Flexes and rotates leg medially; extends thigh	Hamstring nerve

TABLE 7-11   Muscles of the Foot

MUSCLE	ORIGIN	INSERTION	ACTIONS	INNERVATION
Tibialis anterior	Tibial lateral condyle	Base of 1st metatarsal; cuneiform	Dorsiflexion and inversion of foot	Deep peroneal nerve
Peroneus tertius	Fibula	Bases of 4th and 5th metatarsals	Dorsiflexion and inversion of foot	Deep peroneal nerve
Extensor digitorum longus	Lateral condyle of tibia; anterior surface of fibula	2nd and 3rd phalanges of four lateral toes	Dorsiflexion and eversion of foot; extension of toes	Deep peroneal nerve
Gastrocnemius	Lateral and medial femoral condyles	Calcaneus via Achilles tendon	Plantar flexion of foot	Tibial nerve (branch of sciatic nerve)
Soleus	Fibular head and shaft; tibial posterior surface	Calcaneus via Achilles tendon	Plantar flexion of foot	Tibial nerve
Flexor digitorum longus	Tibial posterior surface	Distal phalanges of four lateral toes	Plantar flexion and inversion of foot; flexion of four lateral toes	Tibial nerve
Tibialis posterior	Tibial lateral condyle and posterior surface; fibular posterior surface	Tarsal and metatarsal bones	Plantar flexion and inversion of foot	Tibial nerve
Peroneus longus	Tibial lateral condyle; head and shaft of fibula	First cuneiform; base of 1st metatarsal	Plantar flexion and eversion of foot	Superficial peroneal nerve
Peroneus brevis	Fibular lateral surface	5th metatarsal	Plantar flexion and eversion of foot	Superficial peroneal nerve

CHAPTER SUMMARY

- Muscles give the body shape and work with the skeletal system to aid in body movement.

- The three types of muscle tissue are: skeletal, smooth, and cardiac.

- Skeletal muscles are also called voluntary muscles. They attach to bones and are consciously moved. Cells are long, narrow, and multinucleated, and the tissue is striated.

- Smooth muscles are also called involuntary muscles, since they are not under the control of the individual. The tissue is not striated, the cells are shorter and narrower as compared to skeletal muscle cells, and the cells are spindle-shaped with one centrally located nucleus. The muscle is found in the wall of the stomach, intestines, urinary bladder, blood vessels, and uterus. They function in churning food, pushing food forward through the intestines, emptying the urinary bladder, and constricting the arteries.

- Cardiac muscle tissue is the only muscle tissue in the body that has striations but is composed of smooth muscle. The cells form a network of branches that are joined end to end. The intercalated disk marks the junction where one cell joins another. The cells have only one nucleus. The muscle contracts and relaxes to pump the blood through the heart and into the blood vessels.

- Nerve impulses that generate from the frontal lobes of the cerebrum travel along motor nerves to the skeletal muscle fibers, stimulating them to contract.

- Muscle sense is the brain's ability to provide the individual with the unconscious sense of where the muscles and parts of the body are during movement.

- Stretch receptors work with the sensory receptors to sense the changes in the length of a muscle as it stretches. These sensory impulses travel to the brain where the impulses are interpreted, aiding in the person's unconscious sense of the body.

- The impulses from muscle sense are coordinated by the parietal lobes of the cerebrum and this is integrated with the unconscious muscle sense that is coordinated by the cerebellum.

- The origin is the end of the skeletal muscle that is attached to the immovable part of a bone. The insertion is the end of the muscle that is attached to the movable part of the bone.

- The action of every muscle when a joint is bent is that the insertion is pulled toward the origin.

- The muscle that does most of the work of flexing and contracting is referred to as the prime mover or agonist. It is the muscle primarily responsible for producing an action.

- Muscles that contract and assist the prime mover are called synergists.

- Antagonistic muscles resist the prime mover's action and work to cause action in the opposite direction.

- Fascia is a type of fibrous connective tissue. There are three types: deep, subcutaneous, and subserous. Deep fascia surrounds muscles to hold them together and provide support. Subcutaneous fascia is a continuous layer of connective tissue over the entire body located between the skin and deep fascia. Subserous fascia is located between the internal layer of the deep fascia and the serous membranes.

- Deep fascia forms fascial compartments, which are individual groups of muscles that contain nerves and blood vessels surrounded by fascia. A complication that can occur, called compartment syndrome, is the abnormal accumulation of fluid in a compartment. It is treated by performing the surgical procedure called fasciotomy.

- Tendons are a dense fibrous connective tissue that consists of parallel fibers kept together by the tenosynovium. The fibers of the tendon merge with the periosteum of bone to attach muscle to bone. Athletes and active individuals often experience tendonitis and tenosynovitis.

- Aponeuroses are a special type of fascia that binds muscle to muscle. An example is the aponeurosis of the external abdominal oblique muscle.

- Ligaments are a fibrous tissue consisting of parallel collagenous bundles that bind bone to bone to form joints.

- The epimysium is a connective tissue that surrounds skeletal muscles. Inward extensions of the epimysium are called the perimysium, which divides the muscle tissue into sections called fascicles. Each muscle fiber in the fascicle is surrounded by endomysium.

- A skeletal muscle fiber is actually a single muscle cell. Each fiber is covered by a membrane called the sarcolemma, which is electrically polarized, and underneath the sarcolemma is the sarcoplasm, which contains the nuclei and mitochondria. The muscle fiber is further broken down into myofibrils, which are composed of myofilaments.

- There are two kinds of myofilaments: myosin or thick filament, and actin or thin filament. The two filaments produce the striations in the skeletal and cardiac muscle. The myofibrils are further broken down into sarcomeres, the functioning unit of the myofibril.

- The striation pattern is broken down in the following manner. I band (light band) composed of actin myofilaments are attached to the Z lines, which are in the center of the I band. Sarcomeres occupy the region between the Z lines. The A band (dark band) consists of myosin filaments. The actin and myosin filaments overlap in the A band. In the center of the A band is the H zone, which consists of myosin filaments. In the center of the H zone is the M line, which consists of proteins that hold the myosin filaments in place. Connectin also holds the myosin filaments in place.

- Cross-bridges project outward from the myosin filaments toward the actin myofilaments, which contain a binding site for the cross-bridges to attach to.

- Actin myofilaments contain two proteins: tropomyosin and troposin. The two molecules regulate the actions of myosin and actin in muscle contractions.

- The sarcoplasmic reticulum (SR) is a complex system of tubules and sacs that surround each myofibril. The SR stores and releases calcium ions; therefore, it regulates the calcium ion concentration within myofibrils.

- Transverse tubules (T-tubules) are attached to the surface of the SR. They have openings to the surface of the skeletal muscle fiber and contain extracellular fluid. Each T-tubule is located between two transverse cisternae, which act as a reservoir for extracellular fluid. The T-tubules and cisternae are referred to as a triad and this marks the region where myosin and actin myofilaments overlap.

- The contraction and relaxation of muscle occur according to the sliding filament theory.

- When a muscle contracts the sarcomeres shorten, but the actin and myosin filaments do not change length. The filaments slide past one another. The I bands and H zones narrow, and the Z lines move closer together, shortening the sarcomere.

- Skeletal muscle fibers are innervated by motor neurons that extend from the spinal cord. The myoneural junction indicates the region where an axon touches a muscle fiber. The motor end plate is the membrane of the muscle fiber at this junction. There is only one motor end plate, but several branches of the axon allow the motor neuron to connect to several muscle fibers. The motor neuron and muscle fibers are called a motor unit.

- The synaptic cleft is the small area of space between an axon and motor end plate. The ends of the axons contain mitochondria and synaptic vesicles, which contain the neurotransmitters.

- Acetylcholine (ACh) is the primary neurotransmitter of motor neurons. ACh is synthesized in the cytoplasm of motor neurons and stored at the end of the axons in the synaptic vesicles. When an action potential travels to the end of an axon, the vesicles release ACh into the synaptic cleft and the ACh binds to the receptor sites of the motor end plate to stimulate the muscle fiber. The electrical muscle impulse causes the muscle cell membrane to transmit the impulse in all directions along the length of the muscle cell.

- The SR releases calcium ions that diffuse from the cisternae into the cytosol of the muscle fiber.

- The calcium ions bind to the troponin, change their conformation, and change the position of the tropomyosin, causing the cross-bridge linkages to form between the myosin cross-bridges and actin filaments.

- When the nerve impulses stop, relaxation begins. The ACh is broken down by acetylcholinesterase (AChE). The calcium pump causes the transfer of calcium ions back into the SR. The cross-bridge linkages break.

- ATP supplies the needed energy for the action of myosin and actin filaments. But ATP must be regenerated.

- Creatine phosphate regenerates ATP from ADP and phosphate. ATP is broken down to ADP, and the energy from creatine phosphate molecules transfers to the ADP molecules to convert them back to ATP. However, this is not sufficient to sustain a high level of muscle activity. Therefore, muscle fibers depend on cellular respiration of glucose as a source of ATP.

- The process of glycolysis is anaerobic and releases a few ATP molecules. The breakdown of glucose is aerobic and produces a large number of ATP molecules.

- The oxygen molecules released from hemoglobin supply the needed oxygen for aerobic respiration.

- Myoglobin is another pigment that provides oxygen to the muscles.

- When the muscles are active they switch to the anaerobic phase of cellular respiration to create energy and the outcome is anaerobic threshold.

- During anaerobic conditions, glucose is broken down into the end product lactic acid, which travels to the liver. The hepatocytes form glucose from lactic acid, which requires ATP. During active exercise oxygen is used to synthesize ATP for muscle contraction, not to synthesize ATP for converting lactic acid to glucose. Therefore, a person develops oxygen debt.

- Muscle fatigue develops due to the buildup of lactic acid in the muscle.

- A myogram is a recording of a contraction of a muscle.

- A single contraction is called a twitch.

- The latent period is the delay between the application of the stimulus to the muscle and the time the muscle contracted. The period of contraction is when the muscle pulls at its attachments and the period of relaxation is when the muscle assumes its normal length. If two rapid stimuli are transmitted to the muscle, it will twitch only in response to the first stimulus. The brief period the muscle cannot respond is called the refractory period.

- Tonus is a partial sustained contraction within the muscle fibers and is important in the body's ability to maintain a normal posture without fatigue.

- Slow-twitch fibers are type I and always oxidative.

- Fast-twitch fibers are type II and are either glycolytic or oxidative.

- Most of the muscles of the body are a combination of fiber types.

- Cells are shorter and have a single, centrally located nucleus. The cells are elongated and taper at both ends.

- Myofibrils contain actin and myosin and are randomly arranged.

- Smooth muscle fibers do not contain T-tubules and the SR is not well developed.

- There are two types of smooth muscles: multiunit and visceral. Visceral smooth muscle is the most common type located in the walls of hollow organs. There are two layers of visceral: the outer is longitudinal and the inner is circular, allowing the organ to change shape and size.

- Visceral smooth muscle consists of spindle-shaped cells that lie next to each other. This allows the visceral smooth muscle to respond as a single element when one fiber is stimulated by a nerve impulse, and it has a domino effect in that it stimulates the other fibers.

- Some visceral muscles can spontaneously repeat contractions, which is called rhythmicity.

- Together the domino effect and rhythmicity cause peristalsis.

- Multiunit smooth muscles are separate, independent units that work separately from each other.

- The contraction of smooth muscle is the same as skeletal muscle contraction in many ways but there are key differences. Smooth muscle fibers do not contain troponin, but use the protein called calmodulin. ACh along with norepinephrine is required by smooth muscle, and the two neurotransmitters either stimulate contraction in some smooth muscles or inhibit contraction in others. Hormones affect smooth muscle. The stretching of smooth muscle fibers stimulates contractions. Smooth muscle contracts and relaxes slower than skeletal muscle, but can sustain the contractions longer using the same amount of ATP as skeletal muscle.

- Cardiac muscle cells are arranged end to end to form fibers that are interconnected.

- Muscle cells have a centrally located single nucleus, and have actin and myosin filaments.

- The endomysium is located between the muscle fibers and is well supplied with capillaries and lymphatics.

- In cardiac muscle the T-tubules are well developed and the cells contain a large number of mitochondria. The T-tubules are wider than those in skeletal muscle and release a large amount of calcium ions into the SR when stimulated. The T-tubules lie at the Z line, not the A or I bands. Therefore, there is only one level of T-tubules per sarcomere.

- The SR in cardiac muscle has smaller compartments and cisternae are not present. The SR contains longitudinal sarcotubules that store calcium, but not as much as what skeletal muscle fiber can store.

- To compensate for less storage of calcium, the cardiac muscle cells rely on a supply of extracellular calcium ions. The contraction of the heart muscle relies on both extracellular and intracellular calcium ions. Calcium aids in controlling the strength of heart contractions and allows the cardiac muscle fibers to contract for a longer period as compared to skeletal muscle fibers.

- Cells are joined at each end by intercalated disks. This cellular connection allows for the rapid transfer of impulses from cell to cell causing the whole cardiac muscle to respond to the stimulation in an all-or-nothing manner.

- The contraction of the cardiac muscle is referred to as myogenic. The rate of contractions is controlled by the nerve impulses of the autonomic nervous system.

- ECG is used to record the rhythmic pattern of a person's heartbeat.

- EMG records the electric activity in a skeletal muscle and the recording is called an electromyogram. The data are used to aid in diagnosing neuromuscular pathologies.

- EMG is performed by applying electrodes to the skin or inserting a needle electrode intramuscularly.

- EMG also measures the muscle action potential induced by voluntary muscle contraction.

- EMG has shown that with minimal voluntary activity a few motor units discharge and, as the voluntary activity is increased, additional motor units are involved. This is called recruitment of motor units.

- Muscle tissue and tendon are slow healing and do not tolerate suturing well.

- Surgery is performed on tendon injuries as soon as possible to avoid atrophy of the tissue.

- Fibroblasts begin the process of repair when a tendon is injured. When the two ruptured ends of the tendon are approximated, initial healing is with scar tissue, which is eventually replaced with new tendon fibers.

- The most popular type of suture material for tendon repair is stainless steel. Other types include polyester, polypropylene, and nylon. Suturing technique is important to avoid interference with the gliding mechanism and keep sutures from slipping. The figure-of-eight and Bunnell techniques are often used.

- The goal is to incise muscle in the direction of its fibers to avoid disrupting the nerve and blood supply. The surgeon will incise the muscle with either sharp or blunt dissection.

- When opened in the direction of its fibers, muscle does not require suturing, only fascia does.

- The best type of suture to use if the muscle must be closed is stainless steel and polypropylene.

- Muscle cells do not regenerate, since they do not develop through mitosis. However, myofibrils can regenerate. Skeletal muscle fibers are derived from myosatellite cells, which are a source of myoblasts that fuse to form new skeletal muscle fibers.

- Smooth muscle cells have the ability to regenerate through mitosis. In addition, new smooth muscle cells are generated from pericytes.

- The response of all three types of muscle tissue to increased functional demands is enlargement or hypertrophy of the existing fibers.

- Cardiac muscle cells that die are not replaced, since they do not have the ability to develop by mitosis. Furthermore, there are no types of cells, such as the myosatellite cells, that can aid in regeneration. The affected portion of the myocardium is replaced with ineffective fibrous scar tissue, which does not have the ability to contract.

- Every surgical specialty must deal with the incision and healing of muscles.

- The surgical technologist must also have the general anatomic and physiologic knowledge of the major muscles of the body in order to assist the surgeon. This knowledge will aid the surgical technologist in properly preparing for the surgical procedure.

CRITICAL THINKING QUESTIONS

1. EMG and muscle biopsy are performed on a patient with muscular dystrophy. What will EMG demonstrate and what are the common findings of a muscle biopsy?
2. Why is it advantageous that the muscles of the iris of the eye are multiunit smooth muscles?
3. What two muscles combine to form the calf muscle?

4. When a surgeon is performing a hemorrhoidectomy, what nerve does she or he want to ensure is not damaged and why?

5. Achilles tendon contracture is a pathologic shortening of the Achilles tendon due to a congenital anomaly or muscular adjustment to a physical process, such as happens when joggers land on the balls of their feet instead of their heels. Some individuals will experience "foot drop" due to the contracture. What is foot drop? What muscles and nerve are affected?

REFERENCES

Cormack, D. H. (2001). *Essential histology* (2nd ed.). Philadelphia: Lippincott Williams & Wilkins.

Ethicon Products Worldwide. (2002). *Wound closure manual.* Somerville, NJ: Ethicon, Inc.

Ganong, W. F. (1993). *Review of medical physiology* (16th ed.). Norwalk, CT: Appleton & Lange.

Weinstock, D., Andrews, M., & Cray, J. V. (Eds.). (1998). *Professional guide to diseases* (6th ed.). Springhouse, PA: Springhouse Corporation.

8

NERVOUS SYSTEM

CHAPTER OUTLINE

CHAPTER OBJECTIVES

After completing the study of this chapter, you should be able to:

1. Describe the structure and function of the neuron.
2. Compare and contrast the divisions of the central nervous system.
3. Describe the relevant anatomy and physiology associated with structures of the brain and spinal cord.
4. Describe the blood supply of the brain.
5. Compare and contrast the various neoplasms of the central nervous system.

KEY TERMS

all-or-none response	cerebrum	microglial cells	repolarization
astrocytes	dendrite	multipolar neurons	resting potential
autonomic nervous system (ANS)	depolarization	myelin sheath	Schwann cells
axon	diencephalon	neuroglial cells	somatic nervous system (SNS)
basal ganglia	ependymal cells	neuron	synapse
bipolar neurons	gray matter	Nissl bodies	synaptic cleft
brainstem	hypothalamus	nodes of Ranvier	unipolar neurons
central nervous system (CNS)	limbic system	oligodendroglial cells	ventricles
cerebellum	membrane excitability	peripheral nervous system (PNS)	white matter
cerebral cortex	meninges	reflex	
	mesencephalon		

Case Study 1

Melissa is the on-call surgical technologist employed by St. David's General Hospital. She has been called out by the evening supervisor to clip a cerebral aneurysm on a patient who has recently sustained a subarachnoid hemorrhage.

1. What is a subarachnoid hemorrhage?

2. What is a cerebral aneurysm?

3. How will the aneurysm be approached and repaired?

4. How is this problem diagnosed?

INTRODUCTION

The nervous system is the body's control and communication center. It serves to organize incoming data into useful information that can be used for internal functions (homeostasis) and, by interpreting external dangers and initiating movement, physical activities necessary for survival ("fight or flight"). As the seat of reasoning, the brain generates thoughts for higher levels of behavior, and serves to control behaviors that are against preestablished social norms. This chapter will describe the major divisions of the nervous system, and the organs and accessories that comprise them.

BASIC STRUCTURE AND FUNCTION: THE NEURON

The high degree of organization of the central nervous system (CNS) is related to the types of cells that make up the system, and their many connections. The nerve cell (**neuron**) is designed to transmit various levels of information from one cell to another, modifying the message through amplification or dampening, depending on the urgency of the message. There are three main types of neuron, with further classifications described later:

- Sensory neurons (also called afferent neurons), which emerge from the sensory organs of the body (such as the skin) and transmit impulses back toward the brain or spinal cord
- Motor neurons (also called efferent neurons), which carry impulses away from the brain or spinal cord to the muscles and glands of the body
- Associative neurons (also called interneurons), which carry impulses from sensory neurons to motor neurons

The neuron shares many of the internal organelles of other body cells, with the exception of extensions of cytoplasm that receive incoming impulse information and sends information out of the cell again after processing (Figure 8-1). In addition, the neuron has an extensive rough endoplasmic reticulum (ER, see Chapter 2). This rough ER has attached ribosomes that are called **Nissl bodies**, or chromatophilic substances. These structures synthesize significant amounts of protein within the neuron.

The neuronal extension that receives information is called a **dendrite**, and cells may have several, one, or none according to their function. Dendrites are typically short and branched. The extension that transmits the impulse away from the cell is called the **axon**, and each cell has only one. Axons begin as slight enlargements of the cell body, called an axonal hillock. They tend to be long, and branch at their end in extensions called axon terminals, which make contact with the dendrites of other neurons.

Neurons with many dendrites and one axon are called **multipolar neurons**, and most of the neurons of the brain and spinal cord are of this type. Neurons with only one dendrite and one axon are called **bipolar neurons**, which function as receptor cells in special sense organs. Bipolar neurons are found only in the inner ear, the olfactory area of the nose, and the retina of the eye. Most sensory neurons are **unipolar**, meaning that they have only one extension from the cell body that branches to serve as both an axon (which enters the brain or spinal cord) and a peripheral dendrite (which connects to parts of the body).

The axon is covered by an insulating material called the neurilemma, also known as the **myelin sheath** (Figure 8-2). This sheath is similar in function to the insulating plastic of an electrical wire: it speeds up the electrical signal and prevents it from interacting with

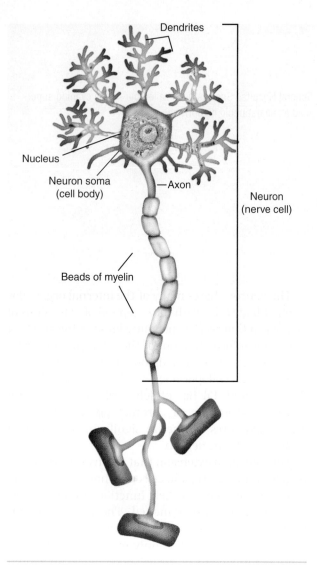

Dendrites

Nucleus

**Neuron soma
(cell body)**

Axon

**Neuron
(nerve cell)**

Beads of myelin

FIGURE 8-1   A neuron

TABLE 8-1	Types of Neuroglia
TYPE	**DESCRIPTION**
Astrocytes	Star-shaped cells that function in the blood–brain barrier to prevent toxic substances from entering the brain
Oligodendroglia	Provide support and connection
Microglia	Involved in the phagocytosis of unwanted substances
Ependymal cells	Form the lining of the cavities in the brain and spinal cord
Schwann cells	Located only in the peripheral nervous system and make up the neurilemma and myelin sheath

gaps allow ions to flow freely from extracellular fluid to the axons, assisting in the development of action potentials for nerve transmission (to be described in detail in subsequent text).

Neuroglial Cells

In addition to neurons, nervous tissue is also made up of another type of specialized cell called **neuroglial cells**. These cells do not transmit impulses like the neurons, but instead insulate, support, and protect the neurons.

Astrocytes are a type of neuroglial cell that is shaped like a star (hence the name). These cells serve as a part of the blood–brain barrier (described later), which helps to prevent certain substances from entering the brain. **Oligodendroglial cells** are shaped like smaller astrocytes, and provide support by forming rigid connections between neurons. These cells also produce myelin for insulation of the axons of the brain and spinal cord. **Microglial cells** protect the neurons through phagocytosis (engulfing and destroying foreign materials that can harm the cells).

other signals. The fatty substance that makes up the myelin sheath is produced by specialized structures called **Schwann cells** (also known as neurolemmocytes) that surround the axon at specific sites. Gaps in the myelin sheath are called **nodes of Ranvier**. These

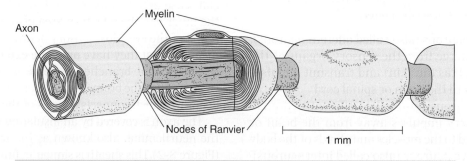

Axon

Myelin

Nodes of Ranvier

1 mm

FIGURE 8-2   A section of an axon from the peripheral nervous system with its myelin sheath, a fatty substance made by Schwann cells

Ciliated **ependymal cells** are designed to help move cerebrospinal fluid (CSF) through the CNS, whereas others are specialized to produce CSF within the walls of the ventricles. Schwann cells, described previously, produce protective myelin sheaths.

Cell Membrane Potential

Nerve cells generate electrical impulses through a process called **membrane excitability**. The membrane that separates the cytoplasm on the inside of the cell from the extracellular fluids on the outside of the cell separates two areas of different chemical composition. Positively charged sodium (Na^+) ions are in greater concentration outside of the cell. Positively charged potassium (K^+) ions are in greater concentration on the inside of the cell. In addition, the inside of the cell has negatively charged chloride (Cl^-) ions that give the cell an electrical component of a positive charge on the outside and a negative charge on the inside. This electrical component is called the **resting potential**, and in addition to simple diffusion of ions across the cell membrane, is maintained by a sodium–potassium pump located in the cell membrane that uses active transport to maintain the flow of ions across the membrane from higher to lower concentrations (Figure 8-3). This restores the cytoplasm and extracellular fluid to their original electrical state after an action potential occurs.

When a neuron is properly stimulated, the permeability to the Na^+ changes, and Na^+ ions rush across the membrane to the inside of the cell. This briefly causes the inside of the cell to become more positive than the outside (called **depolarization**). This brief change of charge is called the action potential, which moves in one direction down the nerve fiber in a self-propagating wave of depolarization.

Once the impulse is discharged, the K^+ ions that rushed into the cell are moved though the channel gates to the outside of the cell. This causes a **repolarization** of the membrane. After repolarization, the sodium–potassium pump begins to pump out the Na^+ ions that rushed across the cell membrane to the inside of the cell, and pull in the K^+ cells that rushed to the outside, thereby restoring the resting potential with a negative charge on the inside of the cell (Figure 8-4). The wave of depolarization down the length of the nerve fiber is followed immediately by a wave of repolarization. Once a sufficiently significant stimulus initiates an electrical response, the nerve impulse that is generated through depolarization never varies in strength. This is known as the **all-or-none response**.

Synapse

The **synapse** is an area between the terminal branches of an axon and the ends of a branched dendrite. The axon branch and the dendrite branch never actually touch one another, and the small space between the two is called the **synaptic cleft**. An electrical impulse traveling to the end of the axon causes chemical messengers called neurotransmitters to be released from synaptic vesicles in the terminal ends of the axons. These neurotransmitters (usually acetylcholine; the autonomic system utilizes epinephrine) travel across the synaptic cleft to the postsynaptic neuron, unlocking special gates (in a lock-and-key fashion) to accept the neurotransmitter and initiate another response. Once the transmission has been made, special enzymes within the synaptic cleft break down the neurotransmitter so that it does not unintentionally create a new transmission. Although there are many different neurotransmitters, the best understood are dopamine, serotonin, and the endorphins (in addition to those described in the preceding text).

Reflex Arcs

An involuntary reaction to an external response is called a **reflex**. If we place our hand on a hot stove, we recoil automatically. This reflex serves to protect us from injury by decreasing reaction time that would be required if we made a conscious decision that required interpretation by the brain. A reflex arc is the pathway that describes the reflex. Autonomic or somatic reflexes (as they are also called) involving skeletal muscles are controlled by the spinal cord. The reflex arc has the following components:

- a sensory receptor on the skin
- an afferent neuron
- associated neurons within the spinal cord
- an efferent neuron
- an effector organ (one that responds, such as a muscle)

The best known reflex is the one initiated by a reflex hammer to an area just below the knee (also known as the patellar tendon reflex). The blow from the hammer (stimulus) stimulates stretch receptors within the quadriceps femoris muscle. The impulse is transmitted via sensory neurons to the spinal cord, where it is interpreted. The impulse then travels to a motor neuron (the response) back to the muscle, which contracts and extends the leg involuntarily (Figure 8-5).

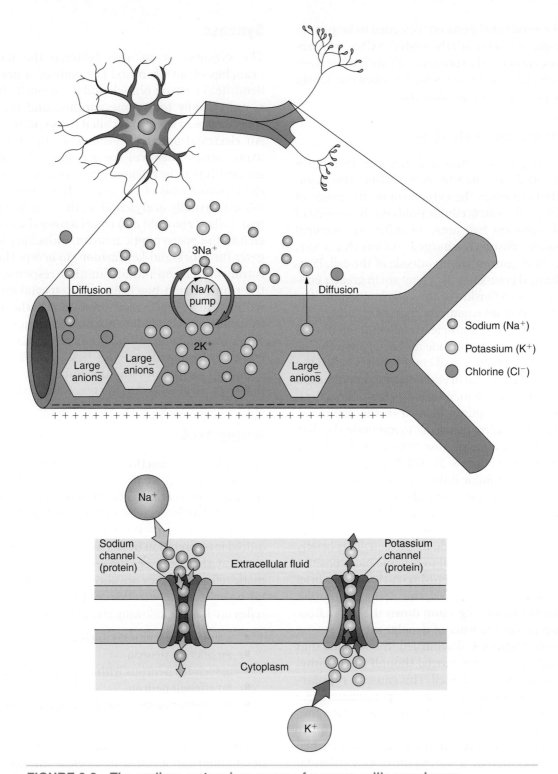

FIGURE 8-3 **The sodium–potassium pump of a nerve cell's membrane**

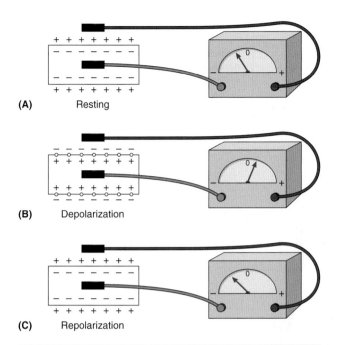

FIGURE 8-4   Sequence of events in membrane potential and relative positive and negative states: (A) Normal resting potential (negative inside, positive outside); (B) Depolarization (positive inside, negative outside); and (C) Repolarization (negative inside, positive outside)

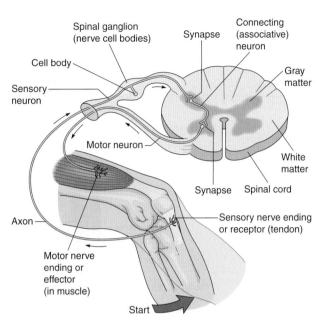

FIGURE 8-5   In this example, tapping the knee (patellar tendon) results in extension of the leg, producing the knee jerk reflex

Other well-known reflexes include coughing when choking occurs, sneezing to expel foreign particles from the nasal cavity, yawning to bring more oxygen into the body, and vomiting to expel toxic substances from the gastrointestinal tract.

DIVISIONS OF THE NERVOUS SYSTEM

The nervous system of the human body is divided into two systems: the **central nervous system (CNS)**, composed of the brain and spinal cord; and the **peripheral nervous system (PNS)**, composed of the nerves that link the various parts of the body to the CNS (Figure 8-6).

The PNS includes the cranial nerves, which originate from the brain, and the spinal nerves, which originate from the spinal cord. The primary functions of the nervous system are:

1. Sensory: The nervous system detects alterations of internal and external stimuli.
2. Integrative: Sensory information is analyzed and appropriate behaviors are selected in response.
3. Motor: The appropriate behaviors are implemented.

Divisions of the Peripheral Nervous System

The PNS can be divided into the **somatic nervous system (SNS)** and the **autonomic nervous system (ANS)**. The SNS connects the CNS to skin and skeletal muscles via the cranial and spinal nerves, initiating voluntary responses. The ANS connects the CNS to visceral organs via the cranial and spinal nerves, initiating involuntary responses. The ANS can be subdivided into the sympathetic and parasympathetic divisions. A sympathetic response prepares the body to deal with emergencies through the expenditure of energy (the "fight or flight" response), whereas a parasympathetic response restores homeostatic balance and conserves energy.

THE BRAIN

The human brain weighs slightly less than 3 pounds and is composed of approximately 100 billion neurons that communicate with each other through electrochemical pulses. These complex interactions are ultimately responsible for all human physical and mental functions.

Neurons are the same as other body cells except that they are specialized to gather and evaluate information from the internal and external environment, and then coordinate a response to that information.

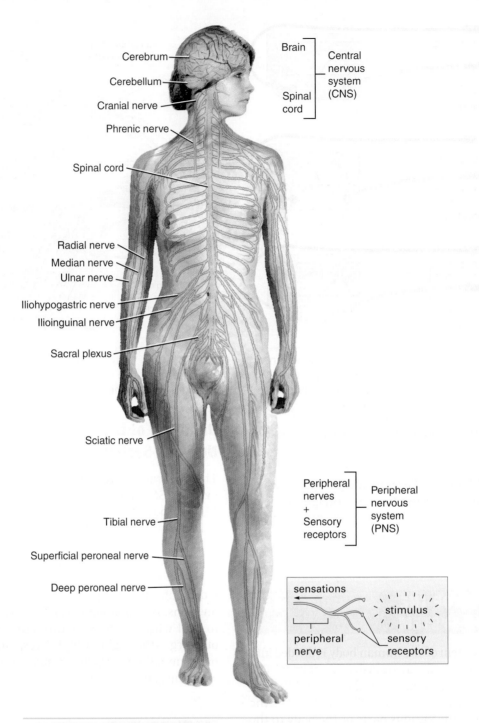

FIGURE 8-6 The peripheral nervous system connects the central nervous system to structures of the body

When sectioned, the brain reveals areas of white and gray contrast. The gray coloration, also known as **gray matter**, is a collection of large numbers of cell bodies. Examples of gray matter include the cerebral cortex on the surface of the brain and the basal ganglia deep within the brain. The white coloration, also known as **white matter**, is a collection of bundles of axons, covered in the protective sheath of myelin, leading away from the cell bodies through the brain. White matter consists of association fibers, which transmit impulses between specific locations in the same hemisphere; commissural fibers, which transmit impulses between specific locations between hemispheres; and projection fibers, which transmit information back and forth between the cerebrum and deeper brain structures and the spinal cord.

Meninges

Three layers of protective tissue called the **meninges** cover the brain and spinal cord. The outermost layer, referred to as dura mater, is composed of tough fibrous connective tissue. The dura mater extends between the cerebral hemispheres within the longitudinal fissure and is referred to as the falx cerebri. Dura mater also extends between the cerebellar hemispheres and is referred to as the falx cerebelli. The dural extension between the cerebrum and the cerebellum is called the tentorium cerebelli. In certain areas, the dura mater separates and creates channels for venous blood from cranial veins. These channels are called dural sinuses.

The dura mater of the spinal cord does not attach directly to the bones of the vertebrae, but creates a space between bone and dura called the epidural space. The middle meningeal layer is a thin, weblike membrane lacking blood vessels called the arachnoid mater.

The innermost layer is the pia mater; it contains blood vessels and nerves for the nourishment of the underlying neural tissue. The space created between the arachnoid mater and the pia mater is referred to as the subarachnoid space, an area that contains CSF (Figure 8-7).

Cerebral Cortex

The **cerebral cortex** is a layer of neurons on the surface of the brain that is approximately 2–4 mm thick. These neurons are specialized for specific functions, and are distributed across layers in the cortex. Approximately 25% of the cortical neurons are located in definite regions and are in charge of processing specific stimuli and motor responses. The great majority of cortical neurons, however, have associative properties; that is, they integrate information from various portions of the brain into cohesive patterns. For example, the association areas of the parietal lobe process somatosensory data from the skin, muscles, tendons, and joints with data related to body posture and movements. These stimuli are integrated with stimuli from hearing and visual brain centers, allowing a conscious thought to be formulated about precise body location. The cerebral cortex represents the most recent evolutionary addition to the CNS, and ultimately separates humans from lower mammals.

Cerebrum

The **cerebrum** represents the largest portion of the human brain. Its surface is covered with convolutions (gyri) that are separated by shallow depressions (sulci) and deep grooves (fissures). The cerebrum is divided into separate halves, or hemispheres, by a prominent central groove called the longitudinal fissure. The transverse fissure separates the cerebrum from the cerebellum.

Each hemisphere has important functional distinctions; for instance, the left hemisphere generally handles speech functions, whereas the right hemisphere

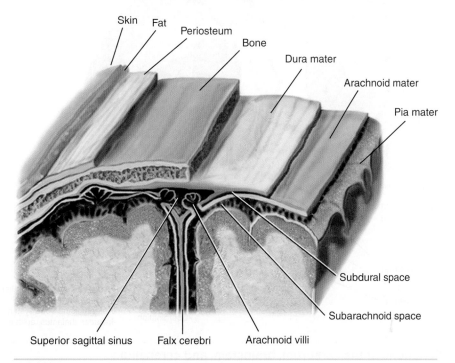

Skin   Fat   Periosteum   Bone   Dura mater   Arachnoid mater   Pia mater

Superior sagittal sinus   Falx cerebri   Arachnoid villi   Subdural space   Subarachnoid space

FIGURE 8-7   Meninges and related structures

deals with nonverbal, intuitive behaviors. Although the hemispheres share common functions of sensory integration and contralateral motor control, one hemisphere almost always "dominates" the other. For 90% of the population, the left hemisphere is the dominant hemisphere because it controls verbal, computational, and analytical skills (Figure 8-8).

The two hemispheres are connected by a thick bundle of commissural nerve fibers referred to as the corpus callosum and anterior and posterior commissures. These structures allow for communication between the brain halves.

The cerebrum is divided by sulci and fissures into specific lobes, each with complex functions and named for the cranial bone that covers it. The anterior portion of the cerebrum is called the frontal lobe. Its posterior boundary is the central sulcus, also known as the fissure of Rolando, and its lateral boundary is the lateral sulcus, or fissure of Sylvius. Just posterior to the frontal lobe is the parietal lobe, separated from the frontal lobe by the fissure of Rolando. The occipital lobe forms the posterior region of the cerebrum, and has no clear demarcation from

the parietal lobe. The temporal lobe lies just inferior to the frontal lobe and is separated from it and the parietal lobe by the fissure of Sylvius.

The association areas of the frontal lobes are responsible for the elaboration of thinking, planning, problem solving, and judgment of consequences of behavior. The motor areas of the frontal lobes, located in the precentral gyrus just anterior to the central sulcus, control voluntary muscle movements. The parietal lobes contain sensory areas, located in the postcentral gyrus just posterior to the central sulcus, which are responsible for the sensation of touch, proprioception, temperature, and pain. The association areas of the parietal lobes help to interpret sensory information, make sense of speech, and formulate words with emotional content. The sensory areas of the temporal lobes are primarily responsible for hearing, and the association areas are used to understand speech, read printed words, and recall visual memory and music.

The sensory areas of the occipital lobes are responsible for vision, and the association areas integrate visual patterns with other sensory stimuli.

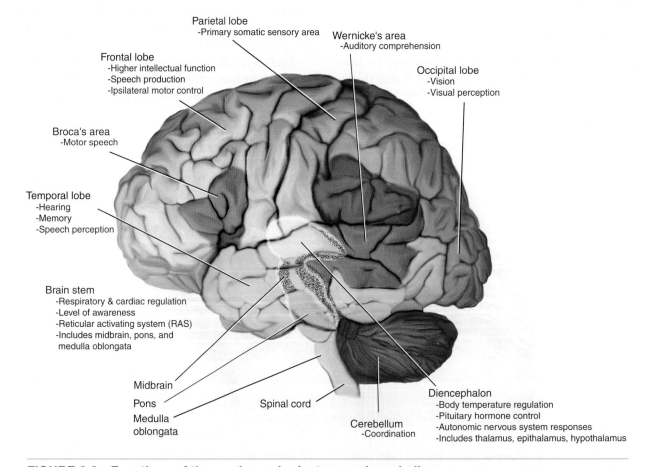

FIGURE 8-8 **Functions of the cerebrum, brainstem, and cerebellum**

Ventricles and Cerebrospinal Fluid

Within the brain are a series of interconnected canals and cavities called **ventricles**. The first two ventricles are referred to as the lateral ventricles (right and left). The two large ventricles, which are located in each cerebral hemisphere, connect to the smaller third ventricle, located between the halves of the thalamus, by way of the interventricular foramen (foramen of Monro). The third ventricle connects to the even smaller fourth ventricle, located in the brainstem anterior to the cerebellum, by way of the cerebral aqueduct (aqueduct of Sylvius). The fourth ventricle is continuous with the central canal of the spinal cord.

The ventricles are filled with a clear, colorless fluid containing small amounts of protein, glucose, lactic acid, urea, and potassium, as well as a relatively large amount of sodium chloride. The fluid, known as CSF, helps to support and cushion the brain and spinal cord, and stabilizes the ionic concentration of the CNS. It also acts to filter the waste products of metabolism and other substances that diffuse into the brain from blood.

Approximately 800 ml of CSF is produced each day by specialized capillaries that project from the medial walls of the lateral ventricles and the roofs of the third and fourth ventricles. These specialized capillaries are called choroid plexuses, and they create CSF by filtration of blood plasma. The lateral ventricles, however, produce the largest amount of CSF. From the lateral ventricles, CSF flows through the interventricular canal into the third ventricle. From the third ventricle, CSF flows through the aqueduct of Sylvius into the fourth ventricle, where a small portion enters the subarachnoid space through the fourth ventricular wall. CSF flows from the fourth ventricle into the central canal of the spinal cord and around the cord's surface, eventually surrounding the brain and spinal cord. The CSF is reabsorbed by fingerlike projections of the arachnoid that project into the dural sinuses called arachnoid villi. This reabsorption occurs at approximately the same rate that CSF is formed, allowing for a constant CSF pressure (Figure 8-9).

A blockage may occur in the narrow connections between the ventricles, and drainage of CSF into the

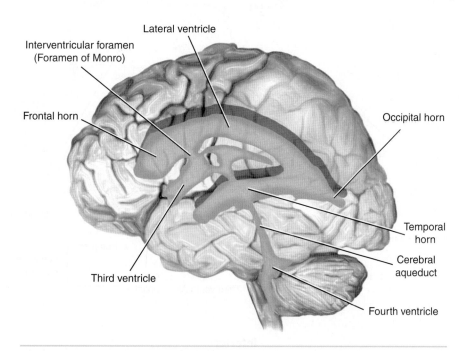

Lateral ventricle

Interventricular foramen
(Foramen of Monro)

Frontal horn

Occipital horn

Temporal horn

Cerebral aqueduct

Third ventricle

Fourth ventricle

FIGURE 8-9   Ventricular system

subarachnoid space may be impeded. The obstruction could be caused by a tumor, scarring due to inflammation, injury, subarachnoid hemorrhage, or a congenital abnormality.

As CSF is manufactured, it accumulates within the ventricles and causes the cavities to expand and compress nervous tissue. This condition is known as hydrocephalus. If hydrocephalus occurs in an infant whose fontanels have not yet closed, the cranium can grow to an extreme size.

Basal Ganglia

The **basal ganglia** are a collection of nuclei (gray matter) embedded deep within the white matter of the cerebral hemispheres. They act with the cerebellum to modify movement from moment to moment. The cerebellum and basal ganglia receive information that is sent out from the motor cortex, which is located in the precentral gyrus of the frontal lobes. The information is modified and sent back to the motor cortex via the thalamus (Figure 8-10).

The output of the cerebellum is excitatory, whereas the output of the basal ganglia is inhibitory. The balance between these three systems allows for smooth, coordinated movement.

The largest structure of the basal ganglia of the brain is the corpus striatum, which consists of the caudate nucleus and the lenticular nucleus. The

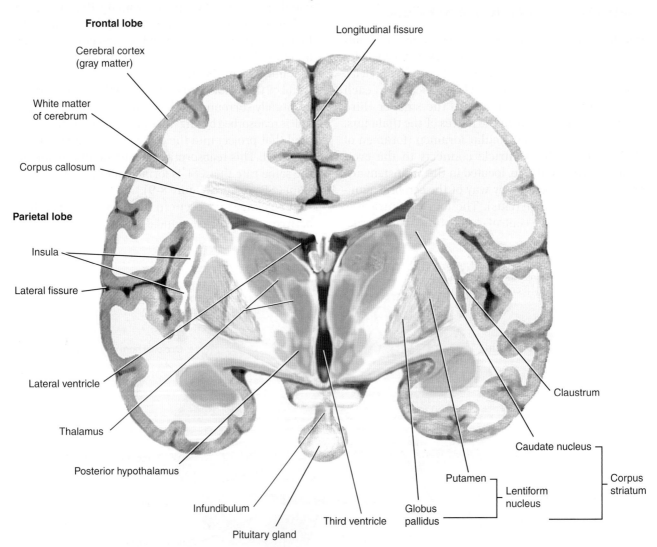

FIGURE 8-10   Frontal view of basal ganglia

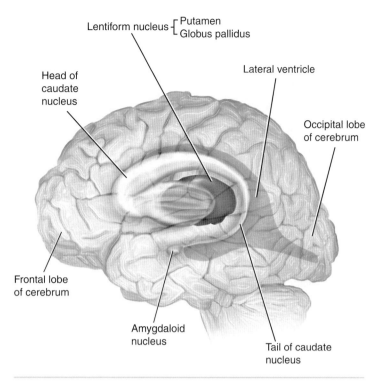

FIGURE 8-11   External view of the corpus striatum (caudate nucleus and lenticular nucleus)

lenticular nucleus is subdivided into the putamen and globus pallidus. Other structures of the basal ganglia include the substantia nigra and subthalamic nuclei (Figure 8-11).

Lesions within the basal ganglia produce disorders of movement. Typically, disorders fall into one of two categories: unwanted movements and difficulty with intended movements. Parkinson's disease is a result of the gradual loss of dopamine-producing nuclei within the substantia nigra. The three symptoms typically associated with Parkinson's are tremor at rest, rigidity (a result of the simultaneous contraction of extensors and flexors), and bradykinesia (the inability to initiate a movement).

Limbic System

The **limbic system** refers to a ring of gray matter nuclei on the inner border of the cerebrum that forms a border around the brainstem. The limbic system commands certain behaviors that are necessary for the survival of all mammals, such as the ability to distinguish between favorable or unfavorable outside stimuli, or the need to protect and care for offspring. The limbic system is also responsible for a portion of memory formation, emotional expression, and some aspects of personal identity.

The structures of the limbic system include the parahippocampal and cingulate gyri within the cerebral hemispheres, the hippocampus on the floor

BOX 8-2
Stereotactic Cranial Surgery

Stereotactic cranial surgery, used in conjunction with computed tomography, allows a probe to be guided to a specific location within the brain with minimal damage to normal neural tissue. Intracranial masses (e.g., tumor, hematoma, and abscess) and vascular malformations (arteriovenous malformations) can be successfully treated using stereotactic techniques. Biopsy of intracranial tumors for treatment planning has been the primary focus of this technique, but stereotactic techniques are currently being utilized for the surgical treatment of movement disorders such as Parkinson's disease.

Stereotactic surgery requires the placement of a rigid head-mounted frame, whose purpose is to provide a marker system during computer imaging, as well as a rigid platform for mounting instruments during surgery.

The marker set is visualized with the respective imaging modalities and provides a coordinate system within which targets appearing in the images may be localized.

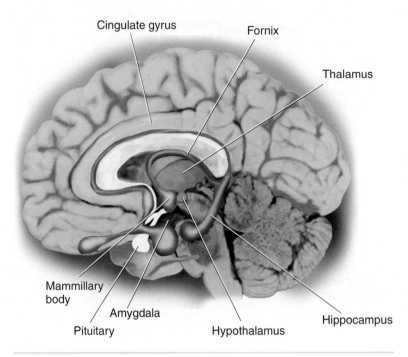

Cingulate gyrus

Fornix

Thalamus

Mammillary
body

Amygdala

Pituitary

Hypothalamus

Hippocampus

FIGURE 8-12   The limbic system

of the lateral ventricle, the dentate gyrus, the amygdala, the septal nuclei, the mammillary bodies, the anterior nucleus of the thalamus, and the olfactory bulbs (Figure 8-12).

Cerebellum

The **cerebellum** is the second-largest structure of the brain and is located posterior to the medulla oblongata and inferior to the cerebrum's occipital lobe. The cerebellum is separated from the cerebrum by the transverse fissure and the tentorium cerebelli. This structure acts to coordinate skeletal muscle movement by comparing input from the motor cortex of the frontal lobe with proprioceptive feedback from the extremities, and correcting any perceived problems. The cerebellum is also partly responsible for learning new motor tasks, such as throwing or catching a ball.

The structure of the cerebellum is similar to that of the cerebrum. Both consist of two hemispheres of approximately the same size. Both have convolutions (although the convolutions of the cerebellum are much smaller), an outer cortex of gray matter, inner white matter, and islands of gray matter nuclei within the white matter. Unlike the cerebrum, however, the cerebellum controls functions ipsilaterally.

The two hemispheres of the cerebellum are separated by a layer of dura mater called the falx cerebelli, and joined by a structure called the vermis. The cere-

bellum communicates with other structures of the CNS via the inferior, middle, and superior cerebellar peduncles. Input to the cerebellum is received via the spinocerebellar pathways, the inferior olive, and the pons, which transmits impulses from the cerebrum. The three deep nuclei of the cerebellum are the fastigial, interposed, and dentate nuclei. The dentate and interposed nuclei are concerned with voluntary movement; the fastigial nucleus is concerned with balance.

Diencephalon

The **diencephalon** is located between the midbrain and the cerebrum. It is composed of gray matter nuclei and surrounds the third ventricle. The primary structures of the diencephalon include the thalamus, hypothalamus, posterior pituitary gland, and pineal gland.

The thalamus acts as a relay station to the cerebral cortex for all sensory data from the cerebellum, brainstem, spinal cord, and other parts of the cerebrum. The thalamus decides which sensory data will make its way to the cortex for further action and interpretation, and then channels the data to the appropriate location. This structure of the diencephalon also produces a general awareness of the sensations of pain, touch, and temperature.

The **hypothalamus** is a collection of nuclei located just inferior to the thalamus. It regulates homeostasis of the body through coordination of activities of the ANS. It releases neurosecretory substances that stimulate the anterior pituitary gland to release hormones; therefore, the hypothalamus serves as a link between the endocrine system and the nervous system.

The hypothalamus also regulates emotional and behavioral patterns through connections with the limbic system. Other important functions of the hypothalamus include the following:

1. Glandular secretion control for the gastrointestinal tract
2. Wakefulness and arousal regulation
3. Control of water balance
4. Control of electrolyte balance
5. Hunger and thirst regulation
6. Regulation of body temperature
7. Regulation of heart rate and arterial blood pressure

Mesencephalon

The midbrain, or **mesencephalon**, is a section of the brainstem located between the diencephalon and the pons. It contains tracts of white matter and gray matter nuclei. The white matter tracts that connect the cerebral cortex with the pons, medulla, and spinal cord are called the cerebral peduncles. Other important structures of the midbrain include the following:

1. The superior cerebellar peduncles, which connect the mesencephalon with the cerebellum
2. The corpora quadrigemina, which serve as reflex centers for eye, head, and neck movement in response to visual stimuli, as well as movement of the head and trunk in response to auditory stimuli
3. The substantia nigra, which controls subconscious muscle movement (dopamine-producing neurons within this structure may degenerate, resulting in Parkinson's syndrome)
4. Red nuclei, which coordinate muscular movements in conjunction with the basal ganglia and cerebellum

Brainstem

The **brainstem** connects the diencephalon to the spinal cord and consists of the following:

1. The medulla oblongata, which forms the inferior portion of the brainstem, begins at the foramen magnum and ends at the inferior border of the pons. It contains all ascending and descending tracts (white matter) that connect the brain with the spinal cord. Five of the 12 cranial nerve nuclei are located in the medulla. The medulla also contains the nuclei responsible for breathing rhythm, heart rate, and blood pressure.
2. The pons, which lies superior to the medulla and anterior to the cerebellum, connects the brain with the spinal cord and other brain parts. The pons also contains the nuclei for 4 of the 12 cranial nerves, as well as nuclei that work with the medulla for the regulation of breathing.
3. The midbrain, located just inferior to the thalamus, contains a center for visual reflexes, such as movement of the head and eyes (Figure 8-13).

SPINAL CORD

The spinal cord is a column of nervous tissue that begins at the level of the foramen magnum and terminates at the level of the first and second lumbar disks. It runs within the vertebral canal of the vertebral column as a continuation of the medulla oblongata of the brainstem.

The spinal cord is protected by the same three meningeal coverings as the brain (dura, arachnoid, and pia mater). Its function is to conduct impulses and serve as a spinal reflex center.

When cross-sectioned, the cord reveals central areas of gray matter (shaped somewhat like a butterfly) surrounded by white matter. The anterior extensions (the wings of the butterfly) of gray matter are called the ventral horns, and the posterior extensions are called the dorsal horns. A bridge of gray matter called the gray commissure connects the left and right ventral and dorsal wings (Figure 8-14).

The white matter of the cord consists of longitudinal nerve tracts that are axons from cell bodies located throughout the CNS. The ascending nerve tracts carry information from the body to the brain, and the descending tracts carry information from the brain to the body.

At the level of the first lumbar vertebra, a collection of spinal roots descends from the inferior spinal cord, resembling the hairs of a horse's tail. These nerves are known collectively as the cauda equina.

BLOOD SUPPLY

The internal carotid artery, branching from the common carotid artery, provides the brain with most of its blood. It divides into the anterior cerebral artery,

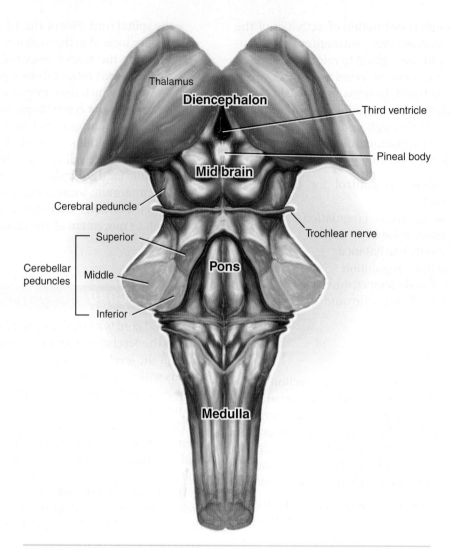

FIGURE 8-13   The brainstem

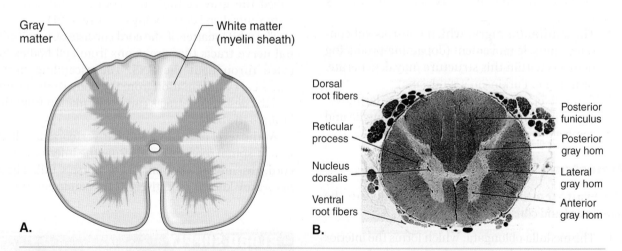

FIGURE 8-14   Cross sections of the spinal cord (B is from *Atlas of Microscopic Anatomy: A Functional Approach: Companion to Histology and Neuroanatomy* by R. Bergman, A. Afifi, and P. Heidger, 1999. www.vh.org/Providers/Textbooks/MicroscopicAnatomy.html. Reprinted with permission.)

which supplies blood to the medial surface of the cerebrum, and the middle cerebral artery, which supplies blood to the lateral surface of the cerebrum.

Posteriorly, the two vertebral arteries unite to form the single basilar artery, which divides to form the posterior cerebral arteries. The posterior cerebral arteries serve the occipital and temporal regions of the cerebrum.

The posterior cerebral arteries are connected to the internal carotid arteries by the posterior communicating arteries, forming the posterior portion of the circle of Willis. This circle is a ring of arteries that give rise to the various branches supplying blood to the brain. The anterior communicating artery connects the anterior cerebral arteries, forming the anterior portion of the circle (Figure 8-15).

The spinal cord receives its blood supply from the median anterior spinal artery, which arises from the vertebral arteries, and paired posterior spinal arteries from the posterior inferior cerebellar arteries. Below the cervical level, the cord receives additional blood from the radicular arteries, which branch from the intercostal and lumbar arteries. The cord is drained by the anterior and posterior spinal veins.

CRANIAL NERVES

There are 12 pairs of cranial nerves, and with the exception of the 1st and 2nd, all originate in the brainstem. They are designated by Roman numerals that indicate the order in which they arise from the brainstem (from the front to the back). The cranial nerves can be divided into sensory (originating in the lateral brainstem), motor (originating in the medial brainstem), or mixed nerves (both sensory and motor).

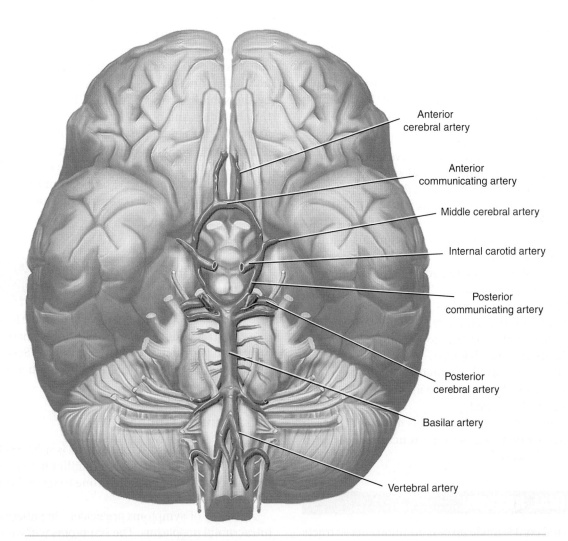

Anterior cerebral artery

Anterior communicating artery

Middle cerebral artery

Internal carotid artery

Posterior communicating artery

Posterior cerebral artery

Basilar artery

Vertebral artery

FIGURE 8-15   Circle of Willis

The nerves are described as follows:

I   Olfactory: entirely sensory; conveys impulses related to smell.

II   Optic: entirely sensory; conveys impulses related to sight.

III   Oculomotor: mixed; movement of levator palpebra superioris eyeball and upper lid; also conveys impulses about sense of position; its parasympathetic functions cause constriction of the pupil.

IV   Trochlear: mixed; movement of superior oblique eyeball; sensory: controls impulses related to muscle sense.

V   Trigeminal: mixed; has three branches called ophthalmic, maxillary, and mandibular, as follows:

  ▪ ophthalmic: sensory; sensation from skin in upper eyelid, eyeball, lacrimal glands, region above orbit, nasal cavity, side of nose, forehead

  ▪ maxillary: sensory; sensation from skin in mucosa of nose, portion of pharynx, upper region from orbit to lip, upper teeth, palate, mouth

  ▪ mandibular: mixed; sensory: sensation anterior two thirds of tongue, lower teeth; motor: chewing mandibular muscles, cheek

VI   Abducens: mixed; proprioception: lateral rectus muscle; motor: movement of eyeball.

VII   Facial: mixed; controls muscles for facial expression; conveys impulses related to taste; parasympathetic division controls tear and salivary glands.

VIII   Vestibulocochlear: sensory; controls equilibrium and hearing.

IX   Glossopharyngeal: mixed; controls swallowing and the sense of taste.

X   Vagus: mixed; controls skeletal muscle movements in the pharynx, larynx, and palate; parasympathetic functions control viscera in the thorax and abdomen.

XI   Accessory: mixed; originates from the brain and spinal cord; controls swallowing and movements of the head.

XII   Hypoglossal: mixed; controls muscles of speech and swallowing; sensory functions deal with muscle sense.

SPINAL NERVES

The spinal cord is made up of continuous nerve tracts and cell columns that can be divided into segments, each of which gives rise to a pair of spinal nerves. There are 31 of these spinal nerve roots: 8 cervical, 12 thoracic, 5 lumbar, 5 sacral, and 1 coccygeal. At each segment, a root arises from the dorsal and ventral portions of the spinal cord and combines into one spinal nerve that exits outward from the vertebral canal through the intervertebral foramen. The ventral root deals with motor stimuli from the brain to the body, and arises from the axons of the motor neurons within the ventral horn (gray matter) of the spinal cord. The dorsal root arises from the gray matter dorsal horn. It handles sensory information from the body and is easily identified by an enlarged portion of the root called the dorsal root ganglion.

With the exception of the thoracic nerves, branches of the spinal nerves unite to form networks that combine fibers from neighboring nerves. These networks are called plexuses. The primary plexuses are the cervical, brachial, lumbar, and sacral plexuses. The cervical plexus is formed on either side by the first four cervical nerves (C1–C4) with contributions from C5. These supply the skin and muscles of the head, neck, and top of the shoulders. Branches of the cervical plexus also combine with fibers from the 11th and 12th cranial nerves. The brachial plexus is formed by the spinal nerves C5–C8 and T1, and innervates the shoulders and upper limbs. The lumbar plexus is formed by the spinal nerves L1–L4. It innervates the anterolateral abdominal wall, external genitals, and portions of the lower extremities. The sacral plexus is formed by the spinal nerves L4–L5 and S1–S4 and innervates the buttocks, perineum, and lower extremities (Figure 8-16).

NEOPLASMS OF THE CENTRAL NERVOUS SYSTEM

The nervous system is vulnerable to damage from primary and secondary neoplasms. Primary neoplasms arise from neural tissues or the meninges. Secondary neoplasms are metastatic lesions from other parts of the body.

Intracranial Tumors

Although the cause of brain tumors is still largely unknown, some patients with a familial history of tumors are known to be more prone to several types of intracranial tumors.

A variety of symptoms are evident in patients with intracranial neoplasms. The symptoms will vary with the size and location of the tumor. The following are

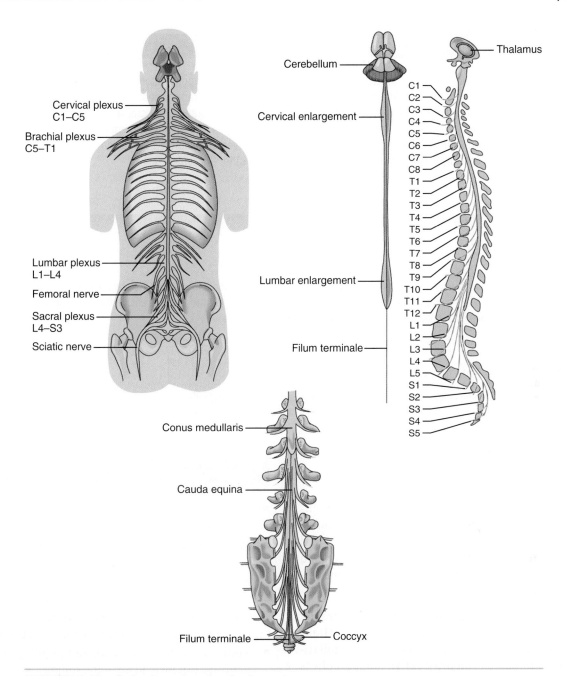

FIGURE 8-16   Spinal cord and spinal nerves

among the symptoms experienced by most patients with intracranial tumors:

1. Compression: Tumors on the surface of the brain compress the brain itself, as well as surrounding cranial nerves. Compression of these nerves will cause specific symptoms:

   - Optic nerve (II)—vision loss
   - Ocular muscle nerves (III, IV, VI)—loss of eye movement
   - Trigeminal nerve (V)—numbness in the face
   - Facial nerve (VII)—weakness in the face

   - Accessory nerve (XI)—loss of function in the trapezius muscle
   - Hypoglossal nerve (XII)—loss of movement of the tongue

2. Destruction: Tumors destroy brain tissue, and function in those parts of the brain is lost. This destruction of neural tissue may cause impairment, such as the loss of speech or comprehension (aphasia). Other symptoms may include loss of sensation, coordination, or mental abilities.

IMPLICATIONS FOR THE SURGICAL TECHNOLOGIST

An understanding of the anatomy and physiology of the nervous system is imperative for those who choose the neurosurgery specialty. As technology for the treatment of intracranial neoplasms and other anomalies increases, the understanding of functions of the CNS and the associated structures must increase accordingly. The surgical technologist will assist with surgical procedures of the head and spine, as well as various peripheral nerve procedures. Stereotactic procedures for treatment of intracranial neoplasm or movement disorders are becoming increasingly common, as are other minimally invasive techniques (such as endoscopes) for the same.

Case Study 2

Morris is a 51-year-old male who has been suffering from visual disturbances and ataxia. An MRI of the brain reveals hydrocephalus with a third ventricular mass of approximately 3 cm. The neurologist is certain that the mass is causing the hydrocephalus, and asks a neurosurgeon to evaluate the possibility of removal through a ventriculoscope.

1. What is hydrocephalus?

2. Why would a mass in the third ventricle cause hydrocephalus?

3. What is a ventriculoscope, and why is it the preferable treatment for this condition?

3. Irritation: Tumors may irritate the cerebral cortex, resulting in seizures.

4. Increased intracranial pressure: As tumors increase in mass, intracranial pressure increases. Symptoms include nausea, vomiting, and headaches. If intracranial pressure reaches a high enough level, the patient may become unconscious.

Tumors are diagnosed with computed tomography (CT) and magnetic resonance imaging (MRI). High-resolution MRI allows the detection of very small tumors (see Chapter 21, Figure 21-14). Radiography is still used because it shows bone erosion and tumor calcification. Cerebral angiography is used to show the vascularity of tumors and aids in determining the type of tumor.

Benign tumors can usually be excised totally through craniotomy. These tumors include craniopharyngiomas, epidermoids, dermoids, hemangiomas, meningiomas, acoustic neuromas, and pituitary microadenomas. Malignant tumors, such as the astrocytomas or gliomas, usually cannot be totally excised, but as much tumor as possible is removed. Glioblastoma multiforme tumors are excised when there is only one tumor, but not when there are multiple tumors or the patient has a short life expectancy.

CHAPTER SUMMARY

- The nervous system is the body's control and communication center.

- The nerve cell (neuron) is designed to transmit various levels of information from one cell to another.

- There are three main types of neuron, with further classifications described later: sensory neurons, motor neurons, and associative neurons.

- Neuroglial cells do not transmit impulses like the neurons, but instead insulate, support, and protect the neurons.

- Nerve cells generate electrical impulses through a process called membrane excitability.

- Na^+ ions are in greater concentration outside of the cell. K^+ ions are in greater concentration on the inside of the cell.

- The inside of the cell has negatively charged Cl^- ions that give the cell an electrical component of a positive charge on the outside and a negative charge on the inside (called the resting potential).

- The resting potential is maintained by a sodium—potassium pump located in the cell membrane that uses active transport to maintain the flow of ions across the membrane from higher to lower concentrations.

- When a neuron is properly stimulated, the permeability to the Na^+ changes, and Na^+ ions rush across the membrane to the inside of the cell. This briefly causes depolarization (called the action potential) that moves in one direction down the nerve fiber in a self-propagating wave of depolarization.

- Once the impulse is discharged, the K^+ ions that rushed into the cell are moved though the channel gates to the outside of the cell. This causes a repolarization of the membrane.

- After repolarization, the sodium—potassium pump begins to pump out the Na^+ ions that rushed across the cell membrane to the inside of the cell, and pull in the K^+ cells that rushed to the outside, thereby restoring the resting potential with a negative charge on the inside of the cell.

- The synapse is an area between the terminal branches of an axon and the ends of a branched dendrite.

- An electrical impulse traveling to the end of the axon causes chemical messengers called neurotransmitters to be released from synaptic vesicles in the axons' terminal ends.

- These neurotransmitters travel across the synaptic cleft to the postsynaptic neuron, unlocking special gates to accept the neurotransmitter and initiate another response.

- An involuntary reaction to an external response is called a reflex. It serves to protect us from injury by decreasing reaction time that would be required if we made a conscious decision that required interpretation by the brain.

- The nervous system of the human body is divided into two systems: the central nervous system (CNS), composed of the brain and spinal cord; and the peripheral nervous system (PNS), composed of the nerves that link the various parts of the body to the CNS.

- The PNS includes the cranial nerves, which originate from the brain, and the spinal nerves, which originate from the spinal cord. The primary functions of the nervous system are: (a) sensory—the nervous system detects alterations of internal and external stimuli; (b) integrative—sensory information is analyzed and appropriate behaviors are selected in response; and (c) motor—the appropriate behaviors are implemented.

- The PNS can be divided into the somatic nervous system (SNS) and the autonomic nervous system (ANS).

- The SNS connects the CNS to skin and skeletal muscles via the cranial and spinal nerves, initiating voluntary responses. The ANS connects the CNS to visceral organs via the cranial and spinal nerves, initiating involuntary responses

- The ANS can be subdivided into the sympathetic and parasympathetic divisions.

- A sympathetic response prepares the body to deal with emergencies through the expenditure of energy (the "fight or flight" response), whereas a parasympathetic response restores homeostatic balance and conserves energy.

- The white coloration, also known as white matter, is a collection of bundles of axons, covered in the protective sheath of myelin, leading away from the cell bodies through the brain.

- Three layers of protective tissue called the meninges cover the brain and spinal cord: dura mater, arachnoid mater, and pia mater.

- The cerebral cortex is a layer of neurons on the surface of the brain that is approximately 2–4 mm thick. These neurons are specialized for specific functions and are distributed across layers in the cortex.

- The cerebrum represents the largest portion of the human brain. It is divided into separate hemispheres by a central groove called the longitudinal fissure.

- Within the brain are a series of interconnected canals and cavities called ventricles.

- The first two ventricles are referred to as the lateral ventricles and are located in each cerebral hemisphere. They connect to the smaller third ventricle by way of the interventricular foramen. The third ventricle connects to the even smaller fourth ventricle by way of the cerebral aqueduct. The fourth ventricle is continuous with the central canal of the spinal cord.

- The basal ganglia are a collection of nuclei embedded deep within the white matter of the cerebral hemispheres. They act with the cerebellum to modify movement from moment to moment.

- The limbic system commands certain behaviors necessary for the survival of all mammals, such as the ability to distinguish between favorable or unfavorable outside stimuli, or the need to protect and care for offspring.

- The cerebellum acts to coordinate skeletal muscle movement by comparing input from the motor cortex of the frontal lobe with proprioceptive feedback from the extremities, and correcting any perceived problems.

- The diencephalon (located between the midbrain and the cerebrum) is composed of the thalamus, hypothalamus, posterior pituitary gland, and pineal gland.

- The thalamus acts as a relay station to the cerebral cortex for all sensory data from the cerebellum, brainstem, spinal cord, and other parts of the cerebrum.

- The hypothalamus regulates homeostasis of the body through coordination of activities of the autonomic nervous system.

- The midbrain, or mesencephalon, is a section of the brainstem located between the diencephalon and the pons.

- The brainstem connects the diencephalon to the spinal cord and consists of the following: medulla oblongata, pons, and midbrain.

- The spinal cord is a column of nervous tissue that begins at the level of the foramen magnum and terminates at the level of the first and second lumbar disk.

- There are 12 pairs of cranial nerves, and with the exception of the 1st and 2nd, all originate in the brainstem: olfactory, optic, oculomotor, trochlear, trigeminal, abducens, facial, vestibulocochlear, glossopharyngeal, vagus, accessory, and hypoglossal.

- The spinal cord is made up of continuous nerve tracts and cell columns, which can be divided into segments, each of which gives rise to a pair of spinal nerves.

- There are 31 of these spinal nerve roots: 8 cervical, 12 thoracic, 5 lumbar, 5 sacral, and 1 coccygeal.

- The primary plexuses are the cervical, brachial, lumbar, and sacral plexuses.

CRITICAL THINKING QUESTIONS

1. Blood in the CSF removed by a lumbar puncture is usually indicative of what condition?
2. Stereotactic craniotomy is preferable to open craniotomy for what reasons?
3. Besides cervical laminectomy, describe another approach for removal of a ruptured cervical disk.
4. What would happen if the corpus callosum of the brain was severed?
5. In certain instances, a small artery may compress the trigeminal nerve, causing extreme pain in the areas of the face that this innervates. What procedure (and approach) can treat this condition?

BIBLIOGRAPHY

Adams, R. D., & Victor, M. (Eds.). (1993). *Principles of neurology* (5th ed.). New York: McGraw-Hill.

Allen, M. B., & Miller, R. H. (Eds.). (1995). *Essentials of neurosurgery: A guide to clinical practice.* New York: McGraw-Hill.

Anthony, C. P., & Thibodeau, G. A. (1979). *Textbook of anatomy and physiology* (10th ed.). St. Louis: C. V. Mosby.

Association of Surgical Technologies, Inc. (2004). *Surgical technology for the surgical technologist: A positive care approach* (2nd ed.). Clifton Park, NY: Thomson Delmar Learning.

Grabowski, S. R., & Tortora, G. J. (1996). *Principles of anatomy and physiology* (8th ed.). New York: Harper-Collins.

Hasselkus, B. R. (1974). Aging and the human nervous system. *American Journal of Occupational Therapy, 28*(1), 16–21.

Hole, J. W. (1987). *Human anatomy and physiology* (4th ed.). Dubuque, IA: W. C. Brown.

Kim, M. J. (1987). Physiologic responses in health and illness: An overview. *Annual Review of Nursing Research, 5,* 79–104.

O'Toole, M. (Ed.). (1997). *Miller–Keane encyclopedia & dictionary of medicine, nursing, and allied health* (5th ed.). Philadelphia: W. B. Saunders.

Sanders, T., & Scanlon, V. C. (1995). *Essentials of anatomy and physiology* (2nd ed.). Philadelphia: F. A. Davis.

Scott, A., & Fong, E. (2004). *Body structures and functions* (10th ed.). Clifton Park, NY: Thomson Delmar Learning.

Shepard, G. M. (1988). *Neurobiology* (2nd ed.). New York: Oxford University Press.

Solomon, E. P., Schmidt, R. R., & Adragna, P. J. (1990). *Human anatomy & physiology* (2nd ed.). Ft. Worth, TX: Saunders.

9

THE SENSES

CHAPTER OUTLINE

CHAPTER OBJECTIVES

After completing the study of this chapter, you should be able to:

1. Compare and contrast receptors and sensations.
2. Describe the anatomy and physiology associated with the sense of sight.
3. Describe the anatomy and physiology associated with the sense of hearing and equilibrium.
4. Describe the anatomy and physiology associated with the sense of taste.
5. Describe the anatomy and physiology associated with the sense of smell.

KEY TERMS

accommodation	eustachian tube	nyctalopia	rods
aqueous humor	Golgi tendon organs	optic chiasma	sclera
auricle	incus	Pacinian corpuscles	sensations
cerumen	iris	perception	sensory adaptation
chemoreceptors	labyrinths	photopigments	somatic senses
choroid coat	lens	photoreceptors	stapes
ciliary body	macula lutea	presbyopia	static equilibrium
cochlea	malleus	projection	stretch receptors
cones	Meissner's corpuscles	referred pain	taste buds
conjunctiva	muscle spindles	refraction	tympanic membrane
cornea	nociceptors	retina	vitreous humor
dynamic equilibrium			

INTRODUCTION

The special senses are the organs and accessories that are related to vision, hearing, taste, smell, and equilibrium. Changes in the environment stimulate sensory receptors to initiate impulses that travel along sensory pathways to specific and specialized areas for processing and interpretation.

RECEPTORS AND SENSATIONS

There are many different types of sensory receptors but they do have a few things in common. Each receptor is more sensitive (has a low threshold) to a specific kind of environmental change but is less sensitive to others. Based on their sensitivities, five general types of receptors are recognized:

1. Receptors sensitive to changes in chemical concentration are called **chemoreceptors**. The sensations of smell and taste fall into this category.
2. Pain receptors (**nociceptors**) detect tissue damage.
3. Receptors sensitive to temperature changes (thermoreceptors) respond to temperature differences.
4. Mechanoreceptors respond to changes in pressure or movement.
5. Photoreceptors in the eyes respond to light energy.

Sensations

Sensations are feelings that occur when the brain receives sensory impulses from the peripheral nervous system (PNS). The arriving impulses are relatively the same (electrical waves), so it is the brain's interpretation that makes them seem different and unique. The brain uses the information about the location of origin of the arriving impulse to brand the sensation, and the result depends primarily on the area of the cerebral cortex that accepts the impulse (these areas of the cortex are designed to interpret the sensory information; those reaching the temporal lobe are interpreted as "sounds," and those reaching the occipital lobe are interpreted as "sight"). **Perception**, then, is the conscious awareness of sensation after interpretation. Once interpreted and perceived, the sensation is stored as a local memory. The strength of recall depends on the intensity of the sensation.

At the same time the sensation is being formed, the brain uses a process called **projection** to send the sensation back to its point of origin so the person can pinpoint the area of stimulation. A burn on the hand is identified as just that, rather than a general pain "somewhere."

Sensory Adaptation

Persistent stimulation of receptors causes sensory impulses to be sent at decreasing rates until receptors fail to send impulses entirely. This process is called **sensory adaptation**, and unless there is a change in strength of the stimulus, no impulses are triggered. If you put your hand into a bowl of hot water, it seems unbearable at first, but becomes comfortable after a short period of time.

Receptors vary in degree of adaptation. Those associated with pressure, touch, and smell adapt quickly (after a short while, you adapt to a strong odor in a kitchen). Receptors that deal with pain and body position adapt much slower.

SOMATIC SENSES

Somatic senses are those that involve receptors associated with the skin, muscles, joints, and visceral organs. Those associated with changes occurring at the body surface are called exteroceptive senses, and include touch, pressure, and temperature. Those associated with changes occurring in body position as relayed by muscles and tendons are called proprioceptive sensations. Those associated with changes occurring in visceral organs (of the thorax and abdomen) are called visceroceptive senses.

Touch and Pressure Senses

Sensations of touch result from sensation of tactile receptors located in the skin of just beneath it. Sensations of pressure result from stimulation of receptors in deeper tissues. Each sensation is triggered by a degree of displacement of the tissues involved, and can be classified as crude or discriminative. Three types of receptors detect touch and pressure:

1. The free ends of sensory nerve fibers in the epithelial tissues are associated with both touch and pressure.
2. **Meissner's corpuscles** are egg-shaped receptors for discriminative touch (light touch). They are also utilized when a person wants to judge the texture of something. They are a mass of dendrites enclosed by connective tissue sheaths surrounding two or more nerve fibers. They are found in the dermal papillae of the skin, and are abundant in hairless areas that are very sensitive to touch (eyelids, lips, clitoris, tip of the penis, palm, fingertips, and soles).
3. **Pacinian corpuscles** are large structures of connective tissue and cells that detect deep pressure or vibrations. They are located in subcutaneous tissues, deep submucosal tissues (under mucous membranes), and serous membranes. They can be found around joints, tendons, and muscles; and in the mammary glands, external genitalia, and pancreas and urinary bladder.

Temperature Senses

Thermal sensations are perceptions of degrees of warmth and coolness (extreme heat or cold are experienced as pain). Temperature receptors include two groups of free nerve endings located in the skin: heat receptors and cold receptors. The heat receptors are sensitive to temperatures above 25°C (77°F), and become unresponsive above temperatures of 45°C (113°F, when pain receptors kick in and report the sensation of burning). Cold receptors respond to temperatures between 10°C (50°F) and 20°C (68°F). If temperatures are below 10°C, a freezing sensation is reported by pain receptors. Both heat and cold receptors adapt quickly.

Sense of Pain

Pain receptors consist of free nerve endings that are stimulated when tissues are damaged. They serve to protect the body by signaling damage and identifying changes that may cause long-term damage. For medical professionals, pain helps to diagnose specific diseases or malfunctions of the body. These receptors (called **nociceptors**) are widely distributed throughout the skin and internal tissues.

Tissue injury releases chemicals called prostaglandins and kinins that stimulate nociceptors. Pain persists after initial tissue injury because these chemicals linger and there is little to no adaptation for these types of receptors.

Pain impulses are processed in the gray matter of the dorsal horn of the spinal cord and conducted to the thalamus, hypothalamus, and cerebral cortex of the brain. A person becomes aware of pain when impulses reach the thalamus, but the cerebral cortex judges the intensity and location of the pain. Other areas of the brain regulate the flow of pain impulses from the spinal cord and can trigger the release of enkephalins and serotonin, which inhibit the release of pain impulses in the spinal cord. Endorphins (morphinelike chemicals) released in the brain provide natural pain control.

Pain can be either acute or chronic, depending on its speed of onset and duration. Acute pain occurs very rapidly, and is typically not felt in deeper tissues of the body. It is often described as a sharp or stabbing pain. Acute pain fibers are thin, myelinated fibers that carry impulses rapidly and cease when the stimulus stops.

Chronic pain has a slower onset, and builds slowly in intensity over a period of seconds or minutes. It is often described as burning, aching, or throbbing. Chronic pain fibers are thin, unmyelinated fibers that conduct impulses slowly and continue sending impulses long after the stimulus stops (Table 9-1).

Visceral pain receptors are the only receptors in the viscera that produce sensations. The response of pain receptors is quite different from those associated with surface tissues. Typically, localized stimulation of the viscera does not evoke much of a response, but widespread stimulation may elicit a strong response. Stretching of visceral tissues or a decrease in blood flow (accompanied by lower tissue oxygen concentration) elicits the most painful responses.

A characteristic of visceral pain is that it often seems to come from somewhere other than its actual

TABLE 9-1	Acute Versus Chronic Pain	
	ACUTE	**CHRONIC**
Time Span	Less than 6 months	More than 6 months
Location	Localized, associated with a specific injury, condition, or disease	Difficult to pinpoint
Characteristics	Often described as sharp, diminishes as healing occurs	Often described as dull, diffuse, and aching
Physiologic Signs	■ Elevated heart rate ■ Elevated BP ■ Elevated respirations ■ May be diaphoretic ■ Dilated pupils	■ Normal vital signs ■ Normal pupils ■ No diaphoresis ■ May have loss of weight
Behavioral Signs	■ Crying and moaning ■ Rubbing site ■ Guarding ■ Frowning ■ Grimacing ■ Complains of pain	■ Physical immobility ■ Hopelessness ■ Listlessness ■ Loss of libido ■ Exhaustion and fatigue ■ Complains of pain only when asked

origin. The most frequently cited example is the pain that radiates down the left arm during myocardial infarction. This is called **referred pain**, and it occurs because of common nerve pathways: the two areas are served by the same segment of the spinal cord (Figure 9-1). The left arm and the area of skin over the chest enter spinal cord segments T1–T5, and so pain from the heart is experienced in both of these areas simultaneously.

Stretch Receptors

Stretch receptors are proprioceptors that deal with sensations from the lengthening and stretching muscles. The two main types are Golgi tendon organs and muscle spindles.

Muscle spindles are located in muscles near the origin of the tendons that serve them. Each spindle is composed of 3–10 specialized muscle fibers called intrafusal muscle fibers, enclosed in a connective tissue sheath. The central region of the spindle has few or no actin or myosin filaments, but the ends do contain a few. Extrafusal muscle fibers are skeletal muscle fibers that surround the muscle spindle.

With no actin or myosin filaments, the central portion of the spindle cannot contract. But there are two types of afferent (sensory) fibers inside the spindle: Type Ia fibers are large, rapidly conducting fibers with dendrites that wrap around the central area of the

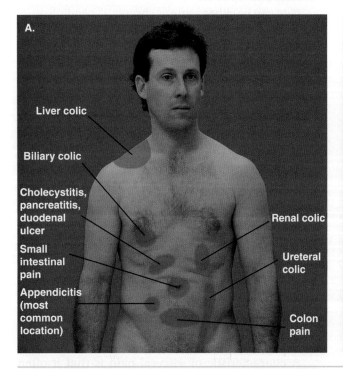

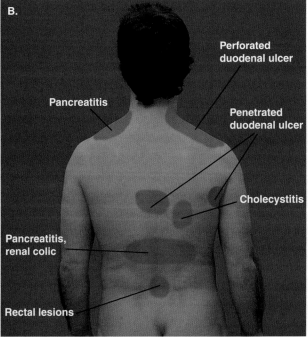

FIGURE 9-1   Areas of referred pain. (A) Anterior view (B) Posterior view

intrafusal fiber. When stretched, the spindle stimulates the dendrites, which send a nerve impulse toward the spinal cord. Type II fibers have dendrites located on either side of the type Ia dendrites. They also send impulses to the spinal cord when the central region of the spindle is stretched.

Muscle spindles respond to the rate and degree of length change in a skeletal muscle. The information is transmitted to the cerebrum via the spinal cord for perception of limb position, and to the cerebellum for coordination of muscle contraction.

Golgi tendon organs are found in tendons at the point of attachment to their respective muscles, and are stimulated by increased tension in the skeletal muscle. Sensory impulses from these receptors produce an inhibiting reflex for muscle contraction (the opposite of the stretch reflex). This tendency to inhibit contraction of the muscle helps to prevent the muscle from pulling away from its insertion point, and also helps to maintain posture.

SENSE OF SIGHT

The eye, protected by the skeletal orbit that encases it, is the primary organ of sight. Accessory organs, namely the lacrimal apparatus, eyelids, and extrinsic muscles, aid the eye in its function.

The upper and lower eyelids (palpebrae) are composed of four layers: skin, muscle tissue, connective tissue, and conjunctiva. The skin of the eyelid is the thinnest in the body. The eyelids protect the eye from foreign objects and excessive sunlight, shade the eyes during sleep, and lubricate the eye during blinking.

The orbicularis oculi muscle of the eyelid acts as a sphincter that contracts and closes the eyelid, while fibers of the levator palpebrae superioris muscle contract to raise the eyelid. The connective tissue of the eyelid helps to give it form, and secretes oily secretions from sebaceous glands (called tarsal glands) that keep the eyelids lubricated and prevent them from sticking together. An infection of this gland creates a growth on the eyelid called a chalazion.

The **conjunctiva** is a thin mucous membrane composed of stratified columnar epithelium. The palpebral conjunctiva lines the inner surface of the eyelids (where it is quite thick) and folds back to become the bulbar conjunctiva, which covers the anterior surface of the eyeball (where it is very thin). Infection of this mucous membrane causes a condition called conjunctivitis, also known as "pink eye." Because this structure is transparent, the vessels beneath it are clearly visible, and, when dilated, a person is said to have "bloodshot eyes."

The lacrimal apparatus is a group of structures designed to produce and drain lacrimal fluid (tears) from the eye. It consists of a lacrimal gland (about the size and shape of an almond) that secretes tears, and a series of excretory lacrimal ducts that carry the tears to the surface of the conjunctiva of the upper lid. From here, the tears pass medially over the surface of the eyeball where they enter two small openings called lacrimal puncta. They pass into two small ducts called lacrimal canals that lead to the nasolacrimal sac and nasolacrimal duct. From there they pass into the nasal cavity for drainage. This is the reason your nose runs when you cry. In addition to lubrication, tears contain an enzyme called lysozyme, which serves to protect the eye from bacteria and potential infection.

The extrinsic muscles of the eye arise from the bones of the orbit and attach to tendons that insert them into the sclera (the tough outer surface of the eyeball) (Figure 9-2). These six muscles move the eye in various directions (laterally, medially, superiorly, and inferiorly) through stimulation from the cranial nerves that supply them (III, IV, and VI). Movement in any direction requires coordination from each of the muscles (Table 9-2). When the muscle on one side contracts, the muscle (or muscles) on the other must relax. Because the motor units of these muscle fibers are small in size and number, they can be moved with great speed and precision.

Two check ligaments (the lateral and medial check ligaments) limit the movement of the lateral and medial rectus. The motor units of these eye muscles contain the smallest number of muscle fibers (5–10) of any muscle in the body. Because of this, the eyes move together so that they are aligned when looking at something.

Structure of the Eye

The eye is a fluid-filled hollow sphere with three distinct layers, or tunics (Figure 9-3): the outer tunic, the middle tunic, and the inner tunic.

The outer tunic is the transparent **cornea** at the front of the eye that serves as the window by focusing light rays that enter. It covers the colored iris. The cornea contains few cells and no blood vessels (hence its transparency) but does contain many nerve centers, which make it susceptible to pain sensations.

The cornea is continuous with the **sclera**, the tough, white portion of the eye. It provides protection,

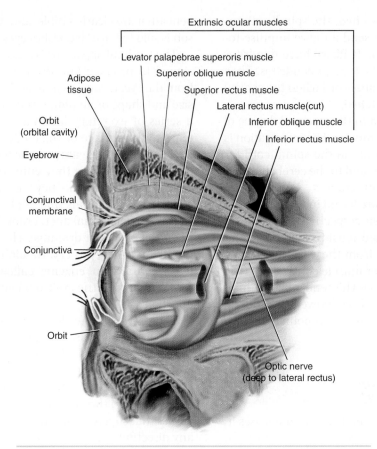

Extrinsic ocular muscles

Levator palapebrae superoris muscle
Superior oblique muscle
Superior rectus muscle
Lateral rectus muscle(cut)
Inferior oblique muscle
Inferior rectus muscle

Adipose tissue

Orbit (orbital cavity)

Eyebrow

Conjunctival membrane

Conjunctiva

Orbit

Optic nerve (deep to lateral rectus)

FIGURE 9-2 Extrinsic eye muscles

gives the eyeball its shape, and serves as an attachment site for the extrinsic muscles described previously. The back of the sclera receives the optic nerve and a few blood vessels, and attaches to the nerve's dura mater.

The middle tunic is also known as the vascular tunic and includes the choroid coat, the ciliary body, and the iris. The **choroid coat** is highly vascular, is the posterior portion of this tunic, and lines most of the internal portion of the sclera. The many vessels of the choroid provide nourishment to the posterior segment of the retina. It also contains melanocytes, which produce melanin and give it a dark brown color; this helps it to absorb excess light and keeps the inside of the eyeball dark.

The **ciliary body** is the thickest part of the middle tunic, extends forward from the choroid, and forms a ring around the front of the eye. The body consists of the ciliary processes (protrusions or folds on the interior surface of the body) and muscle. The ciliary muscle contracts and relaxes to alter the shape of the lens, depending on the amount of light that enters, for near or far vision.

The **lens** is a round, elastic, and transparent structure composed mostly of intercellular material and proteins called crystallins. The body of the lens lies directly behind the iris. Suspensory ligaments attached to its margins pull the lens outward, altering its normal globular shape to a more flattened one. When these ligaments are relaxed, the shape becomes rather convex (meaning that the lens surface bulges outward) to view things that are close to the face. This increase in the surface curvature is called **accommodation**. Accommodation through relaxation of the suspensory ligaments is a function of the ciliary

TABLE 9-2	Muscles of the Eye
MUSCLE	**EYE MOVEMENT**
Superior rectus	upward and toward the midline
Inferior rectus	downward and toward the midline
Medial rectus	toward the midline
Lateral rectus	away from midline
Superior oblique	downward and away from the midline
Inferior oblique	upward and away from the midline

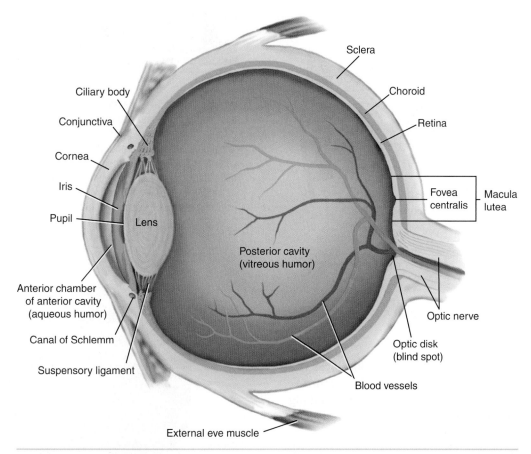

FIGURE 9-3   Internal view of the eye

muscles. When distant objects are viewed, the ciliary muscle is relaxed (and thus, the lens is flattened; the suspensory ligaments controlled by the ciliary muscle are taut in all directions). As people age, the lens loses some of its elasticity and accommodation suffers. This condition, called **presbyopia**, prevents viewing of objects at a close range and requires bifocals or magnifying glasses to see closer, smaller objects.

The **iris** is the colored portion of the eyeball. It is a thin diaphragm composed mostly of connective tissue and smooth muscle fibers, and lies between the cornea and the lens. It serves to divide the space between these two structures (called the anterior cavity, which is filled with aqueous humor) into the anterior chamber (between the cornea and the iris) and the posterior chamber (between the iris and the lens).

The second cavity (and the largest) of the eyeball is the posterior cavity. It lies between the lens and the retina and contains a jellylike substance called **vitreous humor**. This fluid contributes to intraocular pressure and allows the eyeball to maintain its shape (it keeps it from collapsing). The vitreous humor, unlike the aqueous humor, is not replenished: it is formed early in the womb and is never replaced.

The epithelium of the ciliary body secretes a watery substance called **aqueous humor** into the posterior chamber, where it passes through the pupil into the anterior chamber. There, it surrounds the cornea and lens and helps to maintain the shape of this portion of the eye. The fluid leaves the anterior chamber through the scleral venous sinus called the canal of Schlemm.

The iris has a circular and radial set of muscle fibers that constricts the pupil, meaning that it narrows the circular opening through the center of the iris that lets light through to the interior of the eye. The circular set of muscle fibers acts as a sphincter: when they contract, the pupil gets smaller and less light is allowed to enter. The radial set of muscle fibers contract to increase the diameter of the pupil, allowing more light to enter.

The inner tunic (also known as the nervous tunic) consists of the **retina**, a rather complex structure that contains the **photoreceptors** (visual receptor cells that are actually modified neurons) that senses the light entering the eye. This complex system of nerves sends impulses through the optic nerve back to the brain, which translates these messages into images that we see.

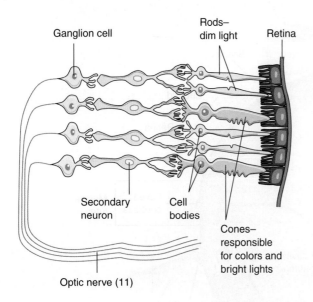

FIGURE 9-4 Diagram of visual neurons showing rods and cones

The retina has a pigmented epithelial layer that prevents light from being reflected back into the eye. It contains vitamin A for the synthesis of visual pigments (described in detail later). The sensory layer of the retina is made of photoreceptors.

There two types of photoreceptors: One group has long thin projections at their ends, and is therefore referred to as **rods**. The cells of the other group have short, blunt projections and are referred to as **cones**. Each retina has about 6 million cones and 120 million rods. Rods are important for seeing shades of gray in dim light, and for seeing general shapes or outlines. Cones provide color vision in bright light, and enable a person to see sharp images (Figure 9-4).

In the central region of the retina lies a yellowish spot called the **macula lutea**. Within the center of this structure lies a small depression called the central fovea. This region of the retina is the area of highest visual acuity, and contains only cones. Just medial to the fovea centralis is the optic disk. In this region, the nerves of the retina merge with the optic nerve. Because this region has no rods or cones, it is referred to as the eye's blind spot.

Photopigments

Both rods and cones contain light-sensitive **photopigments**: colored proteins that change their structure in response to the absorption of light and initiate the events that lead to the receptor potential. There are three different types of photopigments for cones; therefore, there are three different types of cones. The single pigment for rods is rhodopsin.

BOX 9-1

Retinal Detachment

When a tear occurs, the liquid in the vitreous cavity may pass through the tear and get under the retina, separating it from the back wall (choroid) of the eye. This separation is called a retinal detachment (Figure 9-5). Vision is lost wherever the retina becomes detached. A patient may notice a dark shadow, or a veil, coming from one side, above, or below. Eventually the entire retina will detach and all useful vision in the eye will be lost.

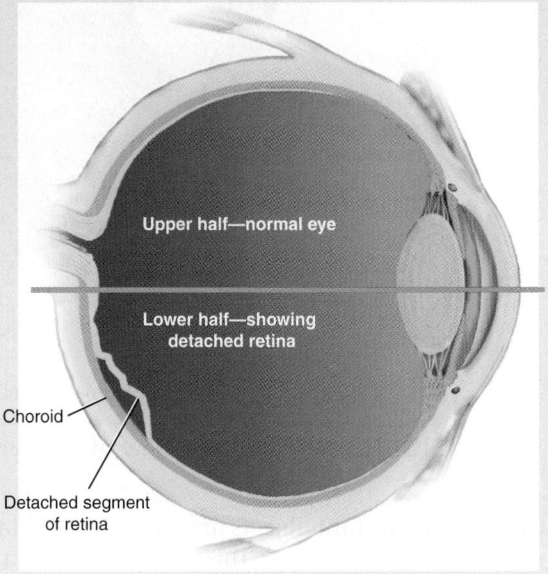

FIGURE 9-5 Retinal detachment

All visual photopigments contain two parts: opsin, a glycoprotein, and retinal, a derivative of vitamin A. The plant pigments called carotenoids (which give carrots their orange color) supply vitamin A, and good vision depends on an abundance of this nutrient. Deficiencies lead to poor night vision (**nyctalopia**) due to an inability to synthesize proper amounts of rhodopsin.

Retinal is the light-absorbing portion of all the visual photopigments. There are four different opsins, one for each cone photopigment and one for rhodopsin. Rhodopsin absorbs blue to green light effectively, whereas the three cone photopigments absorb blue, green, or yellow-orange light.

Rhodopsin breaks down into proteins called scotopsin and retinene (which is synthesized from vitamin A) when light strikes it. As these proteins degenerate, the permeability of the rod cell membrane alters and a potential is generated. The strength of the potential is related to the intensity of the light that strikes the photoreceptors, and the stimulus spreads to adjacent neurons in the retina, which transmit the action potential to the brain for processing.

Visual Pathways

As the axons of the ganglion cells of the retina leave the eye, they converge to form the large optic (II) nerve. These nerves eventually cross at the base of the brain (just in front of the pituitary gland) in a formation referred to as the **optic chiasma**. Some of the nerve fibers cross over and transfer sides (those on the nasal side), whereas some stay on the same side (those on the temporal side).

The nerve fibers continue into the posterior portion of the thalamus of the brain, an area called the lateral geniculate body. From there, the fibers enter nerve tracts that "radiate" to the occipital lobe of the brain (hence their name, optic radiations). Some fibers continue from the lateral geniculate nucleus to the brainstem, where they contribute to simultaneous eye movements and control of visual reflexes.

Summary of Sight

Now that the anatomy of the eye and the functions of its components have been discussed, we can summarize the way that vision operates (Figure 9-6). The human eye functions somewhat like a camera;

that is, it receives and focuses light on a photosensitive receiver, the retina. The light rays are bent (called **refraction**) and brought to focus as they pass through the cornea and the lens. Refraction occurs when light waves pass at an oblique angle from a medium of one optical density (e.g., air) into a medium of another different optical density (the cornea of the eye). When light arrives to the eye, its waves are refracted by the convex surface of the cornea, then again by the convex surface of the lens, and then once more by the fluids in the chambers of the eye.

The shape of the lens can be changed by the action of the ciliary muscles so that clear images of objects at different distances (and of moving objects) are properly focused on the retina (although the image is upside down and reversed from left to right). Once an image is focused on the retina, stimulated photoreceptors alter the light signal into receptor potentials. This propagated wave eventually reaches specific areas of the brain for interpretation.

SENSE OF HEARING

The ear is a sense organ that is designed to pick up and amplify sound waves for eventual interpretation by the temporal lobe of the brain. The inner ear plays a pivotal role in the maintenance of equilibrium by sending messages to the cerebellum about the position of the head.

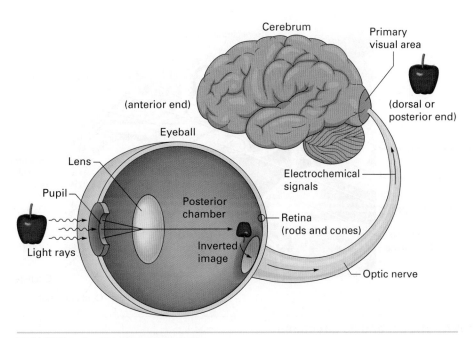

FIGURE 9-6   Pathway of vision

The ear has external, middle, and inner sections (Figure 9-7). The external ear consists of the pinna (auricle) and the external auditory canal (meatus). The **auricle** is the part of the ear that is visible on each side of the head. The pinna consists of flexible cartilage covered by thick skin.

The external auditory canal is shaped like an "S," and extends from the pinna to the **tympanic membrane**. It passes through the auditory meatus of the temporal bone. It collects the sound waves that travel down the external auditory meatus. It is covered with epithelium, and is lined with sebaceous or ceruminous glands that secret a waxlike substance called **cerumen** (earwax).

The middle ear (tympanic cavity) is a mucous membrane–lined, air-filled space located within the temporal bone that houses the auditory ossicles. The middle ear wall has two openings: the tympanic antrum opens posteriorly into the mastoid sinus, and the **eustachian tube**, or pharyngotympanic tube, connects the middle ear to the nasopharynx. The eustachian tube serves to equalize air pressure within the middle ear with that of the external atmosphere.

The middle ear houses three small bones called the auditory ossicles, designed to both transmit and amplify sound waves. They are named according to their shape: the **malleus** (hammer), **incus** (anvil), and **stapes** (stirrup). Each has movable synovial joints,

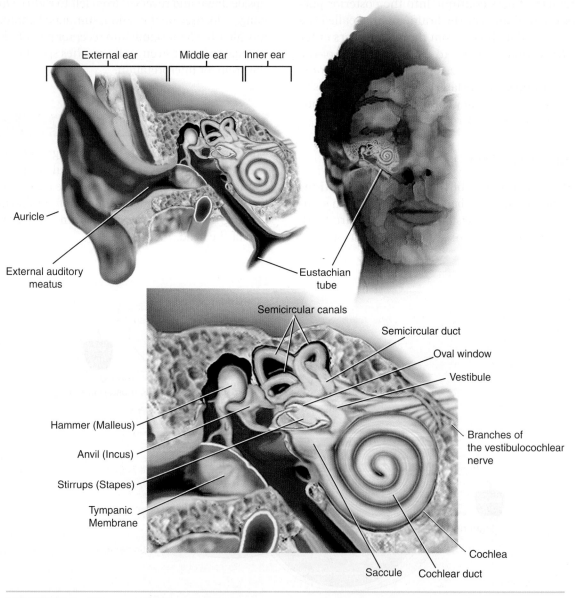

External ear   Middle ear   Inner ear

Auricle

External auditory
meatus

Eustachian
tube

Semicircular canals

Semicircular duct

Oval window

Vestibule

Hammer (Malleus)

Anvil (Incus)

Stirrups (Stapes)

Tympanic
Membrane

Branches of
the vestibulocochlear
nerve

Cochlea

Saccule   Cochlear duct

FIGURE 9-7   The ear and its structures

Otitis media is a very common acute inflammation of the middle ear, usually initiated by blockage of the eustachian tube causing an accumulation of fluid, which would normally be drained into the nasopharynx. The cardinal symptom of otitis media would be the patient's complaint of severe ear pain. The main sign of otitis media, observed by the clinician using the otoscope, is an inflamed, tense tympanic membrane (Figure 9-8). Generally, there is no permanent loss of hearing, if the condition is treated immediately with systemic antibiotics. Decongestants may also assist in opening the eustachian tube, thereby facilitating drainage of the middle ear cavity. The tympanic membrane may rupture spontaneously or may require surgical incision. This procedure is called myringotomy.

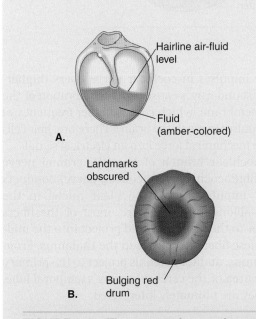

Hairline air-fluid level

Fluid (amber-colored)

A.

Landmarks obscured

Bulging red drum

B.

FIGURE 9-8   The tympanic membrane in the presence of otitis media. (A) Serous otitis media; (B) acute purulent otitis media. Hyperemic means there is increased blood within the vessels.

with ligaments that connect the ossicles to the wall of the middle ear. Small skeletal muscles control their movement.

The handle of the malleus is connected to the tympanic membrane, while its head articulates with the body of the incus. The incus, then, articulates with the

body of the stapes, which rests on the oval window of the inner ear (described later). When sound waves enter the external auditory canal, they stimulate the tympanic membrane to vibrate. The tympanic membrane then vibrates the malleus, which vibrates the incus and then the stapes. The stapes vibrates the fluid inside the oval window of the inner ear.

The inner ear (also called the labyrinth) is made up of a membranous labyrinth inside a bony (osseous) labyrinth. **Labyrinths** are a series of canals and chambers located within the petrous portion of the temporal bone. Between the two labyrinths is a fluid called perilymph, which fills the spaces of the bony labyrinth. Endolymph is a fluid inside the membranous labyrinth.

The osseous labyrinth houses three membrane-lined compartments: the vestibule, the semicircular canals, and the cochlea. The vestibule contains two sacs called the utricle and saccule. These sacs are connected by the endolymphatic duct.

The **cochlea** houses the organ of hearing; the semicircular canals function in equilibrium. Within the cochlea, the oval window leads to the upper compartment, called the scala vestibuli. A lower compartment, the scala tympani, leads to the round window. The cochlear duct lies between these two compartments and is separated from the scala vestibuli by the vestibular membrane, and from the scala tympani by the basilar membrane. The organ of Corti, housing receptors called hair cells, lies on the basilar membrane. Hair cells possess hairs that extend into the endolymph of the cochlear duct. Above the hair cells lies the tectorial membrane, which touches the tips of the stereocilia.

Physiology of Hearing

The auricle directs sound waves into the external auditory canal, and these sound waves then strike the tympanic membrane (Figure 9-9). The tympanic membrane moves back and forth in response to changes in pressure (slowly in response to low-frequency sounds, and faster in response to high-frequency sounds). Loudness is determined by the intensity of the sound waves.

The malleus is connected to the central area of the eardrum, and it begins to vibrate in response to the tympanic membrane's vibrations. The vibration is transferred from the malleus to the incus, and then on the stapes.

The in-and-out movement of the stapes pushes the oval window in and out as well, which sets up waves of fluid pressure in the cochlea's perilymph. The oval window pushed inward into the perilymph of the scala vestibuli and the pressure waves that incur, are

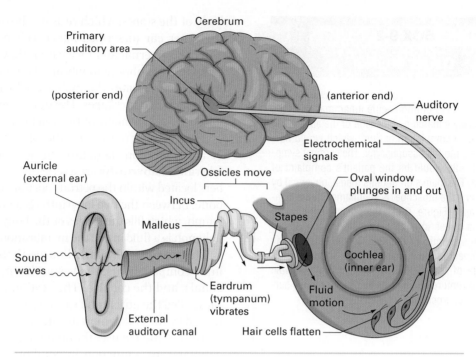

FIGURE 9-9 Pathway of hearing

transmitted from the scala vestibuli to the scala tympani and eventually to the round window. The round window bulges outward into the middle ear.

The pressure waves alter the walls of the scala vestibuli and the scala tympani, and also push the vestibular membrane back and forth, causing the pressure of the endolymph inside the cochlear duct to alternately increase and decrease. These alternating pressure gradients within the endolymph move the basilar membrane. As the basilar membrane vibrates, it causes the hair cells of the spiral organ to move against the tectorial membrane. The movement of the microvilli opens ion channels, which produce depolarizing receptor potentials that lead to the generation

of nerve impulses in cochlear nerve fibers (higher-intensity sound waves cause a greater vibration of the basilar membrane, which causes higher frequency of nerve impulses to reach the brain). Therefore, hair cells convert a mechanical force into an electrical signal.

The cochlear branch of the VIII cranial nerve (the vestibulocochlear, or acoustic nerve) conducts auditory impulses to the cochlear nuclei in the medulla oblongata. From here, most of the fibers cross over to the other side and project into the midbrain. These fibers terminate in the thalamus. From the thalamus, auditory signals project to the primary auditory area of the cerebral cortex's temporal lobe, where they are ultimately interpreted.

BOX 9-3

Deafness

Deafness is defined as any reduction of hearing, and is categorized as follows: conduction-type deafness, sensorineural deafness, central deafness, mixed-type deafness, functional deafness, congenital deafness, and neonatal deafness. Conduction-type deafness occurs when there is an interference with the transmission of sounds from the external or middle ear, preventing sound waves from entering the inner ear. Sensorineural deafness is also referred to as "nerve deafness" and involves the cochlear portion of the inner ear or the cochlear division of the vestibulocochlear nerve (in

some cases, it may include both). Central deafness involves the acoustic center of the cerebral cortex. Mixed-type deafness involves both the conduction system and the nervous system. Functional deafness (sometimes called "selective" deafness) is psychogenic, with no conduction or nerve problem identified. Congenital deafness is present at the time of birth. Its cause may be hereditary or may be due to the mother's exposure to disease or toxic drugs during the pregnancy. Neonatal deafness, which occurs at the time of birth, is caused by prematurity, trauma, or Rh incompatibility.

SENSE OF EQUILIBRIUM

The sense of equilibrium consists of two parts: static and dynamic equilibrium. The organs of static equilibrium help to maintain the position of the head when the head and body are still. The organs of dynamic equilibrium help to maintain balance when the head and body suddenly move and rotate (Figure 9-10).

Static Equilibrium

The organs of **static equilibrium** are located within the bony vestibule of the inner ear, inside the utricle and saccule (expansions of the membranous labyrinth). A macula, consisting of hair cells and supporting cells, lies inside the utricle and saccule. The hair cells contact gelatinous material holding otoliths. Gravity causes the gelatin and otoliths to shift, bending hair cells and generating a nervous impulse. Impulses travel to the brain via the vestibular branch of the vestibulocochlear nerve, indicating the position of the head.

Dynamic Equilibrium

The three semicircular canals detect motion of the head, and they aid in balancing the head and body during sudden movement. The organs of **dynamic** equilibrium are called cristae ampullaris, and are located in the ampulla of each semicircular canal of the inner ear. Hair cells extend into a dome-shaped gelatinous cupula. Rapid turning of the head or body generates impulses as the cupula and hair cells bend, which are interpreted and modified by the brain to maintain specific positions for the body. Mechanoreceptors associated with the joints, and the changes detected by the eyes also help maintain equilibrium.

SENSE OF TASTE

Taste buds are the special organs of taste. They occur primarily on the surface of the tongue and are located within tiny, numerous elevations called papillae. They are also found in fewer numbers on the roof of the mouth and pharynx.

Each taste bud consists of modified epithelial cells (called taste or gustatory cells) that function as receptors. Taste cells contain the taste hairs (microvilli), which are the portions of the taste cell most sensitive to taste reception. A network of nerve fibers is wrapped around each cell, and functions to transmit an impulse to the brain from a stimulated receptor cell.

Chemicals must be dissolved in the fluid (saliva from salivary glands) that surrounds the taste cells in order to be tasted. The sense of taste most likely

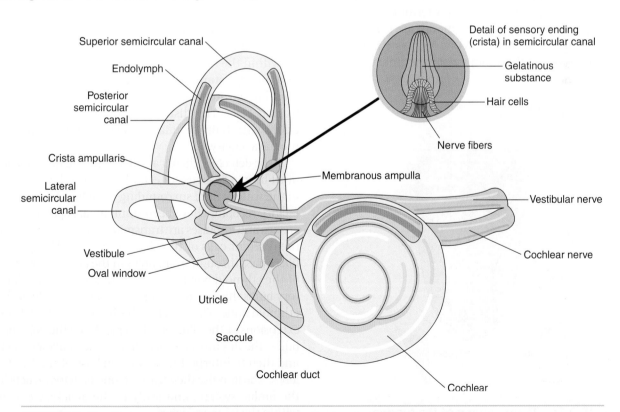

FIGURE 9-10   Enlargement of the ear showing three semicircular canals

results from a taste cell membrane, normally polarized, that becomes depolarized when its cell proteins bind with specific chemicals in food. The depolarization propagates an electrical wave and the generation of sensory impulses on nearby nerve fibers. The strength of the stimulus depends on the chemical concentration in the food.

There are four types of taste buds, each stimulated by a specific and different type of chemical that produces a certain taste sensation. The taste sensations are sweet, sour, salty, and bitter. Some recognize two other taste sensations: alkaline and metallic. Each of the taste sensations that we experience arises from one of the primary sensations or from a combination of two or more of them.

Specific taste receptors are concentrated in different areas of the tongue (Figure 9-11). Sweet receptors are plentiful near the tip of the tongue, and are stimulated by polysaccharides and sugars. Sour receptors occur along the lateral edges of the tongue, and are stimulated by acids. Salt receptors are abundant in the tip and upper portion of the tongue, and are stimulated by ionized inorganic salts. Bitter receptors are at the back of the tongue, and are stimulated by a variety of organic compounds and, to a lesser degree, inorganic compounds.

Taste impulses from the anterior two thirds of the tongue are relayed to the brain via the facial (VII) nerve. Taste impulses from the posterior one third of the tongue and the back of the mouth are transferred via the glossopharyngeal (IX) nerve. Taste impulses from the base of the tongue and the pharynx are transmitted via the vagus (X) nerve. The impulses from these nerves are transmitted first to the medulla oblongata, and from there they are relayed to the thalamus and then to the gustatory cortex of the cerebrum's parietal lobe.

SENSE OF SMELL

The olfactory senses (smell) can give us great pleasure or intense revulsion, and can easily evoke intense memories. It is believed that humans can distinguish among approximately 10,000 chemicals, but recent research has suggested that olfactory receptors are stimulated by a more limited number and combination of olfactory qualities.

The nerve pathways for the sense of smell are directly connected to older, more primitive areas of the brain (the limbic system) that are associated with memory and basic primal instincts, such as aggression, sexual urges, or hunger. For example, a whiff of perfume can bring up intense memories of an old girlfriend from years past, or the smell of burning wood can evoke memories of a Boy Scout camping trip. Smell is also an important component for attraction and sexuality.

The olfactory senses and taste operate together to aid in food selection. In fact, smell accounts for 90% of what we think of as taste. This is easily proved by pinching the nose when eating, and attempting to discern different tastes.

Within the nasal cavity is a patch of tissue the size of a postage stamp with specialized olfactory receptors (bipolar neurons) and supporting columnar epithelial cells. The distal ends of the neurons have knobs with hairlike cilia that extend from them into the nasal cavity.

To be detected, chemicals that enter the nasal cavity must be in a gaseous state, and must then be dissolved in the watery fluid surrounding the cilia. Once the olfactory receptors have been stimulated, depolarization ensues and impulses are transmitted along the axons of the receptor cells of the olfactory nerves. These axon fibers pass through small holes in the cribriform plates of the ethmoid bone and lead to neurons in the olfactory bulbs that lie on either side of the crista galli of the ethmoid bone. The olfactory bulbs are enlarged distal extensions of the olfactory (I) nerve. From the olfactory bulbs, the impulse is transmitted to the olfactory tract, and then to interpreting centers in base of the frontal lobes. The impulse then travels along olfactory tracts to the limbic system, and lastly to the olfactory cortex within the temporal lobes.

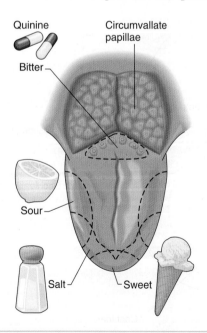

FIGURE 9-11   Taste regions of the tongue

IMPLICATIONS FOR THE SURGICAL TECHNOLOGIST

The surgical technologist assists in surgical procedures on the eyes, ears, and nose, and a sound understanding of the anatomy and physiology of the organs of the senses is imperative for proper patient care.

Surgical patients must be shielded from pain during the procedure, through general, spinal, epidural, or local anesthesia. The surgical technologist must have a solid understanding of the physiologic pathways for pain because they often deal with the medications necessary for pain transmission blockage, and often assist the anesthesia provider with administration of anesthetic.

Procedures for the eye include cataract removal, corneal transplantation, and various types of surgical treatment for glaucoma. The optic nerve is often treated surgically with optic nerve fenestration. Strabismus repair includes recession and resection procedures and adjustable suture surgery. Vitreoretinal procedures include focal laser for wet macular degeneration, laser for diabetic retinopathy, macular hole surgery, vitrectomy, and retinal detachment repair.

Tumors of the VIII cranial nerve (vestibulocochlear) called acoustic neuromas are frequently removed surgically, and the surgical technologist frequently assists with these procedures. An understanding of the ossicles of the middle ear is essential when performing ossicular chain reconstruction (either removal of diseased ossicles with replacement by prosthesis or ossicular transposition) or stapedectomy (removal of the stapes with replacement by prosthesis). The tympanic membrane is often dealt with surgically during tympanoplasty and myringotomy for pressure equalization (PE) tube placement.

The nose is often surgically altered or repaired during plastic procedures for aesthetic purposes (called rhinoplasty). Nasal septal reconstruction, submucous resection, or septoplasty is used to repair the septum of the nose.

Case Study 2

Alicia is a senior surgical technology student who is preparing for her first eye procedure. The procedure is a vitrectomy, and the eye surgeon is explaining what he is going to do and what Alicia needs to know to properly assist with the delicate procedure.

1. What is a vitrectomy?

2. Which common conditions of the eye require vitrectomy?

3. How is the procedure performed?

CHAPTER SUMMARY

- The special senses are the organs and accessories that are related to vision, hearing, taste, smell, and equilibrium.

- Based on their sensitivities, five general types of receptors are recognized:

  1. Receptors sensitive to changes in chemical concentration are called chemoreceptors.
  2. Pain receptors (nociceptors) detect tissue damage.
  3. Thermoreceptors respond to temperature differences.
  4. Mechanoreceptors respond to changes in pressure or movement.
  5. Photoreceptors in the eyes respond to light energy.

- Sensations are feelings that occur when the brain receives sensory impulses from the peripheral nervous system (PNS). Perception is the conscious awareness of sensation after interpretation.

- Sensory adaptation occurs when persistent stimulation of receptors causes sensory impulses to be sent at decreasing rates until receptors fail to send impulses entirely.

- Somatic senses are those that involve receptors associated with the skin, muscles, joints, and visceral organs.

- Sensations of touch result from sensation of tactile receptors located in the skin or just beneath it.

- Sensations of pressure result from stimulation of receptors in deeper tissues.

- Three types of receptors detect touch and pressure:
  1. Free ends of sensory nerve fibers
  2. Meissner's corpuscles
  3. Pacinian corpuscles

- Thermal sensations are perceptions of degrees of warmth and coolness.

- Temperature receptors include two groups of free nerve endings located in the skin: heat receptors and cold receptors.

- Pain receptors consist of free nerve endings that are stimulated when tissues are damaged.

- Pain can be either acute or chronic, depending on its speed of onset and duration.

- Acute pain occurs very rapidly, and is typically not felt in deeper tissues of the body. It is often described as a sharp or stabbing pain.

- Chronic pain has a slower onset, and builds slowly in intensity over a period of seconds or minutes.

- A characteristic of visceral pain is that it often seems to come from somewhere other than its actual origin (referred pain).

- Stretch receptors are proprioceptors that deal with sensations from the lengthening and stretching muscles. The two main types are Golgi tendon organs and muscle spindles.

- The eye, protected by the skeletal orbit that encases it, is the primary organ of sight. Accessory organs, namely the lacrimal apparatus, eyelids, and extrinsic muscles, aid the eye in its function.

- The conjunctiva is a thin mucous membrane composed of stratified columnar epithelium.

- The lacrimal apparatus is a group of structures designed to produce and drain lacrimal fluid (tears) from the eye.

- It consists of a lacrimal gland that secretes tears, and a series of excretory lacrimal ducts that carry the tears to the surface of the conjunctiva of the upper lid.

- The extrinsic muscles of the eye arise from the bones of the orbit and attach to tendons that insert them into the sclera the tough outer surface of the eyeball.
  1. The superior rectus moves the eye upward and toward the midline.
  2. The inferior rectus moves the eye downward and toward the midline.
  3. The medial rectus moves the eye toward the midline.
  4. The lateral rectus moves the eye away from midline.
  5. The superior oblique moves the eye downward and away from the midline.
  6. The inferior oblique moves the eye upward and away from the midline.

- The eye is a fluid-filled hollow sphere with three distinct layers, or tunics. They are the outer tunic, the middle tunic, and the inner tunic.

- The outer tunic is the transparent cornea at the front of the eye, which serves as the window by focusing light rays that enter.

- The cornea is continuous with the sclera, the tough, white portion of the eye.

- The middle tunic is also known as the vascular tunic and includes the choroid coat, the ciliary body, and the iris.

- The ciliary body is the thickest part of the middle tunic, extends forward from the choroid, and forms a ring around the front of the eye.

- The ciliary muscle contracts and relaxes to alter the shape of the lens, depending on the amount of light that enters, for near or far vision.

- The lens is a round, elastic, and transparent structure composed mostly of intercellular material and proteins called crystallins.

- The iris is the colored portion of the eyeball.

- The second cavity (and the largest) of the eyeball is the posterior cavity that lies between the lens and the retina and contains a jellylike substance called vitreous humor.

- The epithelium of the ciliary body secretes a watery substance called aqueous humor into the posterior chamber.

- The inner tunic consists of the retina, which contains the photoreceptors that sense the light entering the eye. This complex system of nerves sends impulses through the optic nerve back to the brain.

- There two types of photoreceptors: rods, which have long thin projections at their ends, and cones, which have short, blunt projections.

- Both rods and cones contain light-sensitive photopigments: colored proteins that change their structure in response to the absorption of light and initiate the events that lead to the receptor potential.

- The ear is a sense organ that is designed to pick up and amplify sound waves for eventual interpretation by the temporal lobe of the brain.

- The inner ear plays a pivotal role in the maintenance of equilibrium by sending messages to the cerebellum about the position of the head.

- The ear has external, middle, and inner sections.

- The external ear consists of the pinna (auricle) and the external auditory canal (meatus).

- The external auditory canal collects the sound waves that travel down the external auditory meatus.

- The middle ear (tympanic cavity) is a mucous membrane–lined, air-filled space located within the temporal bone that houses the auditory ossicles.

- The middle ear houses three small bones called the auditory ossicles, designed to both transmit and amplify sound waves: the malleus (hammer), incus (anvil), and stapes (stirrup).

- The inner ear (also called the labyrinth) is made up of a membranous labyrinth inside a bony (osseous) labyrinth.

- The cochlea houses the organ of hearing; the semicircular canals function in equilibrium.

- The cochlear branch of the VIII cranial nerve conducts auditory impulses to the cochlear nuclei in the medulla oblongata, then to the thalamus, and then to the temporal lobe.

- The sense of equilibrium consists of two parts: static and dynamic equilibrium.

- The organs of static equilibrium help to maintain the position of the head when the head and body are still.

- The organs of dynamic equilibrium help to maintain balance when the head and body suddenly move and rotate.

- The organs of static equilibrium are located within the bony vestibule of the inner ear, inside the utricle and saccule (expansions of the membranous labyrinth).

- The three semicircular canals detect motion of the head, and they aid in balancing the head and body during sudden movement.

- The organs of dynamic equilibrium are called cristae ampullaris, and are located in the ampulla of each semicircular canal of the inner ear.

- Each taste bud consists of modified epithelial cells that function as receptors.

- Taste cells contain the microvilli that are the portions of the taste cell most sensitive to taste reception. A network of nerve fibers is wrapped around each cell, and function to transmit an impulse to the brain from a stimulated receptor cell.

- There are four types of taste buds, each stimulated by a specific and different type of chemical that produces a certain taste sensation: sweet, sour, salty, and bitter.

- Specific taste receptors are concentrated in different areas of the tongue.

- The nerve pathways for the sense of smell are directly connected to the limbic system, which is associated with memory and basic primal instincts, such as aggression, sexual urges, or hunger.

- Within the nasal cavity is a patch of tissue with specialized olfactory receptors and supporting columnar epithelial cells.

CRITICAL THINKING QUESTIONS

1. What is a submucous resection?
2. What is otitis media, and what is the surgical treatment for this condition?
3. What is the difference between epidural and spinal anesthesia?
4. What is retinal detachment?
5. What is a scleral buckle procedure?

BIBLIOGRAPHY

Anonymous. *Special sense organs—pathways*. The Bioengineering Institute, IUPS Physiome Project. Retrieved May 16, 2005, from http://www.bioeng.auckland.ac.nz/physiome/ontologies/special_sense_organs/pathways.php

Association of Surgical Technologists. (2003). *Surgical technology for the surgical technologist: A positive care approach* (2nd ed.). Clifton Park, NY: Thomson Delmar Learning.

Bienfang, D. C. & Kurtz, D. (1998). Management of functional vision loss. *Journal of the American Optometric Association, 69*(1), 12–21.

Eldredge, D. H., & Miller, J. D. (1971). Physiology of hearing. *Annual Review of Physiology, 33,* 281–310.

Gilbertson, T. A. (1993). The physiology of vertebrate taste reception. *Current Opinion in Neurobiology, 3*(4), 532–539.

Hole, J. W., Jr. (1987). *Human anatomy and physiology.* (4th ed.). Dubuque, IA: W. C. Brown.

Martin, K. A., & Perry, V. H. (1988). On seeing a butterfly: The physiology of vision. *Science Progress, 72*(286, Pt 2), 259–280.

Moore, D. R. (1991). Anatomy and physiology of binaural hearing. *Audiology, 30*(3), 125–134.

Oguchi, Y. (1998). Visual information processing and the mechanism of vision. Clinical application. *Nippon Ganka Gakkai Zasshi, 102*(12), 850–875.

Sanders, T., & Scanlon, V. C. (1995). *Essentials of anatomy and physiology* (2nd ed.). Philadelphia: F. A. Davis.

Scott, A. S., & Fong, E. (1998). *Body structures and functions* (9th ed.). Clifton Park, NY: Thomson Delmar Learning.

Tipton, D. A. (1984). A review of vision physiology. *Aviation, Space, and Environmental Medicine, 55*(2), 145–149.

Tortora, G. J., & Grabowski, S. R. (1996). *Principles of anatomy and physiology* (8th ed.). New York: Harper-Collins.

von Baumgarten, R. (1975). Physiology of smell and taste. *Archives of Otorhinolaryngology, 210*(1), 43–65.

Wade, N. J. (2003). The search for a sixth sense: The cases for vestibular, muscle, and temperature senses. *Journal of the History of the Neurosciences, 12*(2), 175–202.

10

BLOOD

CHAPTER OUTLINE

CHAPTER OBJECTIVES

After completing the study of this chapter, you should be able to:

1. Describe the function of blood and its components.
2. Compare and contrast the formation of different types of blood cells.
3. Compare and contrast blood types.
4. Describe Rh factor and its importance to transfusion.
5. Compare and contrast the methods for blood replacement.
6. Compare and contrast anemia and polycythemia.

KEY TERMS

agglutinin	colloidal osmotic pressure	hemoglobin	pernicious anemia
agglutinogen	(COP)	hemorrhagic anemia	plasma
anemia	eosinophils	hemostasis	pluripotent cells
aplastic anemia	erythrocytes	leukocytes	polycythemia
autologous transfusion	erythropoiesis	mononuclear phagocyte	Rh factor
basophils	granular leukocytes	system (MPS)	thrombin
blood salvage	hemodilution	neutrophils	thrombocytes

Case Study 1

Surgical technologists must be aware of the different materials and techniques for hemostasis. For each situation described, explain which hemostatic technique or substance should be used (if a linear stapler is excluded).

1. Oozing from small cortical vessels in the brain during a craniotomy for tumor removal

2. Severed branch of the pulmonary artery during pneumonectomy

3. Bleeding from omentum during laparotomy for bowel resection

4. Bleeding from tonsil bed during tonsillectomy

INTRODUCTION

Blood is a viscous fluid that is carried away from the heart by arteries and back to the heart by veins. Its color is bright red as it is oxygenated, and it becomes dark red in color when it delivers its oxygen molecules to the tissues. Blood pH is about 7.4, and it accounts for about one thirteenth of our body weight, that is, about five to six liters in a typical adult. Half of this volume is made up of solid cellular components, while the other half is plasma (a mixture of water, proteins, and electrolytes).

FUNCTION OF BLOOD

The complex interaction of its individual components makes it possible for blood to simultaneously serve as a supply system, waste removal system, and regulation system. The main functions of the blood are:

- Supply of oxygen to the organs and tissues
- Removal of carbon dioxide
- Temperature regulation
- Water balance
- Maintenance of acid–base metabolism
- Transport of nutrients and removal of waste products of metabolism
- Transport of messenger substances (such as hormones)
- Immunity activities
- Wound-healing activities

Blood is an important transport medium. For example, oxygen extracted from air in the lungs is carried to all body cells by blood, and carbon dioxide produced by cells is brought from tissues back to the lungs by the blood for exhalation from the lungs.

Blood also transports nutrients from the digestive tract and waste products, such as urea, to the kidneys for excretion. Blood transports hormones from endocrine glands to target tissues.

Blood regulates body temperature by transporting heat from deeper parts of the body to the surface. It maintains water balance, and through the use of buffers such as bicarbonate maintains a constant pH (7.4) of tissues and body fluids.

Blood has clotting factors, which are essential for repair and hemorrhage control after injury, and it has white blood cells, which are necessary for immune defense against pathogens and foreign materials. Through regulation of chemical equilibrium, blood can correct the imbalances that occur in infections, traumatic wounds, poisoning, or various immunity malfunctions.

COMPONENTS OF BLOOD AND PLASMA

Blood is made of two parts: cells and a fluid portion called the plasma (Figure 10-1). The cellular elements of blood are:

1. **Erythrocytes** or red blood cells (RBCs), which function to transport oxygen from the lungs to the tissues, and to assist in transportation of carbon dioxide (CO_2) from the tissues to the lungs.
2. **Leukocytes** or white blood cells (WBCs), which function to protect the body against infection and disease.
3. **Thrombocytes** (also known as platelets), which are important for blood coagulation, necessary for the control of hemorrhage after a vessel has been damaged

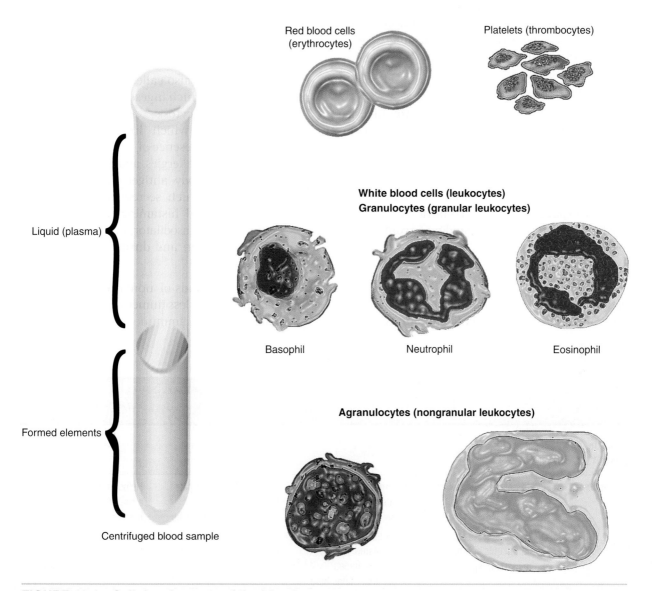

Red blood cells (erythrocytes)

Platelets (thrombocytes)

Liquid (plasma)

White blood cells (leukocytes)
Granulocytes (granular leukocytes)

Basophil   Neutrophil   Eosinophil

Agranulocytes (nongranular leukocytes)

Formed elements

Centrifuged blood sample

FIGURE 10-1 Cellular elements of the blood

Plasma, the yellowish fluid portion of blood, represents 60% of the total of blood (the rest is the hematocrit percentage of packed cells). Plasma is 92% water and 8% proteins (albumin; fibrinogen; and alpha, beta, and gamma globulins) and other substances, such as nonprotein nitrogen. Oxygen and carbon dioxide are the major plasma gases.

Albumin is important for what is called **colloidal osmotic pressure (COP)**, which helps prevent edema and maintains blood pressure by helping to keep fluids within the vascular system.

Fibrinogen is necessary for blood clotting, and the immune globulins are antibodies produced by the immune system in response to invasion by agents such as bacteria, viruses, pollens, molds, or parasites perceived by the body as "foreign." These invading agents are known as antigens. Prothrombin is a globulin that helps blood to coagulate.

The major nonprotein nitrogens (NPNs) of plasma are urea, uric acid, creatine, creatinine, ammonium salts, and amino acids. The blood urea nitrogen (BUN) is 10–20 times that of the plasma creatinine. An elevated BUN : creatinine ratio reflects conditions associated with increased protein breakdown, such as trauma, infection, steroid hormone therapy, or ingestion of a high-protein diet.

Plasma also contains specific organic substances, such as glucose, lipids, enzymes, amino acids, cholesterol, hormones, and clotting factors in organic chemicals. The major inorganic substances are chlorides, carbonates, potassium, calcium, sulfates, and phosphates of sodium and magnesium.

Erythrocytes

Erythrocytes, or RBCs, are nonnucleated round disks that are concave on two sides. They contain a protein called **hemoglobin**, which gives blood its red color and is the method of transport for oxygen molecules from the lungs to the body cells. Hemoglobin also picks up carbon dioxide for transport back to the lungs to be expired, and transports nitric oxide, which regulates blood pressure by expanding or contracting blood vessel walls.

Leukocytes

Leukocytes, or WBCs, play an important role in producing antibodies and in cellular immunity. There are two types: **granular leukocytes**, which have multilobed nuclei, and nongranular (agranular) leukocytes, which have rounded nuclei. The three types of granular leukocytes are:

- **Neutrophils** (also called polymorphonuclear leukocytes), which ingest and destroy bacteria through phagocytosis.
- **Eosinophils**, which increase and become active in the presence of certain infections, infestations, and allergies, and phagocytize the remains of antibody–antigen reactions.
- **Basophils**, which secrete heparin (an anticoagulant) and histamine (an inflammation stimulant and vasodilator) in response to chronic inflammation and during healing from an infection.

There are two kinds of nongranular leukocytes: lymphocytes and the less numerous monocytes, both associated with the immune system. Monocytes,

TABLE 10-1 Characteristics and Functions of the Leukocytes

LEUKOCYTE	WHERE FORMED	TYPE OF NUCLEUS	CYTOPLASM	FUNCTION
AGRANULAR LEUKOCYTES				
1. Lymphocyte	Lymph glands and nodes, bone marrow, spleen	One large, spherical nucleus; may be indented; sharply defined and stains dark blue	Cytoplasm stains a pale blue and contains scattered violet granules	Helps to form antibodies at a site of inflammation; protects against cancer
2. Monocyte (macrophage)	Lymph glands and nodes, bone marrow, spleen	One lobulated or horseshoe-shaped nucleus that stains blue	Abundant cytoplasm that stains a gray-blue	Phagocytosis of cellular debris and foreign particles
GRANULAR LEUKOCYTES				
1. Neutrophil	Formed in bone marrow from neutrophilic myelocytes	Lobulated: contains 1 to 5 or more lobes, stains deep blue	Cytoplasm has a pink tinge with very fine granules	Displays marked phagocytosis toward bacteria during infections and inflammations; contributes to pus formation
2. Eosinophil	Formed in bone marrow from eosinophilic myelocytes	Irregularly shaped with 2 lobes, stains blue, but less deeply than neutrophils	Cytoplasm has a sky-blue tinge with many coarse, uniform, round, or oval bright-red granules	Marked increase during parasitic, worm infections and allergic attacks
3. Basophil (mast cell)	Formed in bone marrow from basophilic myelocytes	Centrally located, slightly lobulated nucleus, stains a light purple and hidden by granules	Cytoplasm has a mauve color with many large deep-purple granules	Phagocytosis; releases heparin and histamine and promotes the inflammatory response

through phagocytosis, ingest nonbacterial foreign substances to help prevent infection.

Thrombocytes

Thrombocytes (also called platelets) are small, round, nonnucleated bodies that adhere to the walls of blood vessels at the site of an injury to plug a defect in the vascular wall. Normal blood count for platelets ranges from 250,000 to 450,000 per cubic millimeter of blood. In fact, the number of platelets increases in any condition in which blood clotting becomes a factor, such as hemorrhagic diseases or injury. The number also increases in infections, iron deficiency, and certain types of cancers.

When a blood vessel is damaged, platelets flow over the roughened area of collagen fibers extruding from the injury, which stimulates the platelets to disintegrate and release various clotting agents that lead to the local formation of thromboplastin. Thromboplastin is a complex substance that requires the presence of calcium ions and prothrombin (a plasma protein synthesized in the liver) to cause coagulation. Platelets also release a substance that causes vasoconstriction to decrease the amount of blood that flows through the area, thereby inhibiting blood loss.

BLOOD FORMATION

Blood cells originate from stem cells in red bone marrow called **pluripotent cells**, a name meaning that they are capable of developing into various types of cells. Pluripotent stem cells give rise to two different types of cells: lymphoid stem cells, which migrate to the lymphatic tissue, and myeloid stem cells, which remain in the bone marrow. These cells then divide by mitosis to produce all the other kinds of blood cells. Each type of blood cell is continuously worn out or consumed and must be continuously replaced.

Erythrocytes are formed in the bone marrow of most bones in a process called **erythropoiesis** (in the fetus, RBCs are formed in the liver). As a person ages, the process is taken over by the short and flat bones, as the red marrow of the long bones is replaced with fat marrow. The lifespan of the average red blood cell is 120 days; after that, it is broken down and removed by the spleen.

Leukocytes are formed in various places: Neutrophils, basophils, and eosinophils are formed in

the bone marrow. Lymphocytes are formed in the thymus, the lymph glands, and other lymphatic tissue. Monocytes are formed in the spleen, liver, lymph nodes, and other organs.

Thrombocytes are synthesized from larger cells called megakaryocytes in red bone marrow. Megakaryocytes have two unique features: They undergo a process known as endomitosis, which allows the nucleus to accumulate many times the normal number of chromosomes. The cytoplasm develops specialized structures that permit fragments to be released. These fragments become platelets.

BLOOD TYPES

In the early twentieth century, an Austrian scientist named Karl Landsteiner classified blood according to differences in different blood samples, observed under a microscope. He noted two distinct chemical molecules present on the surface of the RBCs, labeling one "type A" if only "A" molecules were observed, and the other "type B" if only "B" molecules were observed. If the RBCs had a mixture of both molecules, that blood was called "type AB," and "type O" if the RBCs had neither molecule.

We now know that this marker on the surface of the RBC is a blood protein called **agglutinogen** (antigen). A protein present in blood plasma, known as **agglutinin** (antibody), also indicates blood type: a person with type A blood has *b* antibodies in the blood plasma; type B blood has *a* antibodies; type O blood contains both *a* and *b* antibodies; and type AB contains no antibodies.

It is important that blood types be matched before blood transfusions take place because if two different blood types are mixed together, the blood cells can possibly clump together and create emboli that lead to infarction. Table 10-2 lists compatible blood types. Type O blood can be given in emergency situations because it is most likely to be accepted by all blood types (but even then problems can arise).

Rh Factor

In addition to containing antigens A and B, blood also contains a protein called **Rh factor** ("Rh" is for Rhesus monkey, the animal in which the protein was first identified). The presence of the protein, or lack of it, is referred to as the Rh factor. If the protein is present in blood, the person is said to be Rh positive (Rh+); if absent, the person is said to be

Blood cell		Life span in blood	Function
Erythrocyte	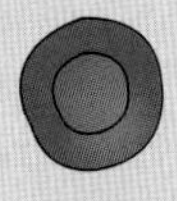	120 days	O_2 and CO_2 transport
Neutrophil	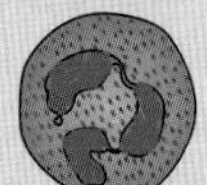	7 hours	Immune defenses
Eosinophil	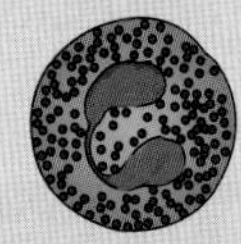	Unknown	Defense against parasites
Basophil	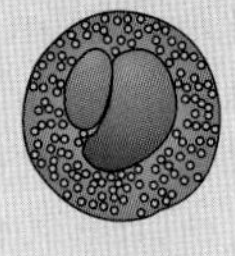	Unknown	Inflammatory response
Monocyte	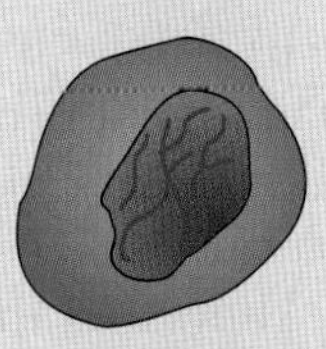	3 days	Immune surveillance (precursor of tissue macrophage)
B Lymphocyte	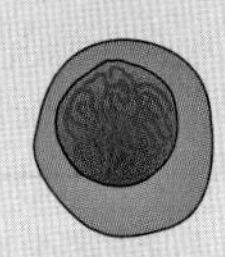	Unknown	Antibody production (precursor of plasma cells)
T Lymphocyte	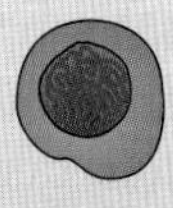	Unknown	Cellular immune response
Platelets	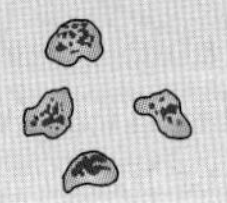	7–8 days	Blood clotting

FIGURE 10-2   The lifespan and functions of blood cells

Rh negative (Rh−). Most North Americans are Rh positive (about 85%).

Neither Rh-positive nor Rh-negative blood contains agglutinins or antibodies in blood plasma, but if an Rh-negative person receives blood from an Rh-positive person, antibodies are formed two weeks after transfusion, causing the antibodies to clump together with the Rh antigen of the blood that is received. Therefore, blood type and Rh factor must be considered when blood is to be transfused to prevent serious problems.

Expectant mothers need to know their blood's Rh factor. A baby can inherit an Rh-positive blood type from the father while the mother has an Rh-negative blood type, producing an Rh-positive child and threat-

---

TABLE 10-2   Compatible Blood Types for Transfusion

- A person with type A blood can donate blood to a person with type A or type AB.
- A person with type B blood can donate blood to a person with type B or type AB.
- A person with type AB blood can donate blood to a person with type AB only.
- A person with type O blood can donate to anyone (and is therefore referred to as a universal donor).
- A person with type A blood can receive blood from a person with type A or type O.
- A person with type B blood can receive blood from a person with type B or type O.
- A person with type AB blood can receive blood from anyone (and is therefore referred to as a universal recipient).
- A person with type O blood can receive blood from a person with type O only.

---

ening the life of the infant. The mother will make antibodies in response to this situation that will attack an Rh-positive baby's blood, causing it to break down the RBCs and creating a condition of anemia (described later). An exchange transfusion of compatible blood may be required for treatment.

HEMOSTASIS

Hemostasis is defined as the arrest of blood that escapes from a blood vessel by either natural or artifical means. For surgical personnel, hemostasis is achieved by artificial means, through the use of hemostatic agents or suture ligatures. Hemostasis is also achieved intraoperatively by the use of thermal cautery or laser. Some patients in need of surgery have congenital or acquired clotting disorders, making the maintenance of hemostasis more difficult.

Natural hemostasis depends on certain mechanisms and on the ability of the blood to clot (Figure 10-3). During the initial phase of hemostasis, vascular spasms, caused by contractions that result from sympathetic nervous system stimulation and the action of serotonin, serve to narrow blood vessels (cause vasoconstriction) and reduce blood flow. Serotonin is a powerful local vasoconstrictor substance released by blood platelets.

Blood usually flows smoothly through the vascular system without cellular adherence to the vessel walls, but when vascular injury occurs following trauma (or certain vascular diseases or surgery) the endothelial cells interact with platelets and clotting factors to form a blood clot at the site of injury. These platelets swell and become sticky, and adhere to the torn vessel. They begin to extrude their contents, including epinephrine, serotonin, and, most important, adenosine diphosphate (ADP) and thromboxane A2. The release of ADP causes more platelets to clump upon the first layer, resulting in an initial thrombus (an aggregation of blood factors that helps aid in hemostasis). This initial thrombus formation may be sufficient to stop the flow of blood in small vessels, but for larger vessels a second, permanent thrombus must be formed.

After the initial white cell thrombus formation, a reaction between plasma and fibrin from the connective tissue of the cells activates clotting factors that cause another set of reactions. Blood coagulation factors (except for calcium, tissue thromboplastin, and fibrin-stabilizing factor) are formed in the liver. Calcium is required for coagulation, and vitamin K is required by the liver for formation of coagulation factor prothrombin, which, in the presence of calcium, catalyzes the formation of the protein enzyme **thrombin**.

Thrombin reacts with fibrinogen and forms fibrin, which has an ability to stabilize blood clots. Over time, fibrin strands form a matrix through the clot to trap RBCs and platelets, forming a stronger plug that can withstand the pressure of blood within the vessel. Another substance, fibrin-stabilizing factor, acts on fibrin threads and forms cross-links between them, thereby adding strength to the fibrin network. The clot formed attaches to the vascular opening, thus preventing blood loss until repair of the opening takes place (Figure 10-4).

The tissue of the damaged vessel can be repaired with new growth once hemostasis is achieved. Damaged endothelial cells activate a plasma plasminogen in the clot to form plasmin, a protein enzyme that begins to degrade the fibrin network in a process referred to as fibrinolysis. The fibrin degradation products, the platelets, and the damaged tissues are then removed by phagocytic cells of the **mononuclear phagocyte system (MPS)**, which is collectively made by the monocytes, mobile macrophages, fixed tissue macrophages, and endothelial cells in the

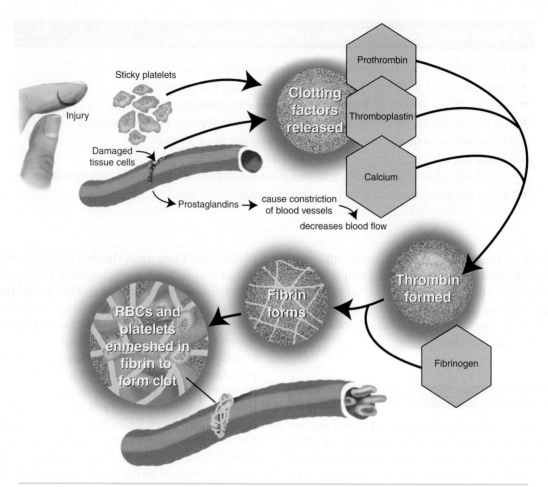

FIGURE 10-3 **The process of clot formation**

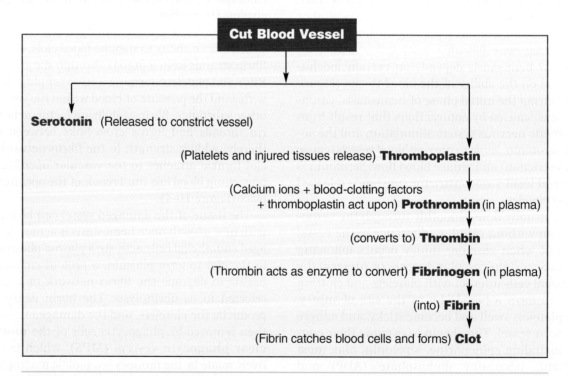

FIGURE 10-4 **Blood clotting process**

BOX 10-1

Hemostatic Agents for Surgical Procedures

Mechanical hemostasis is achieved using any of several instruments or devices to control bleeding until a clot can form. Most perioperative methods of achieving hemostasis involve clamping and/or ligating or clipping the cut vessels with hemoclips, or using electrocautery to achieve hemostasis. Clamps are used to compress the walls of vessels together and also to grasp tissue. Most commonly used is the *hemostat*, a clamping instrument with a fine point that is available with either straight or curved jaws. Special hemostatic clamps are available for differing situations, such as vascular clamps designed to be noncrushing, and do little damage to large vessels.

Ligatures, or *ties* (referred to as "stick ties" when a needle is attached), are strands of material used to tie off blood vessels. Ligatures are made of either natural (animal) tissue or synthetic material and are designed either to dissolve over a period of time or to be incorporated into the patient's own body tissue.

Ligating clips are often used in place of suture ligatures when many small vessels need to be ligated in a short period of time. These clips are made of a nonreactive metal such as titanium or stainless steel or of a plastic material, and come in various sizes, as well as absorbable or permanent varieties. They are applied either from a manually loaded applicator, or from any of several preloaded disposable applicators.

Electrocautery is the most commonly used thermal hemostatic device. This pencil has a small metal loop or tip that passes electric current through the patient to a grounding pad in order to generate intense heat at the site being touched by the tip. The tip of the electrocautery pencil is the active electrode, and current returns to the generator through the grounding pad, which acts as the passive or dispersive electrode.

bone marrow. Blood then passes through the spleen, which is lined with many macrophages that rid the blood of unwanted debris.

BLOOD REPLACEMENT IN SURGERY

Blood transfusions are given to replace blood lost during surgery, trauma, or internal bleeding caused by certain conditions. Transfusions are also used in the treatment of certain cancers (such as leukemia) and to treat different types of anemia (such as sickle cell disease).

Depending on the recipient's needs, a whole-blood transfusion or a blood component may be ordered. Whole blood is usually used in situations in which the patient has lost a large amount of blood. Blood components include RBCs (for the restoration of blood's ability to transport oxygen), WBCs (to restore WBCs lost in certain types of infections), platelets (for patients with blood-clotting disorders), immunoglobulins (to build immunity when antibody levels are low), or fresh frozen plasma (to help with blood clotting; often transfused in patients with liver failure).

For surgery that is planned in advance, patients can donate and store their own blood for transfusion during the procedure (referred to as an **autologous transfusion**). The patient may also ask a friend or family member with the same blood type to donate blood specifically for them (referred to as a direct donation). Stringent screening methods ensure blood transfusions are safe: donors must answer questions about their general health, lifestyle, and any medical conditions that might disqualify them as donors. All donated blood is carefully checked for viral hepatitis, AIDS, syphilis, and other viruses.

Recycling Blood during Surgery

When an operation is expected to involve a large loss of blood, the surgical team may recover the patient's blood and reinfuse it during the surgery. This practice, called intraoperative blood collection, or **blood salvage**, has become increasingly common in surgical procedures in which blood loss is expected to be excessive. Blood salvage may be done using one of two methods: washed or unwashed.

The washed method uses a high-speed centrifuge specifically designed to prevent damage to RBCs. Blood from the wound is suctioned into the centrifuge, which separates it into components. The centrifuge concentrates the RBCs, washes them with a saline solution, and pumps the red cell suspension into an infusion bag for return to the patient. WBCs and platelets do not remain in salvaged blood in useful amounts; therefore, care must be taken to limit the amount of blood reinfused to a patient within a certain time period to prevent clotting problems.

The unwashed method bypasses the centrifuge and collects the suctioned blood into a filtering reservoir. After filtration, the unwashed blood is transferred into a bag for reinfusion.

The choice of blood salvage method is based on the type of surgery. Certain procedures may contribute debris (such as bone chips) to the suctioned blood, so

TABLE 10-3 Hematology Values

Red blood cell (RBC) count	
Male:	$4.3–5.9 \times 10^6$ /mm^3,
	$4.3–5.9 \times 10^{12}$ /L (SI units)
Female:	$3.5–5 \times 10^6$ /mm^3,
	$3.5–5.0 \times 10^{12}$ /L (SI units)
RBC indices	
Mean corpuscular hemoglobin (MCH),	27–33 pg (standard and SI)
Mean corpuscular hemoglobin concentration (MCHC),	33–37 g/dL, 330–370 g/L (SI units)
Mean corpuscular volume (MCV)	76–100 μm^4, 76–100 dL
Hemoglobin	
Male:	13.5–18 g/dL,
	135–180 g/L (SI units)
Female:	11.5–15.5 g/dL,
	115–155 g/L (SI units)
Glycosylated (HbA1-C),	<7.5%, 5–6% (desired)
Hematocrit	
Male:	40–52% (0.40–0.52)
Female:	35–46% (0.35–0.46)
Platelets	$130–400 \times 10^3$ mm^3
White blood cells (leukocytes)	5,000–10,000/mm^3
Neutrophils	50–70%
Segments	50–65%
Bands	0–5%
Basophils	0.25–0.5%
Eosinophils	1–3%
Monocytes	2–6%
Lymphocytes	25–40%
T lymphocytes	60–80% of lymphocytes
B lymphocytes	10–20% of lymphocytes
Bleeding time	1–3 min (Duke)
	1–5 min (Ivy)
Coagulation time (Lee White)	5–15 min
Prothrombin time	10–15 sec (same as control)
Partial thromboplastin time (PTT)	60–70 sec
Thrombin time	Within 5 sec of control
INR recommended range	
Standard therapy	2.0–3.0
High-dose therapy	2.5–3.5
Activated partial thromboplastin time (APTT)	30–45 sec

INR, international normalized ratio.

the surgeon may choose to use the washed (centrifuge) method.

Blood dilution (**hemodilution**) helps to prevent loss of RBCs during a surgical procedure. For this method, the patient has blood removed preoperatively, and is immediately given intravenous fluids to

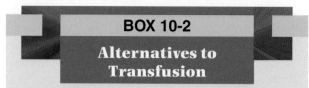

BOX 10-2

Alternatives to Transfusion

Certain religious groups, most notably the Jehovah's Witnesses, do not allow the infusion of blood or blood products. Hospitals often turn these patients away, or they are forced to choose between their religious convictions and their lives. New technologies, referred to as transfusion-free methods, provide these individuals with alternatives to traditional medical and surgical techniques that require transfusions. Blood loss can be minimized through:

- The use of lasers instead of scalpels, and argon beam coagulators for hemostasis
- Intraoperative monitoring of oxygen levels
- Preoperative stimulation of bone marrow to produce red blood cells
- Intraoperative blood salvaging techniques (described previously)
- Hemodilution methods in conjunction with blood salvaging (described previously)
- Intraoperative hypotension anesthesia to lower blood pressure during surgery

make up for the blood that was removed. Any blood the patient loses during the procedure will have been diluted; therefore, fewer red cells will have been lost. Following surgery, the blood that was removed preoperatively is reinfused, providing a good supply of normally concentrated red cells.

ANEMIA AND POLYCYTHEMIA

Anemia is a disease of the blood that is caused by factors that result in destruction or hemolysis of red blood cells, resulting in an abnormally low blood count. Anemia may be caused by the loss or destruction of circulating RBCs or a defective production of RBCs in the bone marrow. Certain anemias force the body to respond to low RBC numbers by increasing cell production in the bone marrow and releasing immature RBCs (polychromatophils) into the blood circulation. With proper staining, these immature cells appear bluish-green cells under a microscope.

Types of Anemia

Hemorrhage caused by trauma or internal bleeding can result in anemia (referred to as **hemorrhagic** anemia). When blood loss is severe, iron is not absorbed rapidly enough to make up for hemoglobin loss, giving rise to a condition called hypochromic anemia.

The lack of production of RBCs (referred to as **aplastic anemia**) may result from an improperly functioning bone marrow. Bone marrow can be destroyed by certain heavy metals, x-rays, or overuse of antibiotics.

Pernicious anemia (or maturation failure anemia) can be caused by the absence of intrinsic factor secreted by the stomach. This intrinsic factor is important for vitamin B12 absorption in the small intestines. Vitamin B12 is essential, as a coenzyme, for DNA synthesis in the bone marrow, and it is important for growth and maturation of RBCs. Under the microscope, a blood smear from a patient with pernicious anemia reveals oversized immature cells with fragile membranes.

Nutritional deficiencies or lack of proteins, copper, iron, and vitamins in the diet can cause anemia. In this case, the bone marrow is normal, but it lacks the building blocks for manufacturing RBCs.

Polycythemia is a clonal stem cell disorder that results in the abnormal increase in the number of circulating RBCs (a three- to fourfold increase in red blood cell count is not uncommon). Its etiology is not fully established, but hypersensitivity to interleukin-3 (a substance that can improve the body's natural response to disease and that enhances the immune system's ability to fight tumor cells) may play a role.

Polycythemia occurs within the age range of 20–80 years, with 60 being the mean age of onset, with clinical features that include headache, weakness, weight loss, and pruritus (itching without visible eruption on the skin). Hemorrhage, thrombosis, and hyperviscosity may be evident at any time. Splenomegaly (enlargement of the spleen), as a result of vascular congestion, is seen in 75% of patients at the time of presentation. Hepatomegaly (enlargement of the liver) is observed in about 30% of cases.

UNIVERSAL AND STANDARD PRECAUTIONS

Universal Precautions, defined by Centers for Disease Control and Prevention (CDC) in 1985, were designed to prevent blood-borne diseases. The surgical technologist is exposed to blood on a daily basis, and must understand and abide by these procedures to remain healthy and to prevent exposure to pathogens (such as HIV and hepatitis B).

Universal Precautions state that all patients should be considered infectious and precautions must be taken to prevent exposure to body fluids, such as blood, semen, and vaginal secretions. These rules do not apply to feces, nasal secretions, sputum, sweat, tears, urine, and vomitus unless blood is visible. Procedures for the minimization of exposure to blood-borne pathogens include the use of personal protective equipment such as gloves, masks, and protective eyewear.

Standard Precautions, written in 1966 by the CDC, combine Universal Precautions and the body substance isolation rules that preceded Universal Precautions. Standard Precautions apply to all body fluids, secretions, and excretions, with the single exception of sweat.

See Table 10-4 for safety precautions in the operating room.

TABLE 10-4 General Safety Checklist

Absolute Prerequisites

Complete the hepatitis B vaccination series.
Use Standard Precautions with all patients.
Use personal protective equipment—appropriate choices.
Wear fluid-resistant headgear when appropriate.
Use adequate eye and face protection.
Use appropriate neck protection. Consider recently shaved skin as being nonintact.
Wear fluid-resistant or fluid-impervious gowns as appropriate to expected exposure risk.
Choose gloves appropriately.
Wear appropriate footwear or shoe covers.
Remove gloves carefully to avoid splatter.
Wash hands with antiseptic soap after removing gloves.
Remove eye protection last.
Remove contaminated personal protective equipment before leaving the room.
Carefully remove and discard mask following each procedure.

Safety Techniques

Wear gloves when handling surgical specimens.
Wear eye protection if container is opened or splashing is anticipated.
Apply dressings and handle drains or packs with clean gloves.
Avoid touching any surface with contaminated gloves.
Avoid touching existing contaminated surfaces.

IMPLICATIONS FOR THE SURGICAL TECHNOLOGIST

The surgical technologist deals with blood on practically every case that is performed during the course of the day. It is important for the surgical technologist to understand Standard Precautions to prevent exposure to blood-borne pathogens, and to closely follow established procedures that minimize risk. Needlestick and blade (sharps) injuries are by far the most common pathways for exposure in this profession, and carry great risks of infection. Intraoperative safety measures established through hospital policy include the establishment of a safety zone between the surgeon and the surgical technologist who is passing instruments. Sharps are laid down carefully within the safety zone and picked up by the other person, instead of being passed directly. In addition, the surgical technologist should never recap hypodermic needles. The best defense against sharps injuries, however, is awareness of the surgical field and anticipation of events that involve sharps. The surgical technologist should be aware of the location of each and every sharp that is used for the procedure.

Case Study 2

Millie is a surgical technologist who is scrubbed in on an emergency splenectomy. The spleen was ruptured during a motor vehicle accident, and the patient is hemorrhaging badly. The cardiac perfusionist on call is quickly setting up a Cell Saver blood salvage device for washed autotransfusion technique.

1. What is the washed technique for autotransfusion?

2. What is the unwashed method for autotransfusion?

3. Why is Cell Saver useful?

CHAPTER SUMMARY

- Blood is a viscous fluid that is carried away from the heart by arteries and back to the heart by veins.

- Blood pH is about 7.4, and it accounts for about one thirteenth of our body weight (five to six liters).

- Half of this volume is made up of solid cellular components, while the other half is plasma (a mixture of water, proteins, and electrolytes).

- The main functions of the blood are: (a) supply of oxygen to the organs and tissues, (b) removal of carbon dioxide, (c) temperature regulation, (d) water balance, (e) maintenance of acid–base metabolism, (f) transport of nutrients and removal of waste products of metabolism, (g) transport of messenger substances (such as hormones), (h) immunity activities, and (i) wound-healing activities.

- Blood is an important transport medium: oxygen is carried to all body cells and carbon dioxide is brought from tissues back to the lungs.

- Blood also transports nutrients from the digestive tract and waste products to the kidneys for excretion.

- Blood transports hormones from endocrine glands to target tissues.

- Blood regulates body temperature and maintains water balance.

- Blood maintains a constant pH (7.4) of tissues and body fluids.

- Blood has clotting factors, which are essential for repair and hemorrhage control after injury.

- Blood has white blood cells, which are necessary for immune defense against pathogens and foreign materials.

- Blood is made of two parts: cells and a fluid portion called the plasma.

- The cellular elements of blood are: (a) erythrocytes or red blood cells, (b) leukocytes or white blood cells, and (c) thrombocytes (also known as platelets).

- Plasma, the yellowish fluid portion of blood, represents 60% of the total of blood.

- Erythrocytes contain a protein called hemoglobin, which gives blood its red color and is the method of transport for oxygen molecules from the lungs to the body cells.

- Leukocytes, or white blood cells, play an important role in producing antibodies and in cellular immunity.

- There are two types of leukocytes: granular leukocytes and nongranular (agranular) leukocytes.

- The three types of granular leukocytes are: (a) neutrophils, which ingest and destroy bacteria through phagocytosis, (b) eosinophils, which increase and become active in the presence of certain infections, infestations, and allergies, and phagocytize the remains of antibody–antigen reactions, and (c) basophils, which secrete heparin and histamine in response to chronic inflammation and during healing from an infection.

- There are two kinds of nongranular leukocytes: lymphocytes and monocytes, both associated with the immune system.

- Thrombocytes adhere to the walls of blood vessels at the site of an injury to plug a defect in the vascular wall.

- Blood cells originate from stem cells in red bone marrow called pluripotent cells.

- Pluripotent stem cells give rise to two different types of cells: lymphoid stem cells, which migrate to the lymphatic tissue, and myeloid stem cells, which remain in the bone marrow.

- Erythrocytes are formed in the bone marrow of most bones in a process called erythropoiesis.

- Leukocytes are formed in various places: Neutrophils, basophils, and eosinophils are formed in the bone marrow. Lymphocytes are formed in the thymus, the lymph glands, and other lymphatic tissue. Monocytes are formed in the spleen, liver, lymph nodes, and other organs.

- Thrombocytes are synthesized from larger cells called megakaryocytes in red bone marrow.

- Landsteiner classified blood according to differences in different blood samples.

- He noted two distinct chemical molecules present on the surface of the red blood cells, labeling one "type A" if only "A" molecules were observed, and the other "type B" if only "B" molecules were observed.

- For a mixture of both molecules he labeled the blood "type AB," and "type O" if the red blood cell had neither molecule.

- In addition to containing antigens A and B, blood also contains a protein called Rh factor.

- The presence of the protein, or lack of it, is referred to as the Rh factor.

- A baby can inherit an Rh-positive blood type from the father while the mother has an Rh-negative blood type, producing an Rh-positive child and threatening the life of the infant.

- Hemostasis is defined as the arrest of blood that escapes from a blood vessel by either natural or artificial means.

- Natural hemostasis depends on certain mechanisms and on the ability of the blood to clot.

- When vascular injury occurs, the endothelial cells interact with platelets and clotting factors to form a blood clot at the site of injury.

- These platelets swell and become sticky, and adhere to the torn vessel. They extrude their contents (epinephrine, serotonin, and adenosine diphosphate [ADP] and thromboxane A2).

- ADP causes more platelets to clump upon the first layer, resulting in an initial thrombus.

- Calcium is required for coagulation.

- Vitamin K is required by the liver for formation of coagulation factor prothrombin, which, in the presence of calcium, catalyzes the formation of thrombin.

- Thrombin reacts with fibrinogen and forms fibrin.

- Fibrin strands form a matrix through the clot to trap RBCs and platelets, thereby forming a stronger plug.

- Blood transfusions are given to replace blood lost during surgery, trauma, or internal bleeding caused by certain conditions.

- Transfusions are also used in the treatment of certain cancers and different types of anemia.

- Whole blood is used in situations in which the patient has lost a large amount of blood.

- Blood components include: (a) red blood cells for the restoration of blood's ability to transport oxygen, (b) white blood cells to restore white blood cells lost in certain types of infections, (c) platelets for patients with blood-clotting disorders, (d) immunoglobulins to build immunity when antibody levels are low, and (e) fresh-frozen plasma to help with blood clotting.

- Patients can donate and store their own blood for transfusion during the procedure (autologous transfusion).

- The surgical team may recover the patient's blood and reinfuse it during the surgery (intraoperative blood collection, or blood salvage).

- Blood salvage may be done using one of two methods: washed or unwashed.

- The washed method uses a high-speed centrifuge specifically designed to prevent damage to red blood cells.

- The centrifuge concentrates the red blood cells, washes them with a saline solution, and pumps the red blood cell suspension into an infusion bag for return to the patient.

- The unwashed method bypasses the centrifuge and collects the suctioned blood into a filtering reservoir.

- Hemodilution helps to prevent loss of red blood cells. The patient has blood removed preoperatively and is immediately given intravenous fluids to make up for the blood that was removed.

- Hemorrhage caused by trauma or internal bleeding can result in hemorrhagic anemia.

- When blood loss is severe, iron is not absorbed rapidly enough to make up for hemoglobin loss, giving rise to a condition called hypochromic anemia.

- The lack of production of red blood cells (referred to as aplastic anemia) may result from improperly functioning bone marrow.

- Pernicious anemia (or maturation failure anemia) can be caused by the absence of intrinsic factor secreted by the stomach.

- Polycythemia is a clonal stem cell disorder that results in the abnormal increase in the number of circulating red blood cells.

- Universal Precautions state that all patients should be considered infectious and precautions must be taken to prevent exposure to body fluids, such as blood, semen, and vaginal secretions.

- Standard Precautions apply to all body fluids, secretions, and excretions, with the single exception of sweat.

CRITICAL THINKING QUESTIONS

1. What is a tie on a pass? What is a tie on a reel?
2. What is the difference between Universal Precautions and Standard Precautions?
3. What liquid coagulant is frequently used with Gelfoam for hemostasis?
4. What is Surgicel and why is it used?
5. What is a bipolar electrosurgery and where is it typically used?

BIBLIOGRAPHY

Anonymous. *Blood and its functions in a nutshell.* Retrieved May 16, 2005, from http://www.vet.purdue.edu/vtdl/tmp/course_work/blood/nutshell/blood_nutshell.htm

Anonymous. *Blood types tutorial.* The Biology Project, University of Arizona. Retrieved May 16, 2005, from http://www.biology.arizona.edu/human_bio/problem_sets/blood_types/Intro.html

Anonymous. *What's your type?* Franklin Institute. Retrieved May 16, 2005, from http://sln.fi.edu/biosci/blood/types.html

Association of Surgical Technologists. (2003). *Surgical technology for the surgical technologist: A positive care approach* (2nd ed.) Clifton Park, NY: Thomson Delmar Learning.

Farley, D. Alternatives to regular blood transfusions. *FDA Consumer.* Retrieved May 17, 2005, from http://www.fda.gov/bbs/topics/CONSUMER/CON284b.html

Hole, J. W., Jr. (1987). *Human anatomy and physiology* (4th ed.). Dubuque, IA: W. C. Brown.

Iveson, R. (1979). Anatomy and physiology: The blood. *Nursing Mirror, 148*(19), 35.

Levy, M. N., & Zieske, H. (1967). A closed circulatory system model. *Physiologist, 10*(4), 419–424.

Magder, S. (1998). The heart: Physiology, from cell to circulation. *New England Journal of Medicine, 339,* 1949–1950.

Murray, D. J., Olson, J., Strauss, R., & Tinker, J. H. (1988). Coagulation changes during packed red cell replacement of major blood loss. *Anesthesiology, 69*(6): 839–845.

Palosaari, S., & Linko, K. (1980). Flow of blood in transfusion systems. *Biorheology, 17*(4), 385–390.

Roberts, A. (1994). Systems of life. Blood: 1. *Nursing Times, 90*(19), 35–38.

Sanders, T., & Scanlon, V. C. (1995). *Essentials of anatomy and physiology* (2nd ed.). Philadelphia: F. A. Davis.

Scott, A. S., & Fong, E. (1998). *Body structures and functions* (9th ed.). Clifton Park, NY: Thomson Delmar Learning.

Tortora, G. J., & Grabowski, S. R. (1996). *Principles of anatomy and physiology* (8th ed.). New York: HarperCollins.

11

THE HEART

CHAPTER OBJECTIVES

After completing the study of this chapter, you should be able to:

1. Evaluate the anatomic development of the heart.
2. Describe the basic anatomy of the heart, including coverings, wall, chambers, and valves.
3. Trace the flow of blood into, through, and out of the heart.
4. Evaluate myocardial infarction.
5. Describe the conduction system of the heart.
6. Describe basic cardiac dysrhythmias and electrocardiogram elements.

KEY TERMS

angina pectoris	coronary artery bypass	fibrous pericardium	pericardium
atria	grafting (CABG)	foramen ovale	primitive heart tube
atrioventricular (AV) node	coronary atherosclerotic	intracoronary thrombolysis	pump oxygenator
atrioventricular (AV) orifice	heart disease	mitral valve	Purkinje fibers
bundle of His	diastole	myocardial infarction (MI)	serous pericardium
cardiac aneurysm	ductus arteriosus	myocardial ischemia	sinoatrial (SA) node
cardiac cycle	ductus venosus	percutaneous transluminal	systole
cardiac output (CO)	electrocardiogram (ECG)	coronary angioplasty	tricuspid valve
chordae tendineae	extracorporeal circulation	(PTCA)	ventricles

Case Study 1

Joanne is a surgical technologist employed by a major cardiac center. She works in the cardiac catheterization lab, and has been called out for an emergency coronary angiogram for a patient with an acute myocardial infarction. The surgeon discovers a lesion in the left anterior descending (LAD) and circumflex arteries.

1. What structure of the heart do the LAD and circumflex arteries serve?

2. Why is this a particularly critical lesion of the coronary artery system?

3. If the lesions are relatively straightforward, what will the cardiologist attempt first for treatment?

4. If percutaneous transluminal coronary angioplasty fails (PTCA), what will the cardiologist do?

INTRODUCTION

The cardiovascular system is made up of the heart (as the organ that pumps blood) and the peripheral vascular system (the arteries, veins, and capillaries that carry blood away from and back to the heart). The cardiovascular system is one part of the circulatory system, which also includes the lymphatic system that returns excess fluid from tissues to the cardiovascular system. The lymphatic system is covered in Chapter 13. In addition, the circulatory system is responsible for the transport of hormones, enzymes, and other important biochemical substances necessary for the proper maintenance and health of the body.

This chapter deals with the heart and its anatomic structures and physiology. The peripheral vascular system, the closed system of vessels that carries blood away from and back to the heart, is covered in Chapter 12.

The surgical technologist must understand the basic anatomy and physiology of the heart in order to properly assist the surgeon with those procedures that repair its pathologic conditions. A basic understanding of the flow of blood through the heart is essential for an understanding of cardiopulmonary bypass, a technique used to stop the heart and divert blood from the body and then back again after oxygenation (described later in Box 11-2). An understanding of basic dysrhythmias is also essential for proper intraoperative patient care, especially if the surgical technologist is employed by a cardiac catheterization laboratory.

THE HEART

The heart plays an essential role within the cardiovascular system as the muscular pump that initiates the circulation of blood, which carries waste substances from cells and to excretory organs for elimination, and vital nutrients and oxygen from the respiratory and digestive organs to cells throughout the body.

Anatomic Development of the Heart

The human heart begins its development just before the end of the third week of gestation. Development begins with the formation of two separate tubes that originate from mesodermal cells called endocardial tubes. One end of each tube represents the eventual arterial component of the heart and the other represents the venous component. Eventually, these two endocardial tubes fuse at specific regions in the center, forming one tube called the **primitive heart tube**. The primitive heart tube has the following five specific regions:

- Ventricle
- Sinus venosus
- Atrium
- Bulbus cordis
- Truncus arteriosus

The bulbus cordis and truncus arteriosus eventually become the pulmonary trunk and aortic arch, whereas the sinus venosus and atrium become the inferior and superior vena cava and atrial chambers. The ventricle becomes, of course, the ventricular chambers. Myocardial contraction begins by the beginning of the fourth week.

By the seventh week, a partition develops to form separate ventricular chambers, as does a wall that separates the right and left atria. An opening between the two atrial chambers, referred to as the foramen ovale, remains until birth. At birth, the foramen ovale closes, leaving a depression in the interatrial septum called the fossa ovalis. Fetal blood secures its oxygen and vital nutrients from maternal blood, thereby bypassing the digestive and respiratory organs. The placenta assumes the function of these organs, interchanging gases, nutrients, and wastes between the fetal and maternal blood.

Two umbilical arteries carry fetal blood to the placenta, and the umbilical vein returns blood with high levels of oxygen and nutrients from the placenta, entering the fetus through the umbilicus and extending branches into the liver. Together, the two umbilical arteries and the one umbilical vein constitute the umbilical cord (Figure 11-1).

The **ductus venosus** is a continuation of the umbilical vein. Only small amounts of blood are shunted to the fetal liver by way of the branches of the umbilical vein. Most of the blood from the placenta is moved through the ductus venosus and into the inferior vena cava.

The **ductus arteriosus** connects the pulmonary artery with the descending thoracic aorta, allowing blood to enter into the fetal circulation without going through the lungs. This structure closes at birth.

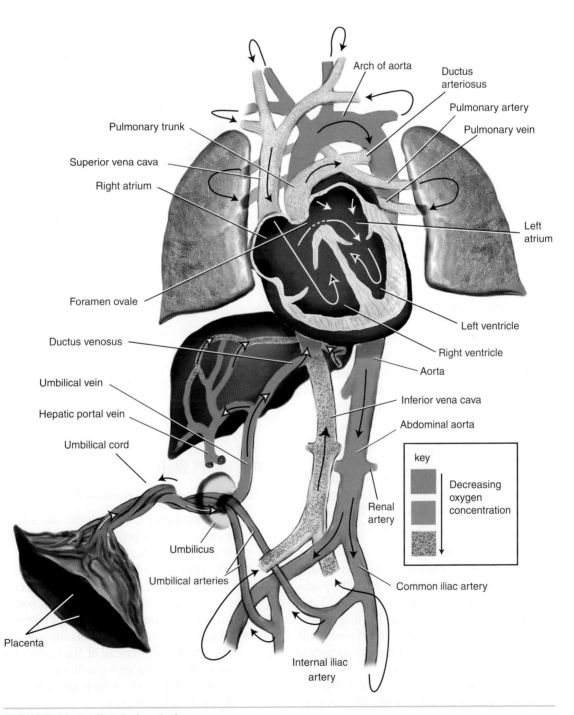

FIGURE 11-1   Fetal circulation

The **foramen ovale** is an opening in the interatrial septum. It is a passageway for blood from the right atrium into the left atrium, and diverts blood from the fetal lungs.

As soon as the umbilical cord is severed, the umbilical arteries and umbilical vein no longer function, and the placenta is expelled shortly after birth. The ductus venosus becomes the ligamentum venosum of the liver, the umbilical vein becomes the round ligament of the liver, and the ductus arteriosus becomes a fibrous cord that helps to stabilize the aorta and pulmonary artery within the thoracic cavity.

After birth—with the elimination of placental circulation, closure of the ductus arteriosus, and a decrease in pulmonary vascular resistance—the right ventricle ejects all of its blood into the pulmonary circulation, and the normal cardiopulmonary circuit is established.

Location of the Heart

The heart is a hollow, muscular organ, and is the approximate size of a man's clenched fist. It is located within the mediastinum, slightly off center of the midline of the thorax, with approximately two thirds of the organ on the left side. The heart sits just posterior to the body of the sternum, between the attachments of the second through sixth ribs, and rests upon the diaphragm.

Posteriorly, the heart sits against the bodies of the fifth through eighth thoracic vertebrae. Within the thorax, the heart lies diagonally, with the distal apex tapering to the left of the midline and the broad, proximal portion lying to the right of the midline.

Coverings of the Heart

The entire heart is enclosed in a loose sac called the **pericardium**, which protects the heart and keeps it from rubbing against the thoracic wall (Figure 11-2). The pericardium consists of two parts:

- **Fibrous pericardium**: a tough, loose-fitting sac that attaches to the large vessels arising from the superior aspect of the heart, the posterior aspect of the sternum, the vertebral column, and the central portion of the diaphragm. It is not, however, attached to the heart itself. The fibrous pericardium is composed largely of white fibrous connective tissue.
- **Serous pericardium**: consists of a parietal layer that lines the inside of the fibrous peri-

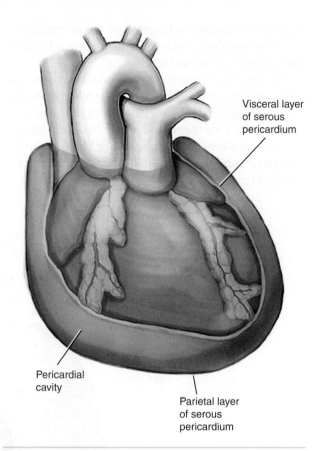

FIGURE 11-2   Pericardium

cardium, and a visceral layer (epicardium) that consists of a thin, serous covering attached to the surface of the heart. Between these two membranes is a potential space called the pericardial cavity, which contains a few drops of serous fluid designed to reduce the friction between the membranes as the heart moves.

The Heart Wall

The wall of the heart is composed of three layers:

- The epicardium, which is the outer layer of the heart, provides protection and is composed of the visceral pericardium.
- The myocardium, which makes up the bulk of the heart wall, is composed of specially constructed cardiac muscle cells that contract and force blood from the heart's chambers.
- The endocardium, which is the inner lining of the heart wall, lines all of the heart's chambers and valves. The endocardium is composed of endothelial tissue, which consists of a single layer of flattened cells.

The Heart Chambers

The heart is divided internally by four chambers, two on the upper half of the heart and two on the lower half. The upper chambers are called **atria** (singular, atrium) and are designed to receive blood from the veins of the body. The lower chambers are called **ventricles** and are designed to pump blood into arteries leading away from the heart (Figure 11-3).

The walls of the atria are relatively thin compared to those of the ventricles, which have a thicker myocardium for pumping blood. The right ventricle has a thinner myocardium than does the left ventricle. The right ventricle pumps blood a short distance to the lungs against moderately low resistance to flow. The left ventricle pumps blood to all other portions of the body against great resistance to flow, and, therefore, needs the extra muscle for increased contractile force.

The chambers of the heart are divided into right and left portions by the septum. The septum between the atria is referred to as the interatrial septum; the interventricular septum separates the ventricles.

The Heart Valves

The atrium on each side of the heart communicates with its corresponding ventricle through an opening called the **atrioventricular (AV) orifice**, which is guarded by an atrioventricular (AV) valve. The atrioventricular orifice between the right atrium and the right ventricle is guarded by the **tricuspid valve**, named for its three leaflike appendages, or cusps.

Fibrous cords called **chordae tendineae** are attached to the cusps on the ventricular side (Figure 11-4). These cords originate from papillary muscles that project outward from the walls of the muscle. The

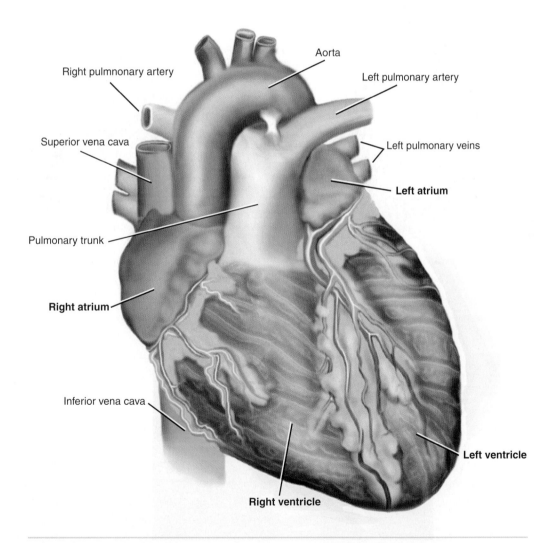

FIGURE 11-3   The human heart (Photo courtesy of Oak Ridge National Laboratory, Oak Ridge, TN)

chordae tendineae prevent the cusps of the valve from folding back into the atrium, causing incomplete closure of the valve and allowing blood back into the atrium.

The cusps fold open when blood pressure is greater on the atrial side, allowing blood to flow passively into the ventricle. When ventricular pressure is greater, the cusps close shut, and the only exit for the blood is across the pulmonary semilunar valve (so called for its three half-moon–shaped flaps), and into the pulmonary trunk. This valve opens as the right ventricle contracts; backflow is prevented when blood backs up against the valve in the pulmonary trunk after the ventricles relax, causing the semilunar valve to close.

Blood from the lungs enters the left atrium and crosses through the AV orifice across the AV valve referred to as the **mitral valve**. This valve has two cusps, and is appropriately named the bicuspid valve. It prevents blood in the left ventricle from backing up into the left atrium, a condition referred to as mitral regurgitation (Figure 11-4).

When the thick walls of the left ventricle contract, the mitral valve closes against the pressure of the blood within the chamber, and blood is ejected into the large artery known as the aorta. At the base of the aorta is another semilunar valve, called the aortic semilunar valve, also consisting of three cusps. This valve prevents blood from flowing back into the left ventricle during ventricular relaxation.

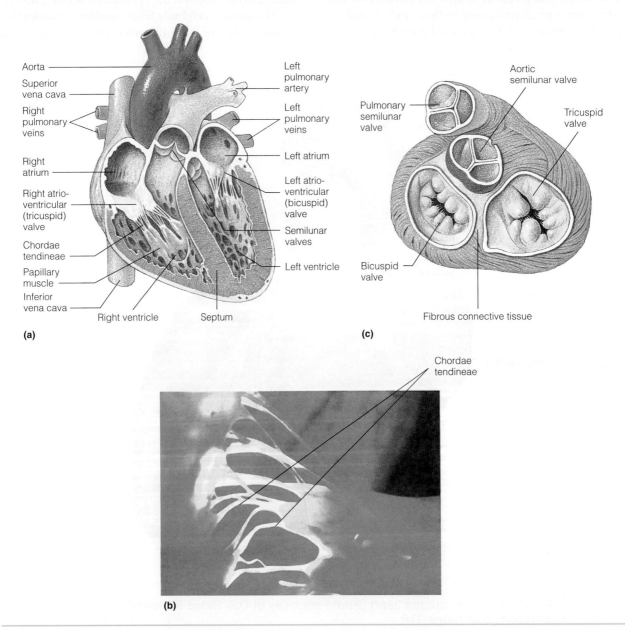

FIGURE 11-4   The heart and its valves

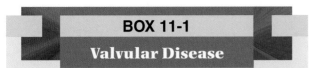

BOX 11-1
Valvular Disease

Disease of the semilunar or AV valves of the heart can lead to stenosis of the valves, a condition that can obstruct the normal flow of blood from one region of the heart to another, or to valvular insufficiency, which can cause a reflux of blood into the area from which the blood was ejected during systole. This reverse flow, usually involving the mitral and tricuspid valves, is known as regurgitation. As the valvular disease progresses, the myocardium enlarges to compensate for insufficient flow, and, unless treated surgically with prosthetic valve replacements, congestive heart failure is bound to ensue.

Rheumatic fever may cause calcium deposition and fibrous tissue formation on the leaflets of the mitral valve. This results in an immobile valve, and the AV orifice between the left atrium and left ventricle becomes progressively narrower. Half of the patients with the disease will develop atrial fibrillation, and blood flow from the atria to the ventricles is not ejected normally because the contraction is eliminated. Blood stagnated in the atria may form thromboses that could result in arterial embolization.

Blood Flow Through the Heart

The right atrium receives blood that is low in oxygen and high in carbon dioxide from two large veins: the superior vena cava brings in venous blood from the upper portion of the body, and the inferior vena cava brings in venous blood from the lower portions of the body. A smaller vein, the coronary sinus, also empties into the right atrium, draining blood from the wall of the heart.

Increased blood pressure in the right atrium causes the tricuspid valve to open, allowing blood to flow somewhat passively into the right ventricle. As blood pressure increases in the right ventricle, the valve closes. Increased pressure within the right ventricle causes the pulmonary semilunar valve to open, and blood is pumped under pressure into the pulmonary artery and on to the lungs for oxygenation. When the right ventricle relaxes, the blood in the pulmonary trunk pushes against the pulmonary semilunar valve and closes it, thereby preventing regurgitation back into the right ventricle.

From the branches of the pulmonary artery, blood enters the capillaries of the alveoli of the lungs. Oxygen and carbon dioxide are exchanged between the blood in the capillaries and the air in the alveoli. The freshly oxygenated blood, which is now low in carbon dioxide, returns to the heart by way of four pulmonary veins and empties into the left atrium. As pressure increases in the left atrium, the atrial wall contracts and the mitral valve opens, moving blood through the left AV orifice and into the left ventricle. As the left ventricle contracts, the mitral valve closes, and blood enters the aorta through the aortic semilunar valve, where it is propelled to the body (Figure 11-5).

Blood Supply for the Heart

The myocardium of the heart receives oxygenated blood for nourishment from two arteries, both of which originate in the ascending aorta, just superior to the aortic semilunar valve (Figure 11-6). The right coronary artery divides into two main branches: the posterior descending artery, which sends branches to both ventricles, and the marginal artery, which sends branches to the right ventricle and right atrium. The left coronary artery divides into two main branches: the anterior descending artery, which supplies blood to both ventricles, and the circumflex artery, which supplies blood to the left ventricle and left atrium.

Both ventricles receive their blood supply from branches of both the right and left coronary arteries. Each atrium receives blood from only a small branch of the corresponding coronary artery. The left ventricle's myocardium receives the most blood, and therefore the most oxygen and nutrients, because of its larger myocardium and increased capacity for pumping.

After blood has nourished the myocardium with oxygen and nutrients and picked up its carbon dioxide wastes, it is delivered back to the right atrium by way of the coronary sinus. The coronary veins that lead into the coronary sinus closely parallel the path of their corresponding arteries.

Coronary Artery Disease

Coronary atherosclerotic heart disease is the most common type of coronary artery disease, and is recognized as the leading cause of death in the industrialized Western world. Each year approximately 1 million Americans die from the disease, and the annual economic costs are staggering, averaging in the tens of billions of dollars.

Risk factors for coronary atherosclerosis include the following:

- Sex: The disease affects more males than females. Female sex hormones are thought to play a role, and estrogen therapy for postmenopausal women is currently being studied.

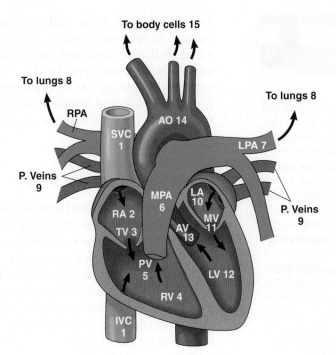

1. Blood reaches heart through superior vena cava (SVC) and interior vena cava (IVC)
2. To right atrium
3. To tricuspid valve
4. To right ventricle
5. To pulmonary valve (semilunar)
6. To main pulmonary artery
7. To left pulmonary artery and right pulmonary artery

8. To lungs—blood receives O_2
9. From lungs to pulmonary veins
10. To left atrium
11. To mitral (bicuspid) valve
12. To left ventricle
13. To aortic valve (semilunar veins)
14. To aorta (largest artery in the body)
15. Blood with oxygen then goes to all cells of the body

AO — Aorta
AV — Aortic valve
IVC — Inferior vena cava
LA — Left atrium
LPA — Left pulmonary artery
LV — Left ventricle
MPA — Main pulmonary artery
MV — Mitral valve
PV — Pulmonary valve
P.VEINS — Pulmonary veins
RA — Right atrium
RPA — Right pulmonary artery
RV — Right ventricle
SVC — Superior vena cava
TV — Tricuspid valve

FIGURE 11-5   Blood flow through the heart

- Race: There is a higher mortality rate among nonwhites.
- Age: Older people are far more likely to be affected.
- Genetics: A familial disposition is thought to have both genetic and environmental origins.
- Hypertension: High blood pressure will accelerate the development of atherosclerosis, particularly if it develops at an early age.
- Cigarette smoking: This is one of the most important risk factors associated with the disease. The negative effects on the cardiovascular system are partially related to nicotine, tar, carbon monoxide, and other harmful components of cigarette smoke.
- Diet: A diet rich in polyunsaturated fats (especially animal fats) contributes to the development of the disease.
- Obesity: Overall, obese people develop atherosclerosis at an earlier age and have more

significant lesions than do those who weigh less. Elevated serum levels of lipids, such as cholesterol, lipoproteins, and triglycerides, directly correlate with the extent and severity of the atherosclerosis. Obese individuals are also more prone to hypertension, diabetes, and glucose intolerance; it is these associated factors that may be the link between obesity and atherosclerosis.

- Clotting factors: Soluble clotting factors, such as thrombin, fibrin, and platelets, play a role in the formation of atherosclerotic lesions.
- Psychosocial influences: Individuals with lower socioeconomic status are more likely to smoke, are more obese, and have higher rates of hypertension than those with higher economic status. Individuals who are under constant pressure to perform, or who can be labeled "overachievers," are more likely to develop atherosclerosis.

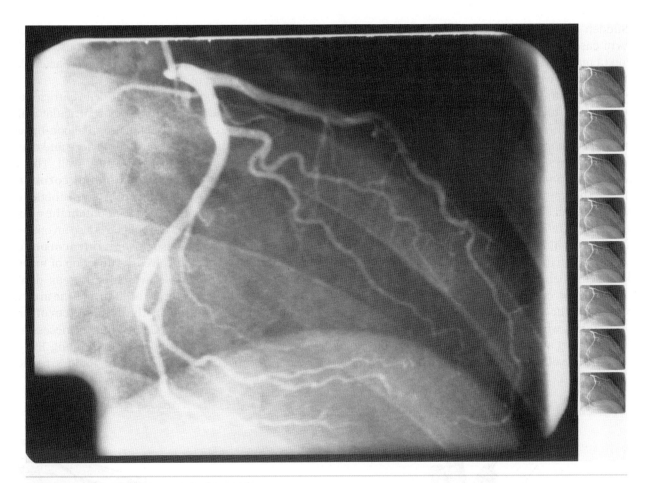

FIGURE 11-6   Coronary arteriography

Progressive, chronic, **myocardial ischemia**, the underlying pathogenic mechanism of coronary atherosclerosis, develops as a result of the progression of narrowing of the lumen of the coronary artery due to atheroma formation (see Chapter 12 for information on atheromas).

It is ischemia that is responsible for the clinical manifestations of coronary atherosclerosis: **angina pectoris**, which occurs when myocardial oxygen demand exceeds supply, and is characterized by substernal or reterosternal "crushing" pain that often radiates to the throat, back, or left arm; acute **myocardial infarction (MI)**, which results in the death of heart muscle tissue; and sudden cardiac death.

Sudden occlusion of the vessel results in acute MI and treatment must be immediate. The area of damage by MI depends on the coronary artery affected and the amount of myocardial tissue served by the artery. For example, an occlusion of the proximal right coronary artery will result in infarction of the right ventricle and posterior wall of the left ventricle; an occlusion of the proximal circumflex branch of

the left coronary system will result in infarction of the lateral wall of the left ventricle; and an anterior ventricular wall infarction is typically caused by occlusion of the proximal left anterior descending artery.

Smaller areas of damage occur in the myocardium when occlusion occurs in one or more distal branches of the coronary arteries. Coronary artery lesions usually occur near the origin and bifurcation of the main coronary vessels, but diffuse involvement throughout the branches is seen in advanced cases. Most lesions occur in the left anterior descending or LAD, artery. The LAD artery accounts for 50% of all atherosclerotic lesions of the coronary system, the right coronary artery accounts for 30–40%, and the circumflex branch of the left coronary system accounts for 15–20% of the lesions.

Within 24 hours of an MI, temperature is elevated and white blood cell count is increased due to myocardial necrosis. Death of the myocardial cells also brings about the release of certain enzymes that enter the bloodstream.

Sudden death from MI occurs in approximately 25% of cases, usually as a result of ventricular fibrillation (a major dysrhythmia in which the walls of the ventricle flutter without coordinated contraction, and blood is not pumped away from the heart), heart block, and asystole (cardiac arrest).

Diagnosis of MI is based on the presenting symptoms and evidence of impaired heart function, which is found by physical examination, electrocardiography, and abnormal serum enzyme levels.

Drug therapy is aimed at reducing myocardial oxygen demand, and includes vasodilators such as nitroglycerin, beta-adrenergic blocking agents, and calcium channel blockers, which inhibit the movement of calcium ions across the cell membranes via the calcium channel.

The cardiac catheterization laboratory, or "cath lab," is often the next stop after the emergency room for the patient who sustains an acute MI. The cardiologist can insert a temporary pacemaker wire into the right ventricle of the heart to stabilize heart rhythm, and can also insert catheters into the coronary arteries for the injection of contrast solutions, which, under fluoroscopy, can outline the coronary artery lesion and the extent of the blockage.

Contrast solution injected into the left ventricle can clearly outline the damage to the left ventricular wall. If necessary, the cardiologist can insert balloon-tipped catheters into the affected coronary artery and compress the atheroma against the artery wall. This is known as **percutaneous transluminal coronary angioplasty (PTCA)**. Placement of a prosthetic intravascular stent (Figure 11-7) to maintain the cylindrical lumen produced by the balloon is also an option.

The cardiologist can also perform **intracoronary thrombolysis**, which involves the injection of an enzyme called streptokinase, which can break down thrombi and thereby enlarge the lumen of the artery.

Surgical intervention in the form of **coronary artery bypass grafting (CABG)** may be necessary. The procedure may not necessarily prolong life or reduce the occurrence of MI, but it does reduce

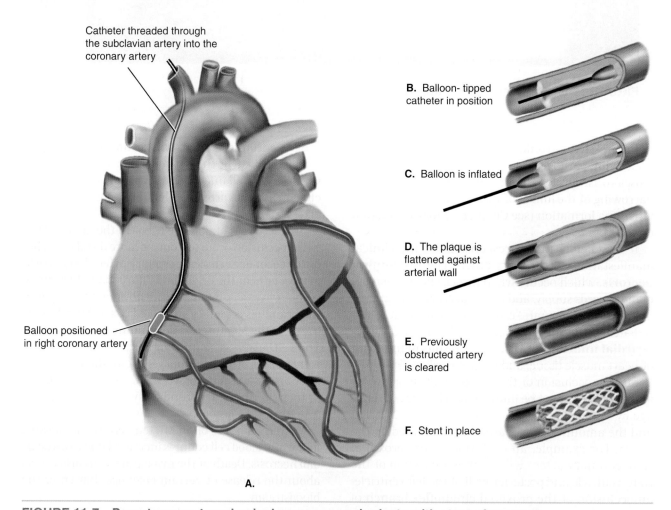

Catheter threaded through the subclavian artery into the coronary artery

Balloon positioned in right coronary artery

B. Balloon- tipped catheter in position

C. Balloon is inflated

D. The plaque is flattened against arterial wall

E. Previously obstructed artery is cleared

F. Stent in place

A.

FIGURE 11-7 **Percutaneous transluminal coronary angioplasty with stent placement**

angina and improve activity tolerance, thereby improving the quality of life. Once damaged, however, the myocardium cannot be repaired.

Complications of MI include the following:

- Myocardial rupture may occur as a result of a softening of the necrotic ventricular myocardium and an increased ventricular pressure. As blood escapes from the ventricle into the pericardial sac, the heart is compressed, interrupting normal rhythm. This potentially lethal condition is known as cardiac tamponade, and is usually treated by pericardiocentesis (insertion of a long needle into the pericardium for drainage of fluid or blood).
- **Cardiac aneurysm**, or a ballooning of the ventricular wall, can be a result of increased ventricular pressure and scar tissue in the ventricular wall formed by massive MIs.

- Heart failure and carcinogenic shock may result. Because of inadequate perfusion of tissues by a failing heart, multisystem organ failure may develop. The most dangerous of these is cerebral ischemia, which may lead to irreversible brain damage. But it is the kidneys that are most often damaged.

The Cardiac Cycle

A single **cardiac cycle** includes everything that occurs within the heart during a single heartbeat. In each cardiac cycle, pressure changes occur as the atria and ventricles alternately contract and relax, and blood flows from areas of higher pressure to those of lower pressure.

As the atria of the heart relax, the ventricles contract, and vice versa. The term **systole** refers to the

---

BOX 11-2

Techniques of Cardiopulmonary Bypass (CPB)

During certain cardiac procedures, the heart must be stopped so that certain surgical techniques can be safely performed (such as the suturing of a venous graft onto a diseased coronary artery). Blood must be diverted around the heart to the rest of the body (Figure 11-8). The **pump oxygenator**, or heart–lung machine, is the apparatus used in cardiac surgery to remove unoxygenated blood from the venous system, oxygenate and filter it, and return the blood to the arterial system. By assuming the roles of the heart and lungs, the pump oxygenator allows the heart to be stopped. It also allows the lungs to be deflated for better exposure of the heart and major vessels. The name heart–lung machine indicates what is required to produce **extracorporeal circulation**: the oxygenation of blood (replacing the function of the lungs) and the pumping of blood (replacing the function of the heart).

The pump oxygenator is relatively simple in design. Venous blood is removed from the body by way of a sterile plastic tube (cannula) that is placed into the right atrium or venae cavae and shunted through an oxygenator.

The oxygenator is equipped with a reservoir and heat exchanger that allows the temperature of the blood to be manipulated as needed. After blood has been oxygenated, a roller pump moves the blood from the reservoir back to the arterial system. Additional pumps are used for removing blood from the operative site (using *cardiotomy suckers* on the operative field) and vented blood from the left ventricle. This blood is added to a reservoir for oxygenation and sent back into the arterial system, thereby preventing blood loss. The placement of cannulas into the right atrium or venae cavae for draining venous blood to the pump oxygenator

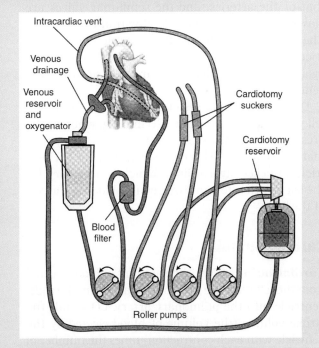

FIGURE 11-8 Cardiopulmonary bypass

and the ascending aorta for the return of arterial blood from the pump oxygenator is referred to as *cannulation*. Before cannulation, a blood thinner called heparin must be administered to prevent clotting.

phase of contraction, and the term **diastole** refers to the phase of relaxation. For a resting heart rate of 75 beats/minute, each cardiac cycle lasts about 0.8 seconds.

After three fourths of the blood within the atria has passively drained into the ventricles through the AV orifice, the walls of the atria contract, forcing the remainder of blood into the ventricles. This contraction is called atrial systole. Contraction of the heart's chambers increases the pressure of the fluid within it. After atrial systole, the walls of the atria relax. This is referred to as atrial diastole. The contraction of the ventricular wall is referred to as ventricular systole, and the relaxation phase of the ventricles is referred to as ventricular diastole. During ventricular systole, pressure within the ventricles rises sharply.

Once blood pressure within the ventricles exceeds the pressure within the atria, the AV valves close, allowing pressure within the atria to build. When ventricular pressure exceeds the pressure within the pulmonary artery and the aorta, the semilunar valves open and blood is pumped into those arteries (ventricular ejection).

As blood leaves the ventricles, pressure falls below that of the arteries, and the semilunar valves are closed by the pressure of blood within the arteries. The lower pressure within the ventricles during ventricular diastole allows the AV valves to open once again, and blood begins to flow from the atria into the ventricles.

During ventricular systole, the pressure within the left ventricle rises to about 120 mm Hg, whereas the pressure within the right ventricle rises to approximately 30 mm Hg. This is a reflection of the left ventricle's thicker myocardium, which is necessary for the left ventricle to pump oxygenated blood to the rest of the body.

Cardiac Output

Cardiac output (CO) is the amount of blood ejected from the left ventricle into the aorta or from the right ventricle into the pulmonary artery. CO equals the stroke volume (the volume of blood ejected by the ventricle with each contraction) times the number of heartbeats per minute. In a typical adult at rest, stroke volume (SV) averages about 70 ml/beat and a heart rate (HR) of 72 beats per minute. Therefore, CO = SV × HR or 70 ml/beat × 72 beats per minute. The result of 5,040 ml/min. or 5.04 L per minute is approximately the total amount of blood volume within the typical adult male.

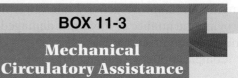

BOX 11-3

Mechanical Circulatory Assistance

Surgical technologists should be familiar with mechanical devices designed for circulatory support after cardiac procedures because they are often implanted intraoperatively. A general understanding of the device and its application is imperative for proper implantation.

Patients may need cardiac support because they are waiting for cardiac transplantation or cannot be weaned from cardiopulmonary bypass (CPB). The mechanical device designed for circulatory support after cardiac procedures is called an intra-aortic balloon pump (IABP). Insertion of the balloon pump may increase cardiac output (CO) to a level that would permit separation from the pump oxygenator (the machine used for CPB) and allow time for the heart to recover. To be completely effective, the IABP must lower left ventricular pressure during systole (when the balloon is deflated), and increase coronary artery circulation during diastole (when the balloon is inflated).

Patients who cannot be separated from CPB by conventional methods or IABP may benefit from the use of a ventricular assist device (VAD). The VAD is designed to boost CO and rest an ailing left ventricle by diverting blood away from the left ventricle, through an artificial pump, and into the aorta for systemic circulation.

For procedures on the descending thoracic aorta, blood flow must be maintained to distal tissues. The use of a heparin-coated impeller flow pump for left ventricular bypass permits work to be done on the descending thoracic aorta and also supplements CO for an ailing left ventricle. Through cannulas inserted into the common femoral artery and left atrium, the pump pulls blood away from the left ventricle and propels it into the aorta.

Cardiac Conduction

Located throughout the heart are specialized areas of tissue that transmit electrical impulses throughout the myocardium for the rhythmical activity of the heart.

The conduction system's key component is the **sinoatrial (SA) node**, which is located in the right atrial wall just inferior to the opening of the superior vena cava. The SA node acts as a natural electrical pacemaker, and so is referred to as the heart's pacemaker. In other words, the cells of this specialized tissue have the ability to excite themselves. The SA node fires an electrical impulse that spreads into the myocardium and stimulates cardiac muscle fibers to contract in a rhythmic manner.

On their own, the autorhythmic fibers in the SA node initiate action potentials 90–100 times per minute, but specific neurotransmitters and hormones can stimulate the autonomic nervous system's parasympathetic division to slow the rate to approximately 75 beats per minute.

The impulse fired by the SA node spreads throughout atrial tissue and down to the **atrioventricular (AV) node**, located in the septum between the two atria. This node provides the only normal conduction pathway between the atrial and ventricular synctium, which are fibers that are interconnected in branching networks that, when stimulated, contract as a unit. The action potential slows considerably at the AV node because the fibers are much smaller, which causes a delay in the impulse. This delay allows time for the atria to empty their contents into the ventricles. From the AV node, the impulse enters the AV bundle, also known as the **bundle of His**. This is the only electrical connection between the atria and the ventricles. The AV bundle enters the upper portion of the septum between the ventricles and divides into left and right bundle branches that course along the septum toward the apex of the heart. It is here that the electrical impulse enters larger-diameter conduction fibers known as **Purkinje fibers**, which spread the action potential to the apex of the left ventricle and upward to the remainder of the ventricular myocardium, resulting in a twisting ventricular contraction.

Parasympathetic and sympathetic nerve fibers for the heart originate within the medulla oblongata of the brainstem, becoming part of the right and left vagus nerves and terminating in the SA node and AV node. The parasympathetic division of the autonomic nervous system is responsible for slowing the heart rate, utilizing a neurotransmitter called acetylcholine to dampen SA and AV nodal activity.

Sympathetic fibers from the brainstem travel to the thoracic region of the spinal cord and reach out to the SA and AV nodes by way of cardiac accelerator nerves, which secrete the neurotransmitter norepinephrine to accelerate heart rate and myocardial contraction.

The body, in its quest for homeostasis, seeks a balance between parasympathetic and sympathetic stimulation of the heart. When the body is at rest and the heart rate is at its average 72 beats/minute, the parasympathetic division is in control. The SA node typically fires at 90–100 beats/minute, so acetylcholine is dampening the node's action through the parasympathetic fibers of the autonomic nervous system.

Cardiac Dysrhythmias

Individuals with heart disease often experience disturbances in normal heart rhythm, which can decrease CO, damage the myocardium, and lead to eventual cardiac arrest. Although these cardiac dysrhythmias can be caused by many factors, including hypoxia, acidosis, electrolyte imbalances, MI, drugs, hypotension, hemorrhage, hypovolemia, or pneumothorax, most are caused by abnormalities in impulse formation, or abnormalities in conduction due to a blockage somewhere along the neural pathway. The following are common dysrhythmias:

- Sinus dysrhythmia, the most common dysrhythmia, is typically found in young adults and the elderly. This dysrhythmia is the physiologic cyclic variation in heart rate related to vagal nerve impulses to the sinoatrial node. It is a benign rhythm that usually requires no treatment.
- Sinus tachycardia, characterized by an atrial and ventricular rate of 100 beats per minute or more, is associated with the ingestion of nicotine, alcohol, or caffeine. It is a normal response to fear, excitement, or physical exertion. The condition is also associated with hyperthyroidism, hypovolemia, and hypotension. Sinus tachycardia is generally benign, but can cause a decrease in CO if there is an underlying myocardial impairment.
- Sinus bradycardia, characterized by an atrial and ventricular rate of 60 beats per minute or less, is considered beneficial because it reduces myocardial oxygen demands. It is often seen in well-conditioned athletes. It can become so slow, however, that CO is reduced, resulting in eventual heart failure if left untreated.

Dysrhythmias originating in the atria include:

- Premature atrial beat
- Atrial tachycardia
- Atrial flutter
- Atrial fibrillation

The premature atrial beat arises from an ectopic focus somewhere within the atria. It is often associated with stress or the consumption of caffeine or nicotine, but may also accompany inflammation or MI. It is considered benign, and treatment usually consists of the omission of tobacco or caffeine from the individual's lifestyle.

Atrial tachycardia is characterized by an atrial rate of 150–250 beats per minute. Symptoms usually involve palpitations and anxiety, but no treatment is necessary unless the atrial rate exceeds 200 beats per minute or the episode continues for an extended length of time.

Atrial flutter involves rapid atrial activity at a rate of 250–350 beats per minute. Generally, as a prevention mechanism, the conduction of each impulse from the atria to the ventricles is blocked by the AV node. Despite this safety control, the ventricular rate may still exceed 150 beats per minute, and could result in a decrease in CO.

Atrial fibrillation is another common dysrhythmia encountered in clinical practice, and involves a rapid and disordered beating of the atria, usually at a rate of 350–600 beats per minute. As in atrial flutter, the atrial impulse to the ventricles is increased, and the ventricular rate is usually 100–180 beats per minute. Without the propulsion of blood from the atria to the ventricles (atrial kick), CO is reduced. CO is also affected by the irregular ventricular rhythm caused by the irregular atrial impulses. Atrial fibrillation may be a chronic or transient condition.

Ventricular dysrhythmias can be classified as benign premature ventricular contractions (PVCs), complex PVCs, or malignant (lethal). A PVC is a contraction of the ventricle that occurs before it is expected in a normal series of cardiac cycles. PVCs that are benign usually are five or less per hour, and are often seen in normal persons in the absence of heart disease. These may be caused by a stretching of the anterior papillary muscle of the right ventricle during mechanical activity.

Complex PVCs (greater than 10–30 per hour) may occur in patients with or without heart disease. Those that occur in patients without heart disease may possibly be due to biochemical abnormalities or patches of myocarditis. Those that occur with left ventricular dysfunction are potentially lethal, and should be treated with antiarrhythmic drugs.

Many are not aware of benign PVCs, and it may be wiser with some individuals not to direct their attention to the ectopic beats if they have no evidence of heart disease because of the anxiety that may be induced. The frequency of PVCs may be reduced by the elimination of caffeine, tobacco, and alcohol. The avoidance of stress factors and frequent exercise are also encouraged. If all general measures fail, and symptoms interfere with the quality of life, antiarrhythmic drugs may be utilized.

Ventricular tachycardia is present when three or more PVCs occur in succession, usually at a rate of 140–250 beats per minute. It is referred to as sustained if it lasts longer than 30 seconds or requires termination because of hemodynamic instability. The nonsustained types last less than 30 seconds and stop spontaneously. The sustained PVCs or nonsustained PVCs with hemodynamic instability are referred to as malignant dysrhythmias, and are usually seen in patients with cardiac disease.

A ventricle is said to flutter when it is contracting regularly, but at a very rapid rate (250–350 contractions per minute). Ventricular flutter presents as regular oscillations on ECG and is likely to be due to damage to the myocardium. Ventricular fibrillation is also characterized by rapid ventricular contractions, but in an uncoordinated fashion.

During this dysrhythmia, small regions of the myocardium contract and relax independently of all other areas. As a result, the myocardium fails to contract as a whole and the walls of the fibrillating ventricle are completely ineffective at pumping blood. Unless this dangerous dysrhythmia is converted by electric shock (defibrillation), death will most certainly ensue. The ventricles can be stimulated to fibrillate by a variety of factors, including ischemia associated with coronary artery obstruction, electric shock, or trauma to the heart.

Dysrhythmias may also be caused by an interference in normal cardiac impulse conduction. These "heart blocks" are impairments of conduction in heart excitation and are influenced by the fact that certain cardiac tissues other than the SA node may act as pacemakers.

For instance, damage to the SA node may cause the AV node to take over the functions of cardiac pacing, in essence functioning as a secondary pacemaker. AV blocks occur in the AV junction tissue (AV node, bundle of His, or the bundle branches). The block is often characterized as first-, second-, or third-degree AV block.

First-degree AV block occurs when conduction time is prolonged but all atrial beats are followed by ventricular beats. This delay could be in the AV node, bundle of His, or any of the bundle branches. Second-degree AV block occurs when some, but not all, atrial beats are conducted to the ventricles. Third-degree AV block can occur in the AV node, bundle of His, or any of the bundle branches. In this type of block, no impulses whatsoever are conducted by the junctional tissues, owing to pathologic factors. This condition may be permanent or paroxysmal, and if syncopal attacks occur in conjunction with bradycardia, it is known as Adams–Stokes disease. This disease is the main indication for use of a permanent cardiac pacemaker.

Electrocardiogram

Each of the dysrhythmias described in the preceding text can be diagnosed with an **electrocardiogram (ECG)**, used to record the electrical activity of the heart. The baseline (also known as the isoelectric line) is a straight line that separates the waves' deflections. Waves are deflected either upward (positive deflection) or downward (negative deflection), and depict the polarization and depolarization of the cells of the myocardium. Deflections and the distance between them are represented by the letters P, QRS, and T, and the types of deflections and their sizes and shapes can tell a cardiologist what is going on in the heart at any given time. The P wave represents atrial depolarization, QRS represents ventricular depolarization, and T represents ventricular repolarization (Figure 11-9). An elevated ST segment (the distance on the line between the S wave and the T wave) often indicates MI, requiring immediate treatment before damage is done to the myocardium.

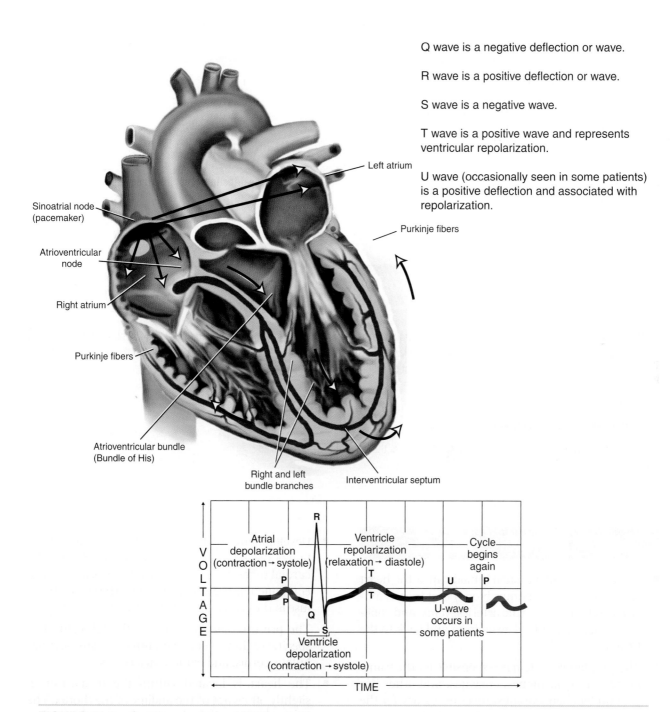

Q wave is a negative deflection or wave.

R wave is a positive deflection or wave.

S wave is a negative wave.

T wave is a positive wave and represents ventricular repolarization.

U wave (occasionally seen in some patients) is a positive deflection and associated with repolarization.

FIGURE 11-9   Cardiac cycle and ECG reading

IMPLICATIONS FOR THE SURGICAL TECHNOLOGIST

The surgical technologist plays a vital role in the surgical interventions for repair of cardiovascular pathologic conditions. In addition, the surgical technologist may assist with cardiac diagnostic procedures performed in the operating room, cardiac catheterization laboratory, or special procedures department.

Diagnostic procedures of the heart include plain x-ray films, computerized axial tomography (CAT) scan, magnetic resonance imaging (MRI), electrocardiography, echocardiography, and cardiac catheterization. In addition to diagnostic coronary arteriograms and ventriculograms performed in the cardiac catheterization laboratory, the surgical technologist often assists in PTCA and permanent pacemaker insertion in the special procedures department (and occasionally in the OR).

Surgical procedures for repair of congenital heart defects include correction of atrial and ventricular septal defect, patent ductus arteriosus, aortic coarctation, tetralogy of Fallot, and transposition of the great arteries.

Surgical procedures for the repair of pathologies of the adult heart and great vessels include:

- Heart transplantation
- Pericardiectomy/pericardial window
- Thoracic aortic aneurysmectomy (TAA)
- Mitral valve replacement
- Aortic valve replacement
- CABG

These are complex procedures that require extensive training for the surgical technologist in the scrub role or first-assist role.

Case Study 2

Dr. Jenkins is beginning a procedure to implant a cardiac pacemaker. Gene is the surgical technologist who is assisting him. The patient has bradycardia, which causes weakness and dizziness. Gene has set up the back table and Mayo tray with the proper supplies and instruments, and calls the radiologic technologist to drape the fluoroscope.

1. What is bradycardia?

2. How does a pacemaker work?

3. In what part of the heart is the lead placed? Where is the generator usually placed?

CHAPTER SUMMARY

- The cardiovascular system is made up of the heart (as the organ that pumps blood) and the peripheral vascular system (the arteries, veins, and capillaries that carry blood away from and back to the heart).

- The circulatory system is responsible for the transportation of hormones, enzymes, and other important biochemical substances necessary for the proper maintenance and health of the body.

- Development of the heart begins with the formation of two separate tubes that originate from endocardial tubes. One end of each tube forms arterial components; the other, venous. These two tubes fuse in the center, forming the primitive heart tube.

- The primitive heart tube has the following five specific regions: ventricle, sinus venosus, atrium, bulbus cordis, and truncus arteriosus.

- The heart is located within the mediastinum, slightly off center of the midline of the thorax. The heart is enclosed in a loose sac (pericardium) that protects it and keeps it from rubbing against the thoracic wall. The pericardium consists of two parts: fibrous pericardium and serous pericardium.

- The wall of the heart is composed of three layers: epicardium, myocardium, and endocardium.

- The heart's upper chambers are called atria and are designed to receive blood from the veins of the body. The lower chambers are called ventricles and are designed to pump blood into arteries leading away from the heart.

- The chambers of the heart are divided into right and left portions by the septum. The septum between the atria is the interatrial septum; the interventricular septum separates the ventricles.

- The atrium communicates with its corresponding ventricle through an opening called the atrioventricular (AV) orifice, which is guarded by an atrioventricular valve. The tricuspid valve sits between the right atrium and the right ventricle.

- Fibrous cords called chordae tendineae are attached to the cusps on the ventricular side, and prevent the cusps of the valve from folding back into the atrium.

- Blood from the lungs enters the left atrium and crosses through the AV orifice across the AV valve referred to as the mitral valve.

- When the left ventricle contracts, the mitral valve closes and blood is ejected into the large artery known as the aorta. At the base of the aorta is another semilunar valve called the aortic semilunar valve.

- The flow of blood through the heart is as follows:

1. The right atrium receives blood from the superior vena cava and the inferior vena cava. Increased blood pressure in the right atrium causes the tricuspid valve to open, allowing blood to flow somewhat passively into the right ventricle.
2. As blood pressure increases in the right ventricle, the valve closes.
3. Increased pressure within the right ventricle causes the pulmonary semilunar valve to open, and blood is pumped under pressure into the pulmonary artery and on to the lungs for oxygenation.
4. When the right ventricle relaxes, the blood in the pulmonary trunk pushes against the pulmonary semilunar valve and closes it, preventing regurgitation back into the right ventricle.
5. From the branches of the pulmonary artery, blood enters the capillaries of the alveoli of the lungs.
6. Oxygen and carbon dioxide are exchanged between the blood in the capillaries and the air in the alveoli.
7. The freshly oxygenated blood, which is now low in carbon dioxide, returns to the heart by way of four pulmonary veins and empties into the left atrium.
8. As pressure increases in the left atrium, the atrial wall contracts and the mitral valve opens, moving blood through the left AV orifice and into the left ventricle. As the left ventricle contracts, the mitral valve closes, and blood enters the aorta through the aortic semilunar valve, where it is propelled to the body.

- The myocardium of the heart receives oxygenated blood for nourishment from two arteries: the right coronary artery and the left coronary artery, which divides into two main branches—the anterior descending artery and the circumflex artery.

- Coronary atherosclerotic heart disease is the most common type of coronary artery disease, and is recognized as the leading cause of death in the industrialized Western world.

- It is ischemia that is responsible for the clinical manifestations of coronary atherosclerosis: angina pectoris, myocardial infarction (MI), and sudden cardiac death.

- Treatments for atherosclerosis include percutaneous transluminal coronary angioplasty (PTCA), intracoronary thrombolysis, and coronary artery bypass grafting (CABG).

- A single cardiac cycle includes everything that occurs within the heart during a single heartbeat. The term systole refers to the phase of contraction, and the term diastole refers to the phase of relaxation.

- Cardiac output (CO) is the amount of blood ejected from the left ventricle into the aorta or from the right ventricle into the pulmonary artery. CO equals the stroke volume times the number of heartbeats per minute.

- The cardiac conduction system coordinates the events of the cardiac cycle; its key component is the sinoatrial (SA) node. The SA node is referred to as the heart's pacemaker.

- The impulse fired by the SA node spreads throughout atrial tissue and down to the AV node, located in the septum between the two atria. This node provides the only normal conduction pathway between the atrial and ventricular synctium.

- From the AV node, the impulse enters the AV bundle, also known as the bundle of His. This is the only electrical connection between the atria and the ventricles.

- The AV bundle enters the upper portion of the septum between the ventricles and divides into left and right bundle branches that course along the septum toward the apex of the heart, where larger diameter conduction fibers known as Purkinje fibers spread the action potential to the apex of the left ventricle and upward to the remainder of the ventricular myocardium, resulting in a twisting ventricular contraction.

- Individuals with heart disease often experience disturbances in normal heart rhythm, which can decrease cardiac output, damage the myocardium, and lead to eventual cardiac arrest.

- The following are common dysrhythmias: sinus dysrhythmia, sinus tachycardia, and sinus bradycardia.

- Dysrhythmias originating in the atria include premature atrial beat, atrial tachycardia, atrial flutter, and atrial fibrillation.

- Each of the dysrhythmias described in the preceding text can be diagnosed with an electrocardiogram (ECG), used to record the electrical activity of the heart.

- Wave deflections are represented by the letters P, QRS, and T. The P wave represents atrial depolarization, QRS represents ventricular depolarization, and T represents ventricular repolarization.

CRITICAL THINKING QUESTIONS

1. Describe the pathway that an embolism from the great saphenous vein of the leg would take before lodging in the pulmonary artery?
2. Why is atrial fibrillation dangerous? Is it more dangerous than ventricular fibrillation?
3. What is a "beating heart" off-pump cardiac procedure?
4. Where are the proximal saphenous vein grafts placed for a CABG? Why are they placed there?
5. What is mitral valve regurgitation?

REFERENCES

Anthony, C. P., & Thibodeau, G. A. (1979). *Textbook of anatomy and physiology* (10th ed.). St. Louis, MO: C. V. Mosby.

Association of Surgical Technologists. (2003). *Surgical technology for the surgical technologist: A positive care approach* (2nd ed.). Clifton Park, NY: Thomson Delmar Learning.

Boettcher, W., Merkle, F., & Weitkemper, H. H. (2003). History of extracorporeal circulation: The conceptional and developmental period. *Journal of Extra-Corporeal Technology, 35*(3), 172–183.

Cassmeyer, V. L., Long, B. C., Phipps, W. J., & Woods, N. F. (Eds.). (1991). *Medical-surgical nursing concepts and clinical practice* (4th ed.) St. Louis, MO: Mosby Year Book.

Damjanov, I. (1996). *Pathology for the health-related professions* (1st ed.). Philadelphia: W. B. Saunders.

Gazes, P. C. (1990). *Clinical cardiology* (3rd ed.). Philadelphia: Lea & Febiger.

Grabowski, S. R., & Tortora, G. J. (1996). *Principles of anatomy and physiology* (8th ed.). New York: HarperCollins.

Hole, J. W. (1987). *Human anatomy and physiology* (4th ed.). Dubuque, IA: W. C. Brown.

O'Toole, M. (Ed.). (1997). *Miller–Keane encyclopedia & dictionary of medicine, nursing, and allied health* (5th ed.). Philadelphia: W. B. Saunders.

Sabiston, D. C., Jr. (1997). *Textbook of surgery. The biological basis of modern surgical practice* (15th ed.). Philadelphia: W. B. Saunders.

Sanders, T., & Scanlon, V. C. (1995). *Essentials of anatomy and physiology* (2nd ed.). Philadelphia: F. A. Davis.

Scott, A., & Fong, E. (2004). *Body structures and functions* (10th ed.). Clifton Park, NY: Thomson Delmar Learning.

12

PERIPHERAL VASCULAR SYSTEM

CHAPTER OBJECTIVES

After completing the study of this chapter, you should be able to:

1. Discuss the relevant vessels of the peripheral vascular system.
2. Compare and contrast the structure of an artery and a vein.
3. Describe the mechanisms that regulate blood pressure.
4. Describe the etiology of atherosclerosis and arterial embolism and their treatments.
5. Compare and contrast bypass grafting and endarterectomy.

KEY TERMS

angiography	blood pressure	Doppler probe	tunica intima
arterial embolism	blood pressure gradient	endarterectomy	tunica media
arteries	capillaries	phleborheography	vasoconstriction
arterioles	central venous pressure	plethysmography	vasodilation
atheromas	(CVP)	resistance	veins
atherosclerosis	claudication	tunica adventitia	venules

Case Study 1

Mrs. Johnson is a 72-year-old diabetic woman who presents to the emergency room with the following symptoms: (a) pain in the calves when walking that is alleviated by rest, and (b) large right toe that is purple in color.

1. What is the most likely diagnosis?

2. How should Mrs. Johnson's diagnosis be confirmed?

3. If an embolism is discovered, how will it be treated?

INTRODUCTION

The peripheral vascular system refers to a closed system of blood vessels that transports blood away from the heart to the body's tissues, and then back again to the heart. The surgical technologist must understand the anatomy of the vessel and the names and locations of the major vessels in order to properly repair them.

BLOOD VESSELS

Arterial blood is pumped by the heart through a large system of blood vessels called **arteries**; therefore, arterial blood refers to blood that is transported away from the heart to the tissues of the body. The arteries are large in size as they leave the heart, but begin subdividing into progressively smaller arteries as they move into various regions of the body. These arteries grow progressively smaller until they become **arterioles**, which in turn become **capillaries**. Capillaries are microscopic vessels designed to exchange nutrients and wastes between the blood and tissue fluid around the cells in specialized areas called capillary beds. After this exchange, capillaries unite to form **venules**, the smallest of veins. These venules, in turn, unite to form progressively larger blood vessels called **veins**, which eventually become the superior and inferior venae cavae, the largest of veins. Veins, then, are designed to transport blood back to the heart (Figure 12-1).

Arterial blood pumped away from the left ventricle of the heart enters the aorta, the largest of the arteries, and begins its trip through the progressively smaller arteries toward the arterioles, which become capillaries. Wastes, nutrients, O_2, and CO_2 are exchanged, and then venous blood begins its trip back to the heart in the venules, which grow progressively larger to become veins. Venous blood is then emptied into the inferior and superior venae cavae, and deposited into the right atrium of the heart.

STRUCTURE OF THE ARTERY AND THE VEIN

The wall of an artery consists of three layers called tunics (Figure 12-2). The outer layer is called the **tunica adventitia** and consists of connective tissue. This layer attaches the artery to the surrounding tissues and also contains tiny vessels called vasa vasorum that nourish the cells of the arterial wall.

The middle tunic is called the **tunica media** and is the thickest of the three layers of the arterial wall. This layer includes elastic fibers and smooth muscle fibers that completely encircle the artery. The smooth muscles in this layer are innervated by sympathetic branches of the autonomic nervous system. Impulses from these nerves can cause the smooth muscles to contract, resulting in a narrowing of the lumen, which is the channel for blood flow within the vessel. This process is referred to as **vasoconstriction**. The inhibition of the impulses from the autonomic nervous system allows the smooth muscles to relax, resulting in an increase of the diameter of the lumen. This is referred to as **vasodilation**. Vasoconstriction results in a rise in blood pressure, whereas vasodilation results in a decrease in blood pressure.

The inner tunic is called the **tunica intima** and is composed of a lining of endothelium. This layer is in contact with the blood; the lining of this layer must be smooth so that platelets can flow without being damaged.

The walls of arterioles are very thin, and consist of only a layer of simple squamous epithelium surrounded by a small amount of smooth muscle and connective tissue.

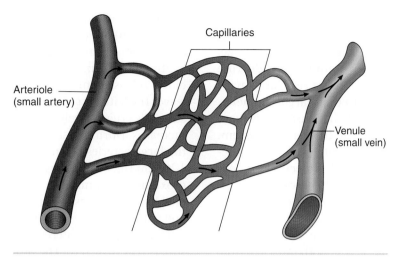

FIGURE 12-1   Arteries deliver oxygenated blood to capillaries, and, once the oxygen has been extracted, blood is returned to the venous system

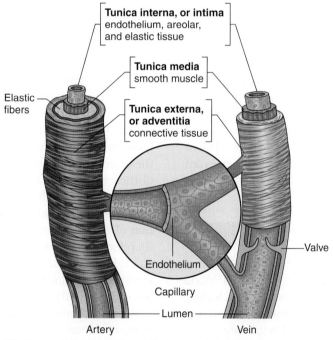

(A) Types of blood vessels and their general structure

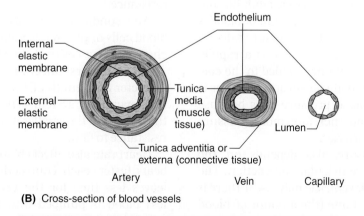

(B) Cross-section of blood vessels

FIGURE 12-2   Different types of blood vessels and their cross-sectional views

The epithelial layer of the capillaries is very thin as well, and contains openings or pores where two adjacent epithelial cells overlap. These pores vary in size, depending on their location. Within the endocrine and digestive systems, the pores are very large, with increased permeability due to their larger diameter. The pores of the capillaries of the muscular system, however, are very small. Within the nervous system, the brain has capillaries with tightly packed endothelial cells, comprising a system of protection for delicate neurons called the blood–brain barrier.

Veins are composed of the same three layers as arteries, but there are differences in their relative thickness. The middle layer of the venous wall is poorly developed, with far less smooth muscle tissue. The tunica adventitia is the thickest layer of the vessel, consisting of collagen and elastic fibers, whereas the tunica intima of the vein is much thinner than that of the artery. The lumen of a vein, however, is larger than that of an artery.

Blood pressure within a vein is low and venous blood must work against gravity in most regions of the body on its trip back to the heart. Therefore, the veins are equipped with flaplike valves made of thin layers of tunica intima that close if blood begins to back up in a vein. Veins pass between groups of skeletal muscles, and when these muscles contract, blood is pushed upward in the vein toward the heart. When the skeletal muscles relax, the vein's valves prevent the blood from moving back away from the heart.

BLOOD PRESSURE

Blood pressure is the force that blood exerts against the internal walls of blood vessels. Arterial blood pressure is dependent on many factors, including blood volume, the strength of a ventricular contraction, resistance, blood viscosity, and heart rate. Blood pressure is dependent on the volume of blood within the cardiovascular system. The average adult has approximately 5 L of blood. If a large amount of blood is lost due to hemorrhage, the blood pressure falls; in fact, a true indication of hemorrhage is a rapidly falling blood pressure. If volume is added to the cardiovascular system by blood transfusion or water is retained in the body, blood pressure rises because there is more fluid, and therefore more pressure against the walls of the arteries.

Arterial blood pressure also depends on the strength of the heart's ventricular contraction. The cardiac output of the left ventricle may rise if there is an increase in stroke volume (the amount of blood ejected by the left ventricle into the aorta with one contraction) or an increase in the heart rate, as long as resistance remains the same. The strength of the contraction, then, is directly related to the amount of blood released into the arterial system. As blood leaves the left ventricle and enters the aorta, its pressure falls progressively as the distance from the heart increases. During systole, the blood pressure within the large arteries of an adult rises to approximately 120 mm Hg; during diastole, the pressure falls to approximately 80 mm Hg. As blood enters the arterioles, pressure drops to approximately 35–40 mm Hg, and in the capillaries the pressure is about 15 mm Hg.

Once blood has entered into the venae cavae, pressure is very near zero. The **blood pressure gradient** for the entire systemic circulation is the difference between the mean blood pressure within the aorta and the mean blood pressure within the venae cavae as they enter the right atrium of the heart. For example, if pressure within the ascending aorta is 120 mm Hg, and pressure within the superior vena cava is 2 mm Hg, the systemic pressure gradient is 118 mm Hg. Without a pressure gradient between the arterial and venous system, blood will not circulate.

Resistance is the hindrance of blood flow within the cardiovascular system due to the friction of blood against the walls of the vessel. It must be overcome by blood pressure for blood to flow. Most resistance is in the arterioles, capillaries, and venules, simply because of their small size. The larger the vessel, the lower the resistance to blood flow because less blood comes into contact with the walls of the vessel. The vasoconstriction of arterioles increases vascular resistance, and therefore raises blood pressure. As the arterioles constrict, blood pressure rises as blood backs up into the arteries, and blood pressure increases to force the blood through the smaller diameter of the arterioles.

Resistance also depends on the viscosity, or thickness, of blood. The cells and proteins within the blood plasma increase its viscosity, and therefore its resistance.

Any condition that alters the concentration of blood cells or plasma proteins, such as hemorrhage, changes the viscosity of the blood.

Other factors affecting resistance include the diameter and length of the blood vessels within the cardiovascular system. The greater the length of the vessel and the smaller its diameter, the greater the resistance to flow.

Heart rate also affects blood pressure. As the heart beats faster, each contraction of the left ventricle leaves less time for the ventricle to refill, and so less blood is pumped into the aorta for systemic circulation. With a decreased cardiac output, arterial blood volume is decreased, and blood pressure is lowered. A change in heart rate will affect the blood pressure only if that change corresponds to an increase or decrease in the stroke volume.

Venous blood pressure, as mentioned previously, is much lower than arterial pressure. As blood approaches the right atrium of the heart, its pressure is near zero. Venous return to the heart does not rely, then, on cardiac output, but rather on other factors. As skeletal muscles contract, they squeeze the blood inside the veins upward against gravity. Many veins, especially those in the arms and legs, have semilunar valves that catch the blood moving toward the heart, preventing backflow. In addition, respiratory inspiration squeezes blood from the abdominal veins upward toward the heart by pushing the diaphragm against the abdominal organs, which creates a decrease in thoracic cavity pressure and an increase in the pressure within the abdomen. As a result, a large volume of blood moves from the compressed abdominal veins into the veins of the thoracic cavity.

Venous blood pressure within the right atrium is referred to as **central venous pressure (CVP)**. CVP is of importance because of the effect it has on the pressure within the large peripheral veins. If the heart is beating weakly, CVP increases and blood backs up into the venous system, causing the pressure within the system to rise. If the heart beats strongly, CVP is low as blood enters and leaves the heart efficiently. Other factors that lead to an increase in CVP are tricuspid regurgitation or an increase in systemic blood volume.

THE ARTERIAL SYSTEM

The aorta, which is the largest artery in the body, begins as the ascending aorta, ascending from the left ventricle of the heart. Just beyond the aortic semilunar valve are the left and right aortic sinuses, which are small dilations of the aorta that precede the only branches of the ascending aorta, the left and right coronary arteries. The aortic sinuses contain the aortic bodies, which are specialized receptors within the epithelial lining that function to control blood pressure and oxygen and carbon dioxide concentrations.

The coronary arteries, as explained previously, supply the myocardium with oxygenated blood. They lie within a groove that encircles the heart called the atrioventricular sulcus. Branches of the left coronary artery are the anterior interventricular artery (also

known as the anterior descending artery), which supply both ventricles, and the circumflex artery, which serves the left atrium and the left ventricle. Branches of the right coronary artery are the posterior interventricular artery (also known as the posterior descending artery), which supplies both ventricles, and the marginal artery, which serves the right atrium and right ventricle.

Three major arteries emerge from the aortic arch: the brachiocephalic artery (also known as the innominate artery), the left common carotid artery, and the left subclavian artery.

The brachiocephalic artery supplies the blood to the tissues of the arm and head, and is the first branch of the aortic arch, veering to the right. Near the junction of the sternum and the right clavicle, the brachiocephalic artery bifurcates into the right subclavian artery, which leads into the right arm, and the right common carotid artery, which serves the brain and the right side of the neck and head.

The left common carotid and the left subclavian arteries are the second and third branches of the aortic arch, and serve the same function as their counterparts on the right side. Just beyond the left subclavian artery, the aorta becomes the descending aorta. The portion of the descending aorta that lies above the diaphragm is known as the thoracic aorta, which passes downward from the 4th through 12th thoracic vertebrae; that portion below the diaphragm is known as the abdominal aorta.

Branches of the descending aorta supplying the thoracic wall are the superior phrenic arteries and the posterior intercostal arteries. Branches supplying the viscera of the thorax are the bronchial, pericardial, mediastinal, and esophageal arteries.

In the abdominal aorta, branches serve the abdominal wall and the abdominal viscera. The visceral branches include the celiac artery, which is a thick, short artery that immediately divides into three arteries: the left gastric, splenic, and common hepatic arteries.

The common hepatic artery has three main branches: the hepatic artery proper (left and right hepatic branches), which serve the liver and gallbladder; the gastroduodenal artery, which serves the stomach, the body of the pancreas, and the duodenum; and the right gastric artery, which serves the stomach.

The splenic artery has three main branches: the left gastroepiploic artery, which serves the stomach; the pancreatic artery, which serves the tail of the pancreas; and the polar arteries, serving the spleen.

The left gastric artery serves the lesser curvature of the stomach and the esophagus. The inferior phrenic arteries supply blood to the inferior surface of the diaphragm and adrenal glands.

The superior mesenteric artery is an unpaired vessel arising anteriorly from the abdominal aorta, just below the celiac trunk. This vessel branches to supply numerous abdominal organs: the pancreas and duodenum are served by the inferior pancreatico-duodenal artery; the small intestine is served by the ileal and jejunal intestinal arteries; and the cecum, appendix, and ascending and transverse colons of the large intestine are supplied by the ileocolic, right colic, and middle colic arteries.

The suprarenal artery is a paired artery that serves the adrenal glands, which are also well supplied by branches of the renal and inferior phrenic arteries. The renal arteries pass laterally from the aorta to each kidney and also serve a small portion of the adrenal glands.

In the male, the right and left gonadal arteries are referred to as the testicular arteries; they arise from the aorta and pass through the body wall by way of the inguinal canal to serve the testes. In the female, the arteries are referred to as the ovarian arteries; they arise from the aorta and pass into the pelvis to supply the ovaries.

The inferior mesenteric artery is an unpaired vessel arising anteriorly from the abdominal aorta, just above the bifurcation of the aorta. This vessel supplies lower abdominal organs, including the descending and sigmoid colons of the large intestine (left colic and sigmoid arteries) and the rectum (superior rectal artery).

The lumbar arteries arise from the posterior surface of the aorta and serve the spinal cord and its meninges, as well as various muscles and skin of the lumbar region of the back.

The middle sacral artery is a small, unpaired vessel that supplies the sacrum, coccyx, and rectum.

The abdominal aorta bifurcates into the left and right common iliac arteries at the level of the fourth lumbar vertebra. These arteries divide inferiorly into two main branches: the right and left external iliac arteries, and the right and left internal iliac arteries.

The internal iliac arteries are the principal blood supply for the pelvis and perineum. Their branches include the iliolumbar and lateral sacral arteries, which serve the pelvic wall and muscles; the middle rectal artery, which serves the internal pelvic organs; the vesicular arteries (superior, inferior, and middle), which serve the urinary bladder; the superior and inferior gluteal arteries, which supply the buttocks; the obturator artery, which supplies the upper medial thigh muscles; and the internal pudendal artery, which supplies the external genitalia and is responsible for blood engorgement of the female genitalia and penile erections in men.

The external iliac arteries become the femoral arteries as they exit the pelvic cavity and cross the inguinal ligament.

Two branches arise from the external iliac arteries: the inferior epigastric artery, which serves the skin and abdominal wall muscles, and the deep iliac circumflex artery, which supplies the muscles of the iliac fossa.

The femoral arteries, which pass fairly close to the anterior surface of the upper thigh, send branches back into the pelvic region to supply the genitals and lower abdominal wall. Branches include the medial and lateral femoral circumflex arteries, which supply muscles in the proximal thigh and encircle the femur; and the deep femoral artery (profundis femoris), which is the largest branch of the femoral artery and serves the hip joint and hamstring muscles of the thigh.

The femoral artery continues down the medial and posterior side of the thigh at the back of the knee joint, where it becomes the popliteal artery. The popliteal artery supplies a few small branches to the knee joint, and then divides into two branches. The first branch, the anterior tibial artery, serves the anterior aspect of the leg, and, at the ankle, becomes the dorsalis pedis artery, which serves the ankle and dorsum of the foot. The second branch, the posterior tibial artery, continues down the posterior side of the leg between the knee and the ankle. The posterior tibial artery sends off a large branch called the peroneal artery, which supplies the peroneal leg muscles. At the ankle, it bifurcates into the lateral and medial plantar arteries, which supply the bottom of the foot. The lateral plantar artery joins with the dorsal pedis artery to form the plantar arch.

Arterial blood supply for the left upper extremity begins at the aortic arch, where the left subclavian artery originates. The right subclavian artery branches from the brachiocephalic artery. The subclavian arteries pass laterally deep to the clavicle, and as they enter the axillary region, they become the axillary arteries. As the axillary arteries enter the brachial region of the arm, they become the brachial arteries, which continue along the medial side of the humerus. The major branch of the brachial artery is the deep brachial artery, which serves the triceps muscle. At the end of the elbow, the brachial artery divides into the medial ulnar and lateral radial arteries. The largest branch of the radial artery is the radial recurrent artery, which supplies the elbow. The branches of the ulnar artery are the anterior and posterior ulnar recurrent arteries. The ulnar and radial arteries pass inferiorly to the palm, where branches fuse to form palmar arches. From these arise palmar digital arteries, which supply the fingers and thumb.

Blood for the head and neck originates from the two common carotid arteries that pass along either side of the trachea in the neck. The right common carotid originates from the brachiocephalic artery, and the left common carotid arises directly from the aortic arch. Small branches of the common carotid artery supply the larynx, thyroid gland, anterior neck muscles, and lymph glands.

The common carotid artery bifurcates into the internal and external carotid arteries at the superior border of the larynx. The external carotid artery supplies structures in the neck and head area external to the skull. The main branches include the superior thyroid artery, which serves the hyoid muscles, larynx and vocal cords, and the thyroid gland; the ascending pharyngeal artery; the lingual artery, which supplies the tongue and sublingual salivary gland; the facial artery, which supplies the palate, chin, lips, and nose; the occipital artery, which serves the posterior scalp, the meninges of the brain, and the posterior neck muscles; and the posterior auricular artery, which supplies the ear.

Near the mandibular condyle, the external carotid divides into the superficial temporal artery, which serves the parotid salivary gland; and the maxillary artery, which supplies the teeth and gums, muscles of mastication, nasal cavity, eyelids, and meninges of the brain.

The internal carotid and the vertebral arteries supply blood to the brain. The internal carotid artery enters the base of the skull through the carotid canal of the temporal bone. After arising from the subclavian arteries, the paired vertebral arteries enter the skull through the foramen magnum. Once inside the skull these two arteries unite to form the single basilar artery. The two internal carotid arteries and the basilar artery unite in a circular arrangement at the base of the brain near the sella turcica called the circle of Willis. This circle is formed by the union of the anterior cerebral arteries, which branch from the internal carotid arteries, and the posterior cerebral arteries, which branch from the basilar artery. The posterior communicating arteries connect the posterior cerebral arteries and the internal carotid arteries. The anterior cerebral arteries are connected by the anterior communicating artery.

BOX 12-1
Sutures for Peripheral Vascular Anastomoses

Typical suture gauges for peripheral vascular anastomoses are:

- Aorta: 3-0 or 4-0
- Iliac: 4-0 or 5-0
- Femoral: 5-0 or 6-0
- Popliteal: 5-0 or 6-0
- Posterior tibial: 6-0 or 7-0
- Common carotid: 6-0
- Internal carotid: 6-0 or 7-0
- Brachial: 6-0 or 7-0
- Subclavian: 6-0
- Radial or ulnar: 6-0 or 7-0

Suture for peripheral vascular procedures includes polypropylene, Dacron, polyester, and PTFE (polytetrafluoroethylene) materials. Double-armed sutures on swaged needles are used for anastomoses. Silk ties and silk and polypropylene suture ligatures are frequently used.

THE VENOUS SYSTEM

The dural sinuses are blood channels that receive blood from the cerebral, ophthalmic, cerebellar, and meningeal veins of the brain. These include the superior sagittal sinus, inferior sagittal sinus, straight sinus, and basilar plexus, which are all unpaired sinuses of the brain. The paired sinuses include the cavernous, superior petrosal, inferior petrosal, occipital, transverse/lateral, and sigmoid sinuses.

The veins of the brain include the superior cerebral vein, inferior and medial veins, the great cerebral vein of Galen, and the superior and inferior ophthalmic veins. The veins that receive blood from these numerous sinuses and veins within the brain are the right and left internal jugular veins. Therefore, the internal jugular veins drain the brain and the meninges, as well as the deep regions of the face and neck. These veins course downward, beneath the sternocleidomastoid muscle and alongside the common carotid artery in the neck, and eventually empty into the right and left subclavian veins. The union of the internal jugular and the subclavian veins creates the brachiocephalic, or innominate veins.

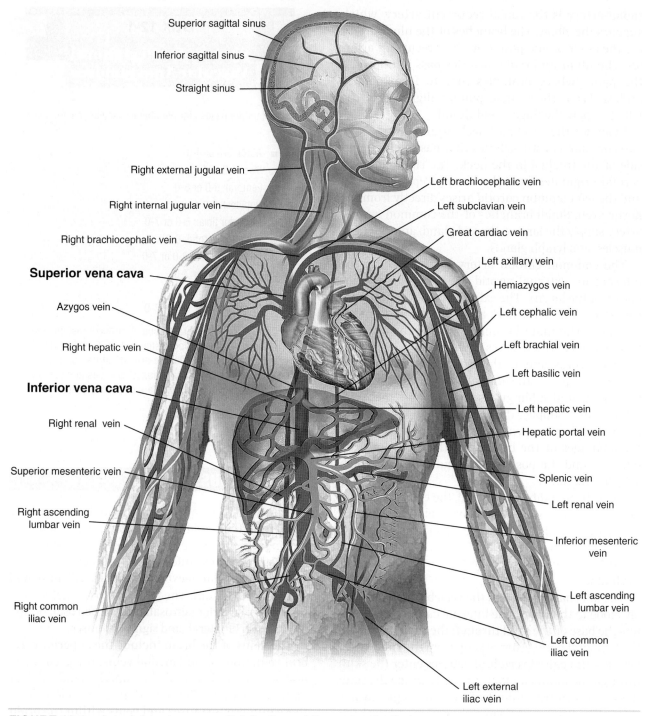

Superior sagittal sinus

Inferior sagittal sinus

Straight sinus

Right external jugular vein

Right internal jugular vein

Right brachiocephalic vein

Superior vena cava

Azygos vein

Right hepatic vein

Inferior vena cava

Right renal vein

Superior mesenteric vein

Right ascending lumbar vein

Right common iliac vein

Left brachiocephalic vein

Left subclavian vein

Great cardiac vein

Left axillary vein

Hemiazygos vein

Left cephalic vein

Left brachial vein

Left basilic vein

Left hepatic vein

Hepatic portal vein

Splenic vein

Left renal vein

Inferior mesenteric vein

Left ascending lumbar vein

Left common iliac vein

Left external iliac vein

FIGURE 12-3   Arterial and venous distribution of the upper body

The brachiocephalic veins then merge into a single superior vena cava, which enters into the right atrium of the heart.

The right and left external jugular veins course downward laterally alongside the internal jugular vein and superficial to the sternocleidomastoid muscle. These veins drain the parotid glands and superficial structures of the face and scalp, eventually emptying into the right and left subclavian veins.

The right and left vertebral veins descend through the transverse foramina of the cervical vertebra alongside the vertebral arteries. These veins drain deep structures of the neck, including the vertebrae, and eventually empty into the subclavian veins.

The superficial tissues of the upper extremities are drained by the cephalic and basilic veins. The cephalic vein courses along the lateral side of the arm from the hand to the shoulder, eventually emptying into the axillary vein. Just beyond the axilla, the axillary vein becomes the subclavian vein.

The basilic vein passes upward along the medial side of the arm and merges with the brachial vein just below the head of the humerus to form the axillary vein. The deep tissues of the upper extremity are drained by the radial, ulnar, and brachial veins, which course upward within the same regions as their counterpart arteries. The radial veins receive blood from the dorsal metacarpal veins; the ulnar veins receive blood from the palmar venous arch; and the brachial veins join into the axillary veins.

The abdominal and thoracic walls are drained by tributaries of the brachiocephalic and azygos veins. The right and left brachiocephalic veins, as mentioned earlier, are formed by the union of the subclavian and internal jugular veins. The brachiocephalic vein drains the head, neck, arms, and upper thorax. The left brachiocephalic vein is the entry point for the thoracic duct of the lymphatic system. The thoracic duct enters the right brachiocephalic vein at the junction of the right internal jugular and subclavian veins. The azygos vein receives the ascending lumbar, hemiazygos, accessory azygos, and bronchial veins in the thorax, as well as certain intercostal and subcostal veins that drain the muscles of the thoracic wall. The azygos originates in the dorsal abdominal wall and courses superiorly to the right side of the vertebral column to join the superior vena cava. Blood from the abdomen and pelvis enters the inferior vena cava for return to the right atrium of the heart. The inferior vena cava, however, does not drain the veins of the spleen, pancreas, gastrointestinal tract, or gallbladder.

The blood from these organs is drained into the hepatic portal vein, which is formed by the union of the superior mesenteric vein and the splenic vein (Figure 12-4). The superior mesenteric vein drains blood from the small intestine and the splenic vein drains blood from the spleen. The hepatic portal vein transports the blood to the liver.

In the liver, the blood, which contains absorbed nutrients of digestion, enters capillaries called hepatic sinusoids, which filter the blood through the hepatic liver cells. This venous pathway is called the hepatic portal system.

Bacteria that is present in the portal vein is filtered by the phagocytic action of the Küpffer cells within the hepatic sinusoids. After passing through the hepatic sinusoids, blood is carried through a series of merging vessels into the hepatic veins, and eventually makes its way back to the inferior vena cava.

As the inferior vena cava ascends through the abdomen, it picks up other tributaries from the abdomen. These include the left and right renal veins from the kidney, the suprarenal veins from the adrenal glands, the inferior phrenic veins, and the gonadal veins from the ovaries or testicles.

The veins of the lower extremities are divided into two groups: the superficial group and the deep group. The deep veins of the lower extremities have the names of their corresponding arteries. The anterior and posterior tibial veins drain blood from the deep veins of the foot. At the knee, these veins unite to form the popliteal vein, which continues upward into the thigh and becomes the femoral vein, which drains blood from the deep femoral vein and lateral-medial circumflex veins in the upper thigh. As the femoral vein approaches the inguinal ligament, it receives blood from the great saphenous vein, the longest vein in the body. Near its junction with the femoral vein, the great saphenous vein receives blood from the upper thigh, groin, and lower abdominal wall.

At the level of the sacroiliac joint, the external iliac vein merges with the internal iliac vein, which carries blood away from the reproductive, urinary, and digestive organs, and becomes the common iliac vein. The left and right common iliac veins merge at the level of the fifth lumbar vertebra to form the inferior vena cava.

ATHEROSCLEROSIS

Vascular abnormalities involving the extremities increase in frequency with age and are a major cause of disability in the United States. Although peripheral manifestations are frequently symptoms of a generalized, systemic disease, the peripheral problem itself demands solution for the well-being of the patient. Reconstructing an occluded peripheral artery will not cure the patient of atherosclerosis, but it will mitigate a major problem for the patient.

The signs and symptoms of peripheral arterial disease are determined by the location and degree of vascular obstruction, the rapidity with which this obstruction develops, and the presence or absence of collateral channels.

The term **atherosclerosis**, from the Greek *athere*, meaning gruel or porridge, and *scleros*, meaning hard, describes a condition that involves the formation of an

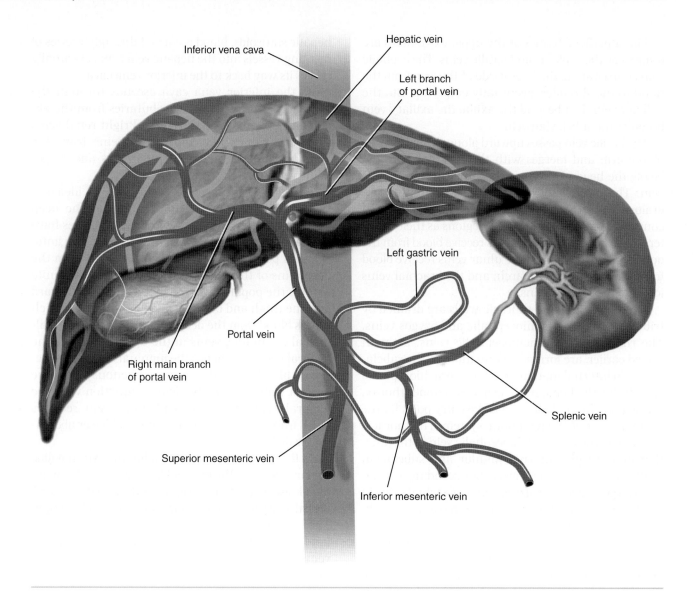

Inferior vena cava

Hepatic vein

Left branch of portal vein

Left gastric vein

Portal vein

Right main branch of portal vein

Splenic vein

Superior mesenteric vein

Inferior mesenteric vein

FIGURE 12-4   Portal and hepatic veins

atheroma in the intima of medium and large arteries (Figure 12-5).

Atheromas are the prototypical lesions of atherosclerosis, and consist of a soft central region composed of lipids and cellular debris covered by a tough layer of fibrous tissue. Calcium salts are eventually deposited into the arterial walls and the atheromas, resulting in a hardening of the artery. The result of the atherosclerotic process is a reduction of blood flow to the target tissues.

The atheroma is also highly thrombogenic, launching small pieces, or thrombi, into the bloodstream. These pieces can become lodged in smaller vessels such as cerebral or coronary arteries and may completely

occlude the lumen of the vessel with subsequent infarction.

The first step in the formation of the atheroma is believed to be an injury to the endothelial lining of the arterial wall. Blood platelets and lipoproteins are deposited into the injury as a repair mechanism, and growth factors released from the platelets stimulate the growth of new smooth muscle tissue in the arterial wall.

Changes in the metabolism of the smooth muscle cells promote the accumulation of cholesterol and other lipids within the cell's cytoplasm, which, when leaked across the cell membrane into the interstitial spaces, attract scavenger macrophages. The

AFFECTED SITE   **COMPLICATION**

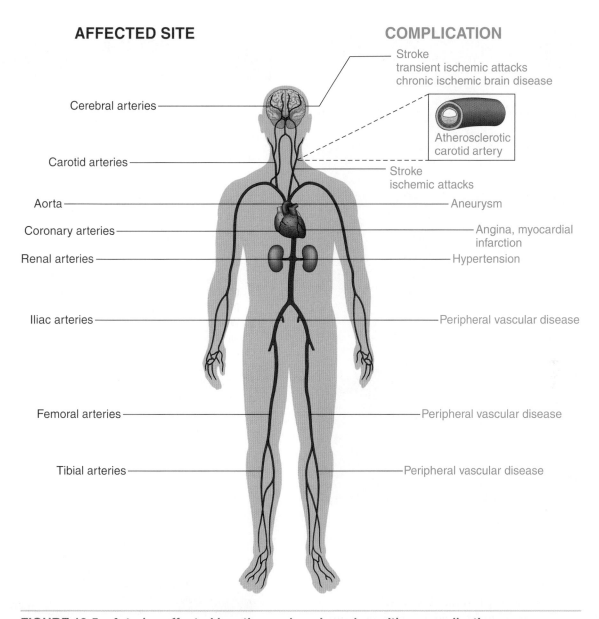

FIGURE 12-5   Arteries affected by atherosclerosis and resulting complications

macrophages secrete biologically active substances that cause further damage to the arterial wall. Eventually, collagen is deposited into the lesion and scar tissue begins to form, narrowing the lumen of the artery (Figure 12-6).

The two main areas of early peripheral involvement are the aortic bifurcation and the distal superficial femoral artery at the adductor canal. The process may then progress to involve other portions of the arterial system.

Diagnostic procedures and tests for the evaluation of peripheral vascular disease include:

- **Plethysmography**: an instrument for determining and registering variations in the amount of blood flowing through an extremity; especially useful for patients with diffuse small vessel arterial disease
- **Doppler probe**: an ultrasonic device used to identify and assess vascular status of peripheral

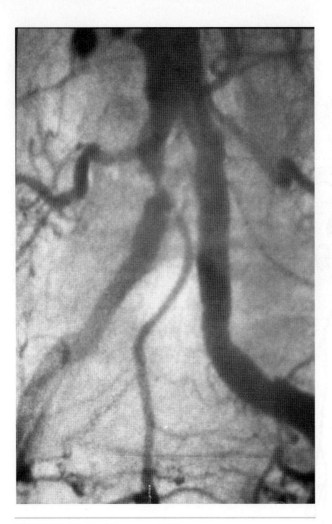

FIGURE 12-6   Stenosed iliac artery

arteries and veins by magnifying the sound of the blood moving through the vessel

- **Phleborheography**: a device used for diagnosis of deep vein thrombosis
- Computerized axial tomography, magnetic resonance imaging, and ultrasonography for the detection and evaluation of carotid artery atherosclerosis or thoracic or abdominal aortic aneurysm
- **Angiography**: the injection of contrast solutions through specialized catheters to outline the vascular system under x-ray; the gold standard for the diagnosis and evaluation of vascular disease

ARTERIAL EMBOLISM

A sudden loss of circulation to an extremity is usually an indication of **arterial embolism**. In addition to

Synthetic grafts used to bypass peripheral arterial obstructions are made of various materials, including:

- Knitted polyester (Dacron): Knitted polyester (Dacron) grafts are porous for rapid tissue in-growth. However, this porosity also allows blood to seep through the material, requiring preclotting by the surgical team.
- Knitted velour (Dacron): Knitted velour polyester (Dacron) grafts are uniformly porous for good tissue in-growth. One type has the antibiotic amikacin impregnated into the prosthetic wall, making the graft impervious to leaks and obviating the need for preclotting.
- Woven polyester (Dacron): Woven polyester construction of the Dacron graft is leak-proof and does not need to be preclotted. Because of their inflexibility, however, these grafts are relegated to larger arterial bypass grafting.
- Polytetrafluoroethylene (Gore-Tex, Impra): Expanded (PTFE) can be taken across the knee joint without risk of kinking. The microporous wall of PTFE serves as a lattice framework for tissue in-growth, creating an ultra-thin layer for contact with blood and obviating the need for preclotting. The PTFE graft may have rigid rings built into the prosthetic wall for support.

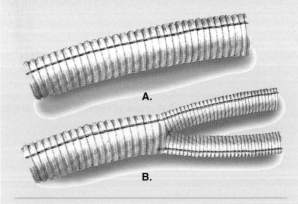

FIGURE 12-7   Vascular grafts (A) tubular; (B) bifurcated

blood clots, emboli may consist of fat, air, or even portions of tumor that circulate through the cardiovascular system until they eventually become lodged in smaller vessels, blocking blood flow to an extremity or organ. Morbidity associated with embolism remains high and consistent at 15–30%, not necessarily because of the ischemic limb but because of the

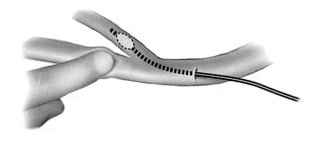

FIGURE 12-8 Insertion of Fogarty catheter

underlying disease that led to the formation of the embolus.

Major emboli lodge at bifurcations or the origin of large branches, at sites of anatomic narrowing, and at sites of pathologic narrowing, such as an atherosclerotic superficial femoral artery. Approximately 80% of peripheral emboli affect the lower limb with the common femoral bifurcation accounting for almost half the cases.

Emboli may originate from the left atrium in patients with atrial fibrillation or from the left ventricle when the endocardium is damaged and the ventricle contracts poorly. Recent studies suggest that 90% of all patients with arterial emboli have an underlying heart disorder, although emboli may also be shed from the aorta to the extremities.

The restoration of peripheral circulation is imperative to prevent loss of limb. Enzymatic lysis of the embolus during angiography may be tried before surgery. The enzyme (urokinase or streptokinase) is delivered through an intra-arterial catheter placed at the proximal extent of the clot. If enzyme therapy is not successful, surgery for the direct removal of the embolus or thrombus is the next option.

Surgical intervention for the removal of emboli (arterial embolectomy) involves an incision made into the affected artery for the removal of thromboembolitic material and the restoration of flow to the extremity. The insertion of a balloon-tipped Fogarty embolectomy catheter into the arteriotomy facilitates the removal of the embolus (Figure 12-8).

BYPASS GRAFTING AND ENDARTERECTOMY

Surgery remains the treatment of choice in most patients with disabling **claudication** (severe pain in the muscles of the lower leg caused by poor circulation), pain during rest, or gangrene. Bypassing the occlusion with a synthetic or biologic graft and endarterec-

tomy are the two basic reconstructive procedures utilized today. **Endarterectomy**, which is the excision of the thickened, atheromatous tunica intima of an artery, has certain advantages over bypass grafting (Figure 12-9). The patient's own vessels are preserved, little or no foreign material is introduced, and the procedure is more sound hemodynamically. However, extensive endarterectomy below the hypogastric level carries a high complication and failure rate. Endarterectomy is most often performed on the carotid artery.

Arterial bypass grafting is the popular alternative to endarterectomy. Biologic or synthetic grafts are required to bypass vascular obstruction or to reconstruct vessels.

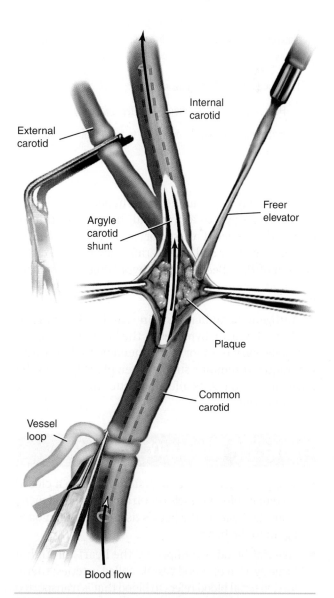

External carotid

Internal carotid

Freer elevator

Argyle carotid shunt

Plaque

Common carotid

Vessel loop

Blood flow

FIGURE 12-9 Carotid endarterectomy

IMPLICATIONS FOR THE SURGICAL TECHNOLOGIST

The surgical technologist frequently assists with various diagnostic and invasive surgical procedures used to treat pathology of the peripheral vessels. Arteriograms are often necessary to identify the location and extent of an arterial blockage and are typically performed in the hospital's special procedures department. Occasionally, a postoperative arteriogram is performed in the OR after repair of an occluded vessel. Surgical intervention for the removal of emboli (arterial embolectomy) requires knowledge of the anatomy and skill in the insertion of a balloon-tipped Fogarty embolectomy catheter to facilitate the removal of the embolus. Peripheral vascular procedures to repair occluded vessels are often performed on diabetic patients who may require special intraoperative care, especially if they are unstable. Surgical repair of diseased peripheral vessels typically involves either peripheral vessel angioplasty or bypass grafting or endarterectomy.

Case Study 2

Hank is a 54-year-old man who presents to the ER in shock with a significant drop in blood pressure. His abdomen is grossly distended, he is pale, and his breathing is shallow. He complains of severe pain in his back and abdomen. His wife reports that he has smoked three packs of cigarettes per day for 30 years.

1. What is the likely diagnosis?

2. How should this condition be treated surgically?

3. Is there a less invasive approach to treatment of this condition?

Grafts may be straight or Y-shaped. One end of the graft is sewn to a proximal, healthy portion of either the affected vessel or another vessel altogether. The other end of the graft is sewn to the distal portion of the affected vessel, bypassing the obstruction and serving as a substitute conduit for blood flow.

Autogenous saphenous vein remains the material of choice for distal bypasses of the lower extremity. It is pliable, easy to tailor, and amenable to fine suture technique. It remains supple when placed across the knee joint, and resists infection better than any other graft material.

CHAPTER SUMMARY

- The peripheral vascular system refers to a closed system of blood vessels that transports blood away from the heart to the body's tissues, and then back again to the heart.

- Arterial blood is pumped by the heart through a large system of blood vessels called arteries; therefore, arterial blood refers to blood that is transported away from the heart to the tissues of the body.

- These arteries grow progressively smaller until they become arterioles, which in turn become capillaries. Capillaries unite to form venules, the smallest of veins.

- Venules, in turn, unite to form progressively larger blood vessels called veins, which eventually become the superior and inferior venae cavae, the largest of veins. Veins, then, are designed to transport blood back to the heart.

- The wall of an artery consists of three layers called tunics. The outer layer is called the tunica adventitia and consists of connective tissue.

- The middle tunic is called the tunica media and is the thickest of the three layers of the arterial wall.

- The inner tunic is called the tunica intima and is composed of a lining of endothelium.

- Veins are composed of the same three layers as arteries, but there are differences in their relative thickness.

- Blood pressure is the force that blood exerts against the internal walls of blood vessels.

- Arterial blood pressure is dependent on many factors, including blood volume, the strength of a ventricular contraction, resistance, blood viscosity, and heart rate.

- The blood pressure gradient for the entire systemic circulation is the difference between the mean blood pressure within the aorta and the mean blood pressure within the venae cavae as they enter the right atrium of the heart.

- Resistance is the hindrance of blood flow within the cardiovascular system due to the friction of blood against the walls of the vessel.

- Resistance also depends on the viscosity, or thickness, of blood. The cells and proteins within the blood plasma increase its viscosity, and therefore its resistance.

- Venous blood pressure within the right atrium is referred to as central venous pressure (CVP). CVP is of importance because of the effect it has on the pressure within the large peripheral veins.

- The term atherosclerosis describes a condition that involves the formation of an atheroma in the intima of medium and large arteries.

- Atheromas (the prototypical lesions of atherosclerosis) consist of a soft central region composed of lipids and cellular debris covered by a tough layer of fibrous tissue.

- A sudden loss of circulation to an extremity is usually an indication of arterial embolism, which may be a blood clot, fat, air, or even portions of tumor that become lodged in smaller vessels, thereby blocking blood flow to an extremity or organ.

- Endarterectomy is the excision of the thickened, atheromatous tunica intima of an artery.

- Arterial bypass grafting involves the use of biologic or synthetic grafts to bypass vascular obstruction or to reconstruct vessels.

CRITICAL THINKING QUESTIONS

1. Why is polypropylene considered the best suture material for arterial anastomosis?
2. Why should sutures for arterial anastomosis be double-armed (needles at both ends)?
3. What is peripheral vessel angioplasty?
4. When a vessel is isolated by the surgeon during peripheral vascular grafting, what is the procedure and instrument order that the surgical technologist must know?
5. What is considered to be the gold standard for diagnosis of peripheral vascular disease?

BIBLIOGRAPHY

Anthony, C. P., & Thibodeau, G. A. (1979). *Textbook of anatomy and physiology* (10th ed.). St. Louis, MO: C. V. Mosby.

Association of Surgical Technologists, Inc. (2004). *Surgical technology for the surgical technologist: A positive care approach* (2nd ed.). Clifton Park, NY: Thomson Delmar Learning.

Carter, D. C., & Dudley, H. (Eds.). (1985). *Rob & Smith's operative surgery* (4th ed.). St. Louis, MO: C. V. Mosby.

Cassmeyer, V. L., Long, B. C., Phipps, W. J., & Woods, N. F. (Eds.). (1991). *Medical-surgical nursing concepts and clinical practice* (4th ed.). St. Louis, MO: Mosby Year Book.

Cormier, J. M., & Ward, A. S. (1986). *Operative techniques in arterial surgery* (1st ed.). Chicago: Precept Press.

Damjanov, I. (1996). *Pathology for the health-related professions* (1st ed.). Philadelphia: W. B. Saunders.

Edwards, W. H. (Ed.). (1976). *Vascular surgery* (1st ed.). Baltimore: University Park Press.

Grabowski, S. R., & Tortora, G. J. (1996). *Principles of anatomy and physiology* (8th ed.). New York: HarperCollins.

Harvey, A. M., Johns, R. J., McKusick, V. A., Owens, A. H., & Ross, R. S. (Eds.). (1988). *The principles and practices of medicine* (22nd ed.). East Norwalk, CT: Appleton & Lange.

Hole, J. W. (1990). *Human anatomy and physiology* (4th ed.). Dubuque, IA: Wm. C. Brown.

O'Toole, M. (Ed.). (1997). *Miller–Keane encyclopedia & dictionary of medicine, nursing, and allied health* (5th ed.). Philadelphia: W. B. Saunders.

Sanders, T., & Scanlon, V. C. (1995). *Essentials of anatomy and physiology* (2nd ed.). Philadelphia: F. A. Davis.

Scott, A., & Fong, E. (2004). *Body structures and functions* (10th ed.). Clifton Park, NY: Thomson Delmar Learning.

13

LYMPHATIC SYSTEM

CHAPTER OBJECTIVES

After completing the study of this chapter, you should be able to:

1. Describe the functions of the lymphatic system.
2. Identify primary lymphatic circulatory pathways.
3. Describe how lymph fluid forms.
4. Describe the functions of lymph fluid.
5. Describe the major functions of a lymph node.
6. Identify the primary locations of lymph node groups in the body.
7. Describe the pathology of lymphatic obstruction.
8. List the functions of the thymus and spleen.
9. Describe specific and nonspecific defenses.
10. List examples of specific and nonspecific defenses.
11. List the types of immunoglobulins, their origin, and their actions.
12. Describe the differences between the primary and secondary immune responses.
13. Describe the differences between active and passive immunity.
14. Explain an allergic reaction and its relationship to the immune system.
15. Explain transplanted tissue rejection and its relationship to the immune system.
16. Explain autoimmunity and its relationship to the immune system.
17. Describe the mechanisms of HIV and how it causes AIDS.
18. Explain why it is important for the surgical technologist to understand the anatomy and physiology of the lymphatic system.

KEY TERMS

abscess	antigen	artificial passive acquired	complement
adenoids	antigen–antibody complex	immunity	complement cascade
agammaglobulinemia	antigenic determinants	attenuation	differential white blood cell
agranulocytes	antiserum	cell-mediated immunity (CMI)	count
AIDS-related complex (ARC)	artificial active acquired	chemotaxis	edema
antibodies	immunity	chylomicrons	goblet cells

Case Study 1

A surgical technologist has been working in surgery for five years. Three to five weeks ago she began experiencing itchy skin, mild diarrhea, and red, teary eyes while working in the surgery department. As time went on, the symptoms became worse including severe urticaria, difficulty breathing, palpitations, flushing, nausea, and abdominal pain. Eventually she had to quit her job as a surgical technologist.

1. Based on the above information, what most likely happened to this surgical technologist?

2. What are the two types of allergic responses that have been identified?

3. Which immunoglobulin is involved in the reaction?

4. What has research shown to be the primary cause of the reaction?

5. What precautions are taken by the surgery department when a patient who has this condition must undergo a procedure?

INTRODUCTION

The lymphatic system can be viewed as a subsystem of the circulatory system, but due to its functions, which are very much different from those of the heart and circulatory vessels, it must be studied separately. However, its intimacy with the circulatory system cannot be overlooked, since the lymph vessels return tissue fluid to the blood and protect the body against the invasion of foreign material. The lymphatic system consists of the lymph fluid, lymph nodes, lymph vessels, spleen, thymus, and tonsils (Figure 13-1).

LYMPH FLUID

Lymph fluid, or simply lymph, is the tissue fluid that enters and travels through the lymph vessels. The tissue fluid that remains in the interstitial spaces, now

called lymph fluid, is returned to the circulatory system via the lymphatic vessels. To understand how lymph fluid is formed, **plasma** and its role must be understood. Plasma is the straw-colored portion of blood in which the blood cells and platelets are suspended. It is made up of water, electrolytes, proteins, glucose, fats, and gases; it carries the cellular constituents of blood through the circulatory system, and transports nutrients and wastes from the tissues. The composition of plasma is the same as that of lymph. This is important because the plasma maintains the osmotic pressure within the blood capillaries, which facilitates the exchange of fluids between the capillaries and the tissues.

The flow of plasma into the interstitial spaces exceeds the reabsorption by the blood capillaries, resulting in the formation of interstitial fluid, which increases the hydrostatic pressure somewhat, forcing the interstitial fluid to enter into the lymphatic

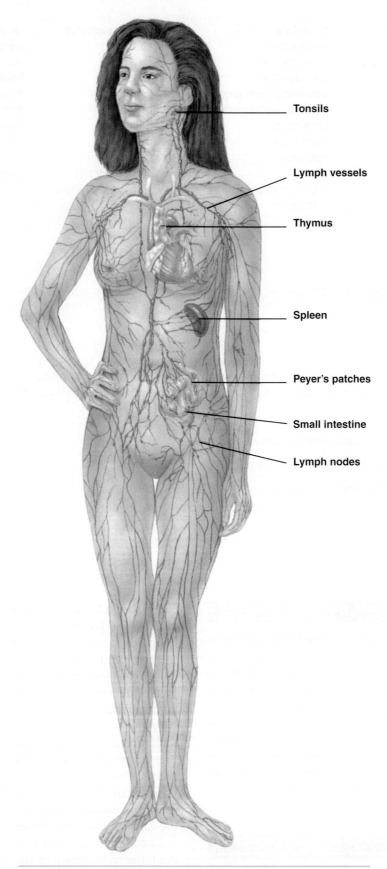

Tonsils

Lymph vessels

Thymus

Spleen

Peyer's patches

Small intestine

Lymph nodes

FIGURE 13-1   The vessels and organs of the lymphatic system

capillaries. This process of lymph formation prevents the abnormal accumulation of interstitial fluid, referred to as **edema**.

LYMPH VESSELS

The system of lymph vessels begins with the smallest dead-end vessels, called **lymph capillaries**, which are located throughout the tissues of the body. They extend into the interstitial spaces, forming networks that travel parallel to the blood capillaries. The wall of the lymphatic capillaries is a single layer of squamous epithelial cells. Due to the high permeability of the walls of the lymph capillaries, they are responsible for the initial collection of tissue fluid; the fluid from the interstitial space enters the capillaries and is now the lymph fluid (Figure 13-2).

The lymph capillaries join to form larger lymph vessels, much like capillaries join to form arterioles, which join to form arteries. The structure of the larger lymph vessels is comparable to veins; the smooth muscle layer of the vessels constricts and contains valves to prevent regurgitation of the lymph. The wall of lymphatic vessels consists of three layers: the inner endothelial layer, the middle smooth muscle layer with elastic fibers, and the outer connective tissue layer. The contraction of the skeletal muscles aids in moving the lymph fluid forward. The lymphatic vessels are compressed by the muscles, causing the lymph fluid to move toward a collecting duct. Breathing also aids in the movement of lymph fluid. During inhalation low pressure is created in the thoracic cavity and at the same time the contraction of the diaphragm increases the pressure in the abdominal cavity. The net effect is the squeezing of lymph fluid from the abdominal lymphatic vessels and into the thoracic vessels.

The lymph travels back to the blood flow to become plasma. Refer to Figures 13-3 and 13-4 as you read the following outline of the flow of lymph. The lymph vessels in the lower part of the body join anterior to the second lumbar vertebra and to the right of the aorta to form a dilation at the beginning of the **thoracic duct** called the cisterna chyli. The cisterna chyli marks the junction of the two lumbar lymphatic trunks and intestinal lymphatic trunk to form and empty into the thoracic duct. The thoracic duct continues in a superior direction while other lymph vessels from the upper body connect to and empty lymph into the duct. The thoracic duct travels upward beside the aorta, through the diaphragm, and then ascends anterior to the vertebral column

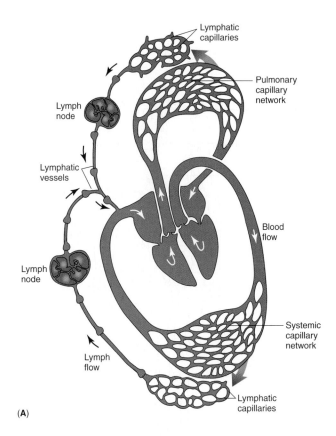

(A)

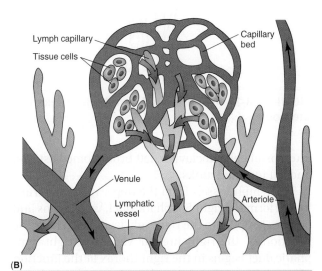

(B)

FIGURE 13-2   (A) Diagrammatic view of lymphatics transporting fluid from interstitial spaces to the bloodstream. (B) Lymph capillaries begin as blind-end tubes next to tissue cells and blood capillaries

and through the mediastinal space. The lymph vessels from the upper left quadrant of the body join the thoracic duct, which eventually joins the left subclavian vein near the junction of the left jugular vein to empty lymph into the subclavian vein. The thoracic duct drains lymph from the intestinal, lumbar,

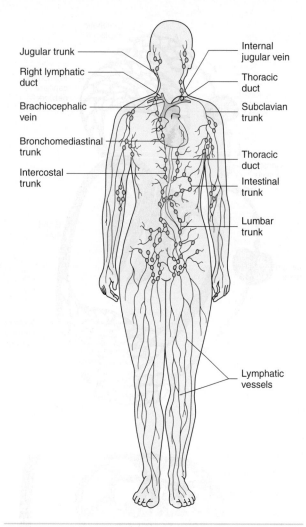

FIGURE 13-3 **The principal lymphatic trunks of the body**

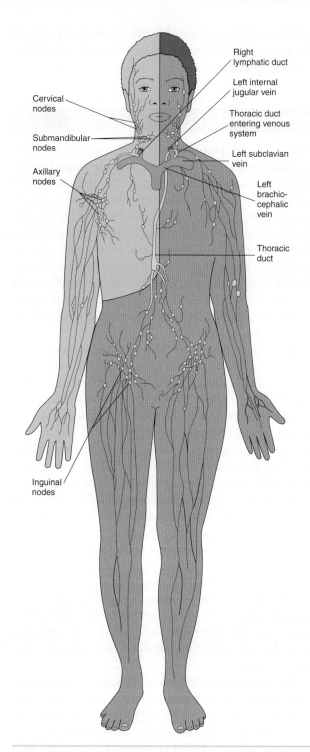

FIGURE 13-4 **Lymphatic trunks pass their lymph into two main collecting ducts, the thoracic duct and the right lymphatic duct. These ducts empty into the left and right subclavian veins, respectively**

intercostal, left subclavian, left bronchomediastinal, and left jugular trunks.

The lymph vessels from the upper right quadrant join to form the right lymphatic duct, which joins and empties lymph into the right subclavian vein near the junction of the right jugular vein. The right lymphatic duct begins in the right thorax at the junction of the right jugular, right subclavian, and right bronchomediastinal trunks. Valves in both subclavian veins allow lymph to enter, but not to regurgitate into the lymph vessels or allow blood to flow back into the lymph vessels.

A specialized type of lymph capillary is called the **lacteal**. Lacteals are found in the villi of the small intestine. They are dead-end capillaries responsible for absorbing the fat-soluble nutrients as an end product of digestion. Bile salts are required for the absorption of fatty acids and fat-soluble vitamins such as A, D, E, and K. When absorbed, the fatty acids combine with glycerol to form triglycerides, including cholesterol and protein, and this combination is called a **chylomicron**. The chylomicrons are absorbed and transported by the lacteals to the major lymph vessels. See Chapter 15 for further information.

LYMPH NODES AND NODULES

Lymph nodes and **nodules** are a group of lymphatic tissue (Figure 13-5). Lymph nodes have three major functions:

1. Filtering pathogens and other foreign material from lymph before it empties into the blood circulatory system
2. Monitoring the level of body fluid
3. Hematopoietic function in that nodes produce lymphocytes, macrophages, and monocytes

Nodes are larger than nodules. The indented portion of a node is called the hilum and is the area where the blood vessels and nerves connect with it. The lymphatic vessels that travel to a node transporting lymph are referred to as **lymphatic afferent vessels** and enter at separate areas on the convex surface of the node. The vessels that exit from the node at the hilum are referred to as **lymphatic efferent vessels**.

Each lymph node is surrounded by a capsule of connective tissue (Figure 13-6). Within the node are germinal centers that represent the area of activity in which lymphocytes and macrophages are dividing. Inside the node, the outer portion next to the capsule are the cortical nodules, which are light-colored; the inner portion is a darker-colored portion called medullary

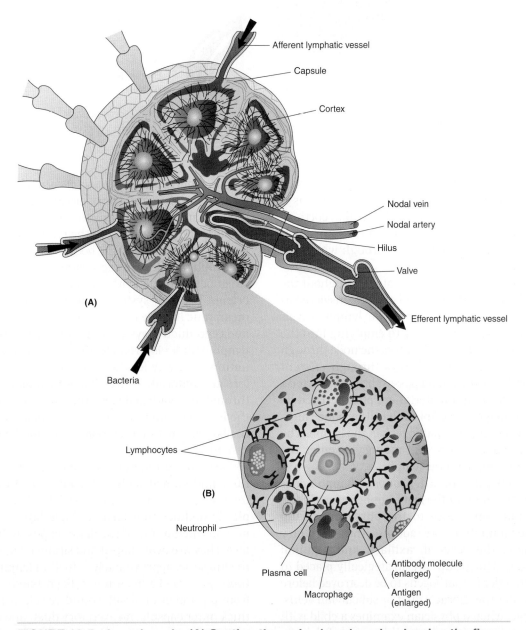

(A)

Afferent lymphatic vessel
Capsule
Cortex
Nodal vein
Nodal artery
Hilus
Valve
Efferent lymphatic vessel
Bacteria

(B)

Lymphocytes
Neutrophil
Plasma cell
Macrophage
Antibody molecule (enlarged)
Antigen (enlarged)

FIGURE 13-5   Lymph node. (A) Section through a lymph node, showing the flow of lymph. (B) Microscopic detail of bacteria being destroyed within the lymph node

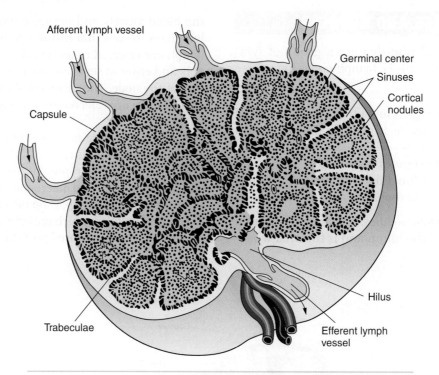

FIGURE 13-6 Internal anatomy of a lymph node showing germinal centers and sinuses

cords. The rest of the node contains closely packed lymphocytes, trabeculae that are inward extensions of the capsule, and three sinuses: subcapsular, cortical, and medullary. The trabeculae and sinuses form a network of chambers and channels through which the lymph circulates.

Groups of lymph nodes are located throughout the lymph circulatory pathway, and can be considered as specialized filters of the body. The lymph travels through the nodes on the way to emptying into the subclavian veins. The lymph enters the node through afferent lymph vessels and exits through efferent lymph vessels. As the lymph passes through, bacteria and any other foreign material are phagocytized by fixed macrophages. Fixed plasma cells produce antibodies in reaction to the pathogens in the lymph. The antibodies, lymphocytes, and monocytes enter the bloodstream along with the lymph.

As previously mentioned, groups of lymph nodes are located throughout the body, but because of their location and importance to the physician during physical examination, we address three primary groups here: the cervical, axillary, and inguinal lymph nodes. The groups are strategically placed in the body in order for pathogens to be destroyed before they can enter the thoracic duct or subclavian veins. For example, when a physician examines a child with a sore throat he or she palpates the region of the cervical nodes, which, if enlarged, may indicate strep

throat, wherein *Streptococcus pyogenes* bacteria have invaded the pharynx. The nodes are enlarged because the fixed macrophages are attempting to destroy the bacteria in the lymph from the pharynx; basically, a battle is taking place in the body.

Lymph nodules are aggregations of lymph cells located beneath the epithelial layer of mucous membranes. The body systems that are lined with mucous membrane include the respiratory, digestive, urinary, and reproductive systems. Again, the location of the lymph nodules is strategic, since body openings are a natural pathway for the entry of bacteria and other foreign material. If the bacteria make their way through the epithelial layer, the fixed macrophages in the lymph nodules are ready to combat and destroy the bacteria before they reach the blood circulatory system.

Particular groups of lymph nodes have been identified and named such as **Peyer's patches** and the tonsils. Peyer's patches are a specialized group of lymphatic nodules that form a single layer within the mucous membrane of the ileum opposite the mesentery. They are oval-shaped and situated lengthwise in the intestine, approximately $\frac{1}{2}''$ to $4''$ in length. Usually there are 20–30 in number. Each patch is formed from a number of small, round vesicles that have a thick outer capsule, no excretory duct, and contain a white-colored secretion (Gray, 1991). The function of the patches is not known.

The **palatine tonsils** are located on each side of the pharynx. The pharyngeal tonsils, better known as the **adenoids**, are located on the posterior wall of the pharynx, and the **lingual tonsils** are located at the base of the tongue. The lingual tonsils form a rounded projection, which contains an opening that leads into a cavity surrounded by lymphoid tissue. The anatomic location of the three tonsils is important, since the pharynx is a common pathway for pathogens contained in inhaled air and ingested food. Children often experience chronic infections of the palatine tonsils and adenoids, causing pain and difficulty in breathing. In this situation, a tonsillectomy and adenoidectomy (T & A) surgical procedure is performed to remove the structures.

LYMPHEDEMA

As previously mentioned, the continuous exchange of fluid between the interstitial spaces into the blood and lymphatic capillaries maintains the normal volume of interstitial fluid. However, pathologic conditions that obstruct the movement of the fluid cause the abnormal accumulation within the interstitial spaces, resulting in edema, also called lymphedema. The causes of lymphedema include:

1. Obstruction of a lymphatic vessel
2. Overproduction of interstitial fluid due to increased capillary blood pressure
3. Abnormal uptake of fluid by the lymphatic capillaries due to traumatic or surgical wounds

Lymphatic vessels may be blocked by tumors or inflammation (**lymphadenitis**). The pressure on the vessels created by the obstruction decreases the flow of lymph. Diagnosis of the obstruction is confirmed by performing a lymphangiography. The usual course of treatment is antibiotics; occasionally surgery on the involved lymph vessels to correct the obstruction and promote drainage is required in extreme situations, but this has seen limited results.

The abnormal uptake of fluid is usually the result of surgery and radiation therapy. It is often seen after breast surgery such as a mastectomy, and affects the arm on the side where the mastectomy was performed. The axillary lymph nodes are removed with the breast, since the lymphatic vessels are often responsible for the transport of cancerous cells to other sites in the body, a process called **metastasis**. However, removing the lymph nodes and associated vessels can prevent drainage from the upper limb, leading to lymphedema of the arm. Postoperative instructions to the patient to prevent lymphedema include placing the arm above the heart while resting, regular exercise of the arm, and avoiding activities that can lead to infection of the hand or arm on the affected side. Infection significantly increases the chance of lymphedema developing. In addition, health care providers should avoid taking the blood pressure and drawing blood samples from the arm that is on the affected side.

BOX 13-1

Sentinel Lymph Node Biopsy

The lymph vessels of the breast drain into the axillary lymph nodes, and in some individuals into the sternal lymph nodes and the supraclavicular lymph nodes. The sentinel lymph node biopsy is a technique developed as an alternative to axillary lymph node dissection. It was developed as a method to determine if breast cancer cells have spread to the lymph ducts or nodes in the axilla without having to perform the long-standing method of axillary lymph node dissection. Research has shown that the lymph ducts of the breast usually drain to one lymph node first before draining into the rest of the axillary lymph nodes. This first lymph node is referred to as the sentinel lymph node. Lymph node mapping is used to identify the sentinel node by using a combination of a radioactive dye and a blue dye to stain the lymph tissue a bright blue color for identification by the surgeon. Negative sentinel lymph node results have consistently shown that there is a 95% chance or more that the remaining axillary lymph nodes do not have cancer cells. This prevents the patient from having to undergo the more invasive axillary lymph node dissection.

On the day of the procedure, the radioactive dye is injected into the area of the breast where the tumor is located and around the areola of the nipple. The patient waits a few hours and returns to the Nuclear Medicine Department to have photos taken, which will reveal the pathways the dye traveled as it exited the breast tissue. This aids the surgeon in identifying the sentinel lymph node. The patient is then taken to the operating room, where the procedure begins with the surgeon injecting the blue dye. A small incision is made in the area of the axillary lymph tissue. A sterile handheld probe is used to measure areas that contain the radioactive dye. The lymph nodes that have taken up the radioactive dye and the blue dye are excised; usually one to three nodes are removed. The nodes are sent to the Pathology Department where the pathologist examines the nodes under the microscope to determine if the sentinel node contains cancer cells. The incision is closed, the placement of a wound drain is not required, and the patient can go home that day. Physical therapy is also not required. If the sentinel node is negative for cancer cells, the patient does not require an axillary lymph node dissection; positive results indicate otherwise.

Pregnancy is a factor that increases venous pressure, causing a domino effect of increased capillary pressure and overproduction of interstitial fluid. The resulting lymphedema is seen in the ankles and feet of the pregnant female. Treatment is aimed at decreasing the venous pressure, and is accomplished by having the woman lie on her left side to improve venous flow, since the inferior vena cava is situated to the right of the midline of the body. When an individual is sitting, the legs should be positioned above the heart level to aid in the flow of fluid toward the head.

SPLEEN AND THYMUS ORGANS

The **spleen** is a soft, highly vascular organ, slightly oval in shape and located between the stomach and diaphragm in the left hypochondriac region or upper left quadrant of the body (Figure 13-7). The tissue of the spleen is highly friable. The lower ribs aid in protecting the organ; however, it is the number one organ injured in motor vehicle accidents (MVAs). The spleen has a hilum located on the medial side through which the splenic artery enters and the splenic vein exits. It is an organ of the lymph system because it contains lymphoid nodules. However, the spleen filters the blood much like the lymph nodes filter lymph.

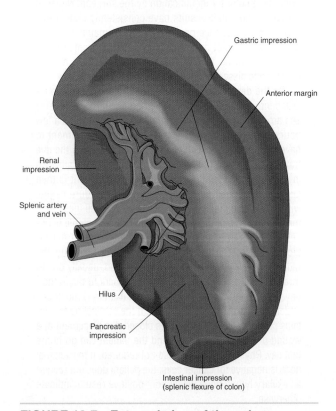

Gastric impression

Anterior margin

Renal
impression

Splenic artery
and vein

Hilus

Pancreatic
impression

Intestinal impression
(splenic flexure of colon)

FIGURE 13-7   External view of the spleen

There are two types of tissue within the spleen: white pulp and red pulp. The white pulp is located throughout the organ as roundish groups of splenic nodules that are analogous to the lymph nodules and contain lymphocytes. The rest of the spleen consists of red pulp that contains hundreds of erythrocytes, lymphocytes, and macrophages.

In the fetus, the spleen produces erythrocytes. After birth the functions of the spleen include hematopoiesis, storage of blood, destruction of dead erythrocytes and platelets, and defense. It is a hematopoietic organ because it produces lymphocytes, monocytes, leukocytes, and fixed plasma cells in reaction to infections. The fixed plasma cells produce antibodies to fight the antigens. Fixed macrophages are located in the spleen that phagocytize pathogens and other foreign material as blood flows through the organ. In traumatic situations wherein the individual sustains severe hemorrhage, the spleen releases the stored blood to aid in compensating for the blood loss. In less than 60 seconds, the spleen can release enough blood to increase the volume from 350 ml to 550 ml.

The blood capillaries within the red pulp are very permeable. The older or dead erythrocytes are able to enter the capillaries and then move on into the venous sinuses of the spleen. This allows the macrophages, which are also within the sinuses, to remove the dead cells and thus keep the circulatory system cleaned of debris.

When the spleen must be surgically removed, a procedure called a **splenectomy**, obviously the individual can live without the organ. However, because the organ is an important site of antibody production and plays an important role in the body's immune system, the person is more prone to certain bacterial infections.

The **thymus** gland is located in the mediastinal region and extends superiorly into the neck to the inferior edge of the thyroid gland and inferiorly to the fourth costal cartilage. It consists of two lateral lobes bound together by connective tissue that encloses the entire organ to form a capsule. The lobes differ in size and the gland is approximately 5 cm long and 4 cm wide. The lobes are further broken down into lobules separated by thin connective tissue.

The activity of the thymus is dependent on the hormone called **thymosin**. The T cells, the function of which is discussed more fully later in this chapter, are produced by the thymus and are important in the cell-mediated immune system. The thymus begins development in the embryo and weighs approximately 12 grams before birth. By puberty, the organ will weigh about 35 grams. After an individual has gone through puberty the organ diminishes in size, and in an elderly person it appears as small piece of yellowish tissue covered by a thin layer of fat.

BODY DEFENSES: FIRST LINE OF DEFENSE

The first line of defense of the body includes the external and internal barriers presented by the skin, mucous membranes, and secretions. The following information pertaining to the body's three lines of defense does not all directly relate to the lymphatic system. However, to fully understand the role of the lymphatic system it is important to discuss all three lines of defense and their physiologic mechanisms.

Skin

The unbroken skin prevents microbes from entering the body. When the skin is damaged, as it is when the surgeon makes the initial skin incision for a procedure, an opening is immediately created for the invasion of microbes such as *Staphylococcus aureus*. Burns, cuts, and scratches are other examples of broken skin that allow microbes to penetrate the body. In certain areas of the planet, a simple scratch can lead to devastating illness if an individual is not from that part of the world and has not built an immunity to the unique microbial environment.

The skin further aids the body by secreting lactic acid from the sweat glands and fatty acids from the sebaceous glands that either kill or inhibit the growth of bacteria. The low-pH environment of the skin also inhibits the growth of the microbes.

The two layers of the skin, the outer epidermis and inner dermis, are constructed in such a way as to provide a barrier that is rarely penetrated by most microbes as long as it remains intact. The dermis is a thick layer of tough connective tissue. The epidermis is thinner, but the epithelial cells are closely knit with little or no space between the cells. The very top layer of the epidermis is dead epithelial cells and is covered by a protein called keratin. However, fungi can hydrolyze keratin, thereby resulting in the fungal infection called athelete's foot.

The sebaceous glands are located in the skin and produce sebum. Sebum prevents the hair from drying out and also forms a thin protective layer on the surface of the skin. A component of sebum is unsaturated fatty acids that inhibit the growth of some pathogenic bacteria and fungi (Tortora, Funke, & Case, 2001). The fatty acids also cause the skin pH to be between 3 and 5, which probably aids in inhibiting the growth of microbes.

The sweat glands, also located in the skin, are responsible for perspiration. Perspiration helps keep body temperature normal, eliminates some body wastes, and washes away microbes from the skin surface. Perspiration contains lysozyme, which is an enzyme that can break down gram-positive bacterial cell walls (O'Toole, 1992). Lysozyme is also a component of tears, saliva, and certain tissue fluids.

Mucous Membranes

Mucous membranes line the respiratory, gastrointestinal, and genitourinary tracts. Specialized epithelial cells, called **goblet cells**, line the membrane and secrete mucus. Some pathogens survive and even thrive because of the moist environment provided by the mucus. When a sufficient number of the microbes are present, they invade the host. An example of such a pathogen is *Treponema pallidum*.

However, the mucus can also catch microbes and not allow them to penetrate farther into the respiratory or gastrointestinal tracts. Another mechanism found in the respiratory tract is the cilia. The cilia trap inhaled dust, dirt, and pathogens. The cilia line the tract and move in a synchronous, wavelike motion, moving inhaled dust, debris, and microbes forward to the pharynx to be expelled by the host through sneezing or coughing of phlegm.

The mucous membrane lining of the genitourinary tract is flushed out by the flow of urine. The flushing action prevents microbial stasis and consequent colonization of the tract.

The stomach contains glands that produce the highly acidic gastric juice. The pH is approximately 1.2–3.0 (Tortora et al., 2001) and consists of hydrochloric acid and mucus. The high acid level usually assures that microbes cannot survive. Exceptions include the toxins produced by *Clostridium botulinum* and *S. aureus*, which survive the gastric juice. Another important exception is *Helicobacter pylori*, which survives by neutralizing the acid and allowing bacteria to grow. *H. pylori* has been determined to be a major contributor to the cause of stomach and duodenal ulcers.

BODY DEFENSES: SECOND LINE OF DEFENSE (CIRCULATORY AND CHEMICAL DEFENSES)

If pathogens are able to penetrate the body past the first line of defense, they encounter the second line of defense: the elements found in the circulatory system, including phagocytes, complement, other blood proteins, interferon, fever production, iron balance, and the body's response to injury or infection (called the inflammatory response).

Phagocytes

Phagocytosis is the second line of defense put forth by the human body. Phagocytosis is the process of surrounding and ingesting another microbe or foreign particle. The cells responsible for this action are called phagocytes, all of which are leukocytes (white blood cells).

When an infection in the human body occurs, the number of leukocytes increases. If a patient presents with signs and symptoms that indicate that they have appendicitis, blood will be drawn from the patient and the surgeon will most likely order a **differential white blood cell count** to be completed in the laboratory. The count is a percentage of each type of white blood cell (WBC) that is present in a sample of 100 WBCs (O'Toole, 1992).

There are two categories of leukocytes: **granuloctyes** and **agranulocytes**. When placed under a light microscope after staining, large granules can be seen in the cytoplasm of granulocytes. Based on how the granules stain, granulocytes are placed into three categories:

- Neutrophils that stain with a mixture of acidic and base dyes and are colored a light lilac
- Eosinophils that are dyed with eosin, an acidic dye, and stain red or orange
- Basophils that are stained with methylene blue and, therefore, stain a bluish color (The function of basophils is not fully understood, but they are important in the process of inflammation that will be discussed later.)

Neutrophils are motile and effective phagocytes that are active in the beginning stages of an infection. They are also the most abundant and efficient phagocytes. They leave the bloodstream to enter the infected area and begin the process of destroying the invading microbes.

Eosinophils can also leave the bloodstream, but their major role is the production of toxic proteins to fight parasites, such as helminths. The eosinophil attaches to the surface of the parasite and secretes peroxide ions, which kill them. During an infection by a parasitic worm, for example, the number of eosinophils greatly increases. Eosinophils play a more efficient phagocytic role during the allergic response.

Agranulocytes do not have granules in the cytoplasm; however, they cannot be seen with the light microscope after staining (Tortora et al., 2001). The two

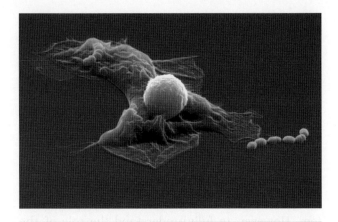

FIGURE 13-8 Scanning electron micrograph of human macrophage and lymphocytes (Reprinted with permission of Cells Alive)

types of agranulocytes are **monocytes** and **lymphocytes** (Figure 13-8). Monocytes do not become phagocytic until they exit the bloodstream and enter the body's tissues where they mature into macrophages. The increase in macrophages and lymphocytes within the lymph nodes causes them to swell during an infection (Tortora et al., 2001). As the blood and lymph fluid travel through body organs that contain macrophages, the microbes are removed by phagocytosis. Lymphocytes are not phagocytes but are important in the specific defense of the body called the immune response, discussed later in the chapter.

Macrophages develop from monocytes during the inflammatory response to an infection. There are two types of macrophages. Those that exit the bloodstream and travel to the infected region are called wandering macrophages, and those that remain in tissues and body organs to trap foreign material are called fixed macrophages or histiocytes.

Fixed macrophages are located in the tissues of the **reticuloendothelial system (RES)**. This nonspecific system refers to the collection of phagocytic cells (including macrophages) that line the sinusoids of the spleen, lymph nodes, bone marrow, intestines, liver (Küpffer cells), and brain (microglia). The main function of the RES is removal and destruction of foreign debris and microbes, excess cellular secretions, and dead leukocytes, erythrocytes, and body tissue (O'Toole, 1992).

Phagocytosis

The granulocytes, in particular the neutrophils, are most active during the initial stages of a bacterial infection. In the later stages, the macrophages become the most dominant phagocyte, destroying the remaining living and dead bacteria. During fungal and viral infections, macrophages are the most dominant phagocyte during all stages of the infection (Tortora et al., 2001).

The process of phagocytosis is divided into four parts: chemotaxis, adherence, ingestion, and digestion. **Chemotaxis** refers to the attraction of phagocytes to microbes, which is due to chemicals from injured tissue cells, peptides, and other microbial products. Motile bacteria contain receptors in the cell wall that sense the chemical stimuli, and once detected, the information is transmitted to the flagella. If the signal is favorable, the bacteria will move toward the chemical stimulus. The chemical attraction is not understood, but it is known to be the result of lymphokines that are produced by T lymphocytes and the activation of complement.

The phagocyte attaches to the microbe by first adhering to its surface. Adherence can either take place in a fairly simple manner or be difficult. Some bacteria, such as *S. pyogenes,* contain a protein called M protein that makes it difficult for phagocytes to attach to the microbial surface. Another barrier is slippery mucoid capsules that surround bacteria, as occurs with *Haemophilus influenzae* type b.

Antibody molecules secrete a serum protein that can coat a bacterial cell and promote the attachment of phagocytes to the pathogens. The process of coating is called opsonization and the antibody molecules are referred to as **opsonins**.

After the phagocyte is able to adhere to the pathogen, the process of ingestion can begin. The phagocyte extends "false feet" called pseudopods, which surround the microbe. The phagocyte's membrane indents (invaginates). The pseudopod's sides meet to completely surround the pathogen, and the resulting sac is called a **phagosome** (Koneman, Allen, Janda, Schreckenberger, & Winn, 1997).

The last step of the process is digestion. The phagosome releases itself from the plasma membrane and enters the cytoplasm. As previously discussed, the cytoplasm contains lysosomes that contain enzymes. When the phagosome and lysosomes make contact, they form a single structure called a phagolysosome. The enzymes are now able to destroy the bacteria. This digestive process is called degranulation because the granules in the granulocytes are used and decrease in number (Grover-Lakomia & Fong, 1999). After the bacteria have been digested, the phagolysosome is called a residual body, and the leftover contents cannot be digested. This residual body moves through the cytoplasm to the edge of the phagocyte and releases the wastes to the outside of the cell.

Blood Proteins: Complement

Complement is a group of 25–30 enzymatic serum proteins found in blood plasma that constitute the "complement system" (O'Toole, 1992). The name is derived from the fact that they complement the action of antibodies in immune and allergic reactions. The complements circulate in the plasma in an inactive form until needed in the antibody–antigen reaction that is part of the third line of defense. Complement is a nonspecific defense mechanism, since it binds to different antigen–antibody immune complexes. Once it binds to the complex, it becomes activated and performs the following functions:

1. Increases the inflammatory response.
2. Attaches to the antibody to assist in the lysis of the antigen.
3. Aids in neutralizing the toxins of some types of microbes.
4. Attracts phagocytes (chemotaxis) to the region.

There are 11 proteins, labeled as C1–C11. Complement aids in the lysis of bacterial cells through the process called **complement cascade**. This is a highly complex biochemical process involving C1–C9, in which one complement interacts with another in a specific sequence called the complementary pathway. The sequence is C1, 4, 2, 3, 5, 6, 7, 8, 9 (Anderson, 1998). The sequence causes an accumulation of fluid that continues until the lysis of the cell membrane occurs and the cell ruptures.

Iron

The virulence of bacteria increases when free iron is present. Many pathogenic bacteria use iron for the synthesis of exotoxins. Leukocytes produce **interleukin-1 (IL-1)**, which, among other functions discussed later, stimulates the liver to store iron, thereby depriving the pathogen of necessary free iron.

Within the body, iron is tightly bound to iron transport proteins called transferrin, ferritin, and lactoferrin (Ingraham & Ingraham, 2000). Again, this deprives pathogens of the needed iron supply. However, some pathogens obtain the iron needed for survival by producing and releasing their own iron-binding proteins called siderophores. The iron binds to the siderophores and the pathogen takes up the siderophores to gain the iron. *Neisseria meningitidis,* the microbe responsible for causing meningitis, has receptors on the cell surface that bind directly to the iron transport proteins. The cell can then take up the proteins along with the attached iron atoms (Ingraham & Ingraham, 2000).

Inflammatory Response

A defensive response to a bodily injury is called inflammation or inflammatory response. The four signs of inflammation are pain, heat, redness, and swelling (edema). Pain is caused by tissue nerve damage, pressure exerted by edema, or toxins; heat and redness, also associated with inflammation, are caused by an increase in blood flow to the affected area; and swelling (edema) is due to a buildup of fluid in the surrounding tissue spaces.

Inflammation is a necessary and beneficial response of the body. It is responsible for three primary processes:

1. Destroying the invasive substance and removing it and any products produced by the substance.
2. Limiting the extent of the infection by "walling off" the substance and the by-products. For example, if an individual has a brief episode of appendicitis and the appendix bursts, the patient will not immediately exhibit signs of inflammation and infection due to the formation of an abscess, which has been walled off. This wall is the body's attempt to isolate the infection by forming a connective tissue wall that inhibits the ability of the pathogens to penetrate deeper into the surrounding tissue (Burton & Engelkirk, 1996).
3. Repairing and/or replacing damaged tissue (Tortora et al., 2001).

The process of inflammation occurs in three stages: vasodilation, phagocyte migration, and tissue repair. **Vasodilation** refers to the dilation, or increase in diameter, of blood vessels, which aids in increasing the blood flow to the area of damage. Vasodilation also increases the permeability of the blood vessels, allowing the host defensive agents that normally travel in the bloodstream to pass through the vessel wall and enter the damaged tissue. Three primary chemicals that are released by damaged cells are responsible for vasodilation: histamine, kinins, and prostaglandins.

Histamine is found in mast cells located in connective tissue, platelets, and basophils. Histamine is released from the injured cells that contain it and has a direct effect on the blood vessels. **Kinins** are found in plasma, the liquid, straw-colored portion of blood. Kinins cause vasodilation and an increase in the permeability of blood vessels. They also play a part in chemotaxis by attracting neutrophils to the damaged tissue. **Prostaglandins** are also released by damaged cells. They increase the action of histamine and kinins and aid phagocytes as they travel through the blood vessel walls (O'Toole, 1992).

Vasodilation also allows the quick delivery of blood-clotting substances to the injured area through permeability. The blood clot that forms in the area of damage inhibits microbes and/or toxins from spreading throughout the body. The result is the formation of an **abscess**. Abscesses (pus) are a combination of body fluids and dead cells that tend to collect in a cavity. Pathogens that cause abscess formation are called pyogenic bacteria and include staphylococci, which typically produce a yellowish-green–colored pus. *Pseudomonas aeruginosa* produces a bluish-colored exudate, caused by the pigment pyocyanin, which is produced by the bacteria (Burton & Engelkirk, 1996).

As neutrophils and monocytes travel to the area of injury, they attach to the inner endothelial lining of the blood vessels. Once the blood vessels dilate, the phagocytes are able to leave the vessels by passing through the endothelial cells to the injured tissue. The phagocytes can begin the process of eliminating the pathogens.

The last stage of inflammation is tissue repair, in which the tissue replaces the damaged or destroyed cells. Repair actually begins during the first phase of inflammation but obviously cannot be complete until all pathogens and other substances have been removed and are no longer causing tissue damage.

The extent to which tissue can regenerate depends on the type of tissue. For example, skin can easily regenerate depending on the amount of damage. The liver can also regenerate but not as easily. However, cardiac tissue cannot regenerate. When an individual has a severe myocardial infarction, a large amount of cardiac tissue can be damaged and the person will be incapacitated.

Fever

Inflammation is an example of a response to a local area of injury. Fever, an abnormally elevated body temperature, is an example of a systemic reaction. A frequent cause of fever is a viral or bacterial invasion.

The hypothalamus is a portion of the diencephalon of the brain, forming the floor and part of the lateral wall of the third ventricle. Its somatic functions include sleep, appetite, and temperature. The development of a fever occurs in the following steps:

1. When phagocytes ingest bacteria, lipopolysaccharides located in the cell wall are released, inducing the phagocytes to release IL-1.
2. The presence of IL-1 tells the hypothalamus to release prostaglandins, which elevate the temperature, thereby causing fever.

For example, as the body is invaded by a pathogenic bacterium, the body temperature rises. The physiologic response is shivering and an increased rate of metabolism, all of which contribute to an increase in body temperature. Even though the temperature is higher, a person experiences chills and the skin is cold and clammy. Until IL-1 is eliminated the elevated body temperature will continue.

As the infection is brought under control within the body, vasodilation and sweating begin. These are two heat-losing processes that signify that the body temperature is falling. This phase of the fever is called crisis.

Fever is a defensive mechanism, but only up to a certain point, because IL-1 increases the production of T lymphocytes. A moderate fever is beneficial because only a few bacteria can survive the temperature and usually only for a short period. Also, the elevated body temperature increases the effect of interferons. The action of interferons is not completely understood as related to fever, but is it believed that interferons decrease the amount of iron, thereby inhibiting the growth of microbes. However, fever that is unchecked can be debilitating and life-threatening if not controlled.

Interferons

Interferon is a protein that is produced when leukocytes, T lymphocytes, and fibroblasts are infected. They enter the host's surrounding cells and inhibit the synthesis of proteins that viruses need for multiplication (Burton & Engelkirk, 1996). Hence, they "interfere" with viral replication. Interferon is a highly potent natural antiviral agent that results in an inhibition of the spread of infection, which allows other host defenses to more effectively fight the disease.

Interferons are not pathogen specific, meaning that they are effective against a variety of pathogens and not just the pathogen that stimulated their production. However, interferons are species specific, meaning that they are effective only in the species of animal that produced them. Therefore, human interferon is effective only for humans.

There are three classifications of interferons: alpha, beta, and gamma. Alpha and gamma interferons are produced by T-cell lymphocytes; beta interferon is produced by fibroblasts (Ingraham & Ingraham, 2000). There are many different types of interferons: 13 alphas, 5 betas, and an unknown number of gamma interferons. The alpha and beta interferons are the most powerful (Ingraham & Ingraham, 2000). Interferons are not classified according to function, but rather by their genetic and chemical makeup.

Interferons perform functions other than fighting viral infections. They also regulate cell motility and division, activate macrophages, and reject transplanted tissue (Koneman et al., 1997).

Cells that have been infected by a virus are stimulated to produce interferons. The interferons exit from the cell and enter healthy cells, causing them to produce antiviral proteins (AVPs) or **translation inhibitory protein (TIP)**. The TIP blocks the translation of viral RNA and, therefore, inhibits the spread of the infection and protects the surrounding cells. Most types of viruses stimulate the production of interferon.

Recently, interferons were thought to be a highly effective agent in the fight against viral diseases and cancer. With use of recombinant DNA technology, large amounts of interferon have been produced. But the results have been disappointing; the interferon was highly toxic and ineffective against many cancers and viral diseases. Instances of effective uses include treatment of rare leukemias and some chronic viral infections, such as herpes and hepatitis (Ingraham & Ingraham, 2000).

BODY DEFENSES: THIRD LINE OF DEFENSE (IMMUNITY)

The third line of defense is the immune response. In this type of immunity, antibodies are produced by lymphocytes that bind with microbes to inactivate and destroy them. These **humoral antibodies** are found in the lymph fluid, plasma, and other body secretions. Formation of the antibodies is stimulated by the presence of specific pathogens. Therefore, the individual develops immunity to that particular disease because of the circulating antibodies that are effective against the pathogen that causes the disease.

Acquired Immunity

Immunity is a resistance to a disease brought about by production of specific antibodies that protect against pathogens that caused the initial disease. Two primary types of acquired immunity are active acquired immunity and passive acquired immunity, each of which has the subcategories natural and artificial.

Individuals who have had a specific infection have partial or total resistance to reinfection by the disease. The antibodies are produced by the stimulated lymphocytes, and this is referred to as **natural active acquired immunity**. Resistance to the disease may be permanent, as is the case with the mumps or measles, or temporary, as with influenza. There is no immunity gained against reinfection by some diseases, such as tuberculosis or gonorrhea.

Artificial active acquired immunity is the second type of actively acquired immunity, and it is gained by vaccination. The vaccine contains a sufficient number of pathogens to cause the person to form antibodies against that particular pathogen.

Vaccines are made from inactivated or living pathogens or from the toxins they secrete. Vaccines created from living microbes are the most effective but must be prepared from a harmless microbe that is closely related to the pathogen, or weakened pathogens that in the laboratory have had genetic changes that render them nonpathogenic. This laboratory process of weakening pathogens is called **attenuation**. Pasteur developed the attenuated vaccine for rabies, and Sabin developed the attenuated oral vaccine for polio. The smallpox vaccine is a weakened live vaccine, since it is derived from the cowpox virus, which causes a mild infection in cattle and humans.

Dead pathogens that have been killed by chemicals or heat are also used to make vaccines. These vaccines can be manufactured more easily and faster, but are less effective when compared to live vaccines and produce a shorter period of immunity. Vaccines produced in this manner are used to vaccinate against whooping cough, cholera, Rocky Mountain spotted fever, plague, and many types of respiratory diseases.

A third type of vaccine, used to prevent diphtheria and tetanus, is the **toxoid vaccine**. Toxoid vaccine is prepared from exotoxins that are inactivated by chemicals or heat. The vaccine is injected to cause the formation of antibodies that neutralize the exotoxins that the pathogens secrete. A serum that contains specific antibodies is called an **antiserum**. An antiserum that contains antibodies against toxoids is called an antitoxin.

Passive acquired immunity differs from active immunity in that antibodies formed in one person are transferred to another person. Because the person who received the antibodies did not produce them, the immunity is temporary. Passive acquired immunity has two subcategories: **natural passive acquired immunity** and **artificial passive acquired immunity**.

In natural passive acquired immunity, antibodies present in the bloodstream of a pregnant female cross the placenta to reach the fetus. In addition, the colostrum, which is secreted for a few days after birth, contains maternal antibodies that are passed on to the infant. Artificial passive acquired immunity is created by transferring antibodies from an immune person to a susceptible person.

ANTIGENS AND ANTIBODIES: PRELIMINARY INFORMATION

An **antigen** is any foreign substance that enters the body and stimulates the production of antibodies or, in other words, is immunogenic (antigens are also referred to as immunogens). Antigens can be formed from many types of biochemical substances, but the most well known are foreign protein antigens. Antigens have one or more sites, called **antigenic determinants**, to which antibodies and/or lymphocytes can bind. Antigens, then, are a foreign substance that the body does not recognize as being part of itself, thereby stimulating the production of antibodies.

Antibodies are glycoproteins produced by B lymphocytes (B cells). Antibodies bind to the receptor site of the specific antigen that stimulated their production. A bacterium has several antigen-determinant sites on its cell membrane, cell wall, capsule, and flagella that stimulate the production of the antibodies.

Antibodies are placed in a class of proteins called **immunoglobulins (Ig)**. The term antibody is used to refer to the specific type of immunoglobulin involved in the immune response. Immunoglobulins are also found in the lymph fluid, colostrum, tears, and saliva.

The type and number of antibodies produced in reaction to the presence of antigens depend on the:

1. Site of antigen stimulus
2. Number of antigens
3. Type of antigen and its action
4. Number of times an individual is exposed to the antigen

After the person has been exposed to the antigen, there is a delayed response in the production of antibodies, which is called the lag phase. During the lag phase, the antigen is involved with macrophages, T cells, and B cells. Some antigens require only B cells.

Eventually B cells develop into larger plasma cells that can produce antibodies by protein synthesis. This first step of the immune response is called the primary response. When the number of antigens declines, the number of antibodies in the bloodstream also declines as the plasma cells die. Other B cells become **memory cells**, which can be stimulated to produce antibodies quickly when the body is exposed to the same antigen again. The production of antibodies following subsequent exposures to the antigen is called the secondary response. This explains why titer counts are performed to measure the concentration of antibodies present, and booster shots are given to return the antibody concentrations to the level of the secondary response. For protection against the hepatitis B virus (HBV), it is strongly recommended that surgical personnel receive the three-shot HBV series and have titer counts with booster shots performed at the correct intervals. In fact, HBV vaccination is required in many institutions for all health care personnel. The primary and secondary responses are discussed in additional detail later in the chapter.

Persons who are born without the ability to produce antibodies have no gammaglobulin in their blood. This condition is called **agammaglobulinemia**. Obviously, these individuals are susceptible to all types of infections, which can prove fatal. One surgically successful treatment for this condition is a bone marrow transplantation. The precursor leukocytes transferred to the patient then become lymphocytes, which eventually become implanted in the lymph nodes. These become capable of being stimulated by antigens to produce antibodies.

Some patients, such as those who will be undergoing an organ transplantation procedure, are immunosuppressed after receiving immunosuppressive drug therapy. One of the most devastating immunosuppressive diseases is HIV infection, which destroys the helper T cells that are required for the processing of T-dependent antigens and are also important in the cell-mediated responses. These patients are open to all types of secondary infections, some of which are highly uncommon in humans.

COMPONENTS OF THE IMMUNE SYSTEM AND TYPES OF ANTIBODIES

The cells involved in the immune system develop in the bone marrow. Three types of lymphocytes develop from lymphoid stem cells in the bone marrow: B cells, T cells, and natural killer (NK) cells. Several of the stem cells migrate to the thymus gland to differentiate into one of the four types of T cells: helper T cell, suppressor T cell, cytotoxic T cell, and delayed-hypersensitivity T cell. The differentiation of the T cells in the thymus begins shortly before birth. The T cells are not involved in humoral antibodies but are involved in the cell-mediated immune response and control of the production of antibodies.

The stem cells that do not migrate to the thymus differentiate in the lymphoid regions of the intestine and liver. The B cells (named for the bursa lymphoid area of birds) originate from those two regions. B cells migrate to the lymphoid tissues and produce antibodies that circulate in the lymph system and bloodstream, provid-

ing **humoral immunity**. B cells live only about one to two weeks. When stimulated by an antigen, the B cells are capable of quickly mass-producing antibodies.

Antibodies are Y-shaped structures and, as mentioned previously, are a type of immunoglobulin. Antibodies circulating in the bloodstream are referred to as humoral or circulating antibodies. Five classes of antibodies are designated as IgA, IgD, IgE, and IgM. Table 13-1 provides a summary of the functions of each immunoglobulin.

BOX 13-2
Organ Transplant

Organ transplantation, although one of the most complicated surgical procedures, have progressed from being headline news to routine procedures in some large hospitals. However, organ transplantations often illustrate how the immune system goes awry and works against the body. In some instances the cells of the organ recipient do not recognize the tissue of the donor organ as self and attack and destroy the transplanted tissue. This reaction is referred to as a tissue rejection reaction.

Tissue rejection occurs when there is a significant antigenic difference between the cell surface molecules of the recipient's body tissues and those of the donor tissue. Therefore, a key to a successful organ transplantation is finding an organ with cell surface molecules that match the cell surface molecules of the recipient as closely as possible to reduce the chances of rejection. This explains why family members and relatives who are not far removed are the ideal donors, since their tissue will be as antigenically similar as possible to the recipient's. The best types of transplanted tissue include:

1. Isograft: Tissue is taken from a genetically identical twin.
2. Allograft: Tissue is taken from an individual who is not genetically identical to the recipient, but of the same species. This includes a family member such as a brother and sister or relatives such as first cousin and uncle.
3. Xenograft: Tissue is taken from a different species. Pigs are often used for transplant purposes in the human.

Immunosuppressive drugs are used to reduce the possibility of organ rejection by suppressing the formation of the recipient's antibodies, thereby inhibiting the cellular- and humoral-mediated responses. However, the use of the drugs is a delicate balance, since the suppressed immune system leaves the patient prone to contracting infectious diseases, such as a common cold, which are normally not dangerous to healthy individuals but can be life-threatening to the patient.

TABLE 13-1 Functions of Antibodies

ANTIBODY CLASS	FUNCTIONS
IgA	Protects mucous membranes and internal body cavities against infection. Known as the secretory antibody, since it is found in the saliva, colostrum, tears, bloodstream, and intestine. Prevents pathogens from adhering to mucosal surfaces.
IgD	Function not well understood. Controls antigen stimulation of B cells. May be involved in determining which antibody type a plasma cell produces. Found on surface of B cells and in bloodstream.
IgE	Is the cause of allergies, anaphylaxis, drug sensitivity, and immediate hypersensitivity in skin test reactions. Cause of rash or hives in allergic reactions, runny nose and itchy eyes of hay fever, asthma, and shock in anaphylaxis.
IgG	Most abundant and smallest of the antibodies. Attaches to phagocytes and complement, making it easier for bacteria to be destroyed by phagocytes or lysed by complement. Crosses the placental barrier. Protects against disease. Found in the bloodstream and lymph fluid.
IgM	Largest antibody. First antibodies formed in response to infection. Especially lethal against gram-negative bacteria. Activates complement. Increases the process of phagocytosis. Found in the bloodstream and lymph fluid.

HUMORAL IMMUNITY

The process of antibody production involves a complex series of events that are not completely understood. The components involved are T cells, B cells, and macrophages. The following is a summary of the steps of antibody production.

1. Bacteria invade the body and are ingested by macrophages.
2. Antigens that are present on the surface of macrophages are presented to helper T cells.
3. The helper T cells are sensitized by the exposure to the antigens and stimulate the production of antibodies by B cells. The helper T cells are not capable of producing the antibodies.
4. The level of antibodies is maintained by the helper T cells inducing the B cells to produce antibodies and the suppressor T cells inhibiting antibody production.
5. Some B cells are stimulated to differentiate into plasma cells, also called large B cells.
6. Antibodies are rapidly produced in great numbers until the plasma cells die.
7. Each plasma cell will produce only one type of antibody, the type that will bind with the antigen that was responsible for initiating the activation of the B cell.
8. B cells that did not become plasma cells and some T cells remain as memory cells to respond to future exposure to the same antigen.
9. An **antigen–antibody complex** is formed by the combination of an antibody with an antigen. When the complex is formed, complement is activated to lyse invading bacterial cells, neutralize toxins, and increase phagocytosis.

CELL-MEDIATED IMMUNITY

Antibodies cannot enter cells, even those with intracellular pathogens. However, **cell-mediated immunity (CMI)** relies on macrophages and T cells to control chronic infections. CMI controls, but does not eliminate, the cause of the infection.

The herpes virus travels through the body fluids from a lysed cell to infect the next normal cell. While moving through the body fluids, the virus is exposed to the antibody–complement complex and is destroyed, thus controlling the viral infection. However, when the virus is established inside the body cell, the CMI response is able to destroy the infected cells. If the virus is not entirely destroyed, it can become latent in the nerve ganglion cells of the body.

CMI is composed of helper T cells that work with B cells to start the antibody response. As a reminder, the suppressor T cells ensure that the cytotoxic T cells are not too abundant and that the immune response is effective but not destructive to the body.

NK cells and cytotoxic T cells are effective in destroying pathogens inside infected cells. Examples include infected liver cells that are killed during hepatitis infections. The decrease of helper T cells impairs the functions of both the humoral and CMI. For a general overview of the body's defense systems, see Figure 13-9. Table 13-2 provides a summary of the various types of T cells and their actions.

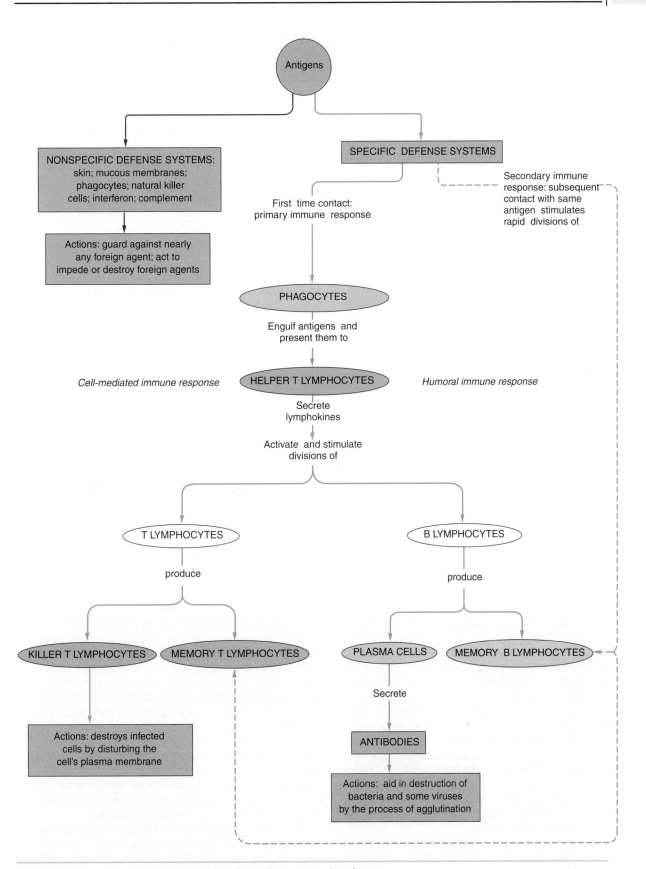

FIGURE 13-9   Overview of the body's defense mechanisms

TABLE 13-2 T Cells

NAME	ACTIONS
Cytotoxic T cell	Recognizes antigens that cancerous cells or virally infected cells have on their surface. The T cell is activated when it combines with an antigen. The T cell then enlarges its clone of cells. After binding to the surface of the cancerous or viral cell, the T cell releases the protein called perforin, which creates openings, thereby destroying the infected or cancerous cell.
Helper T cell	Mobilizes the immune system to prevent a bacterial infection. Once the T cell makes contact with an antigen and the antigen combines with the receptor sites on the T cell, it becomes activated. Once activated, the T cell stimulates the B cell to produce antibodies that are specific to the antigen.
Memory T cell	Produced on initial exposure to an antigen.
Natural killer cell	NK cells also use perforin to kill tumor cells.

PRIMARY AND SECONDARY IMMUNE RESPONSES

When T cells or B cells are activated after contact with the specific antigen that is responsible for starting the activation, the actions of the cells are called the primary immune response. During the response, plasma cells release the antibodies IgM and IgG into the lymph. The antibodies are transported to the blood circulatory system and then throughout the body to aid in destroying the antigen. The production and release of antibodies by the plasma cells will often continue for weeks.

BOX 13-3

Latex Allergy

Latex is manufactured from the natural rubber obtained from the rubber trees that grow in the tropical areas of the earth. In 1979 a British medical journal reported the first latex allergy patient, a lady who had a reaction to the rubber used to manufacture household cleaning gloves. Only about 1% of the population exhibits latex allergy. However, health care providers represent the largest group of individuals who are latex-sensitive. A large number of items used in surgery contain latex and the surgical team members who are exposed to these products on a daily basis become sensitized. What complicates matters is that many of the items containing latex do not have this indicated as an ingredient on the packaging, including shoe covers, tape, elastic bandages, and the electrode pads placed on the patient's chest that are connected to leads to the electrocardiogram machine.

There are two types of latex allergy responses: Type I and Type IV. Type IV is the less serious of the two and is characterized by a local reaction that can include skin irritation, redness, and itchiness. Type I is a serious reaction that is immunoglobulin E (IgE)–mediated. Type I can lead to respiratory arrest if not promptly treated.

Diagnosis of latex sensitivity is based on history, a physical examination of the patient, and a blood test. The blood test confirms the diagnosis by measuring the IgE antibodies against latex.

Rubber contains proteins that have been identified as being allergenic. Research has shown that water-soluble proteins in latex are the cause of the Type I reaction. The proteins attach to the skin from glove powder absorption, or the allergic reaction could also occur from inhalation of airborne allergens that are bound to the glove powder.

Individuals at risk for latex allergy, besides health care providers, include individuals who have had multiple surgeries and children with spina bifida. The surgical technologist should work with the other surgical team members to provide a latex-free environment for patients who are latex-sensitive. This includes using only nonlatex products; notifying all departments involved in the care of the patient, such as the pharmacy, nursing units, and central sterile supply, so precautions will be taken; and confirming that the patient's chart is properly marked to indicate that the patient is latex-sensitive and that the patient is wearing a red ID bracelet as an alert. Also, the latex-allergic patient should be scheduled as the first case of the day in an OR so that the latex dust from the previous day's surgeries has been removed by the end-of-day cleaning.

Items used in surgery that contain latex include gloves, tourniquets, suction tips, disposable face masks, endotracheal tube, and nasal airway. Manufacturers of these types of items substitute latex with materials such as Nitrile, neoprene, vinyl, and polyvinylchloride.

BOX 13-4

Anaphylactic Reaction

An anaphylactic reaction, also called anaphylaxis, is a severe allergic reaction that can be life-threatening. Drugs such as local anesthetics and antibiotics, the proteins found in latex used to manufacture many health care products, insect bites such as bee stings, and foods, in particular eggs and seafood, are often responsible for causing an anaphylactic reaction. Another common cause of anaphylaxis is penicillin.

The initial signs and symptoms of an anaphylatic attack are mild and include itching, swelling, and some difficulty in breathing. Hives and/or urticaria may be present. However, the reaction can progress rapidly, leading to severe difficulty in breathing due to laryngeal edema and bronchospasm. Another life-threatening occurrence during the reaction is vascular collapse due to dramatic shifts in body fluids causing tachycardia and hypotension. The surgical team must quickly treat the patient by providing a patent airway, treating the symptoms of vascular collapse, and treating for shock, which in itself can lead to death.

Anaphylactic reaction requires that the individual was previously sensitized to the specific antigen causing the reaction. The exposure results in the production of immunoglobulin E (IgE) by plasma cells. The IgE antibodies then bind to the receptor sites on the membrane of mast cells and basophils. Upon reexposure, the antigen binds to IgE antibodies, causing degranulation and the release of histamine and platelet-activating factor from the mast cells. In addition IgG or IgM add to the reaction by activating the release of complement.

At the same time bradykinin and leukotrienes are activated and are responsible for inducing vascular collapse by stimulating the contraction of smooth muscle and increasing vascular permeability. Vascular permeability allows plasma to leak from the circulation to interstitial spaces, which lowers the blood volume, causing hypotension, cardiac dysrhythmias, and hypovolemic shock.

The first drug given to a patient the second they exhibit the beginning signs and symptoms of anaphylaxis is epinephrine. The effects of the drug are bronchodilation to counter the bronchospasm and inflammation, decrease laryngeal spasms, and increase the blood pressure. Individuals who are allergic to bee stings are recommended to carry an "epipen," which has a prefilled, one-dose syringe with epinephrine that can be immediately injected into the thigh if the person sustains a bee sting. The second drug given is a steroid to inhibit the reaction and stabilize the mast cells. Levophed, a vasopressor agent, is given to increase the blood pressure and fluids, such as Ringer's lactate, are administered Intravenously (IV) to maintain the patient's normal circulating fluid volume and electrolytes.

In the period after a primary immune response, some B cells remain dormant and are called memory cells. If the same antigen that stimulated the primary immune response is present again and the B cells encounter the antigen, they respond by rapidly producing IgG in response to the antigen to which they were previously sensitized. The memory B cells combine with the memory T cells to produce the secondary immune response.

During a primary immune response, a laboratory-detectable level of antibodies is usually found in the body fluids within 5–10 days following exposure to the antigen. During a secondary immune response, more antibodies are produced within one to two days. Memory cells live much longer than antibodies; consequently, the secondary immune response can be long-lasting.

ACQUIRED IMMUNODEFICIENCY SYNDROME

In 1981, the Centers for Disease Control and Prevention (CDC) was first alerted that a new epidemic, called acquired immunodeficiency syndrome (AIDS), was at hand. The most noticeable characteristics of the new disease were a vulnerability of those infected to opportunistic infections and a profound decrease in the CD4 T-lymphocyte count. It was also noted that infected homosexual males and intravenous drug users were developing a very rare type of skin cancer called Kaposi's sarcoma.

In 1983, the virus that caused AIDS was isolated and called the **human immunodeficiency virus (HIV)**. By 1985, the chief routes of HIV transmission were identified: blood, sexual contact, and mother to child. The main target cells for the virus were identified as CD4 T lymphocytes and macrophages, and an antibody test was established. Therefore, the disease suppresses the body's natural immune defense system and the individual is prone to many types of bacterial, viral, and fungal infections. There are two possible outcomes of infection with HIV: develop AIDS or develop **AIDS-related complex (ARC)**.

The CDC reports that by 1997, HIV infection was pandemic, with 28 million infections worldwide. Of those infected with HIV, 8 million people will develop AIDS. By 2000, 36 million people were infected; of those, 753,900 cases in the United States were reported to the CDC. To date, it is estimated that 20 million

BOX 13-5

Hemolytic Transfusion Reaction

Hemolytic reaction occurs after a patient receives a blood transfusion of mismatched blood. The most serious reaction occurs from the transfusion of serologically incompatible blood, which is characterized by intravascular agglutination of erythrocytes leading to systemic clustering and destruction of the RBCs and possible development of disseminated intravascular coagulation (DIC). The reactions are due to the attachment of IgG or IgM to the transfused incompatible RBCs.

Transfusion of Rh-incompatible blood causes a less serious reaction, which occurs within approximately two weeks. Rh reactions are most common in women sensitized to RBC antigens by a previous pregnancy and in individuals who have received several transfusions.

The conscious patient will display the following signs and symptoms: fatigue, shortness of breath, chills, fever, tachycardia, nausea, tightness in the chest, hypotension, shock, pulmonary edema, bronchospasm, and heart failure. The reaction can occur within a couple of minutes to hours after the transfusion was given. In the surgical patient who has received general anesthesia, these signs and symptoms will not be evident. Instead, there will be generalized oozing of blood from the mucous membranes at the site of the surgical wound and lowered blood oxygen saturation level due to the inability of the erythrocytes to transport oxygen.

If hemolytic transfusion reaction is suspected, the first step is to immediately stop the transfusion. A blood sample from the patient and the blood bag should be sent to the blood bank to rule out or rule in a mismatch. Treatment includes administering IV normal saline solution. The clamp on the IV line should be left completely open to allow the infusion of a large amount of the saline to combat hypovolemia, administration of IV antihypotensive drugs, corticosteroids administered to reduce inflammation, and mannitol given to aid in maintaining urinary output. If an indwelling Foley catheter

has not been inserted in the patient, one should be in order to monitor urine output as an indicator of kidney function. In some instances, the patient may have to undergo dialysis to remove the mismatched blood from the systemic circulation.

Obviously, hemolytic transfusion reactions can be avoided by not transfusing incompatible blood into the patient. Prior to surgery, if a surgeon believes the patient may need a blood transfusion during the surgical procedure, a blood sample is taken from the patient in order to perform what is called type and cross-match so the patient's blood type and Rh is confirmed. Bags containing the same type of blood are set aside for that patient on the day of surgery. If possible, the patient may donate her or his own blood prior to the procedure, and this further reduces the chances of mistakenly transfusing the wrong blood. During a surgical procedure if it is decided a patient needs a blood transfusion, a blood sample is withdrawn from the patient, sent to the blood bank for type and cross-match, and the correct blood bags are selected. Whether the patient donated blood prior to the procedure, type and cross-match were completed prior to the procedure, or type and cross-match were completed after the surgical procedure started, the same protocol must be followed by the blood bank and surgical team for identifying the correct blood bag(s). An individual from the surgery department will go to the blood bank to pick up the blood bag. The OR person and blood bank technician together will read aloud the information on the blood bag including patient's name, hospital identification number, and blood type. This will be cross-checked with the blood bank's patient information, and the OR person signs a ledger showing they are the one who picked up the blood bag. In the OR, the anesthesia provider and circulating person reconfirm the information on the blood bag with the information in the patient's chart and with information provided by the blood bank prior to starting the transfusion.

BOX 13-6

Autoimmunity

Similar to organ transplant rejections, occasionally the immune system fails the body by not distinguishing between cells that are a normal part of the body and those that are not. When this happens the immune system produces autoantibodies and cytotoxic T cells that attack and damage or destroy the tissues and organs of the body. The autoimmune disorder, and often the name given to the disorder, reflects the

cells that are affected. For example, the cells that line the joints of the body are affected by rheumatoid arthritis and the colon cells are affected by ulcerative colitis.

One explanation for autoimmunity is that the T cells, when maturing in the thymus, do not learn to distinguish self from nonself. Another explanation is that a nonself antigen may resemble a self-antigen, thus confusing the immune system.

people have died of the disease. Homosexual contact and intravenous drug use account for 80% of all cases in men. Heterosexual contact and intravenous drug use account for 84% of cases in women. The transmission of HIV occurs in the following ways:

1. Sexual contact with an infected person; the virus enters through the vagina, penis, or rectum. Oral sex has not been definitively proved as a route of transmission.
2. Sharing hypodermic needles for the injection of drugs. If a noninfected person uses a "dirty" needle that contains the blood and body fluids of an infected person, they will most likely contract the virus.
3. Early in the course of HIV, several individuals, such as the famous tennis professional Arthur Ashe, contracted the virus from the transfusion of contaminated blood because the blood banks refused to test all blood donors even though the CDC advocated the donor test. Arthur Ashe underwent open heart surgery in which he received transfusions of blood contaminated with HIV, and he eventually died of AIDS. However, blood banks did finally adopt the test, and, currently, the possibility of receiving contaminated transfused blood is extremely low.
4. The infected mother passes HIV to the fetus in utero or at birth.

Amazingly, the virus is very weak and does not survive outside the body for more than a few seconds.

HIV belongs to a family of RNA viruses distinguished by possession of a viral reverse transcriptase, which transcribes viral RNA into provirus DNA that is integrated into the host cell's genome. These so-called **retroviruses** are generally host specific and are divided into two subfamilies: oncoretroviruses (with human T-cell lymphotropic virus, HTLV) and lentiviruses (HIV).

HIV is subdivided into two distantly related types, HIV-1 and HIV-2. HIV-1 is the predominant pathogen worldwide, while HIV-2 is endemic in West Africa. It is believed that there was a cross-species infection from a subspecies of chimpanzees living in West Africa. All HIV-1 strains are closely related to a strain of simian immunodeficiency virus (SIV) that affects only certain primates. A primate reservoir for HIV-2 has also been found.

HIV actually hides its attachment sites so that the body's immune system does not recognize the virus as being dangerous; this allows the virus to attack the immune system (Tortora et al., 2001). Just like other viruses, HIV is cell specific, meaning that it attacks only

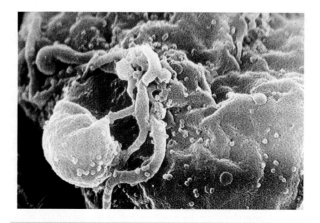

FIGURE 13-10 HIV budding from lymphocyte (Courtesy of the CDC Public Health Image Library)

specific cells, namely the cells in the immune system, the CD4 T lymphocytes. Obviously the lymphocytes have receptor sites for which the HIV attachment sites have an affinity for contact (Figure 13-10).

Initially HIV infection does not produce any symptoms. It is detected by drawing a specimen of the individual's blood and testing it with an HIV antibody test. The HIV antibodies are usually not detectable until one to three months after infection. A positive result indicates the person either is still asymptomatic or may be developing AIDS. There are two types of antibody tests available on the market:

1. Enzyme-linked immunosorbent assay (ELISA). It detects the antibodies but not the virally infected cells.
2. The Western blot test is used as a follow-up test to confirm the results of an ELISA.

In the early stages of AIDS, individuals will experience symptoms that mimic the flu including fever, headaches, enlarged lymph glands, and malaise. The symptoms often disappear and a long incubation period follows, which can last from weeks to years. But the individual is still a carrier and can transmit the virus to another person. During this period the immune system is deteriorating, and eventually the signs and symptoms of AIDS appear. These include: enlarged lymph glands, weight loss, chronic fevers, extreme sweating (diaphoresis) especially at night, severe headaches, extreme fatigue, abdominal cramps, and nausea.

These symptoms are exacerbated by the development of opportunistic infections. The common infections acquired by AIDS patients include:

1. Kaposi's sarcoma
2. Lymphomas

IMPLICATIONS FOR THE SURGICAL TECHNOLOGIST

The surgical technologist is not directly involved in the care of patients with immune system disorders except when they require surgery. However, the surgical procedures that are performed are usually due to complications that the immune system disorder has caused. For example, as previously discussed, a woman who has undergone a mastectomy may develop lymphedema in the arm on the affected side. If all other nonsurgical therapy fails, the patient may have to undergo surgery to reestablish drainage of the axillary region. Another example is AIDS patients. Often the patients are affected internally by Kaposi's sarcoma; in particular, the lesions develop in the esophagus and intestinal tract. Surgery may have to be performed on the esophagus if the patient has severe difficulty in swallowing; or the lesions may cause an obstruction in the colon, in which case a bowel resection is performed to remove the affected portion of colon and reanastomose the two ends.

Understanding the mechanisms of the lymphatic system and their components is important in order to understand the disease processes such as AIDS that affect the system, and to be aware of the preventive measures to take to avoid contracting immune system diseases on both a personal and a professional level. On a professional level, the surgical technologist should know the Standard Precautions that have been established by OSHA to avoid sharps injuries and contact with patients' blood and body fluids. Also, the surgical technologist should know the steps to take if a sharps injury occurs or if any type of contact with blood and body fluids occurs, including blood or body fluids that splash into the eye(s). As always, prevention is the key.

3. Fungal infections; usually candidiasis and histoplasmosis
4. Parasitic infections; usually *Pneumocystis carinii* pneumonia and toxoplasmosis
5. Viral infections; usually cytomegalovirus (CMV) disease, HBV, non-A and non-B hepatitis, and herpes simplex

New **protease inhibitor (PI)** classes of antiretroviral drugs (including saquinavir, ritonavir, and indinavir) inhibit HIV protease and thus interefere with HIV maturation and replication. PIs, used in combination with reverse transcriptase inhibitors, are allowing those infected with HIV to live longer. However, the long-term side effects of the use of these drugs, by themselves and in combination with other new drugs, are just now starting to be seen, such as liver and kidney disorders and effects on the cardiovascular system.

ARC is a term that was developed to describe individuals who contract HIV, but develop conditions other than AIDS. Symptoms range from chronic diarrhea, weight loss, lymphadenopathy, fatigue, and malaise.

Case Study 2

A patient has been brought into the surgery department to undergo a total hip arthroplasty. During the course of the operation the anesthesia provider has decided the individual requires a blood transfusion due to the amount of blood that has been lost during the procedure. The blood is homologous. Within two to three minutes of the start of the blood transfusion, the surgeon notices a generalized diffuse loss of blood at the incision site and the anesthesia provider takes note of a rapid decrease in the blood oxygen saturation level.

1. Based on the above information, what is occurring with this patient?

2. What mistake did the surgical team make to cause this reaction?

3. What immunoglobulins are involved in the reaction and what is their action?

4. What is the first course of treatment?

5. In serious cases, what procedure may the patient have to undergo to correct the incident and stabalize the patient?

CHAPTER SUMMARY

- The lymphatic system is closely linked to the circulatory system, since the lymph is returned to the blood and protects the body against invasion by foreign material.

- It consists of the lymph, lymph nodes, lymph vessels, spleen, thymus, and tonsils.

- Lymph is the fluid that enters and travels through the lymph vessels.

- Plasma is the straw-colored portion of blood and its composition is the same as lymph. Plasma maintains the osmotic pressure within the blood capillaries to facilitate the exchange of fluids.

- The flow of plasma into the interstitial spaces is greater than reabsorption by the blood capillaries, and the end result is the formation of interstitial fluid, which is forced to enter the lymphatic capillaries. This prevents edema.

- Lymph capillaries are the smallest of the vessels that extend throughout the interstitial spaces adjacent to the blood capillaries. They are responsible for the initial collection of tissue fluid.

- Lymph capillaries join to form larger lymph vessels. The larger vessels have three layers: endothelial, smooth, and connective.

- The contraction of skeletal muscles and the act of respiration aids in moving the lymph forward within the vessels. The vessels also contain valves, just like blood vessels, to prevent the regurgitation of lymph.

- Lymph travels back to the blood flow to become plasma.

- The cisterna chyli marks the beginning of the thoracic duct, which travels upward to join the left subclavian vein to empty the lymph. The thoracic duct drains lymph from the intestinal, lumbar, intercostal, left subclavian, left bronchomediastinal, and left jugular trunks.

- The right lymphatic duct joins the right subclavian vein to empty the lymph.

- Lacteals are a specialized type of lymph capillary located in the villi of the small intestine. The chylomicrons are absorbed and transported to the major lymph vessels by the lacteals.

- Lymph nodes and nodules are groups of lymphatic tissue.

- Their functions are to filter pathogens and other foreign material, monitor the level of body fluid, and conduct hematopoiesis.

- Blood vessels and nerves connect with the node at the hilum. Lymphatic vessels that travel to a node are lymphatic afferent vessels; those that exit the node are lymphatic efferent vessels.

- A capsule of connective tissue surrounds a node. The germinal centers within the node represent the area of activity where lymphocytes and macrophages are dividing.

- There are three sinuses in a node: subcapsular, cortical, and medullary.

- There are several groups of nodes located throughout the body. Three important groups are cervical, axillary, and inguinal lymph nodes. As lymph pass through a lymph node group, bacteria and other foreign material are phagocytized by fixed macrophages. Fixed plasma cells produce antibodies, thus the antibodies, lymphocytes, and monocytes enter the blood flow along with the lymph.

- Lymph nodules are collections of lymph cells.

- Other specialized lymph nodes include Peyer's patches and the tonsils. Peyer's patches are located in the ileum. However, their function is unknown.

- There are three groups of tonsils: palatine, pharyngeal or adenoids, and lingual tonsils. A tonsillectomy and adenoidectomy is often performed in children who experience chronic infections of the palatine tonsils and have pain and difficulty in breathing.

- Lymphedema is the abnormal collection of fluid within the interstitial spaces due to a pathology of the lymph system.

- Causes include lymphatic vessel obstruction, overproduction of interstitial fluid due to increased capillary blood pressure, and abnormal uptake of fluid by lymphatic capillaries due to injury.

- Lymphatic vessels are often blocked due to a tumor or lymphadenitis. Diagnosis is by lymphangiography. Treatment is antibiotics; surgery is the last course of treatment to attempt to reestablish drainage.

- The abnormal uptake of fluid is most often due to surgery, such as a mastectomy, and radiation therapy.

- Pregnancy is a primary factor in the increase in venous pressure. The increase in pressure causes an increase in capillary pressure and overproduction of interstitial fluid. The lymphedema is often seen in the ankles and feet of pregnant women.

- The spleen is a highly vascular organ located in the upper left quadrant of the body.

- On the medial side is the hilum where the vein exits and the artery enters.

- The spleen is an organ of the lymphatic system, since it contains lymphoid nodules, but it filters the blood that flows through much like the lymph nodes filter lymph.

- The spleen has two types of tissue: white pulp and red pulp.

- In the fetus, the erythrocytes are produced in the spleen. After-birth functions include: hematopoiesis, storage of blood, destruction of dead erythrocytes and platelets, and defense against bacteria and other foreign invaders.

- Individuals who have undergone a splenectomy tend to be prone to certain types of bacterial infections.

- The thymus gland is located in the mediastinal region.

- It consists of two lobes bound together by connective tissue that encloses the entire organ. The lobes are further broken down into lobules.

- The activity of the thymus is dependent on the hormone called thymosin.

- The thymus produces the T cells.

- With age, the thymus diminishes in size and function.

- The first line of defense of the body is the skin, mucous membranes, and secretions.

- The unbroken skin prevents microbes from entering the body. Once the skin is compromised, such as by a traumatic cut or surgical incision, an opening is created for the invasion of microbes.

- The skin secretes lactic acid from the sweat glands and fatty acids from the sebaceous glands that inhibit the growth of bacteria or kill them.

- The epidermis and dermis layers of the skin are formed in such a way as to provide a difficult barrier for microbes to penetrate.

- Sebaceous glands produce sebum, which prevents hair and skin from drying out and forms a protective layer on the skin surface. The unsaturated fatty acids in the sebum inhibit the growth of some bacteria and establish a pH level that also inhibits bacterial growth.

- The perspiration from the sweat glands washes away microbes from the skin surface and also contains lysozyme, which breaks down the cell walls of gram-positive bacteria.

- Mucous membranes line the respiratory, gastrointestinal, and genitourinary tracts. Goblet cells line the membrane and are responsible for producing mucus.

- The mucus catches microbes to prevent their entrance into the respiratory or GI tracts.

- Cilia are found in the respiratory tract and aid in trapping inhaled dust, dirt, and pathogens.

- The mucous membrane of the GU tract is flushed out by the flow of urine to prevent the colonization of microbes.

- The acidic gastric juice in the stomach kills most microbes.

- Phagocytosis is the process of surrounding and ingesting another microbe or foreign material and is performed by phagocytes, most of which are leukocytes.

- A differential white blood cell count is completed in the laboratory to determine the percentage of each type of white blood cell that is present in the blood specimen. Individuals who exhibit signs of infection often have an elevated number of leukocytes.

- There are two categories of leukocytes: granulocytes and agranulocytes. There are three categories of granulocytes: neutrophils, eosinophils, and basophils.

- Neutrophils are motile and are active in the beginning stages of an infection.

- Eosinophils produce toxins to fight parasites and play an important role during the allergic response.

- There are two types of agranulocytes: monocytes and lymphocytes.

- Monocytes exit the bloodstream and mature into macrophages. The increase of macrophages and lymphocytes within the lymph nodes causes them to swell during an infection.

- There are two types of macrophages: wandering and fixed, also called histiocytes.

- Fixed macrophages are found in the spleen, lymph nodes, bone marrow, intestines, liver (Küpffer cells), and brain (microglia). They remove and destroy foreign debris and microbes, as well as remove excess cellular secretions and dead leukocytes.

- Phagocytosis is divided into four steps: chemotaxis, adherence, ingestion, and digestion.

- Chemotaxis is the attraction of phagocytes to the area of infection.

- The phagocyte attaches to the microbe by adhering to its surface. Antibody molecules secrete a serum protein that coats the bacterial cell to promote the attachment of phagocytes to the pathogen; this is called opsonization and the antibody molecules are called opsonins.

- The process of ingestion begins when the phagocytes extend pseudopods to surround the microbe. The resulting sac is called a phagosome.

- Digestion begins when the phagosome enters the cytoplasm and the lysosomes form a phagolysosome. The enzymes now destroy the bacteria and the phagolysosome is called a residual body with leftover contents that cannot be digested. The residual body releases these contents to the outside of the cell.

- Complement is a group of proteins found in the blood plasma that make up the complement system. It circulates in the plasma until needed during an antibody–antigen reaction. Functions include: increase the inflammatory response; assist in the lysis of antigens; neutralize microbial toxins; and attract phagocytes to area of infection.

- Complement aids in the lysis of bacteria through the process called complement cascade in a specific sequence called the complementary pathway.

- Iron is used by pathogens for the synthesis of exotoxins. Leukocytes produce interleukin-1 (IL-1), which stimulates the liver to store iron and deprive the pathogens of the needed iron.

- Iron also binds to iron transport proteins called transferrin, ferritin, and lactoferrin to deprive the pathogens.

- The four signs of the inflammatory process are pain, heat, redness, and swelling.

- Inflammation is responsible for three processes: destroying the invasive agent; walling of the infection; and repair of damaged tissue.

- There are three stages of inflammation: vasodilation, phagocyte migration, and tissue repair.

- Vasodilation refers to the dilation of the blood vessels to aid in increasing the blood flow to the area of damage and increase the permeability of the vessel wall. The three chemicals responsible for vasodilation are: histamine, kinins, and prostaglandins.

- An abscess is the combination of body fluids and dead cells that collect in a cavity. Pyogenic bacteria cause abscess formation.

- Neutrophils and monocytes travel to the area of injury, leave the blood vessels, and begin the process of phagocytosis.

- The extent of tissue repair is dependent on the type of tissue that has been damaged.

- Fever is a systemic reaction to viral or bacterial invasion.

- The hypothalamus is responsible for the temperature of the body.

- Fever occurs when phagocytes ingest bacteria and the lipopolysaccharides in the cell wall are released, thereby stimulating the phagocytes to release IL-1. IL-1 communicates to the hypothalamus to release prostaglandins, which elevates the temperature causing a fever.

- Infection is brought under control when vasodilation and sweating begins. This phase is called crisis.

- Interferon is a type of protein that is produced during an infection. The interferon enters the host's cells and inhibits the synthesis of proteins that viruses need for multiplying.

- Interferon is not pathogen specific but is species specific.

- There are three classifications of interferon: alpha, beta, and gamma.

- Recently, using DNA recombinant DNA technology, interferon was produced, but it was not an effective agent against viral diseases.

- The immune response is the third line of defense. Antibodies are produced to bind with microbes to inactivate and destroy them.

- Humoral antibodies are located in the lymph and plasma.

- There are two types of acquired immunity: active acquired immunity and passive acquired immunity.

- There are two subcategories of active acquired immunity: natural active acquired immunity and artificial active acquired immunity.

- Natural active acquired immunity: the person has a disease that leaves them with partial or total resistance to reinfection by the same diseases.

- Artificial active acquired immunity: vaccination. Vaccines are made from inactivated pathogens, living pathogens, or toxins that the pathogen secretes. The laboratory process of weakening pathogens for use as a vaccine is called attentuation. Toxoid vaccine is prepared from the exotoxins of the pathogen that are inactivated by chemicals or heat. An antiserum is a serum that contains specific antibodies.

- There are two subcategories of passive acquired immunity: natural passive acquired immunity and artificial passive acquired immunity.

- Natural passive acquired immunity: antibodies are passed from the pregnant female across the placenta to the fetus.

- Artificial passive acquired immunity: antibodies are transferred from an immune person to a susceptible person.

- Antigens stimulate the production of antibodies, since the body does not recognize them as being part of itself.

- Antigenic determinants are sites on the antigen to which antibodies and lymphocytes can bind.

- Antibodies are produced by B cells and are in a class of proteins called immunoglobulins.

- The lag phase is the delayed response in the production of antibodies after antigen exposure.

- The first step of the immune response is called the primary response.

- Subsequent exposures to the antigen are called the secondary response.

- Agammaglobulinemia refers to a condition in which a person is born without the ability to produce antibodies, since they have no gammaglobulin in their blood.

- There are three types of lymphocytes that develop in the bone marrow: B cells, T cells, and natural killer (NK) cells.

- There are four types of T cells that the thymus produces: helper T cell, suppressor T cell, cytotoxic T cell, and delayed-hypersensitivity T cell. T cells are involved in cell-mediated immune response.

- B cells originate from the lymphoid regions of the intestine and liver. They migrate to the lymphoid tissue to produce circulating antibodies, thereby providing humoral immunity. B cells live one to two weeks. They are capable of quickly mass-producing antibodies.

- The five classes of antibodies are: IgA, IgD, IgE, IgG, and IgM.

- The process of antibody production involves T cells, B cells, and macrophages.

- An end result of the process is that some T cells that remain as memory cells to respond to future exposures to the same antigen.

- Another important end result is an antigen–antibody complex formed by the combination of an antibody with an antigen.

- CMI relies on macrophages and T cells to control infections.

- Helper T cells work with B cells to begin the antibody response. NK cells and cytotoxic T cells are also involved in CMI.

- When T cells and B cells are activated, the actions of the cells are called the primary immune response. Plasma cells release IgM and IgG into the lymph, and these antibodies circulate throughout the body to destroy the antigen, which will continue for a long period.

- After the primary immune response some B cells remain dormant and are now called memory B cells, which combine with memory T cells to produce the secondary immune response.

- Memory cells live much longer than antibodies; therefore, the secondary immune response is long-lasting.

- Cases of AIDS were first reported to the CDC starting in 1981, but at that time it was not known what it was or what caused the disease.

- In 1983, HIV was discovered as the cause of AIDS.

- In 1985, the primary routes of HIV transmission were established: blood, sexual contact, and mother to fetus.

- The main target of HIV is CD4 T lymphocytes and macrophages.

- The disease suppresses the body's natural immune defense system and the individual is prone to developing many types of bacterial, viral, and fungal infections, which can be life-threatening.

- There are two possible outcomes of HIV infection: develop AIDS or develop AIDS-related complex (ARC).

- The transmission of HIV occurs through: sexual contact with infected person; sharing of a used hypodermic needle for the injection of drugs; receiving contaminated blood during a blood transfusion; or passing of HIV by the infected mother to the fetus in utero or during birth.

- HIV belongs to a family of RNA retroviruses that is divided into two subfamilies: oncoretroviruses and lentiviruses.

- HIV is subdivided into two related types: HIV-1 and HIV-2.

- HIV hides its attachment sites so that the immune system does not recognize the virus as being dangerous, thereby allowing it to attack the immune system. The CD4 T lymphocytes have receptor sites for which the HIV attachment sites have an affinity for contact.

- Initially no symptoms are present. Antibodies are not detectable until one to three months after infection.

- There are two types of antibody tests: enzyme-linked immunosorbent assay (ELISA); Western blot test.

- HIV has a long incubation period, but the HIV-infected person is still a carrier who can pass on the virus to another person.

- As the immune system deteriorates, the individual develops the severe signs and symptoms of AIDS.

- AIDS patients are prone to opportunistic infections including Kaposi's sarcoma, lymphomas, fungal infections such as candidiasis, parasitic infections such as toxoplasmosis, and viral infections, most commonly CMV and HBV.

- Protease inhibitor classes of antiretroviral drugs have been developed to inhibit HIV protease and interfere with HIV maturation and replication.

- ARC is a term applied to individuals who contract HIV but develop conditions other than AIDS. It is marked by chronic diarrhea, weight loss, fatigue, malaise, and lymphadenopathy.

- Surgical technologists are involved in surgical procedures performed on individuals who have immune system disorders such as AIDS. The surgical procedures are usually performed to correct a pathology caused by the immune system disorder.

- To understand disease processes that affect the lymphatic system and the reasons that surgery is performed due to the diseases, the surgical technologist should understand the mechanisms and components of the system.

- Understanding the system and related diseases provides the surgical technologist additional information as far as the preventive measures to take in surgery to avoid contracting an immune system disease.

- The surgical technologist should know the OSHA Standard Precautions to avoid sharps injuries and contact with the patient's blood and body fluids. Knowing the Standard Precautions also provides the knowledge about what steps to take if a surgical technologist incurs a sharps accident.

CRITICAL THINKING QUESTIONS

1. When a surgeon performs a mastectomy (removal of a breast), why are the axillary lymphatic nodes also removed?
2. When a splenectomy is performed, what other organs and structures can compensate for the functions of the spleen?
3. Discuss the possible reasons that a small group of people in the world who are at high risk for HIV infection do not become infected.
4. Provide an example of a type II immediate hypersensitivity reaction that can occur in the operating room.
5. Why does the strength of the immune response decline in the elderly?

REFERENCES

Anderson, K. N. (Ed.). (1998). *Mosby's medical, nursing, and allied health dictionary* (5th ed.). St. Louis, MO: Mosby-Year Book.

Burton, G. R. W., & Engelkirk, P. G. (1996). *Microbiology for the health sciences* (5th ed.). Philadelphia: Lippincott-Raven.

Gray, H. (1991). *Anatomy, descriptive and surgical.* St. Louis, MO: Mosby-Year Book.

Grover-Lakomia, L. I., & Fong, E. (1999). *Microbiology for health careers* (6th ed.). Clifton Park, NY: Thomson Delmar Learning.

Ingraham, J. L., & Ingraham, C. A. (2000). *Introduction to microbiology* (2nd ed.). Pacific Grove, CA: Brooks/Cole.

Koneman, E., Allen, S., Janda, W., Schreckenberger, P., & Winn, W. (1997). *Color atlas and textbook of diagnostic microbiology* (5th ed.). Philadelphia: J. B. Lippincott.

O'Toole, M. (Ed.). (1992). *Miller–Keane encyclopedia and dictionary of medicine, nursing, and allied health* (5th ed.). Philadelphia: W. B. Saunders.

Tortora, G. J., Funke, B. R., & Case, C. L. (2001). *Microbiology: An introduction* (7th ed.). San Francisco: Benjamin Cummings.

14

RESPIRATORY SYSTEM

CHAPTER OBJECTIVES

After completing the study of this chapter, you
should be able to:

1. List the functions of the respiratory system.
2. Describe the respiratory pathway.
3. Describe the structure and list the functions of the nasal cavity, pharynx, and larynx.
4. Describe the structure and list the functions of the trachea.
5. Describe the structure of the lungs including bronchi and bronchioles.
6. Name the blood and nerve supply to the lungs.
7. State the factors that affect the healing of lung tissue.
8. List optimal methods of achieving wound closure of lung tissue.
9. Describe the layers of the pleural membranes, cellular structure, location, and functions of the serous fluid.
10. Describe the structure and function of the alveoli and pulmonary capillaries, and the role of surfactant.
11. Describe the physiology of inhalation and exhalation and exchange of gases.
12. Explain the processes of oxygen and carbon dioxide transport within the circulatory system.
13. Describe internal respiration.
14. Explain the importance of pressures in relation to breathing and the collapse of the lungs.
15. List and define the pulmonary volumes.
16. Explain the relationship of respiration to maintaining the normal pH level in the body.

KEY TERMS

alveoli	external respiration	nasal mucosa	pulmonary surfactant
apneustic center	hemopneumothorax	nasal septum	recurrent laryngeal nerve
bronchioles	inspiration center	olfactory organ	Sellick's maneuver
chronic obstructive	intercostal muscles	paranasal sinuses	superior laryngeal nerve
pulmonary disease (COPD)	internal respiration	pharynx	tension pneumothorax
diaphragm	larynx	pleural cavity	trachea
emphysema	lobules	pneumotaxic center	vagus nerve
epiglottis	lung	pneumothorax	vocal cords
expiration center	nasal cavities	primary bronchi	
external nares	nasal conchae	pulmonary edema	

Case Study 1

Nancy, CST, is on emergency call in a rural town. On Sunday morning, she is called and asked to get to the hospital surgery department as fast as possible for emergency surgery on a 6-year-old girl who is suffering from acute epiglottitis.

1. What is the usual cause of epiglottitis?

2. What is the epiglottis?

3. What is the respiratory system function of the epiglottis?

4. Why is epiglottitis an extreme emergency situation that requires immediate treatment?

5. Why is the on-call emergency surgery team being called into the surgery department?

INTRODUCTION

The acts of inhaling (inspiration) and exhaling (expiration) facilitate the process of taking in oxygen and getting rid of the waste gas carbon dioxide, which is referred to as respiration. The process of exchanging gases actually occurs on a microscopic level in which the oxygen is eventually transported to all of the tissues of the body that require it for the maintenance of homeostasis. Four terms that apply to all sections of this chapter are defined as follows:

1. Ventilation: movement of air in and out of the lungs; commonly called breathing
2. External respiration: exchange of oxygen and carbon dioxide between the lungs and circulatory system
3. Internal respiration: exchange of oxygen and carbon dioxide between the blood in the circulatory system and the body cells
4. Cellular respiration: the use of oxygen by the cells of the body and the subsequent production of carbon dioxide as the waste gas that must be expelled from the body

STRUCTURE AND FUNCTIONS OF ORGANS OF THE RESPIRATORY SYSTEM

The organs of the respiratory system are commonly divided into the upper respiratory tract, which includes the nose, nasal cavity, pharynx, and sinuses, and the lower respiratory tract, which includes the larynx, trachea, bronchi, lungs, internal lung structures, and ancillary structures (Figure 14-1).

Upper Respiratory Tract

Nose and Nasal Cavity

The outside of the nose is covered by skin, and the structure is supported by bone and flexible cartilage. The **external nares** are the openings through which air enters and exits. Coarse hairs that contain epidermis line the internal portion of the nares and serve as a filtering device, catching large particles that enter with the air that is breathed inward, thus preventing the entrance of tube particles into the respiratory passages and/or lungs.

The air travels through the nares into the two **nasal cavities**, which are separated by the **nasal septum**. The nasal septum is made up of the vomer and ethmoid bones. The lining of the cavities is ciliated epithelium containing goblet cells and is called the **nasal mucosa**. Because of the presence of goblet cells, the nasal mucosa produces mucus. The layer of connective tissue that lies just under the epithelium of the nasal mucous membrane is called the lamina propria. It is attached to the perichondrium of the nasal cartilage and periosteum of the nasal bones. It is highly vascular, so the blood contributes to warming of the incoming air. The air that travels through the nasal cavities is warmed and humidified before it reaches the lungs.

Three curved, shelflike bones project medially from the lateral wall of each nasal cavity. These are the **nasal conchae**, which are covered by nasal mucosa and supported by cancellous bone, and are so named because of the scroll-like appearance of the bones, which mimic the scrolls of a conch shell. The three conchae are the superior, middle, and inferior conchae or turbinates. The lamina propria of the inferior and middle conchae is highly vascular, containing

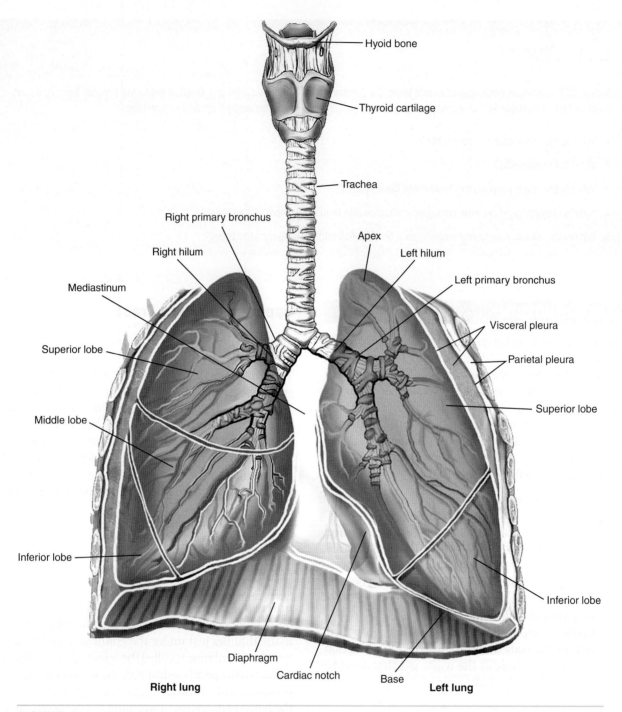

FIGURE 14-1   Trachea, lungs, and related structures

many capillaries. At times, such as when a person has a common cold, the vessels are congested with blood and the conchae become swollen, making it harder to breathe through the nose (commonly referred to as a stuffed-up nose).

Located in the roof or superior portion of each nasal cavity is the olfactory area in which an **olfactory organ** is situated. Within the organ are the olfactory

receptor cells, which are a special type of neuron with a dendrite extending to the surface of the olfactory area and an axon that extends into the lamina propria and farther through the ethmoid bone. The cells detect smells that are inhaled and communicate the information to the brain for interpretation.

There are four **paranasal sinuses** in the nasal cavity: the maxillae, frontal, sphenoid, and ethmoid

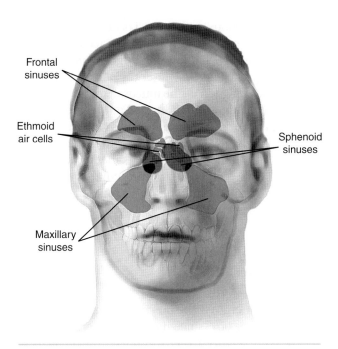

Frontal sinuses

Ethmoid air cells

Sphenoid sinuses

Maxillary sinuses

FIGURE 14-2 **Paranasal sinuses**

(Figure 14-2). Their names indicate their location, since the sinuses are located within the bone of the same name. The sinuses are lined with ciliated epithelium, which is responsible for moving mucus into the nasal cavities. The functions of the sinuses are to make the skull lighter in weight, which facilitates holding up the head for long periods of time, and to provide resonance to the voice.

Pharynx

The **pharynx**, commonly called the throat, is a tubular structure that is approximately 13 cm long in the adult (Figure 14-3). It is posterior to the oral and nasal cavities, extending from the base of the skull and situated anterior to the cervical vertebrae ending at the superior portion of the larynx. It is the only anatomic structure that serves the dual function of conducting air and food. It is primarily innervated by the glossopharyngeal nerve (cranial nerve IX) to aid in the functions of swallowing and secretion of saliva. The pharynx is divided into three sections: the nasopharynx, oropharynx, and laryngopharynx.

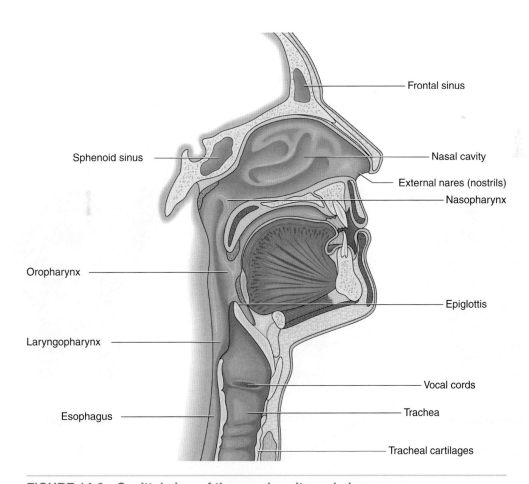

Frontal sinus

Sphenoid sinus

Nasal cavity

External nares (nostrils)

Nasopharynx

Oropharynx

Epiglottis

Laryngopharynx

Vocal cords

Esophagus

Trachea

Tracheal cartilages

FIGURE 14-3 **Sagittal view of the nasal cavity and pharynx**

The superior portion of the pharynx is the nasopharynx, located posterior to the nasal cavities. When swallowing, the soft palate of the mouth elevates to block the nasopharynx and cause food or liquids to travel down toward the stomach. The uvula, which is an extension of the soft palate, can be seen at the back of the oral cavity and is just anterior to the nasopharynx. The adenoids are located on the posterior wall of the nasopharynx and the openings of the two eustachian tubes from the ears are located in the superior portion of the nasopharynx. Most individuals are familiar with the idea of opening their mouths or chewing gum when taking off or landing in an airplane. The eustachian tubes serve to keep the pressure equal in the middle ears; opening the mouth permits air to enter, thus "popping" the ears to keep the pressure equal and allow the eardrums to vibrate.

The oropharynx, as the name implies, is located posterior to the oral cavity. The mucosa consists of stratified squamous epithelium. Located on the lateral walls are the palatine tonsils. The placement of the palatine tonsils, adenoids, and lingual tonsils serves to destroy pathogens that enter the pharynx and prevent further invasion of the mucosal lining.

The laryngopharynx is located at the inferior portion of the pharynx. Its opening leads into the larynx and esophagus. The pharynx as a whole is composed of muscle and lined with mucous membrane. However, the contraction of the muscular wall of the oropharynx and laryngopharynx contributes to the swallowing reflex.

Lower Respiratory Tract

Larynx and Epiglottis

The next structure is the **larynx**, commonly referred to as the voice box, since it contains the vocal cords for speaking (Figure 14-4). It connects the pharynx to

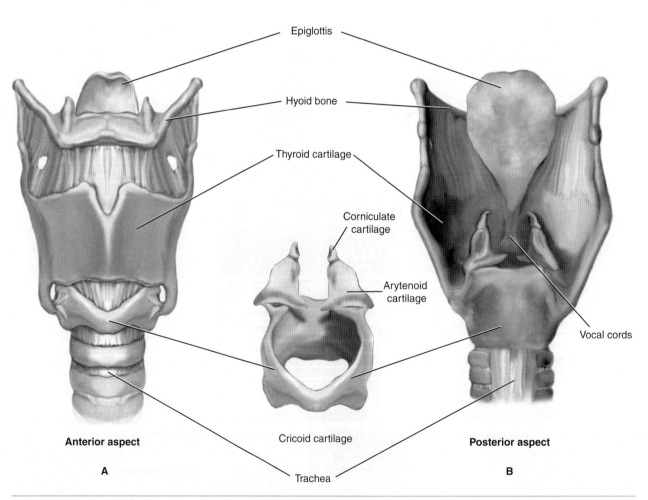

FIGURE 14-4   The larynx: (A) anterior and (B) posterior views.

the trachea and also functions as part of the air passageway. It is lined by mucous membrane that is continuous from the pharynx and on into the trachea. The mucosa is ciliated columnar epithelium, except for the vocal cords, which are composed of stratified squamous epithelium. The cilia move in a smooth, wavelike motion toward the pharynx to push mucus, dust, and microbes upward to be expelled as sputum. The larynx extends to the fourth, fifth, and sixth cervical vertebrae.

To continuously maintain an open airway, the larynx is composed of three single cartilages and three paired cartilages. The cartilages are connected together by ligaments and voluntary muscle. Cartilage is ideal, since it is a firm yet flexible tissue, which prevents the larynx from collapsing but allows free movement of the neck in several directions. The single cartilages are the thyroid, cricoid, and epiglottic. The paired cartilages are the arytenoid, corniculate, and cuneiform.

The thyroid cartilage is butterfly-shaped and is the largest; it is easily palpated on the anterosuperior portion of the neck, often referred to as the Adam's apple. The epiglottic cartilage is the uppermost cartilage. During swallowing, the larynx elevates and the **epiglottis** closes over the opening of the larynx to prevent food from entering. The epiglottic cartilage is the only cartilage of the larynx that is elastic, not hyaline, cartilage. It is attached to the superior border to the thyroid cartilage and supports the epiglottis.

The cricoid cartilage is located inferior to the thyroid cartilage and indicates the lowermost portion of the larynx. The arytenoid cartilages are pyramid-shaped, located superior to and lateral to either side of the cricoid cartilage. The corniculate cartilages are attached to the tips of the arytenoid cartilages and are tiny, cone-shaped cartilages. The corniculate cartilages serve as attachments for muscles that help regulate tension on the vocal cords while speaking and in closing the larynx when swallowing. The cuneiform cartilages are also tiny structures, cylindrical in shape and located between the epiglottic and arytenoid cartilages.

The **vocal cords** contain elastic fibers and are centrally located in the larynx and are situated on either side of the glottis, the opening between the cords. During breathing the vocal cords are closed over the glottis to allow air to pass in and out of the trachea. During speaking, the intrinsic muscles of the larynx stretch the vocal cords across the glottis and exhaled air vibrates the vocal cords, which then produces speech.

The larynx is supplied by motor nerves, which innervate the muscles that contract for voice production. The nerves are as follows:

1. **Vagus nerve** (Cranial nerve X): Innervates the pharynx and larynx.
2. **Superior laryngeal nerve**: Innervates the pharynx, larynx, that cricothyroid muscle. It descends along the side of the pharynx and divides into two branches, the external and internal laryngeal nerves. If damaged, it can result in the loss of the high-pitch tone of voice (McKenney, Mangonon, & Moylan, 1998).
3. **Recurrent laryngeal nerve**: A particularly important nerve that must be positively identified during surgical procedures of the neck such as a thyroidectomy. A branch of the vagus nerve, it enters the larynx at the point where the inferior portion of the thyroid cartilage joins the superior aspect of the cricoid cartilage and is then distributed to all of the muscles of the larynx except the cricothyroid. It eventually joins the superior laryngeal nerve. If injured during surgery, it can result in temporary or permanent hoarseness of the voice due to paresis to one side of the vocal cords. Bilateral nerve damage can result in permanently closed vocal cords, which requires a permanent tracheostomy to maintain an airway (McKenney et al., 1998).

Another important surgical aspect involves the cricoid cartilage. A maneuver referred to as **Sellick's maneuver** or cricoid pressure is performed to reduce the risk of aspiration by a patient undergoing general anesthesia. Cricoid pressure is applied just prior to the induction of anesthesia and is discontinued once the endotracheal tube is in place. The thumb and forefinger are used to apply external pressure to the cricoid cartilage, causing slight blockage of the esophagus between the cricoid and the body of the sixth cervical vertebra. In particular, when a patient requires emergency surgery and they may have recently eaten, the pressure prevents contents of the stomach from regurgitating and possible aspiration occurring.

Trachea and Bronchi

The **trachea**, commonly called the windpipe, is approximately 11 cm long and 2 cm wide, extending from the larynx at the level of the sixth cervical vertebra to where it bifurcates into the two bronchi at the level of the fifth thoracic vertebra (Figures 14-5 and

BOX 14-1

Endotracheal Intubation

Surgical patients who will receive general anesthesia will typically undergo endotracheal (ET) intubation to facilitate the delivery of the anesthetic gases and oxygen, and expiration of carbon dioxide. ET intubation is the insertion of a tube called the tracheal tube, through the mouth or nose, between the vocal cords, and into the trachea. This is performed after the patient has received intravenous drugs that cause the patient to be unconscious. The equipment used consists of a laryngoscope, tracheal tube, stylet, and 10-mL syringe.

The laryngoscope consists of a handle and interchangeable rigid blades that attach to the handle, hence the term rigid laryngoscope. Batteries are inserted into the handle to light the small bulb at the tip of the blade, which helps the anesthesia provider to visualize the back of the throat. A variety of blade sizes are available for adults and pediatric patients. The blades are either straight or slightly curved. The blade must be disinfected between uses so as not to transmit microbes from one patient to the next.

Tracheal tubes are plastic disposable tubes that are formed to contour to the airway passage. The tubes are referred to as being cuffed or uncuffed. The cuff is an inflatable "balloon" that surrounds the tube; when inflated with air it creates a closed airway system that does not allow leakage around the tube. Cuffed tubes are used on adults and uncuffed tubes are used on pediatric patients, since the airway is small and the tube itself closes the airway system.

A flexible, metal stylet is used to modify the contour of the ET tube and stiffen the tube to aid in placement. The stylet is placed within the lumen of the ET tube and removed once the ET tube is in place.

When performing intubation, the patient is placed on the OR table in the supine position. The anesthesia provider will tilt the head slightly backward. The mouth is fully opened and the blade of the laryngoscope is placed within the oral cavity and advanced to the epiglottis. The tip of the blade is used to move the tongue and epiglottis out of the way in order to view the glottis and vocal cords. The ET tube is then inserted into the mouth, and through the glottis between the vocal cords and into the trachea. The syringe with air is attached to a small adjoining tube and is used to inflate the cuff. The laryngoscope is removed and the anesthesia provider uses a stethoscope to listen to breath sounds that ensure the correct placement of the ET tube.

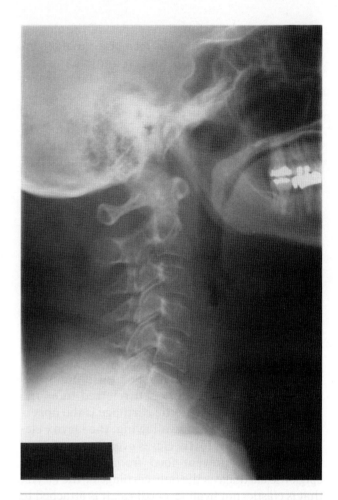

FIGURE 14-5   Lateral projection for upper airway

14-6). The anterior surface of the tube is covered by the isthmus of the thyroid gland; posteriorly it is in contact with the esophagus.

The trachea consists of approximately 20 C-shaped rings of hyaline cartilage, which, as in the larynx, keep the trachea continuously open but flexible. Pos-

teriorly the cartilages are incomplete, which allows the esophagus to expand when food is swallowed. The area between the posterior ends of each ring contains an interlacing network of smooth muscle called the trachealis muscle and fibroelastic connective tissue. The mucosal lining of the trachea contains ciliated columnar epithelium with goblet cells called the respiratory epithelium; the cilia also move toward the pharynx to continuously transport mucus. Large particles that enter with inhaled air are trapped on the mucus; therefore, the mucus is a protective method of keeping the lungs clear and preventing infection by bacteria.

Within the mediastinal space, the trachea bifurcates into the **primary bronchi**. The bronchi enter each lung at the hilum and further divide within the lungs. This branching network is referred to as the bronchial tree (Figures 14-7 and 14-8). The sequence of division is as follows:

1. The trachea bifurcates into the two primary bronchi.

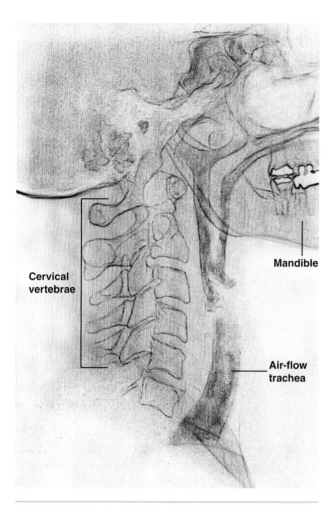

Cervical vertebrae

Mandible

Air-flow trachea

FIGURE 14-6   Lateral projection for upper airway

2. The primary bronchus enters the lung and subdivides into smaller, secondary branches; one branch supplies each lobe of the lung.
3. The secondary bronchi subdivide into segmental (tertiary) bronchi, which supply the segments of the lung.
4. The segmental bronchi subdivide into **bronchioles**, which enter the small compartments of the lung segments called **lobules**, which are the basic units of the lungs.
5. The bronchioles subdivide into smaller, terminal bronchioles, which further divide into alveolar ducts, which terminate at the grapelike clusters of alveoli.

The functions of the bronchi are the same as the trachea. In addition, the structure of the wall of the bronchi is similar in that it contains hyaline cartilage and fibroelastic connective tissue. The bronchi are lined with respiratory epithelium.

The bronchioles are approximately 1 mm or less in diameter. The structure of the wall is different in that it consists of simple epithelium instead of stratified columnar epithelium. They also lack cilia and goblet cells. Bronchioles also do not have cartilage in the wall, but are referred to as being soft-walled. During inspiration the spongy tissue that surrounds the bronchioles expands and the bronchioles are pulled open by this expansion, due to the spongy tissue being attached to the outside of their walls. The wall of the bronchioles contains smooth muscle bundles, which regulate the diameter of the bronchiole lumen.

As previously mentioned, the bronchioles enter into the lobules of the lungs. The bronchioles further subdivide into smaller, terminal bronchioles, which continue to subdivide into respiratory bronchioles. The respiratory bronchioles represent the first structures that deal with the exchange of gases. The respiratory bronchioles terminate in branches that divide into the alveolar ducts. Around each alveolar duct are the round-shaped alveoli that form clusters.

Pleural Membranes, Lungs, and Alveoli

The **pleural cavity** is the space within the thorax that contains the lungs and pleural membranes. The pleural membranes are a delicate serous membrane composed of a single layer of flat mesothelial cells that rest on a thin membrane of connective tissue. The pleural membranes are divided into the visceral pleura and parietal pleura. The parietal pleura lines the thoracic cavity including covering the diaphragm and reflecting over the structures located in the mediastinum. It invaginates at the hilum of the lung to become the visceral pleura (McKenney et al., 1998). The visceral pleura covers the lungs, including the indentations of the fissures of the lobes. Between the two pleura is the narrow pleural space, which contains serous fluid that acts as a lubricant and prevents friction, thereby allowing the pleural membranes to slide over each other as the lungs expand and contract with breathing.

The **lungs** are located on each side of the sternum in the thoracic cavity and consist of a spongy, elastic tissue (Figure 14-9). The right lung is divided by fissures into three lobes and the left lung—due to the position of the heart, in particular the apex being more toward the left side of the thoracic cavity—is divided into two lobes. Each lung is conical in shape; the top, rounded portion is referred to as the apex and extends approximately 3 to 4 cm superior

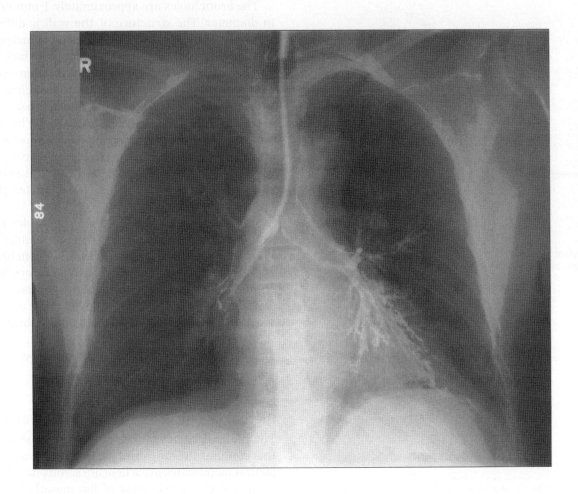

FIGURE 14-7   Posteroanterior view of bronchial tree

to the first rib up to the level of the clavicle. The base of a lung is concave and broad in width. The concave portion rests on the convex surface of the diaphragm, thus moving up with the diaphragm during expiration and moving down during inspiration. The layers of each lung are the external visceral pleura, a subserous layer of areolar tissue that contains elastic fibers, and the parenchyma. The surfaces of the lungs are slightly concave with an indentation for the heart to rest on. Each lung has an average capacity of approximately 5,500–6,000 ml of air.

The arterial blood is supplied to the lungs by the bronchial arteries, which are branches from the thoracic aorta. The bronchial vein is situated at the base of the lung. The blood supply of the bronchial arteries returns via the pulmonary veins to the left atrium

of the heart (Figure 14-10). The lymphatics of the lungs and trachea are as follows:

1. Bronchial glands: Situated around the bifurcation of the trachea and upper portion of the lungs (Gray, 1991). There are approximately 10 to 12 in number.
2. Lymphatics of the lungs: The superficial lymphatics are beneath the pleura and form a minute network on the surface of the lung. The deep lymphatics follow the course of the blood vessels and travel next to the bronchi (Figure 14-11). Both sets of lymphatics end at the upper portion of the lungs in the bronchial glands.
3. Efferent lymphatic vessels: Travel upward next to the trachea and end in the thoracic duct on

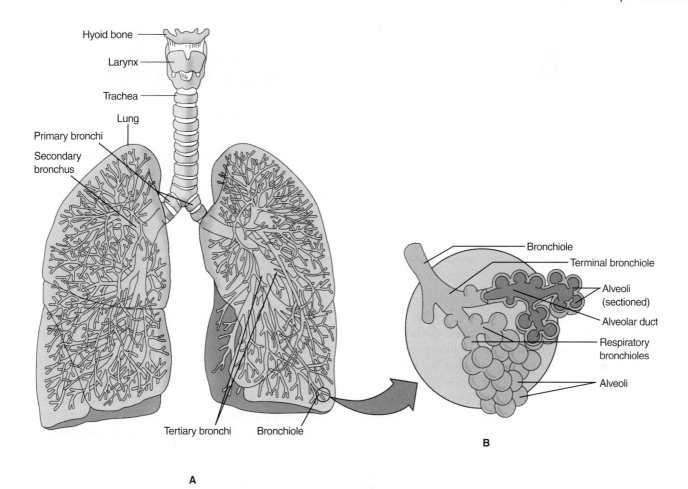

Hyoid bone
Larynx
Trachea
Lung
Primary bronchi
Secondary bronchus
Tertiary bronchi   Bronchiole

A

Bronchiole
Terminal bronchiole
Alveoli (sectioned)
Alveolar duct
Respiratory bronchioles
Alveoli

B

FIGURE 14-8   Bronchial tree: (A) Bronchial divisions, (B) Bronchiole

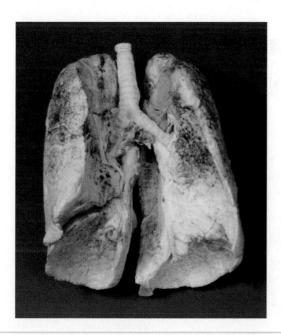

FIGURE 14-9   Human lungs (Courtesy of Oak Ridge National Laboratory, Oak Ridge, TN)

the left side, and right lymphatic duct on the right side (Gray, 1991).

The **alveoli** (singular, alveolus), although they are the smallest structures of the lung, are the hardest-working functional unit (Figure 14-12). It is here that the exchange of gases occurs. New alveoli develop throughout infancy. At approximately age 8, the total number of alveoli, about 300 million, will have developed, and they remain throughout adulthood.

The epithelial covering of the alveolar wall consists primarily of flat interconnected squamous epithelial cells called type I pneumocytes. Each alveolus is surrounded by networks of pulmonary capillaries, but no lymphatics are present. The alveoli and capillaries are supported by a network of elastic and reticular fibers. The capillaries consist of a single layer of endothelial cells, a type of specialized simple squamous epithelial cells. It is commonly recognized that this presents only two cell layers between the air in the alveoli and the blood in the pulmonary capillaries, which contributes to the efficiency of the exchange of gases. The process is efficient; however, what does have to be taken into consideration is that the alveolar–capillary barrier actually has three layers. It appears that the basement membranes of the alveoli and pulmonary capillaries fuse since they are in contact; hence, the three layers consist of the basement membrane of the alveoli, basement membrane of the pulmonary capillaries,

and a thin layer of cytoplasm (Cormack, 2001). However the membrane is very thin, ranging in thickness from 0.2 to 2.5 μm (Cormack, 2001).

Dispersed among the type I pneumocytes are the type II pneumocytes. These cells also have an epithelial covering, but they are distinguished from the type I pneumocytes by their rounded body shape and large nucleus. Within the type II pneumocytes are granules

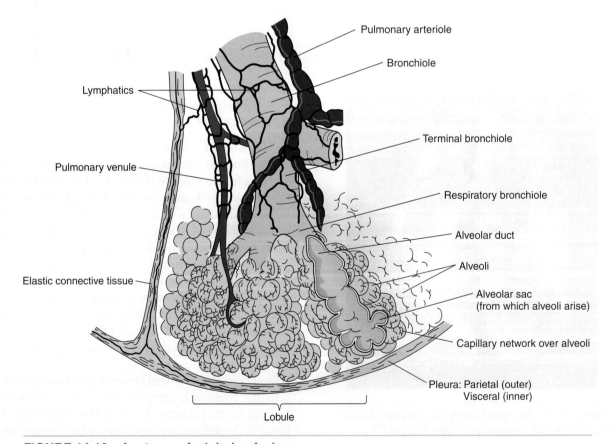

FIGURE 14-10 **Anatomy of a lobule of a lung**

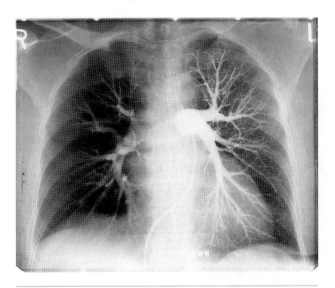

FIGURE 14-11   Pulmonary arteriogram

called lamellar bodies that contain phospholipids. The phospholipid is released to form a thin, filmy layer of fluid called **pulmonary surfactant**, which covers the alveoli to reduce the surface tension forces and aid in the expansion of the alveoli. See Box 14-3 for addi-

BOX 14-3
Pulmonary Surfactant

The alveoli are actually unstable and are comparable to bubbles in that they have a tendency to collapse during expiration due to the surface tension forces. In addition, the inside of each alveolus is lined with a thin layer of fluid, which is necessary for the diffusion of the gases since gas must dissolve in liquid in order to enter or exit a cell. But this fluid can cause the alveolus to stick together upon expiration.

The pulmonary surfactant, which is made up of phospholipids secreted by type II pneumocytes, prevents this collapse of the alveoli. Pulmonary surfactant is actually a mixture of phospholipids, carbohydrates, and proteins. The pulmonary surfactant decreases the alveolar surface tension forces, thereby preventing collapse and allowing inflation of the alveoli.

Pulmonary surfactant is highly essential to newborns. In the fetus, the lungs are filled with amniotic fluid. Upon birth, in order for an infant to starting taking their first breaths of air, pulmonary surfactant must be present to facilitate the expansion of the alveoli. Premature newborns often have undeveloped, immature type II pneumocytes at the time of delivery, which can result in a deficiency of pulmonary surfactant. The result of the deficiency can be respiratory distress syndrome (RDS), which is potentially fatal.

tional important information related to pulmonary surfactant.

Diaphragm

The **diaphragm** is a musculofibrous structure that separates the thoracic cavity from the abdominal cavity. It is elliptical and fan-shaped. It is connected to the anterior surface of the spine from the first to the fourth lumbar vertebrae. Coming off of this attachment are muscular extensions called the right and left crura, crura referring to a structure that resembles a leg. As with any muscle, the origin of the crura is tendons, which serve to attach the muscle to the vertebral bone. The two crura extend upward, forming arms that surround the openings of the aorta and esophagus and insert on the central tendon. If the crura must be approximated with sutures, they should always be placed through the tendinous portion (Skandalakis, Skandalakis, & Skandalakis, 2000).

As the name indicates, the central tendon is located in the central portion of the diaphragm immediately below the pericardium. It consists of three divisions called leaflets, which are separated by slight indentations in the diaphragm tissue. The right leaflet is the largest; the middle leaflet is next largest and is attached to the xiphoid process; and the left leaflet is the smallest.

The anterosuperior surface of the diaphragm is covered by parietal pleura on the right and left sides, and the serous layer of the pericardium covers the central portion (Skandalakis et al., 2000). The posterior surface of the diaphragm is covered by a portion of the peritoneal membrane that lines the abdominal cavity.

The anterior surface is convex on each side to accommodate the pleura and lungs, and slightly more flat in the center to aid in supporting the heart. The posterior surface is concave in order to match the convex surface of the liver.

The major openings in the diaphragm are as follows:

1. Aortic opening: It is the lowest and most posterior opening of the three large openings. In actuality, the course of the aorta takes it behind the diaphragm rather than directly through an opening (Skandalakis et al., 2000). The opening is situated in the midline of the diaphragm, directly anterior to the 12th thoracic vertebra. The aorta, thoracic duct, and azygos vein travel through the opening together.
2. Esophageal opening: The opening for the esophagus is elliptical, located in the muscular portion of

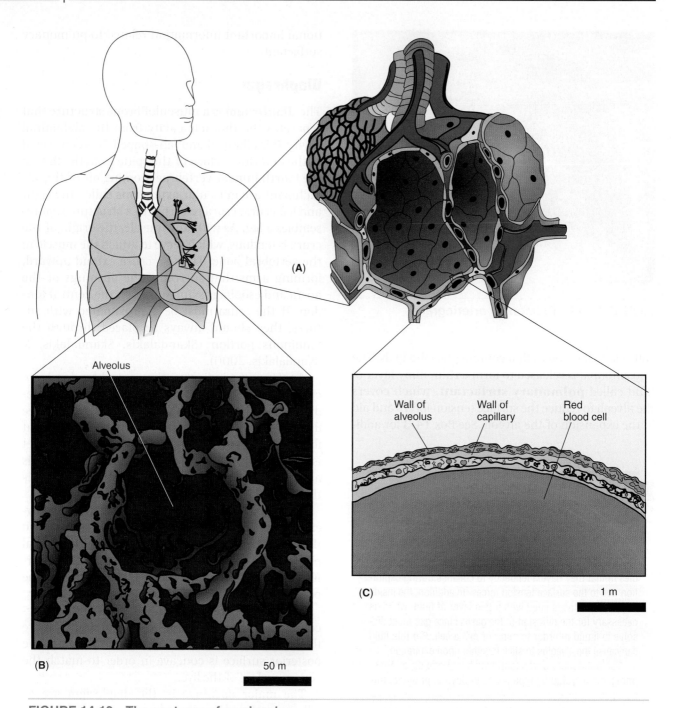

FIGURE 14-12   The anatomy of an alveolus

the diaphragm, and formed by the right and left crura. It is slightly superior to the aortic opening and a little to the left of the midline at the level of the 10th thoracic vertebrae. The esophagus, vagus nerve, esophageal arteries, and veins pass through the hiatus.

3. Inferior vena cava (IVC) opening: The opening for the IVC is slightly superior to the esophageal opening and situated to the right of the midline at the level of the eighth thoracic vertebrae. Its

location is also identifiable, since it is at the junction of the fibers of the right and middle leaflets. The IVC and branches of the right phrenic nerve pass through the hiatus (Skandalakis et al., 2000).

The blood supply to the diaphragm is as follows:

1. Superior surface: branches from the internal thoracic arteries and branches from the thoracic aorta.

2. Posterior surface: inferior phrenic arteries that branch from the aorta.
3. On the superior and posterior surfaces, the veins follow the course of the arteries.

The lymph nodes are located on the superior surface of the diaphragm. They receive drainage from the superior portion of the liver and junction of the esophagus with the stomach. The efferent lymph vessels drain from these nodes to the anterior and posterior mediastinal nodes. The right and left phrenic nerves innervate the diaphragm.

There are several structures located near the esophageal hiatus that the surgeon must be aware of when performing surgical procedures on the hiatus, such as a hiatal hernia repair. These anatomic structures include:

1. thoracic duct
2. lower portion of the esophagus
3. vagus nerve
4. inferior vena cava
5. aorta
6. left inferior phrenic artery and vein
7. left gastric artery and vein

Intercostal Muscles

The **intercostal muscles** are located between the ribs. They are divided into the external intercostal muscles and the internal intercostal muscles. They are the other set of muscles that act with the diaphragm muscle to produce the mechanics of breathing and are the primary structures responsible for the movement of the ribs during respiration.

The surface of the external intercostal muscles and inner surface of the internal intercostal muscles are covered by a thin, but strong layer of fascia called the intercostal fascia. The intercostal muscles are innervated by the intercostal nerves and its numerous branches. There are 11 external intercostal muscles attached to the margins of the ribs. The fibers travel in an oblique direction, downward and forward. The fibers are thicker than the internal intercostal muscle fibers.

There are also 11 internal intercostal muscles, which are located underneath the external intercostal muscles. However, their muscle fibers travel in an oblique fashion, downward and backward. This criss-cross pattern of the intercostal muscle fibers contributes to strength in breathing, in particular during exercise. The external intercostal muscles raise the ribs upward and outward to increase the capacity of the thoracic cavity, whereas the internal

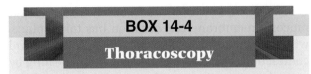

BOX 14-4

Thoracoscopy

Thoracoscopy is a minimally invasive surgical procedure that involves the use of a special scope called a thoracoscope, which is rigid. The thoracoscope is inserted into the thoracic cavity to view the pleura, mediastinal space, thoracic wall, lymph nodes, diaphragm, and pericardium. Special instruments can be inserted to obtain tissue biopsies of the lung(s), mediastinal lymph nodes, or pleura. A camera is attached to the scope so the surgeon can view the thoracic cavity on the monitor (TV screen). The procedure is performed in the operating room and the patient is placed under general anesthesia.

The patient is positioned on the OR table on the nonoperative side referred to as the lateral position. A small incision is made in the intercostal muscles between the sixth and seventh ribs. The thoracoscope is introduced through the incision into the thoracic cavity. Other small incisions may be made according to where biopsies need to be taken, such as between the third and fourth ribs and/or between the fifth and sixth ribs. At the end of the procedure, a chest tube is inserted and hooked up to a closed waterseal drainage system (see Box 14-6) and the incisions closed with suture.

intercostal muscles pull the ribs downward and inward.

Healing of the Respiratory Tract Structures

Healing of the tissues in the respiratory tract has not been well studied in the past. The healing of the trachea and lung have received more attention as compared to other tissues in the respiratory pathway, because of the surgical procedures like tracheostomy or lobectomy. However, the following discussion focuses in brief on the oral cavity, pharynx, trachea, and bronchus.

Oral Cavity

Wounds of the oral mucous membranes generally heal well without suturing. It is thought the slight antibacterial property of human saliva and a constant moist surface contribute to the healing process. When a mucous membrane defect occurs due to an injury, healing will most likely be by contraction or epithelization (Peacock, 1984). Redundant mucous membrane is located in the oral cavity, which contributes to the various jaw and tongue movements that are required for speaking and eating, but also allows healing by wound contraction.

When a wound heals, it can be falsely assumed that mucosal membrane regeneration has taken place, when in fact the surface has healed by wound contraction (Peacock, 1984). In addition, healing by wound contraction rarely causes abnormalities such as malocclusion or temporomandibular joint pathologies.

Even though redundant mucous membrane is located in most portions of the oral cavity, there are some areas where the tissue is attached to the periosteum, which does not allow much shifting of the tissue and therefore healing by wound contraction does not occur. In these areas, the mucous membranes heal by epithelization (Peacock, 1984). Epithelial regeneration will most often properly restore the surface, thus avoiding a skin graft procedure.

Surgical wounds of the oral cavity that penetrate to the surface, such as what occurs during excision of an intraoral tumor, tend to develop orocutaneous fistulas during the first phase of healing. There are two main reasons for the development of the fistula: one is improper approximation of the tissue and the second is the interruption of the blood supply due to the surgical procedure or preoperative radiation therapy of the tumor. It is recommended that a continuous suturing technique not be used in the mucous membrane of the oral cavity (Peacock, 1984). This technique interferes with the blood supply because of an inversion of the mucous membrane. The occurrence of fistulas is reduced by suturing the submucous tissues with interrupted absorbable suture, which results in the everting of the mucous membrane (Peacock, 1984). Next, the mucosal edges are approximated by continuous suture technique.

Pharynx

An important wound healing characteristic of the pharynx is the flexibility of the mucous membrane and its ability to be stretched (Peacock, 1984). Due to this characteristic, a large portion of the pharyngeal mucous membrane can be excised when removing a particularly invasive tumor, leaving enough mucosa to surround a feeding tube. In approximately six weeks postoperatively, the patient's pharyngeal opening will be large enough to permit speaking and swallowing (Peacock, 1984), evidence that tissues need not be transplanted to the area to promote healing of the pharynx if there is enough mucous membrane remaining to enclose a feeding tube.

Trachea

If the trachea loses the ciliated epithelium and underlying tissues, it attempts to heal with scar tissue and epithelium that does not represent the original tissue or is otherwise poorly differentiated. The patient is prone to respiratory complications and infections since the loss of the cilia, which are responsible for the removal of inhaled dust and debris. If an attempt is made to replace the previous normal tissue with an artificial prostheses or it is replaced by scar tissue, cells grow over the surface but will not differentiate into the original ciliated epithelium. This argues for the approximation of the tracheal tissue with suture to allow the regeneration of the ciliated epithelium.

There are two complications in the wound healing of the trachea. The first is the postoperative formation of granulation tissue in the subglottic region following a tracheostomy (Peacock, 1984). If the tracheostomy is not permanent, the presence of the granulation tissue makes it difficult to close. The second is stenosis, caused by wound contraction (Peacock, 1984). The anastomosis of the trachea, in particular if a section has been excised, without tension on the suture, is the primary factor in the prevention of stenosis.

Bronchus, Lung, and Sutures

Regeneration of the bronchial epithelium is comparable in importance to the regeneration of the tracheal epithelium. An example of the importance of the role of epithelium occurs during a lung transplantation procedure. When the donor lung is transplanted two problems occur. First, due to the nature of the surgical procedure, denervation causes the mucus-forming cells in the bronchial epithelium to cease activity; however, the ciliary movement is not affected. Second, at the site of the bronchial anastomosis there is a small area of denuded connective tissue that acts as a barrier to the sweeping forward of bacteria and debris (Peacock, 1984). Consequently, bacterial infections are a major concern with lung transplants.

When a lobectomy or pneumonectomy (removal of a lobe of the lung or removal of the entire lung, respectively) is performed, the bronchial stump closure is of primary concern. Poor suturing technique to approximate the stump or leaving too long of a stump is conducive to the formation of a bronchopleural fistula (Ethicon, 2002). The stump must be tightly closed with interrupted sutures that are placed close together to prevent the escape of air into the thoracic cavity. In addition, the bronchial stump heals slowly, so the preservation of the blood supply to the area of the closure is critical (Ethicon, 2002).

Sutures of choice in the respiratory tract include polypropylene monofilament, since they are less prone to causing tissue reaction, and silk suture. Absorbable sutures are not used, since they will lose their tensile strength, thus permitting air leakage. Nylon suture is not used due to the poor knot-holding characteristic of the suture. More commonly, rather than using suture to close the stump, stapling devices are used, since they achieve maximal, long-term closure with little tissue reaction and small chance of air leakage.

INHALATION AND EXHALATION

Inhalation and exhalation are also called inspiration and expiration, respectively (Figure 14-13). The act of breathing involves the structures of the respiratory tract that have been discussed, the respiratory centers

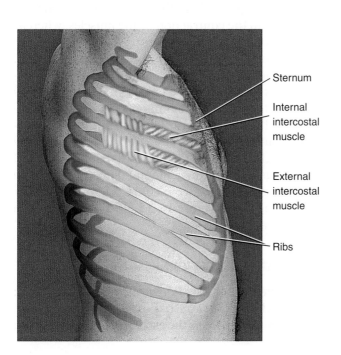

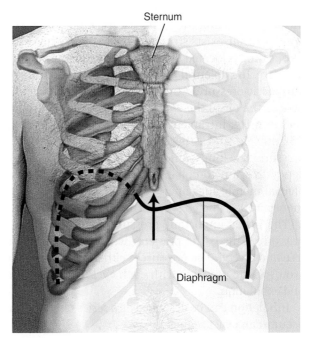

A

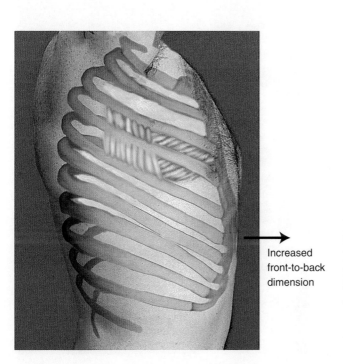

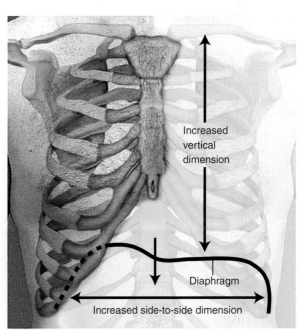

FIGURE 14-13   Thoracic changes during respiration: (A) Expiration, (B) inspiration

of the brain, chemical regulation, and the transport of gases.

Inhalation

Before the sequence of inhalation and exhalation is discussed, the role of the serous fluid between the pleural membranes in relation to pressures must be understood. The serous fluid aids in the adherence of the parietal membrane to the visceral membrane. The pressure that exists in the pleural space where the serous fluid is located is referred to as the intrapleural pressure. Intrapleural pressure is a little less than atmospheric pressure. Atmospheric pressure is the pressure of the air in the environment and at sea level is 760 mm Hg; intrapleural pressure is approximately 756 mm Hg, and is therefore referred to as a negative pressure. The lungs, much like the alveoli, have a tendency to want to collapse, thereby pulling the two pleural membranes apart. The serous fluid prevents the separation and preserves the intrapleural pressure.

The other important pressure is intrapulmonic pressure. This is the pressure within the bronchial tree and alveoli. The pressure is either above or below atmospheric pressure with each cycle of inhalation and exhalation.

Inhalation can be described as a series of steps that occur in an exact sequence:

1. Motor impulses travel from the medulla via the phrenic nerve to the diaphragm and intercostal nerves to the intercostal muscles.
2. The nerve impulses cause the diaphragm to move downward, thereby expanding the thoracic cavity in superior and inferior directions.
3. The intercostal muscles are stimulated to perform the actions as described previously.
4. As the thoracic cavity expands so does the parietal pleura, causing the intrapleural pressure to become increasingly negative. However, as previously mentioned, the serous fluid binds the two pleural membranes allowing the visceral pleura to expand, which then allows the lungs to expand.
5. With the expansion of the lungs, the intrapulmonic pressure decreases below atmospheric pressure, and air enters the nose cavity to travel through the respiratory tract into the alveoli. The air continues to enter until the intrapulmonic pressure equals the atmospheric pressure.

Exhalation

1. Exhalation begins when the motor impulses from the medulla cease.

2. The diaphragm and intercostal muscles relax.
3. As the thoracic cavity returns to normal size, the lungs and alveoli are compressed.
4. The intrapulmonic pressure increases above atmospheric pressure as the air is forced out of the lungs until both pressures are once again equal.

It should be pointed out that inhalation requires energy due to the contraction of the muscles, whereas exhalation is a passive process that releases the air to the atmosphere. However, in instances of singing, playing an instrument such as the trumpet, or blowing out the candles on a cake, exhalation becomes an activity that requires energy due to the contraction of the intercostal muscles. In particular, the internal intercostal muscles are more involved by pulling the ribs down and inward to force air out of the lungs. In addition, abdominal muscles push the diaphragm upward, which aids in forcing more air out of the lungs. Figure 14-14 illustrates the course of respiration.

Exchange of Oxygen and Carbon Dioxide

The exchange of gases is divided into two categories: **internal respiration** and **external respiration**. External respiration is the exchange of gases between

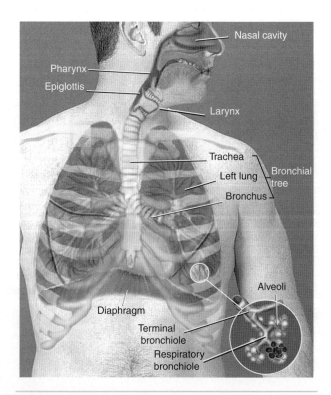

FIGURE 14-14 Pathway of respiration

the air that has been inhaled into the alveoli and the blood in the pulmonary capillaries. Internal respiration refers to the exchange of gases between the systemic capillaries and the tissue cells of the body.

Air that is inhaled contains approximately 21% oxygen and 0.04% carbon dioxide. The exhaled air contains approximately 15% oxygen and 5% carbon dioxide. These numbers display the importance of the retention of oxygen by the body and the ability to rid the body of carbon dioxide.

A basic physiologic principle is that the gas within the body diffuses from an area of greater concentration to an area of lesser concentration, which only makes sense; it is comparable to a roomful of people who are crowded together wherein individuals will seek a room with less people. The concentration of a gas in a particular area of the body such as the alveoli, pulmonary blood, and arterial blood is stated as a value called partial pressure. Partial pressure is measured in millimeters of mercury (mm Hg). It is the pressure exerted by any type of gas that is in a mixture of gases or in a liquid, and is related to the concentration of that gas to the total pressure of the mixture. The initial P is used to designate partial pressure.

Partial pressure is calculated using the following mathematical equation: percentage of the gas in a mixture $\times$ total pressure = P. For example, the concentration of oxygen in the atmosphere is approximately 21% of the total atmospheric pressure and the atmospheric pressure is 760 mm Hg. Using the math formula: $0.21 \times 760 = 160$ mm Hg. Table 14-1 lists the partial pressures of oxygen and carbon dioxide in various parts of the body.

The principle previously stated in which gas diffuses from an area of higher concentration to an area of lower concentration can now be better understood by the following examples based on the values provided in Table 14-1:

1. The inhaled air in the alveoli has a high PO_2 and low PCO_2. This is logical, since the inhaled air, as previously mentioned, is 21% oxygen. The blood in the pulmonary capillaries (venous blood) will be opposite: low PO_2 and high PCO_2.

TABLE 14-1	Partial Pressures	
BODY SITE	PO$_2$ (mm Hg)	PCO$_2$ (mm Hg)
Atmosphere	160	0.15
Air in alveoli	104	40
Venous blood	40	40–45
Arterial blood	95–100	35–45
Body cells	40	50

Thus, during external respiration, oxygen diffuses from the alveoli to the blood, and carbon dioxide diffuses from the blood to the alveoli. The blood that is high in PO_2 returns to the heart to be pumped out by the left ventricle into the aorta and throughout the circulation of the body.

2. Arterial blood has a high PO_2 and low PCO_2. The body cells, due to the use of oxygen during cellular respiration, produce carbon dioxide during this process. Therefore, the body cells have a low PO_2 and high PCO_2. During internal respiration, the oxygen diffuses from the blood to the body cells and carbon dioxide diffuses from the body cells to the blood. Now the venous blood has a low PO_2 and high PCO_2, which the right ventricle of the heart pumps to the lungs to be reoxygenated during external respiration.

Circulatory Transport of Gases

Oxygen is able to bind to the red blood cells (RBCs) or erythrocytes in the circulatory system because of iron that is located in the hemoglobin of the cells. The bond between oxygen and hemoglobin develops in the lungs, where the PO_2 level is high. The bond is not a strong one and, as the blood circulates through the tissues that have a low PO_2 the bond breaks, releasing the oxygen to the tissues. During exercise, tissues such as the muscles will need oxygen; consequently, the lower the oxygen concentration in a tissue, the more hemoglobin will be released.

The majority of carbon dioxide (CO_2) is transported in the plasma; however, it is in the form of bicarbonate ions (HCO_3^-). Carbon dioxide enters the bloodstream and diffuses into the RBCs. The RBCs contain the enzyme carbonic anhydrase, which catalyzes the reaction of CO_2 and water to form carbonic acid (H_2CO_3). The carbonic acid then breaks apart: $H_2CO_3 \rightarrow H^+ + HCO_3^-$. The bicarbonate ions diffuse from the RBCs into the plasma and the hydrogen ions stay in the RBCs. It could be assumed the hydrogen ions would make the RBCs too acidic and cause acidosis; however, the hemoglobin prevents this from happening. An ionic equilibrium is maintained by what is called the chloride shift, wherein chloride ions enter the plasma from the RBCs. The CO_2 can now travel to the lungs because the HCO_3^- entered the plasma. The bloodstream travels to the lungs, which have a low PCO_2, and the above-described reactions are reversed to re-form CO_2, which diffuses into the alveoli to be exhaled.

BOX 14-5

Pulse Oximeter

Pulse oximetry is the noninvasive, continuous measurement of the hemoglobin saturation level in the arterial blood, or simply put, the oxygen level in the circulating arterial blood. It can warn of hypoxemia and improve the outcome of the surgical patient by avoiding hypoxic episodes. Many studies have demonstrated the occurrence of unexpected hypoxemia when a surgical patient is sedated for local anesthesia procedures and postoperatively after waking from general anesthesia. Introduced in the 1980s, pulse oximetry was immediately adopted by all hospitals in the United States and is now a standard of practice.

A small clip is placed on the index finger, large toe, or earlobe. The clip works by passing a light through the tissues to determine the optical density of the blood. It measures the level of oxygen saturation in the arterial blood in percentages; the normal value is 95%–97%. If the patient falls below a certain percentage, usually 90%, an alarm goes off on the pulse oximeter device. The patient will be instructed to take deep breaths to raise the saturation level or 100% oxygen is administered through a mask or nasal cannula.

Nervous System

The nervous system regulation of respiration is located in the medulla and pons, which are portions of the brainstem (Figure 14-15). The medulla is responsible for inspiration and expiration. Within the medulla is the **inspiration center**, rhythmic impulses are produced that travel along nerve routes to the respiratory muscles to stimulate contraction, thereby causing inhalation. To prevent the overextension of the lungs, a reflex called the Hering–Breuer reflex takes place. When an individual inhales, stretch receptors within the bronchi and bronchioles send impulses that travel via afferent fibers of the vagus nerve to the respiratory centers of the medulla and travel back by motor neurons to the respiratory muscles of the thorax. The inflation reflex stops inspiration, stimulates expiration, and prevents overdistension of the alveoli.

As mentioned, stimulation to the inspiration center decreases, the **expiration center** is stimulated causing the respiratory muscles to relax, and exhalation is the result. The stimulation to the inspiration center then begins, causing another cycle of breathing.

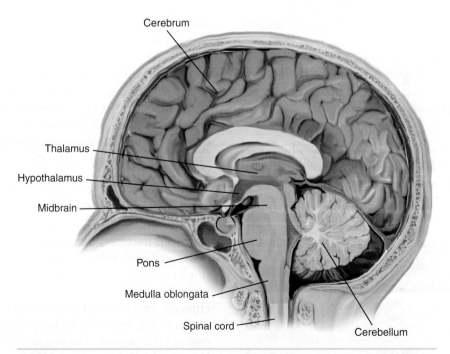

Cerebrum

Thalamus

Hypothalamus

Midbrain

Pons

Medulla oblongata

Spinal cord

Cerebellum

FIGURE 14-15 **Cross section of the brain – the medulla oblongata is the respiratory center**

The pons is responsible for regulating the normal rhythm of breathing. The two centers in the pons are the apneustic center and pneumotaxic center. The apneustic center is a collection of nerve tissue in the posterior portion of the pons that controls the inspiratory rate of respiration. Impulses from the pneumotaxic center interrupt the signals to the apneustic center to aid in exhalation.

Breathing and Blood pH Level

Breathing effects the level of pH in the bloodstream as well as the oxygen and carbon dioxide levels. Chemoreceptors are located in the medulla, aortic bodies, and carotids to detect changes in the pH and blood gas levels. The chemoreceptors in the carotids and aortic bodies detect a decrease in the level of oxygen in the bloodstream. The nerve impulses from the chemoreceptors travel along the vagus and glossopharyngeal nerves to the medulla, which is stimulated to increase the rate and depth of respiration. Consequently, the individual inhales more air into the lungs to deliver more oxygen, which is diffused into the bloodstream for delivery to the tissues of the body.

When an excess of carbon dioxide is present in the bloodstream, the pH is lowered thus making the blood more acidic. The chemoreceptors in the medulla detect changes in pH, in particular decreases leading to acidosis. The medulla is stimulated to increase respirations in order to increase the exhalation of carbon dioxide and bring the level of pH back to the normal.

LUNG CAPACITIES

The capacity of the lungs is measured by various volumes that aid in diagnosing respiratory pathologies and determining if an individual is experiencing the diminished ability for full-capacity breathing that requires treatment. Pathologies such as edema, pneumonia, emphysema, lung cancer, fibrosis, and atelectasis all affect proper respirations. The following are descriptions of the most common pulmonary volumes:

- Tidal volume (TV): The amount of air that is inhaled and exhaled during a normal respiration. The average tidal volume is 500 ml.
- Minute ventilation: The total amount of air inhaled and exhaled in one minute. It is calculate by multiplying tidal volume by respiratory rate. The respiratory rate averages 12 to 20 breaths per minute for the adult. Since the TV is 500 ml,

the minute ventilation is $500 \times 12 = 6,000$ ml or 6 liters of air per minute.
- Inspiratory reserve volume (IRV): The maximum volume of air that can be inhaled beyond the tidal volume. The IRV ranges from 2,000 to 3,000 ml.
- Expiratory reserve volume (ERV): The maximum volume of air that can be exhaled beyond normal exhalation. Normal ERV is 1,000–1,500 ml.
- Vital capacity (VC): The measurement of the amount of air that can be exhaled at the normal rate of exhalation after maximum inhalation; it provides information on the maximum possible breathing capacity. VC is obtained by adding IRV + TV + ERV. VC averages 4,000–5,000 ml.
- Residual volume (RV): The amount of air that remains in the lungs after a maximum expiration. RV averages 1,000–1,500 ml.
- Total lung capacity: Measurement of lung capacity at the end of maximum inhalation. It is obtained by adding functional residual capacity and inspiratory capacity.
- Forced expiratory volume (FEV): The volume of air that can be forcibly exhaled during a set time period such as 30 seconds after a full inhalation.

BREATHING ABNORMALITIES

There are several pathologies that affect the respiratory system and have an effect on the surgical patient. The following are pathologies that illustrate the difficulties the surgical team can encounter when caring for patients with respiratory disorders.

Pulmonary Edema

Pulmonary edema is the accumulation of fluid in the extravascular spaces or alveoli of the lungs. Pulmonary edema is often the consequence of cardiac disorders such as congestive heart failure in which the left ventricle is not working to its fullest capacity. The left ventricle does not pump strongly enough; therefore, the chamber does not fully empty and does not allow the left atrium to pump all of the blood from that chamber into the ventricle. The result is the retrograde flow of blood in the pulmonary veins and capillaries. The blood pressure in the capillaries increases and forces tissue fluid to collect in the extravascular spaces and alveoli of the lungs. Diagnosis of pulmonary edema is obtained by arterial blood gas analysis that shows hypoxia, and respiratory alkalosis and/or acidosis often occurs. Treatment is as follows:

1. Administration of 100% oxygen by face mask or assisted ventilation
2. Diuretic drugs such as furosemide that promote diuresis to aid in ridding the body of excess fluid
3. Drug therapy for treatment of the cardiac disorder

Pneumothorax

Pneumothorax is the abnormal accumulation of air between the parietal and visceral pleura causing the affected lung to collapse. Recall that the intrapleural pressure is below atmospheric pressure. Air that enters the pleural cavity at atmospheric pressure causes the lung to collapse due to the sudden increase in higher pressure.

Spontaneous pneumothorax does not occur due to trauma, but it is often the result of lung diseases such as emphysema. Emphysema weakens the alveoli, leading to their collapse and thus the collapse of the lung.

Traumatic pneumothorax is due to penetrating injuries, such as a knife wound or gunshot wound (GSW). Often the injury is accompanied by the accumulation of blood, and is then referred to as a **hemopneumothorax**. A serious consequence of traumatic pneumothorax is **tension pneumothorax**. When air enters the pleural space it can be trapped and each inhalation traps more air in the pleural space, resulting in positive pleural pressure. This causes the lung to collapse, impair the venous return, and push the heart, great vessels, trachea, and esophagus to the opposite side of the chest, referred to as mediastinal shift. This is a severe life-threatening situation that requires immediate treatment including the insertion of chest tubes and possibly surgery.

Pneumonia

Pneumonia is an acute infection of the lungs that impairs the exchange of gases. The prognosis is most often good for healthy individuals, but for the elderly or individuals who have preexisting conditions, especially respiratory conditions, it can be a life-threatening event.

Pneumonia can be viral or bacterial in origin, but most commonly is caused by *Streptococcus pneumoniae*. Primary pneumonia is the result of inhaling or aspirating the pathogen. The distal airways are involved including the alveoli. Lobar pneumonia is a term used to describe the involvement of an entire lobe of the lung. The bacteria establish within the alveoli and fluid accumulates. Neutrophils migrate to the site of infection to phagocytize the bacteria. Consequently, the alveoli become filled with fluid, bacterial cells, and neutrophils and the exchange of gases is inhibited. Treatment includes antimicrobial drugs such as penicillin G or erythromycin, oxygen, and adequate fluid intake.

Chronic Obstructive Pulmonary Disease

Chronic obstructive pulmonary disease (COPD) is a chronic airway obstruction that occurs secondary to emphysema, asthma, chronic bronchitis, or other respiratory disease, and is usually caused by a combination of disorders. COPD is a common disorder that

---

BOX 14-6

Chest Tubes

Pneumothorax most often requires the placement of chest tubes. Chest tubes are also inserted following a cardiothoracic surgical procedure. The purpose of the tubes is to evacuate air and fluid from the pleural space. When two tubes are used, one is placed in the upper portion of the thoracic cavity to facilitate the evacuation of air; the second is placed posterior to the first tube to facilitate the evacuation of fluids. This arrangement makes sense because air is lighter than fluids. The chest tubes are secured to the skin with suture and connected to the closed water-seal drainage system.

The chest tube is inserted through the intercostal space. A small incision is made and a large clamp is forced through the opening into the pleural space. The clamp is opened to widen the incision and then withdrawn. The chest tube is placed through this opening. It is connected to the "Pleur-evac" system, the three-container closed water-seal drainage system. Fluid from the patient drains through the chest tube into the first collection container, which is connected to the second water-seal container to prevent air from reentering the pleural space and maintains the negative pressure within the thoracic cavity to prevent the lung from collapsing. The third container is the suction chamber, which further aids in the evacuation of air and fluid from the thoracic cavity. The drainage system must be placed below the level of the thoracic cavity to promote the evacuation of air and fluids by gravity and prevent reflux.

must be addressed by the surgical team, in particular the anesthesia provider. The number one predisposing factor to the development of COPD is cigarette smoking. Smoking impairs the movement of the cilia in the respiratory passages and causes inflammation of the airways. The primary sign and symptom is inability to perform strenuous work or exercise, which gradually worsens as the disease progresses and dyspnea becomes the most common sign. Treatment includes stopping smoking, drug therapy, breathing and coughing exercises, regular exercise such as walking if possible, and oxygen therapy if necessary. For severely affected patients, lung volume reduction surgery may be performed to remove the nonfunctioning portion of the lung, which allows the functional portion of the lung tissue to expand and allows the diaphragm to return to its normal anatomic position.

Emphysema

Emphysema often occurs in conjunction with COPD. It is an abnormal, irreversible enlargement of the alveoli due to destruction of the alveolar walls, resulting in decreased elastic recoil of the alveoli. Again, the number one cause of emphysema is cigarette smoking. The irritants in the cigarette smoke damage the alveolar walls and break down the elasticity of the connective tissue that surrounds the alveoli. Macrophages migrate to the affected area and produce an enzyme that further damages the elastin. The body is reacting to the damaged tissue by sending the macrophages and thinks it is helping by getting rid of the tissue, when in actuality it is working against itself.

As emphysema progresses, the permanently damaged lung tissue is replaced by scar tissue, which is fibrous, nonelastic connective tissue that further inhibits the efficient exchange of gases. The oxygen level in the bloodstream decreases and the carbon dioxide level increases, causing the pH level to decrease, which leads to respiratory acidosis.

The common sign of emphysema is that the individual must work to exhale. Because of the loss of alveolar elasticity, which makes normal exhalations an easy, passive process, the person must now work to exhale in order to make room for air when inhaling. The affected individual becomes easily tired from having to constantly work to exhale. Treatment involves continous oxygen therapy at a low-flow setting to avoid hypoxia, and breathing exercises. Lung volume reduction surgery has seen limited use in individuals with emphysema.

IMPLICATIONS FOR THE SURGICAL TECHNOLOGIST

Thoracic surgery involves some of the more complicated procedures that challenge the skills of the surgical technologist and other team members. As evidenced by the information in this chapter, breathing is absolutely vital to all of the processes of the body. Preserving that function is a necessity and speaks to one of the several basic physiologic needs of the individual. Surgery is often performed to preserve the individual's ability to properly breathe. Procedures often performed include:

- thoracotomy
- thoracoscopy
- bronchoscopy
- wedge resection
- lobectomy
- pneumonectomy with or without lung transplantation

To properly assist the surgeon during these types of procedures the surgical technologist must know the anatomy and physiology of the respiratory tract, lungs, and entire thoracic cavity, including the great vessels and heart. Having this knowledge helps the surgical technologist to:

1. Choose the correct instruments and supplies that are specifically developed for thoracic surgery.
2. Aid the surgeon in identifying the anatomy of the thoracic cavity.
3. Correctly orient the endoscope during a thoracoscopy.
4. Understand the pathology and how it affects the tissues of the thoracic cavity, which contributes to decisions related to instrumentation, supplies, and perioperative patient care.
5. Be able to quickly react during emergency thoracic procedures or emergency situations that may arise during thoracic surgery. This includes aiding the surgical team in anticipating and recognizing emergency situations.

Case Study 2

Nancy and the surgical team are finished with the surgical procedure on the patient with epiglottitis. However, the anesthesia provider's pager signals to call the emergency department stat. A 13-year-old patient has been admitted to the ER with possible foreign-body obstruction of the airway that has caused atelectasis of the right lung. The patient is being immediately transported to the surgery department for treatment.

1. Define atelectasis.

2. What other respiratory complications can occur due to atelectasis?

3. What surgical procedure will be performed to treat atelectasis in this patient?

CHAPTER SUMMARY

- Inhaling and exhaling facilitate the process of taking in oxygen and getting rid of the waste carbon dioxide. The process is referred to as respiration.

- The four terms that apply to the overall chapter are ventilation, external respiration, internal respiration, and cellular respiration.

- The upper respiratory tract includes the nose, nasal cavity, pharynx, and sinuses.

- The lower respiratory tract includes the larynx, trachea, bronchi, lungs, internal lung structures, and ancillary structures.

- The nose is covered by skin and supported by bone and cartilage. Air enters through the external nares and coarse hairs line the internal part of the nares to act as filters.

- The two nasal cavities are separated by the nasal septum, which is made up of the vomer and ethmoid bones. The lining of the cavities is ciliated epithelium called the nasal mucosa. The nasal cavity is highly vascular due to the lamina propria, thus the incoming air is warmed.

- The nasal conchae, or turbinates, are curved, scroll-like bones that project medially from the lateral wall of each nasal cavity. The three conchae are the superior, middle, and inferior turbinates.

- The olfactory area that contains the olfactory organ is located in the superior portion of each nasal cavity. Within each organ are the olfactory receptor cells, which detect smells.

- There are four paranasal sinuses: maxillae, frontal, sphenoid, and ethmoid. The names provide their location, since they are located within the bone of the same name. The sinuses move mucus into the nasal cavities by the movement of ciliated epithelium and make the skull lighter in weight.

- The pharynx is a tubular structure that is posterior to the oral and nasal cavities, extending from the base of the skull and situated anterior to the cervical vertebrae. It serves the dual function of conducting air and food. It is divided into three sections: nasopharynx, oropharynx, and laryngopharynx. The pharynx is composed of muscle and lined with mucous membrane.

- The larynx, or voice box, contains the vocal cords. It connects the pharynx to the trachea and serves as part of the air passageway. It is lined by mucous membrane and lined with ciliated columnar epithelium.

- The larynx is composed of three single and three paired cartilages to provide flexibility, but prevent the larynx from collapsing. The single cartilages are thyroid, cricoid, and epiglottic. The paired cartilages are: arytenoid, corniculate, and cuneiform.

- The thyroid cartilage is also referred to as the Adam's apple. During swallowing, the larynx elevates and the epiglottis closes over the opening of the larynx to prevent food from entering.

- The vocal cords are composed of elastin fibers and are centrally located in the larynx on either side of the glottis, the opening between the cords. During breathing, the vocal cords close over the glottis; during speaking, the intrinsic muscles of the larynx stretch the vocal cords over the glottis and exhaled air vibrates the vocal cords to produce speech.

- The motor nerves that are important to the production of the voice include: the vagus nerve, superior laryngeal nerve, and recurrent laryngeal nerve.

- Sellick's maneuver or cricoid pressure is performed to prevent aspiration by a patient undergoing general anesthesia. Slight external pressure is manually produced by placing thumb and forefinger on the cricoid cartilage.

- The trachea, or windpipe, extends from the larynx to where it bifurcates into the two bronchi. The anterior surface is covered by the isthmus of the thyroid gland and posteriorly is in contact with the esophagus.

- The trachea is composed of 20 C-shaped rings of hyaline cartilage that are flexible and keep the trachea continuously open.

- Within the mediastinal space, the trachea bifurcates into the primary bronchi that enter the lung at the hilum and further divide within the lungs; this is referred to as the bronchial tree.

- The sequence of division is: trachea, two primary bronchi, secondary branches, segmental or tertiary bronchi, bronchioles, terminal bronchioles, alveolar ducts, and alveoli.

- The functions of the bronchi are the same as that of the trachea and are lined with respiratory epithelium.

- Bronchioles have a different structure in that they consist of simple epithelium and lack cilia, goblet cells, and cartilage in their wall. The walls of the bronchioles contain smooth muscle bundles to regulate the diameter of the bronchiole lumen.

- The respiratory bronchioles represent the first structures in which the exchange of gases occur. The respiratory bronchioles terminate in branches that divide into the alveolar ducts and surrounding each duct are the grapelike clusters of alveoli.

- The pleural cavity contains the lungs and pleural membranes. The pleural membranes are divided into the parietal pleura and visceral pleura and the space between the two membranes is called the pleural space, which contains serous fluid.

- The lungs are composed of a spongy, elastic tissue. The right lung has three lobes and the left lung two lobes. The lungs are conical in shape; the base is concave and rests on the convex surface of the diaphragm. The layers of the lung are the external visceral pleura, subserous layer of areolar tissue, and parenchyma.

- Arterial blood supply to the lungs are the bronchial arteries that branch from the thoracic aorta. The blood supply from the bronchial arteries returns to the left atrium of the heart via the pulmonary veins.

- The lymphatics of the lungs and trachea are: bronchial glands, superficial lymphatics, deep lymphatics, and efferent lymphatic vessels.

- The alveoli are the primary functional unit of the respiratory system and are responsible for the exchange of gases.

- The covering of the alveolar walls are squamous epithelial cells called type I pneumocytes. Each alveolus is surrounded by pulmonary capillaries that consist of a single layer of endothelial cells.

- The alveolar–capillary barrier has three layers between the air in the alveoli and and the blood in the pulmonary capillaries.

- Type II pneumocytes are round in shape and have a large nucleus. They contain lamellar bodies, which in turn contain phospholipids that release the fluid called pulmonary surfactant.

- The diaphragm separates the thoracic cavity from the abdominal cavity. It is divided into the muscular extensions called crura and central tendon. The central tendon is subdivided into three divisions called leaflets.

- The major openings in the diaphragm include: aortic, esophageal, and inferior vena cava.

- The blood is supplied to the diaphragm from branches of the internal thoracic arteries and branches of the thoracic aorta, inferior phrenic arteries, and the veins that follow the course of the arteries.

- Lymph nodes of the diaphragm are located on the superior surface and receive drainage from the liver and esophagogastric junction.

- The phrenic nerves innervate the diaphragm.

- There are several anatomic structures located near the esophageal hiatus that must be identified during surgical procedures on the hiatus, including the thoracic duct, esophagus, vagus nerve, inferior vena cava, aorta, inferior phrenic artery and vein, and gastric artery and vein.

- The intercostal muscles are located between the ribs and are divided into the external intercostal muscles and internal intercostal muscles. The surface of the muscles is covered by intercostal fascia. The intercostal nerves innervate the muscles. They are the primary structures responsible for the movement of the ribs during respiration.

- The external intercostal muscles raise the ribs upward and outward and the internal intercostal muscles pull the ribs downward and inward.

- The oral mucous membrane tends to heal well without suturing. Healing is by either contraction or epithelization.

- If the oral mucous membrane must be sutured, an interrupted absorbable suture should be used to prevent interference with the blood supply.

- An important healing characteristic of the pharynx is the flexibility of the mucous membrane and ability to be stretched, allowing a large portion of the mucous membrane to be excised while leaving enough mucosa to surround a feeding tube. This prevents having to transplant tissue to the area.

- Wounds to the trachea attempt to heal with scar tissue and epithelium, and due to the loss of the cilia, the patient is prone to respiratory complications and infections. This supports the approximation of the wound with suture to allow for the regeneration of ciliated epithelium.

- There are two complications associated with wound healing of the trachea: postoperative formation of granulation tissue following a tracheostomy and stenosis caused by wound contraction.

- Two complications occur during lung transplantations: denervation causes the mucus-forming cells to cease activity, and at the site of anastomosis is a small denuded area of connective tissue, which presents a barrier to the sweeping forward of bacteria.

- The closure of the bronchial stump is of primary concern to avoid the formation of a bronchopleural fistula. Interrupted sutures must be placed close together to prevent the escape of air into the thoracic cavity, and the preservation of the blood supply is critical.

- Silk suture and polypropylene monofilament suture are commonly used for closure of the bronchial stump. Stapling devices are even more common.

- The serous fluid between the pleural membranes aids in adhering the parietal membrane to the visceral membrane. The serous fluid prevents the separation of the two membranes, thereby preserving the intrapleural pressure.

- The other important pressure is the intrapulmonic pressure.

- Inhalation requires energy and exhalation is a passive process, except in instances of activities like playing a wind instrument or blowing out candles.

- The exchange of gases is divided into internal respiration and external respiration.

- Partial pressure is the concentration of a gas in a particular portion of the body. It is the pressure exerted by any type of gas in a mixture of gases or in a liquid and is related to the concentration of that gas to the total pressure of the mixture. It is calculated as follows: percentage of the gas in a mixture $\times$ total pressure = P.

- During external respiration, O_2 diffuses from the alveoli to the blood, and CO_2 diffuses from the blood to the alveoli. The blood that is high in O_2 returns to the heart to be pumped out by the left ventricle via the aorta to the rest of the body.

- During internal respiration, the O_2 diffuses from the blood to the body cells and CO_2 diffuses from the body cells to the blood. The venous blood that is low in O_2 returns to the right ventricle to be pumped to the lungs for reoxygenation.

- Oxygen binds to the iron that is located in the hemoglobin of the RBCs. The bond is weak and as the blood circulates through the tissues that are low on oxygen the bond breaks, thereby releasing the oxygen to the tissues.

- Carbon dioxide is transported in the form of bicarbonate ions in the plasma. The carbon dioxide enters the RBCS and is broken down into carbonic acid. The carbonic acid is broken apart and the bicarbonate ions diffuse from the RBCs into the plasma. Chloride shift takes place to maintain ionic equilibrium. The carbon dioxide travels to the lungs, since the bicarbonate ions entered the plasma, and within the lungs the reaction is reversed to re-form carbon dioxide, which diffuses into the alveoli to be exhaled.

- The nervous system regulation of the respiratory system is located in the medulla and pons. The medulla is responsible for inspiration and expiration. It has two centers: the inspiration center and the expiration center. To prevent the overdistension of the alveoli and lungs the Hering–Breuer reflex takes place.

- The pons is responsible for regulating the normal rhythm of breathing. It has two centers: the apneustic center and the pneumotaxic center.

- Breathing aids in maintaining the pH level in the bloodstream. Chemoreceptors located in the medulla, aortic bodies, and carotid bodies detect changes in the pH and blood gas levels. The chemoreceptors in the aortic and carotid bodies detect changes in the level of oxygen in the bloodstream. The chemoreceptors in the medulla detect changes in the pH level.

- The capacity of the lungs is measured through the use of various volumes that aid in determining if the individual is experiencing any diminished respiratory values.

- Common pulmonary volumes include: tidal volume, minute ventilation, inspiratory reserve volume, expiratory reserve volume, vital capacity, residual volume, total lung capacity, and forced expiratory volume.

- Pulmonary edema is the abnormal accumulation of fluid in the extravascular spaces or alveoli of the lungs. It is often a secondary disorder to a primary cardiac disorder such as congestive heart failure.

- Pneumothorax is the abnormal accumulation of air between the parietal and visceral pleura causing the affected lung to collapse. Spontaneous pneumothorax is the result of lung diseases such as emphysema. Traumatic pneumothorax is due to traumatic penetrating injuries. If blood also accumulates, the injury is called a hemopneumothorax. A serious complication is tension pneumothorax, which can lead to mediastinal shift.

- Pneumonia is an acute infection of the lungs and is most often caused by a bacterium. Due to the accumulation of bacteria, fluid, and neutrophils in the alveoli, the alveoli become filled and the exchange of gases is inhibited.

- COPD is a chronic airway obstruction that occurs secondary to emphysema, asthma, or other respiratory disorders. The number one predisposing factor for the development of COPD is cigarette smoking. The primary sign is the inability to perform strenuous work or exercise, which worsens as the disease progresses.

- Emphysema is an abnormal, irreversible enlargement of the alveoli due to the destruction of the alveolar walls, resulting in decreased elastic recoil of the alveoli. The body works against itself by sending macrophages to the area of damaged tissue, which releases an enzyme that further weakens the alveolar walls.

- As emphysema progresses, the damaged lung tissue is replaced by nonelastic, fibrous scar tissue that inhibits the exchange of gases. A common sign of emphysema is that the patient must work to exhale and make room for inhaled air.

- Thoracic surgery involves some of the more complicated procedures, since multiple body systems are affected by the surgery.

- The surgical technologist must know and understand the anatomy and physiology of the respiratory system in order to properly assist the surgeon.

CRITICAL THINKING QUESTIONS

1. A patient undergoes a tracheostomy. What are the differences that occur between inhaling air through the normal respiratory route and tracheostomy? What complications could occur due to the breathing of air through the tracheostomy?

2. Based on the information given concerning pulmonary volumes, if a person stops breathing, approximately how long can he or she go without oxygen before experiencing hypoxia and damage to the body's tissues, in particular the brain? Why?

3. Emphysema effects the ability of the lung tissue and alveoli to recoil due to the loss of elasticity. What pulmonary volumes are affected? Why?

4. An individual sustains a gunshot wound to the thorax, entering on the right side and exiting out the back (called a through and through or T & T). The ambulance is on the way, but what can be accomplished for the patient at the site to aid in breathing? Why?

5. Briefly describe sleep apnea and its associated dangers. What surgical procedure is occasionally performed to treat sleep apnea?

REFERENCES

Cormack, D. H. (2001). *Essential histology* (2nd ed.). Philadelphia: Lippincott Williams & Wilkins.

Ethicon Products Worldwide. (2002). *Wound closure manual.* Somerville, NJ: Ethicon, Inc.

Gray, H. (1991). *Anatomy, descriptive and surgical.* St. Louis, MO: Mosby-Year Book.

McKenney, M. G., Mangonon, P. C., & Moylan, J. A. (Eds.). (1998). *Understanding surgical disease: The Miami manual of surgery.* Philadelphia: Lippincott-Raven.

Peacock, E. E., Jr. (1984). *Wound repair* (3rd ed.). Philadelphia: W. B. Saunders.

Skandalakis, J. E., Skandalakis, P. N., & Skandalakis, L. J. (2000). *Surgical anatomy and technique.* New York: Springer-Verlag.

15

DIGESTIVE SYSTEM

CHAPTER OUTLINE

CHAPTER OBJECTIVES

After completing the study of this chapter, you should be able to:

1. Describe the digestive process including the function of digestive enzymes, absorption of nutrients, and formation of feces.
2. List the tissue layers of the wall of the digestive tract.
3. List the surgical anatomic landmarks of the abdomen.
4. List the muscles of the abdomen, their component anatomic parts, incisions, and healing.
5. Explain the functions of the oral cavity, salivary glands, pharynx, esophagus, stomach, pancreas, liver, gallbladder, and large intestine, including anatomic location.
6. Explain the healing characteristics of the major and accessory organs of the digestive tract.

KEY TERMS

acini	Auerbach's plexus (myenteric plexus)	colon	dentin
alimentary canal		common bile duct (CBD)	descending colon
alveolar processes	Bartholin duct	common hepatic duct (CHD)	duct of Santorini
ampulla of Vater	bile	coronary ligament	duct of Wirsung
anal canal	buccal cavity	crown	dysphagia
anal sinuses	calorie	cystic artery	enamel
anus	cardiac sphincter	cystic duct	esophageal hiatus
appendix	cecum	deciduous teeth	esophagus
ascending colon	cholesterol	deglutition	facial nerve
atherosclerosis	chymification	dental pulp	friable

Case Study 1

A 12-year-old girl is brought into the operating room for an appendectomy. The surgeon has made the decision to perform an open appendectomy as opposed to laparoscopic due to the possibility that the appendix is positioned retrocecally. As the procedure progresses and the appendix is exposed, the surgeon asks for hemostatic clamps to place on the mesoappendix and cut with scissors to free the appendix from its attachment to the colon.

1. Explain the term retrocecal in relation to the anatomic position of the appendix.

2. Why does the appendix become inflamed and infected?

3. What are the function(s) of the appendix?

4. Describe the mesoappendix and its function in relation to the appendix.

INTRODUCTION

The digestive system consists of one long tube that begins with the opening to the mouth and ends at the opening of the anal canal (Figure 15-1). It involves organs that serve in a direct role, such as the stomach and intestines, and organs that serve in an accessory role, such as the pancreas and gallbladder. The overall purpose of the digestive system is to digest the food we ingest and remove from the food the substances that are needed by the cells, tissues, and organs of the body to maintain homeostasis.

DIGESTIVE PATHWAY OF FOOD

The process of digestion involves the chemical and mechanical breakdown of food into simpler chemical substances that can then be used by the cells of the body to carry on the processes that maintain homeostasis. The digestive organs and accessory organs carry out the process of digestion, which allows the body's cells to convert the food molecules into adenosine triphosphate (ATP), the chemical energy needed by the cells to perform their work.

The functions of the digestive system include ingestion of food, mechanical and chemical breakdown of food, absorption or breakdown of complex organic nutrient molecules into simple organic molecules that are absorbed into the blood or lymph to be transported to the cells of the body, and the formation and elimination of feces. The digestive system is composed of two groups of organs:

1. The first is the **alimentary canal** or gastrointestinal tract, a long tube that begins with the mouth and ends at the anus. It includes in order from when food enters the mouth: the pharynx,

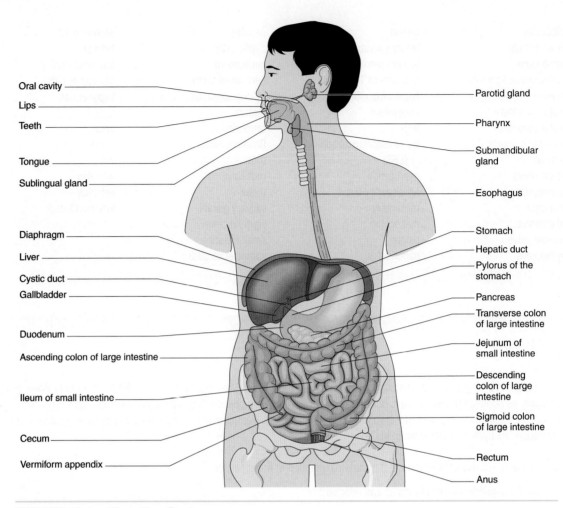

FIGURE 15-1   Digestive System

esophagus, stomach, small intestine, colon, and anal canal.

2. The second group is the accessory organs, which include the salivary glands, liver, gallbladder, and pancreas. These organs contribute digestive secretions that aid in the chemical breakdown of food.

The digestive system originates from the endoderm of the embryo that develops into the alimentary canal. The accessory organs originate as buds from the alimentary canal (Shier, Butler, & Lewis, 2002).

TISSUE LAYERS OF THE INTESTINAL WALL

Each organ varies somewhat in the number and types of tissue layers. The following is the general order of tissue layers, but the description of each organ will include a specific order of the layers. The tissue layers

are referred to as **tunics** or coats. Beginning with the innermost layer:

1. The tunica mucosa is the innermost layer and consists of mucous membrane. The tunica mucosa itself is made up of three layers:

   - The inner layer that is in contact with the contents within the intestine is the epithelial layer.
   - The middle layer is the lamina propria, which is composed of epithelial cells.
   - The outer layer is the muscularis mucosa.

The tunica mucosa in the esophagus is stratified squamous epithelium. In the stomach and intestine, the mucosa is simple columnar epithelium. The functions of the epithelial layer include secretion of digestive enzymes in the stomach and intestine, secretion of mucus to lubricate the passageway for food, and the absorption of nutrients from the breakdown of the food. The lamina propria serves as the middle layer to bind the epithelial layer to the muscularis mucosa and provides the intestine with its lymph and blood supply. Located in the lymph nodes of the lamina propria are macrophages, which travel through the epithelial to phagocytize bacteria and other foreign material. The muscularis mucosa is composed of muscular fibers that form folds and tiny projections to increase the absorptive surface area of the small intestine.

2. The tunica submucosa is the next layer. It is composed of loose areolar connective tissue. It contains many lymphatic and blood vessels that nourish the surrounding tissue and carry away absorbed materials. The mucosal layer is innervated by an autonomic nerve network located in the submucosal layer called **Meissner's plexus**. Parasympathetic impulses increase the release of digestive secretions and sympathetic impulses decrease the secretions.

3. The tunica muscularis is composed of either skeletal muscle or smooth muscle depending on the location in the body. In the mouth, pharynx, and upper third of the esophagus, the tunica muscularis is skeletal muscle in order to allow the act of swallowing. The rest of the alimentary tract consists of smooth muscle that consists of two layers: (a) the inner coat, which is circular that contract to decrease the diameter of the tube, and (b) the outer coat, which consists of longitudinal fibers that, when they contract, cause the tube to shorten. The stomach has three layers of smooth muscle as opposed to the two layers of the other organs. The contractions of the smooth muscle mechaonically break down food, mix the food with digestive secretions that chemically breakdown food, and are responsible for the action of peristalsis that pushes the food through the alimentary canal. Contained in the tunica muscularis is a major nerve supply called **Auerbach's plexus** (also called **myenteric plexus**). Auerbach's plexus is an autonomic nerve network. Parasympathetic impulses increase peristalsis and sympathetic impulses decrease peristalsis. The parasympathetic nerves are the X cranial nerve or vagus nerve. The vagus nerve will be discussed often throughout this chapter. The term vagus means "wanderer" and it lives up to that name.

4. The outer covering of the alimentary tube is the serosa or serous layer. It is composed of visceral peritoneum, which consists of epithelium. The serosa of the superior portion of the esophagus (above the diaphragm) is fibrous connective tissue. Below the diaphragm the abdominal cavity is lined with a fibrous tissue called the **peritoneum**. The parietal peritoneum lines the anterior, lateral, and posterior sides of the abdominal cavity and the inferior diaphragmatic surfaces. The visceral peritoneum is the outside serosal layer of the organs. The parietal peritoneum is innervated by somatic nerves and is responsible for localized pain. The visceral peritoneum is innervated by afferent nerves and transmits a dull sensation of pain. A thin space exists between the mesentery and peritoneum called the peritoneal space. It contains serous fluid, which acts as a lubricant to prevent friction when the organs within the abdominal cavity rub against each other.

The mesentery is a folded extension of the peritoneum. It invests and weaves in and between the organs to hold them in place. The mesentery attaches the small intestine and colon to the posterior abdominal wall. The mesentery also contains the blood vessels, lymph vessels, and nerves that supply the intestines. During colon surgery the mesentery must be divided to free up the portion of intestine to be removed. Consequently, the mesentery must be repaired with suture after the anastomosis of the colon is completed. The repair of the mesentery is also critical to prevent postoperative **herniation** of the intestine. Absorbable suture is commonly used for the repair.

The omental bursa is a cavity in the peritoneum located posterior to the stomach, the lesser omentum, and lower border of the liver, and anterior to the pancreas and duodenum. The **mesocolon** is divided into three folds composed of peritoneal tissue. The ascending mesocolon is the fold that connects the posterior portion of the ascending colon with the posterior wall of the abdomen. The transverse mesocolon is a large fold that connects the transverse colon with the posterior wall of the abdomen. It is formed by two layers of the greater omentum that separate and surround the transverse colon, join behind it, and continue posteriorly to the abdominal wall. This fold contains the blood vessels that supply the transverse colon. The descending mesocolon connects the descending colon to the posterior abdominal wall. The retroperitoneum, also called the retroperitoneal space, is located in the area posterior to the parietal peritoneum and extends from the diaphragm to the pelvis. The retroperitoneum is bounded anteriorly by the peritoneum, posteriorly by the spine, and laterally by the psoas and quadratum lumborium muscles (Caruthers & Price, 2001). There are three regions of the retroperitoneum: anterior

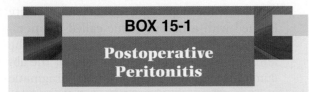

BOX 15-1

Postoperative Peritonitis

Postoperative peritonitis, inflammation of the peritoneum, has many causes, including intraoperative injury to an organ such as the bladder or gastrointestinal (GI) tract that allows spillage of contents. Retained foreign bodies, such as a surgical sponge, can cause severe inflamed adhesions and fibrosis to form until the foreign body is discovered and removed. However, as in the case of spillage of contents from the GI tract, the majority of cases of peritonitis are due to an invasion by bacteria and are usually polymicrobial. Normal peritoneum is thin, glistening, and almost transparent in appearance. When infected, it is reddish and thick in appearance. The appearance of fibrin causes the loops of the intestine to adhere to one another and to the peritoneum ("Acute Peritonitis," 2003). The greater omentum becomes adherent to the intestine, which aids in preventing the spread of the infection. The surgical treatment of peritonitis is centered on three factors: (a) eliminate the source of the infection, (b) reduce the number of bacteria in the peritoneal cavity, and (c) prevent recurrent infection. The operative approach is dependent on the source of the infection and current condition of the patient. Generally speaking, the surgeon will make a skin incision just inferior to the xiphoid process down to the umbilicus to treat severe secondary peritonitis (Bosscha, Vroonhoven, & Werken, 1999). The second goal is achieved by intraoperative peritoneal lavage and aspiration of the lavage fluid along with the purulent exudates and other particles present such as fecal matter. Peritoneal lavage is the process of gently pouring fluids into the peritoneum and aspirating or suctioning the fluids to remove the infectious fluid. Prevention of recurrent infection is attained by planned abdominal procedure or re-laparotomy. Rather than waiting to see if signs of recurrent infection develop, re-laparotomies are performed at intervals in order to evacuate any exudate until it is decided that the peritoneal cavity is clean of bacteria (Bosscha et al., 1999).

pararenal in which the pancreas and portions of the duodenum and colon are located; perirenal where various urologic and vascular structures are located; and posterior pararenal where no organs are located (Caruthers & Price, 2001).

SURGICAL REFERENCE POINTS OF THE ABDOMEN

Landmarks that serve as reference points for the abdominal incisions and muscular attachments include:

1. Xiphoid process: A midline incision is a type of abdominal incision made down the middle of abdomen. The surgeon often begins the incision just below the xiphoid process.
2. Subcostal margin: The subcostal margin is an imaginary line that can be drawn along the lower border of the ribs. A subcostal incision is made along this area to access either the gallbladder on the right side of the body or the spleen or lower portion of the stomach on the left side of the body.
3. Umbilicus: The umbilicus is used as an anatomic landmark for a lower midline incision, which begins just inferior to the umbilicus to just superior to the symphysis pubis.
4. Linea alba: Also used in determining where the midline incision should be made on a patient (see xiphoid process). It is part of the abdominal aponeurosis, which extends from the xiphoid process to the symphysis pubis and includes the umbilicus.
5. Anterior iliac spine: A projection of the ilium of the pelvic girdle that provides attachments for ligaments and muscles.
6. Symphysis pubis: See umbilicus. In addition, a transverse incision called a Pfannenstiel incision, which is used for performing a cesarean section, is made just superior to the symphysis pubis.
7. Groin creases: Groin creases represent lines in the skin. The surgeon, for cosmetic and wound-healing purposes, will attempt to make incisions that follow skin lines. The groin crease is, obviously, in the region of the groin where a skin line has developed due to the movement of the leg and hip.

MUSCLES OF THE ABDOMEN

The following are the muscles of the abdomen that are commonly encountered during surgery and require closure at the end of the procedure:

1. External oblique muscle
2. Internal oblique muscle
3. Transverse abdominis
4. Rectus abdominis

The muscles are covered by a tough, fibrous fascia that varies in thickness with each muscle. The transverse abdominis and both obliques are connected by a special type of tendon called the aponeurosis. The aponeurosis connects in the midline of the body and creates a covering around the rectus abdominis and linea alba.

Surgical Incisions and Healing of the Abdominal Muscles

Muscle tissue and fascia do not endure suturing well and can be slow to heal. Fascia can take up to a year or longer to regain original maximum strength. The surgeon prefers to cut, split, or retract the muscles in the direction of their fibers to prevent interference with the blood supply, preserve the nerve supply, and facilitate healing. When these methods of opening the muscle are used, suturing is not necessary and only the fascia requires closure. When muscle or fascia is closed, either nonabsorbable suture or absorbable suture, which has a longer tensile strength, may be used.

ORAL CAVITY

The first portion of the alimentary canal is the mouth, also called the **buccal cavity**. It is responsible for beginning the process of digestion by mechanical means, breaking the large portions of food into smaller pieces and mixing them with saliva. The action of chewing food is called **mastication**. The mouth is made up of the lips, cheeks, tongue, hard and soft palate, and the teeth (Figure 15-2).

The cheeks form the lateral sides of the mouth, which are continuous anteriorly with the lips. Externally the cheeks are composed of integument and internally of mucous membrane made up of stratified squamous epithelium. The major muscles of the cheek are the buccinator, zygomatic, masseter, and platysma. The lips are externally composed of integument and internally of mucous membrane. They contain skeletal muscles, capillaries near the surface, which provide the lips with their reddish color, and nerve receptors, which help to determine the texture and temperature of food. The orbicularis oris muscle surrounds the outer portion of the lips. During surgical procedures that involve the lips and area around the mouth, the **facial nerve** must be preserved, since it innervates the orbicularis oris. Temporary or permanent damage of the nerve will cause the lips to droop and prevent the individual from forming facial expressions such as a smile. The inner surface of each lip is connected to the middle of the gum by a fold of mucous membrane, respectively, called the superior labial frenulum and inferior labial frenulum. Together, the lips and cheeks aid in keeping food between the lower and upper teeth, and are important in speech.

The **tongue** is a muscular structure that is located on the floor of the mouth. The outside of the tongue is covered by mucous membrane that covers the

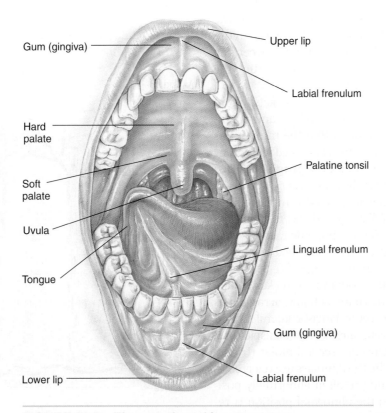

Gum (gingiva)

Upper lip

Labial frenulum

Hard palate

Soft palate

Palatine tonsil

Uvula

Tongue

Lingual frenulum

Gum (gingiva)

Lower lip

Labial frenulum

FIGURE 15-2   The mouth and its structures

inside skeletal muscle. There are two sets of skeletal muscle in the tongue.

1. Extrinsic muscles originate outside of the tongue and insert directly into it. They aid in moving the tongue from side to side and in and out to move food.
2. Intrinsic muscles originate and insert inside the tongue. They are responsible for changing the shape of the tongue to aid in speech and swallowing.

The tongue is connected to the midline of the floor of the mouth by a membranous fold of tissue called the **lingual frenulum** and is supported by attachment to the hyoid bone. The surface of the tongue has small, rough projections called **papillae**. They contain the taste buds, which determine the four tastes: sweet, sour, bitter, and salt.

The **palate** forms the roof of the mouth. It consists of two parts: the hard palate and the soft palate. The hard palate is located in the anterior portion formed by periosteum and mucous membrane, which adhere together and are continuous with the soft palate. The soft palate is located in the posterior portion of the roof of the mouth separating the mouth from the pharynx. The soft palate extends downward, and hanging from the most posterior portion that is continuous from the palate is a cone-shaped structure called the **uvula**. When an individual swallows, the muscles within the soft palate draw it and the uvula upward. This serves to close the opening between the nasal cavity and the pharynx, thereby preventing the food from entering the nasal cavity.

The teeth are located and develop in sockets within the **alveolar processes** of the mandible and maxillary bones. Teeth are unique in that the human has two sets. The **deciduous teeth** (also called temporary or primary teeth) enter through the **gingiva** (gums) between the ages of 6 months and 2 years. There are 20 deciduous teeth, which are located from the midline toward the sides in the following order: central incisor, lateral incisor, cuspid (canine), first molar, and second molar. The **permanent teeth** (also called secondary teeth) begin to appear at about the age of 6–8 years by pushing the deciduous teeth out of their sockets. There are 32 permanent teeth, 16 in each jaw, arranged as follows from the midline: central incisor, lateral incisor, cuspid, first bicuspid (premolar), second bicuspid (premolar), first molar (tricuspid), second molar (tricuspid), and third molar. The third molars are referred to as the wisdom teeth and are often abnormally positioned within the jaws; the abnormal position is referred to as impacted. The impaction can cause pain and misalignment of other teeth when these teeth enter, and they most likely will require removal.

The incisors are used to bite off pieces of food and to cut food. The cone-shaped cuspids grasp and tear food. The top portion of the bicuspids and molar teeth are basically flattened and are used to grind food. Bicuspid means the tooth has two cusps or projections and tricuspid means there are three cusps.

The gums are made of compact fibrous tissue that surrounds the necks of the teeth. At the neck of the teeth the tissue is continuous with the periosteal membrane that lines the alveolar processes.

Each tooth has two main portions—the **crown**, located above the gum, and the **root**, located in the alveolar process of the jaw (Figure 15-3). The area where these two portions meet is called the neck of the tooth. The roots of the teeth are firmly situated within the alveoli and the depressions are lined with periosteum. At the margin of the alveolus, the periosteum is continuous with the fibrous structure of the gum. The root of the tooth is enclosed by two layers—the periodontal ligament and cementum. The outer ligament is composed of collagenous fibers, located between the inner cementum and the bone of the alveolar process to firmly attach the tooth to the jaw. The cementum forms a thin layer terminating at the level of the tooth enamel. Chemically and structurally it is similar to bone.

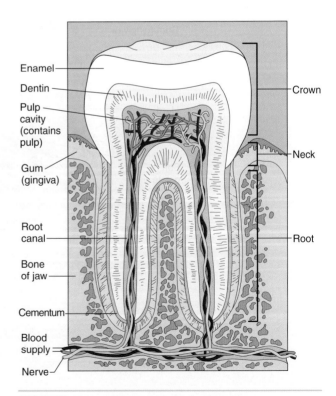

Enamel
Dentin
Pulp cavity (contains pulp)
Gum (gingiva)
Root canal
Bone of jaw
Cementum
Blood supply
Nerve
Crown
Neck
Root

FIGURE 15-3   Structure of the tooth

The next layer that forms the majority of the mass of the tooth is **dentin**. Dentin is a bonelike substance that encloses the pulp cavity and in the crown is located beneath the enamel. The pulp cavity is located in the center of the tooth extending from the root to the crown. Within the pulp cavity is the highly vascular soft substance called the **dental pulp**. The pulp cavity contains the blood vessels and nerves that supply the tooth. The vessels enter the tooth through small tubular extensions called **root canals** that extend upward into the root. At the base of each root canal is a foramen called the apical foramen through which the vessels enter the pulp of the tooth.

Enamel, glossy white in appearance, is the hardest and most compact substance in the body. The enamel is thickest on the crown of the tooth and becomes thinner toward the neck. It consists primarily of calcium salts. With age, the enamel tends to wear away, becoming a concern for the older adult. Also, bacteria are a concern due to their ability to cause dental caries. *Actinomyces, Streptococcus mutans,* and *Lactobacillus* are three of the primary acid-forming microorganisms responsible for the cause of dental caries. For example, a person eats a candy bar but does not brush the teeth soon afterward. The food that is lodged between the teeth provides food for the bacteria. The microbes metabolize the carbohydrates in the food and in the process produce acid byproducts that destroy the enamel, causing a cavity.

SALIVARY GLANDS

The majority of saliva is secreted by the **salivary glands**. However, there are many small glands called buccal glands located throughout the mucosa of the tongue, palate, and cheeks that continuously secrete saliva to keep the inside of the mouth moist. Saliva moistens the food particles to make chewing easier, brings the particles together into a food bolus, and chemically begins the process of digesting carbohydrates. The teeth are protected from saliva because it contains bicarbonate ions, keeping the pH of the saliva neutral, between 6.5 and 7.5. This also aids in protecting the teeth from the acids contained in many foods.

Two types of cells are found in the salivary glands: mucous cells and serous cells. The watery fluid produced by serous cells contains the digestive enzyme called amylase. The enzyme is responsible for breaking down the carbohydrate molecules, starch and glycogen, into disaccharides. Mucous cells, obviously, secrete mucus, which aids in binding the food to form a bolus and lubricates the passageway for food.

The salivary glands are innervated by branches of the sympathetic and parasympathetic nervous systems. The sympathetic nerve impulses stimulate the glands to secrete mucus. Parasympathetic nerve impulses cause the release of the watery fluid. Therefore, when an individual smells, sees, tastes, or thinks about food they consider good, the watery fluid is released. On the other hand, if the food is not considered good, the parasympathetic response is not as active so less saliva is released making swallowing more difficult.

There are three pairs of large salivary glands that are situated outside of the oral cavity, and the saliva they secrete is transported to the cavity via ducts. The three glands are the parotid glands, submandibular glands, and sublingual glands (Figures 15-4 and 15-5).

The parotid gland is the largest of the three glands located on the lateral sides of the face anterior to the external ear. When performing surgery on the parotid, the platysma muscle is retracted in the direction of its fibers and two more layers cover the parotid: fascia and integument. The surgeon will also encounter one to two lymphatic glands that rest on the surface of the parotid. The excretory duct is called **Steno's duct** and its orifice is on the inner surface of the cheek opposite the second molar tooth of the upper jaw. Important vessels to consider when operating on any three of the salivary glands include: external carotid artery, temporal artery, facial artery, sublingual artery, and the facial nerve.

The submandibular gland is located inferior to the jaw. It lies on top of the strap muscles and is also covered by the platysma, integument, and fascia. The facial artery and nerve are both important structures to consider when operating on the parotid and submandibular glands. Both structures are situated within or close to the glands. For example, the facial artery lies in a groove in the posterior, superior border of the submandibular gland. The excretory gland of the submandibular gland is called **Wharton's duct**.

The sublingual gland is the smallest of the three glands. It is located beneath the mucous membrane that covers the floor of the mouth. Each gland is located on either side of the lingual frenulum. The excretory ducts, **Riviniani ducts**, number anywhere from 8 to 20 and open separately into the mouth. One or more of the ducts join to form a single tube that joins the Wharton duct; this single duct is called the **Bartholin duct**.

A common disorder, in particular of the parotid, is the formation of stones that block the ducts. The stones can be one or two large stones to several small

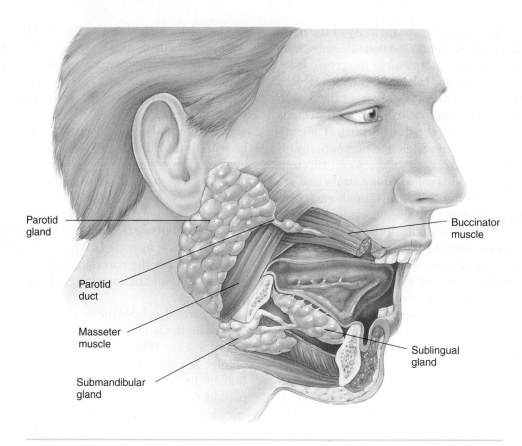

Parotid gland

Parotid duct

Masseter muscle

Submandibular gland

Buccinator muscle

Sublingual gland

FIGURE 15-4 **The salivary glands**

stones that will be located in the gland itself or in the duct. Surgery is performed to either clear the ducts or, if too many stones are present, to remove the gland.

PHARYNX

The pharynx is the only structure that serves as part of both the respiratory and digestive tracts. It is approximately $4\frac{1}{2}$ inches in length and is continuous with the esophagus. There are seven openings into the pharynx: two nares, two Eustachian tubes, a mouth, a larynx, and an esophagus. It has three coats: mucous, muscular, and fibrous. The pharynx is divided into three portions: the nasopharynx, oropharynx, and laryngopharynx. The nasopharynx begins just superior to the soft palate and the nasal cavity opens into the pharynx, providing a passageway for air and secretions (when an individual is crying or has a cold, the saliva and mucus enter at the back of the throat creating phlegm). The auditory tubes from the middle ear open into the nasopharynx. This accounts for a large percentage of infant and adolescent ear infections. Because the auditory tube has not matured and reached full length, microbes from the na-

sopharynx can easily travel through the auditory tube to the middle ear causing an infection and the commonly known "ear ache." The oropharynx is posterior to the soft palate opening into the nasopharynx, and is downward to the superior level of the

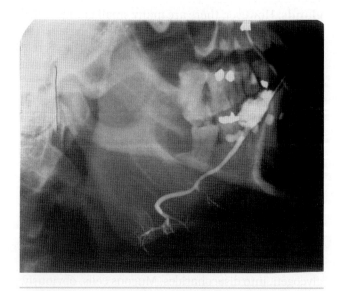

FIGURE 15-5 **Radiologic examination of submandibular ducts**

epiglottis. This also serves as a passageway for food and air. The laryngopharynx is located inferior to the oropharynx, extending from the superior border of the epiglottis to the inferior border of the cricoid cartilage, and serves as the opening to the esophagus.

The muscles of the pharynx are skeletal muscles to voluntarily begin the process of swallowing. There are two layers of pharyngeal muscles, outer longitudinal muscles and inner circular muscles. The inner circular muscles, called constrictor muscles, bring the walls of the pharynx inward during swallowing. The superior constrictor muscles are attached to the bony processes of the skull and mandible, traveling around the upper portion of the pharynx. The middle constrictor muscles are attached to bony processes of the hyoid bone and travel around the middle portion of the pharynx. The inferior constrictor muscles originate from the cartilage of the larynx and travel around the lower portion of the pharynx. Many of the lower muscle fibers of the inferior constrictor muscle are constantly contracted to prevent air from entering the esophagus while breathing.

The role of the pharynx is to begin the process of **deglutition** (swallowing). Once food has entered the mouth, then has been chewed, mixed with saliva, and formed into a bolus, it is forced into the pharynx and the swallowing reflex is initiated. As the swallowing reflex occurs, breathing is temporarily halted. The steps of the swallowing reflex are as follows:

1. The soft palate and uvula rise to prevent food from entering the nasal cavity by closing off the nasopharynx.
2. The larynx and hyoid bone respond by moving upward and forward causing the epiglottis to seal off the glottis to prevent food from entering the trachea.
3. The bolus of food passes through the laryngopharynx and begins to enter the esophagus. The fibers of the lower portion of the inferior constrictor muscles relax, opening the esophagus in preparation to receive the bolus.
4. The superior constrictor muscles begin to contract, stimulating peristalsis to force the food into the esophagus and aid in transporting the food the length of the esophagus. The respiratory passage can now reopen and normal breathing resumes.

Healing of the Oral Cavity

The oral cavity, including the pharynx, is considered a clean area, not sterile, and harbors many types of resident and opportunistic microbes. (The term clean area means that microorganisms are present, whereas sterile means the absence of all microorganisms.) When an infection is not present the oral cavity and pharynx usually heal quickly. Absorbable or nonabsorbable sutures are used by the surgeon. Nonabsorbable suture may be preferred, since it tends to cause less tissue reaction in the buccal mucosa, but obviously requires removal after the healing process is complete.

Periodontitis presents a challenge to the surgeon. The infection is generally moderate to severe. Consequently the surgeon is concerned about preventing the spread of the infection, facilitating the healing of the tissues as quickly as possible, and preserving healthy tissue. Most often the surgeon will prefer to use either a nonabsorbable suture or an absorbable one that has a long absorbable rate and greater tensile strength.

ESOPHAGUS

The **esophagus** is a long, collapsible, muscular tube approximately 25 cm in length that is located posterior to the trachea (Figures 15-6 and 15-7). It provides the passageway for food to the stomach and by wavelike motions, called peristalsis, of the smooth muscle, the food is propelled forward. The esophagus begins at the end of the laryngopharynx and terminates at the **cardiac sphincter** of the stomach. It travels through the space of the mediastinum and passes through the opening in the diaphragm called the **esophageal hiatus**. The general direction of the esophagus is vertical, but it does have two slight curvatures that are important to the surgical team. The first is a curvature to the left at the base of the neck that returns to the midline curve again to the left just before the esophageal hiatus of the diaphragm. The esophagus has three coats: muscular, submucosa, and mucosa. The muscular coat is composed of external longitudinal fibers and internal circular fibers. It is important to note that the lower portion of the esophagus is composed of involuntary muscular fibers. The submucosa connects the mucosa and muscular coats. The mucosa is thick and covered with a layer of squamous epithelium. Mucous glands are located throughout the mucosa and secrete mucus to lubricate the inside of the esophagus to aid in the passage of food.

Just at the point where the esophagus joins the stomach is a layer of circular muscle fibers forming what is called the **lower esophageal sphincter (LES)**. The sphincter is usually contracted to close the entrance to the stomach. When the peristaltic waves

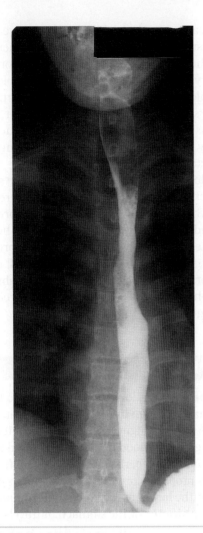

FIGURE 15-6   AP esophagus

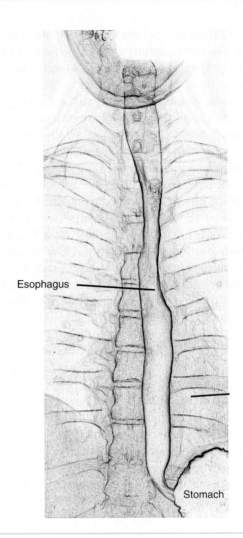

FIGURE 15-7   AP esophagus

of the esophagus reach the stomach, the circular muscle fibers relax to allow the food bolus to enter and close once the food has passed. The contraction prevents the food and gastric juices from reentering the esophagus. A condition commonly referred to as "heartburn" (due to a burning sensation in the chest region) is actually gastric juices passing through the LES and into the esophagus. There are two primary reasons this occurs: One is the weakening of the muscle fibers of the LES and the other is the occurrence of a **hiatal hernia**. A hiatal hernia occurs when the esophageal hiatus has weakened allowing the superior portion of the stomach to protrude into the thoracic cavity. The result is the reflux of gastric juices into the esophagus causing irritation to the inner lining, damage to the cells, and **dysphagia**. Nissen fundoplication is the surgical procedure to correct hiatal hernia, and is commonly performed as a laparoscopic procedure in which a scope is inserted through a small incision into the abdomen to view the area of

surgery. The surgical instruments are also inserted into the abdomen through additional small incisions in order to perform the surgery.

Another esophageal pathology of concern is portal hypertension. Portal hypertension is due to elevated pressure in the portal vein and occurs when the blood flow meets abnormal resistance. The disorder is commonly a result of liver disease such as cirrhosis. As the portal pressure increases, blood backs up into the spleen and enters the venous system, bypassing the liver. The results of portal hypertension are splenomegaly, esophageal varices (dilated veins), and hemorrhoids. In the majority of patients, the first sign of portal hypertension is bleeding from ruptured esophageal varices—dilated veins located in the submucosa of the esophagus. Bleeding is usually severe and life-threatening, requiring surgery to control hemorrhage and prevent hypovolemic shock, shock brought on the by the abnormal loss of blood and body fluids from the body (thus the use of

This surgical procedure is performed to treat gastroesophageal reflux disease (GERD) by wrapping the fundus of the stomach around the cardia to prevent GERD and hiatal hernia. The operation is performed laparoscopically. The patient is placed supine on the operating room table with legs in stirrups. A small needle called the Veress needle is inserted into the abdominal cavity to allow carbon dioxide to be pumped into the cavity and distend the abdominal region. This prevents injury to the abdominal organs when the cannulas are placed into the abdomen, and allows the surgeon to visualize the organs. A cannula is a short tube that is placed through a small skin incision and into the abdomen. Five cannulas are inserted at various positions in the abdomen; the laparoscope and other surgical instruments can be inserted through the cannulas in order to perform the operation. The surgeon creates an opening or window behind the esophagus at the level of the cardiac sphincter of the stomach; while creating this opening the vagus nerve is identified and preserved. The esophageal hiatus is also incised to temporarily widen the opening. The surgeon will then grasp the fundus of the stomach (remember, the fundus is above the level of the cardiac sphincter), bring the fundus through the window, around the esophagus, and place it on the superoanterior portion of the stomach. The surgeon will then repair the enlarged opening of the esophageal hiatus with suture. Another portion of the fundus across from the first portion is grasped and placed opposite. The two segments are sutured or stapled together. This prevents the stomach from slipping back through the esophageal hiatus.

the prefix *hypo-,* meaning below, and the root word *volemic,* meaning volume).

The blood supply of the esophagus is as follows:

1. Esophageal arteries that are branches from the descending thoracic aorta
2. Branches of the inferior thyroid arteries
3. Branches of the gastric and inferior phrenic arteries

Healing of the Esophagus

An important structural feature of the esophagus that influences pathology and surgical procedures is the absence of a serosal layer. The esophagus is easily injured, difficult to repair, and slow healing. The mucosal layer heals slowly and the thick muscular layer does not hold sutures well. Consequently, a high

incidence of failure of esophageal repair has been reported. This affects the choice of surgical procedure and suture to repair the esophagus.

Based on the anatomy described in the preceding text, when a patient is surgically treated for esophageal cancer, the esophagus will be removed en bloc and replaced with a portion of the colon. The colon is ideal for replacement, since it is flexible and peristalsis can be restored with the establishment of the LES.

STOMACH

The stomach is a large muscular pouch that is situated inferior to the diaphragm; the major portion of the organ is located in the upper left abdominal quadrant. It is the primary organ of digestion, performing the process of breaking down the food called **chymification**. When empty it is partially collapsed, but the stomach can greatly expand to accept large amounts of food.

The superior border of the stomach is referred to as the **lesser curvature**. The **lesser omentum** is connected to the lesser curvature and extends to the posterior surface of the liver to hold the stomach in place. A fold of peritoneum called the **gastrophrenic ligament** extends from the diaphragm to the cardia of the stomach to also aid in stabilizing the anatomic postion of the stomach. The inferior border of the stomach is called the **greater curvature**, and the **greater omentum** is attached to this border.

The lesser omentum is derived from the peritoneum, covering the anterior and inferior surfaces of the stomach. In addition, it travels upward from the attachment at the lesser curvature of the stomach to the porta hepatis. At this point it is a double fold of peritoneal tissue that contains the hepatic artery, portal vein, nerves, lymphatic vessels, and bile duct. The duodenum is connected to the liver by the hepatoduodenal ligament, which is formed by the lesser omentum.

The greater omentum is a double fold of peritoneum that doubles back on itself to form four layers. It drapes downward like an apron from the stomach, covering the transverse colon and the majority of the small intestine. It contains adipose tissue, some vessels, and helps to prevent the spread of infection into the peritoneal cavity. During stomach and intestinal surgery, the surgeon will often deliver the greater omentum through the surgical wound onto the sterile drapes for later replacement into the cavity when the procedure has been completed. Sterile sponges that have been soaked in sterile saline will be placed on the omentum to keep it from drying out until placed back into the abdominal cavity.

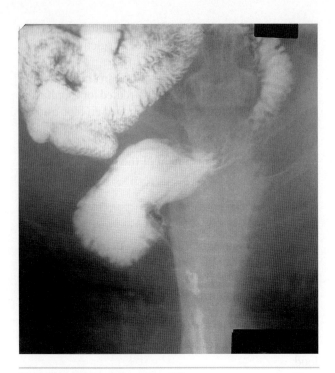

FIGURE 15-8 AP upper GI

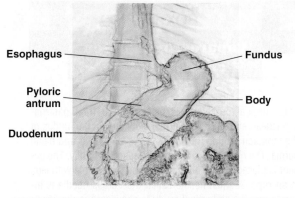

FIGURE 15-9 AP upper GI

The stomach is divided into four regions: cardiac, fundus, body, and pyloric regions (Figures 15-8 and 15-9). The cardiac region is the area around the cardiac sphincter. The fundus is the superior region of the stomach, which is superior to the level of the cardiac sphincter. The body is the primary middle portion of the stomach. The pyloric region, also called the antrum, is the portion that narrows and is funnel-shaped. It connects to the small intestine via the **pyloric sphincter**.

The arterial blood supply is extensive. The following are the arteries: (a) left gastric artery, (b) branches of the celiac artery, (c) branches of the splenic artery, (d) branches of the left gastroepiploic, (e) one branch of the left gastric artery, and (f) gastroduodenal artery. During surgery of the stomach, much time is spent clamping, cutting, and tying off the arterial branches to free up the stomach. The nerve supply consists of branches of the pneumogastric and branches from the sympathetic nerves.

The mucosal and submucosal layers of the stomach form thick folds called **rugae** when the stomach is empty and smooth out when the stomach is full (Figure 15-10). The mucous membrane contains many small openings called gastric pits that are located at the ends of tube-shaped **gastric glands**. The gastric glands contain three kinds of secretory cells:

1. Mucous cells, also called goblet cells, are located near the opening of the gastric gland.

2. Chief cells, also called **peptic cells**, are located deeper in the gastric gland and secrete the gastric enzyme pepsinogen.
3. Parietal cells, also called oxyntic cells, also are located deep in the gastric gland and secrete hydrochloric acid.

Together the secretions of the cells form what is referred to as the **gastric juice**.

Pepsinogen, secreted by the chief cells, is an inactive enzyme. However, when it comes into contact with hydrochloric acid it is converted to pepsin. Pepsin can continue to convert pepsinogen into pepsin. But more important, pepsin is responsible for beginning the digestion of protein.

The muscularis coat of the stomach is composed of three layers of smooth muscle: inner oblique, middle circular, and outer longitudinal. It is important for the surgical team to understand the anatomy of these three layers due to their intimacy with the esophagus and the surgical incisions through the layers. The inner oblique layer is continuous with the circular layer of the esophagus and is thicker in the fundus as compared to the antrum. The middle layer is composed of circular fibers. This is the primary layer involved in gastric emptying. The outer layer is continuous with the longitudinal fibers of the esophageal muscle. It travels to the pylorus and becomes continuous with the longitudinal muscle of the duodenum.

The production of gastric juice is regulated by hormones and nerve stimulation. Within the gastric glands is another type of cells, closely related to the parietal cells, which secrete the hormone somatostatin that inhibits acid secretion. The opposite reaction is caused by acetylcholine (ACh). ACh is released from nerve endings that have been stimulated by parasympathetic impulses from the vagus nerve. ACh inhibits the secretion of somatostatin, thereby stimulating the

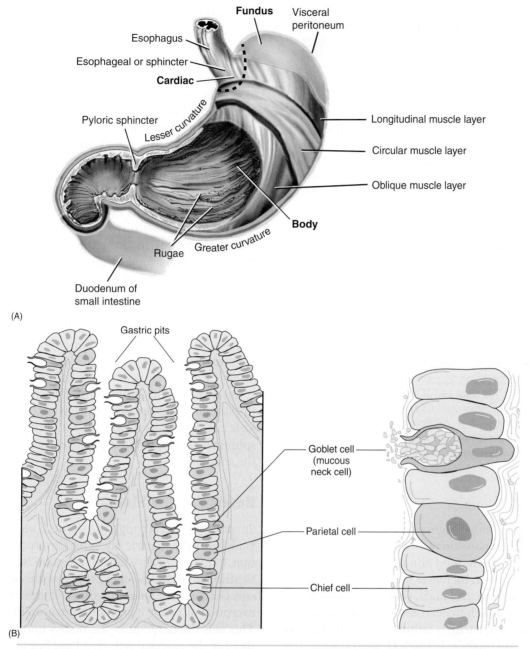

FIGURE 15-10   (A) Parts of the stomach; (B) three types of gastric gland cells that make up the gastric glands that line the stomach

gastric glands to secrete gastric juice. The parasympathetic impulses stimulate two other important reactions. In the pyloric region of the stomach, the impulses stimulate the release of the peptide hormone called gastrin, which in turn stimulates the secretory activity of the gastric glands. The impulses together with the gastrin stimulate the release of histamine from the mucosal cells, which causes additional stimulation of gastric secretion. The three layers of the stomach contribute to the process by contracting, which further breaks up the food into smaller pieces and mixes it with the gastric juice, forming what is called chyme; this process of mixing the food with gastric juice is called chymification.

There are three stages of gastric secretion—cephalic, gastric, and intestinal. The cephalic stage begins when an individual sees, smells, or thinks about food. This stimulates the parasympathetic reflexes of the vagus nerve, which stimulates the release of gastric secretions.

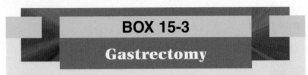

The gastric stage begins when food enters the stomach. The expansion of the stomach wall due to the presence of the food stimulates the release of gastrin, which then increases the stimulation for the release of more gastric juice. Gastrin causes the pH level in the stomach to decrease, and, consequently, the release of gastrin is inhibited. When the pH reaches approximately 1.5 to 1.0, gastric secretion will stop. In order to release hydrochloric acid, hydrogen ions are removed from the bloodstream and replaced with bicarbonate ions. Therefore, after eating food the blood level of bicarbonate ions increases and the urine excretes this excess of ions.

The intestinal stage begins when food exits the stomach and enters the duodenum. As the food travels into the duodenum, the sympathetic reflex is stimulated by acid in the duodenum and inhibits the release of gastric juice in the stomach. The proteins and fats in the food that has entered the duodenum cause the release of the peptide hormone cholecystokinin, which inhibits gastric motility. The fats also stimulate the duodenal cells to release intestinal

somatostatin, which decreases the release of gastric juice.

It is important to understand the action of the vagus nerve in relation to the production of gastric juice. Some individuals who have a chronic condition of producing too much gastric juice or continuous production, which can lead to ulcerations of the stomach tissue, will undergo surgery to remove small portions of the vagus nerve. The surgery is performed after all other nonsurgical treatments have been tried and deemed not effective. Removing some of the vagus nerve reduces the parasympathetic impulses, thereby reducing the release of gastric juice.

In summary, within the stomach the digestive process begins with the mucous secretions in the cardia, allowing food to pass more easily into the stomach. The cells in the fundus secrete hydrochloric acid. The cells in the body of the stomach produce pepsinogen and additional mucous. The antrum is the non–acid-producing area of the stomach, secreting mucus and gastrin. The function of the pylorus is basically an area for the broken-down food to be briefly stored before passing through the pyloric sphincter into the duodenum. Peristaltic waves of the stomach muscles push the chyme toward the pyloric region and as the chyme builds up, the pyloric sphincter relaxes to allow passage of the chyme into the small intestine.

Healing of the Stomach

Surprisingly, even though the stomach secretes strong acids and other gastric juices for the process of digestion, it quickly heals when an infection is not present. Gastrin aids in the healing process of the stomach tissue. Gastrin stimulates mucosal cell growth, with the exception of where it is produced within the stomach. This aids the surgeon in the body's natural replacement of the mucosal cells that have been damaged by disease, trauma, or surgical treatment. The tissues of the stomach usually regain full strength in 14 to 21 days postoperatively. Absorbable sutures are used but can produce a mild tissue reaction; nonabsorbable sutures are used as well.

A common condition that affects the stomach and duodenum is ulcers. Ulcers develop when the inner tissue layers of the stomach or duodenum are damaged by the digestive enzymes and, more specifically, by hydrochloric acid. This is primarily due to two reasons: either the excess production of the acid or the underproduction of mucus that protects the stomach lining. A dangerous condition occurs when the ulceration of the tissue continues and perforates completely through the organ causing the leaking of fluids and digested food into the abdominal cavity, which can lead to life-threatening peritonitis. In addition, hemorrhaging can be severe and life-threatening. A frequently occuring type of ulcer is the peptic ulcer, which is most often found in the duodenum. Three major causes have been identified: (a) infection with *Helicobacter pylori,* (b) use of nonsteroidal anti-inflammatory drugs (NSAIDs), and (c) pathological hypersecretory disorders such as Zollinger–Ellison syndrome. It is not known how *H. pylori* contributes to the formation of gastric or peptic ulcers. NSAIDs promote ulcer formation by inhibiting the secretion of prostaglandins, substances that aid in preventing ulcerations. Treatment ranges from drug therapy to surgery. Surgery is indicated for perforation and presence of GI bleeding and unresponsiveness to nonsurgical treatment. Surgical procedures include vagotomy, pyloroplasty, distal gastrectomy, and small-intestine resection with removal of affected area of duodenum.

PANCREAS

The **pancreas** is the only organ of the body that performs endocrine and exocrine functions (Figure 15-11). In this chapter the exocrine function, the secretion of pancreatic juice, will be discussed. The pancreas is a long gland, approximately 6–7 inches in length, extending horizontally across the abdomen, and is posterior to the parietal peritoneum. It is divided into three portions: head, body, and tail. It is posterior to the great curvature of the stomach with the head resting in the curve of the duodenum and the tail by the spleen. The body is the main portion of the organ.

The internal pancreatic tissue is composed of three types of cells. A group of glandular epithelial cells called the islets of Langerhans are the cells that perform the endocrine functions. The islets of Langerhans are composed of two clusters of cells, one consisting of alpha cells that secrete glucagon and the other beta cells that secrete insulin. The third type of cells, called acinar cells, perform the exocrine function by producing pancreatic juice. They form clusters called **acini** (singular, acinus). Small tubes exit the clusters for the pancreatic juice to travel along and the small tubes unite to eventually form the large duct that runs the length of the pancreas called the **duct of Wirsung**, or pancreatic duct, in which the pancreatic juice collects to travel to the duodenum.

Pancreatic juice consists of hydrolytic enzymes (lipases, proteases, and carbohydrases). The enzymes break down fats, proteins, carbohydrates, and nucleic acids. The specific enzymes and their action are as follows:

1. Pancreatic lipase: breaks down triglyceride molecules into monoglycerides and fatty acids
2. Pancreatic amylase: carbohydrate enzyme that breaks down glycogen molecules into disaccharides
3. Trypsin, carboxypeptidase, and chymotrypsin: enzymes that work together to break down proteins by splitting the bonds between amino acids

The acini also secrete sodium bicarbonate to help maintain an intraluminal pH to protect the duodenal mucosa from the pepsin and gastric acid.

Normally the duct of Wirsung joins the common bile duct and enters the duodenum through the **ampulla of Vater**. The opening of the ampulla of Vater is called the **sphincter of Oddi**. A band of smooth muscle surrounds the sphincter to aid in controlling the release of the pancreatic juice into the duodenum. The surgical team must be aware of the sphincter of Oddi when performing procedures, such as placing a feeding tube in the duodenum, in order to preserve its function. Occasionally a second duct will exist, which extends from the duct of Wirsung and opens separately onto the duodenum, usually about $\frac{1}{2}$ to 1 inch above the ampulla of Vater. This separate duct is

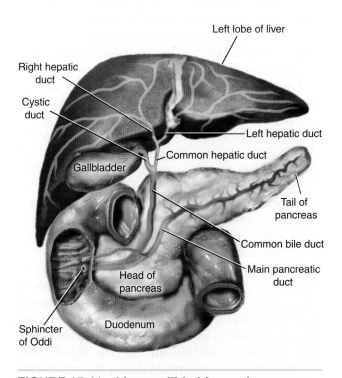

FIGURE 15-11 Liver, gallbladder, and pancreas

Left lobe of liver

Right hepatic duct

Cystic duct

Left hepatic duct

Common hepatic duct

Gallbladder

Tail of pancreas

Common bile duct

Main pancreatic duct

Head of pancreas

Sphincter of Oddi

Duodenum

called the **duct of Santorini**. The surgical team should be prepared for the possibility of two ducts when performing surgery on the pancreas and duodenum in order to identify and preserve both ducts.

The blood supply to the pancreas is extensive and requires much attention from the surgical team. The following is the arterial blood supply: (a) branches of the celiac artery, (b) branches of the superior mesenteric arteries, and (c) branches of the large splenic artery. The pancreatic veins drain into the splenic, superior mesenteric, and portal veins.

The nervous and endocrine systems control the release of pancreatic juice. Parasympathetic impulses stimulate the pancreas to release digestive enzymes. The peptide hormone secretin is released into the bloodstream from the mucous membrane of the duodenum in response to the acidic chyme that enters the duodenum. Secretin stimulates the pancreas to release fluid that contains sodium bicarbonate to neutralize the acid.

The fats and proteins in the chyme also stimulate the release of the hormone cholecystokinin from the mucous membrane of the small intestine. Just as with secretin, cholecystokinin reaches the pancreas via the bloodstream and pancreatic juice is released due to the stimulation by cholecystokinin.

Healing of the Pancreas

Wounds of the pancreas and ducts can heal by either primary or secondary intention. The stroma (supporting tissue) of the pancreas is able to adequately hold the tissue together until tissue tensile strength has returned. Therefore, the pancreas can be repaired using sutures and it will heal by the normal processes of protein synthesis, epithelization, and production of fibrin. The primary concern of the surgeon when the pancreas is healing is the reestablishment of the direction and flow of the pancreatic secretions and physiology of the production of the secretions.

LIVER

The **liver** is the second largest organ of the human body, located inferior to the diaphragm primarily in the right abdominal quadrant and weighing approximately 1,200 and 1,500 grams, which accounts for about 2% of the body weight of the adult. It is protected by several ribs and the organ extends from the level of the fifth intercostal space to the inferior margin of the ribs. The entire liver is covered by a fibrous and serous coat. The serous coat is derived from the peritoneum and underlying is the fibrous coat. This thin coat of connective tissue is called Glisson's capsule.

The liver is divided into two unequal lobes, right and left lobes, by the falciform ligament. The ligament is a fold of visceral peritoneum that not only separates the liver into lobes but attaches the organ to the diaphragm and abdominal wall anteriorly. The liver has two additional small lobes, the quadrate lobe located next to the gallbladder and the caudate lobe located next to the vena cava that are contained in the right lobe. A surgical anatomic landmark, called the porta hepatis, is the region where the right and left lobes meet and blood vessels and ducts enter or exit. On the superior side of the liver, another fold of visceral peritoneum called the coronary ligament anchors the organ to the diaphragm.

The cells of the liver, called **hepatocytes**, form the mass of hepatic lobules. These are the functional units of the liver, which are responsible for the production of **bile**. A duct referred to as the bile canal exits each lobule, and these ducts eventually join to form the right and left **hepatic ducts** that exit the liver. Bile is collected by the bile canals and travels to the hepatic ducts. The right and left hepatic ducts join to form the **common hepatic duct (CHD)**, which then joins with the cystic duct of the gallbladder to form the **common bile duct (CBD)**. The CBD is also joined by the duct of Wirsung from the pancreas. The purpose of the ducts is to allow bile to travel to the duodenum.

The liver is highly vascular and the vessels subdivide numerous times in order to provide the necessary blood supply. Injuries to the liver can produce hypovolemic shock in a short period of time, and, therefore, the surgical team must be prepared to control the bleeding with compression, cautery, and suture. The vessels are the hepatic artery, portal vein, and hepatic vein. The hepatic artery provides all the oxygen supply needed by the liver, carrying 25% of the blood into the liver. The portal vein provides nutrients to the liver and carries the other 75% of the blood to the liver. The area where the hepatic artery and portal vein enter the liver and the CHD exits is called the porta hepatis. The liver is drained by the right and left hepatic veins, which empty into the inferior vena cava.

Vascular openings, called hepatic sinusoids, are located throughout the liver tissue. The hepatic portal vein carries blood from the digestive tract into the liver and brings nutrients to the sinusoids. In addition, the hepatic artery carries oxygenated blood that also contains nutrients and as the blood flows through the liver, it nourishes the hepatocytes via the sinusoids.

The blood in the portal veins can contain bacteria that entered through the intestinal wall. Within the liver, large fixed cells called **Kupffer cells** remove the bacteria by the process of phagocytosis. The Kupffer cells also remove dead erythrocytes and leukocytes.

The nerves that innervate the liver are derived from the hepatic plexus of the sympathetic nervous system, from the pneumogastric nerves, and from the right phrenic. The primary lymphatic drainage is into the portal system.

The surgical team must be aware of the conditions that can produce changes in the anatomic position of the liver. Its position will change according to the position of the body. Therefore, when a patient is placed in the supine position, lying on the back with face up, or lateral position, lying on the side on the surgical table, the liver often recedes beneath the ribs. Disease conditions will change the postion of the liver. A patient with emphysema will have distended lungs and a low diaphragm, which push the liver downward. Tumors of other organs will have an effect on liver position, as well as the buildup of fluid in the thoracic or abdominal cavity due to trauma.

The functions of the liver are numerous. However, it is interesting to note that humans can live without a major portion of the liver. This is advantageous when a segmentectomy or lobectomy is performed to remove a diseased part of the liver. Another important feature of the liver is the ability of limited regeneration, much like the skin. The following is a list of the primary liver functions:

1. It is important in carbohydrate metabolism as it keeps the blood glucose level normal. Liver cells lower the blood glucose level by polymerizing glucose to glycogen and raise the blood glucose level by breaking down the glycogen molecules into glucose.
2. It converts protein and carbohydrate molecules into fat molecules. The blood transports the fat for storage as adipose tissue.
3. It synthesizes cholesterol, lipoproteins, and phospholipids.
4. It stores iron and vitamins A, D, and B_{12}.
5. Iron from the blood combines with the protein called apoferritin in liver cells to form what is called ferritin. The iron is stored in the liver as ferritin until the blood iron concentration has decreased to the level requiring the release of iron from the liver.
6. Most important, the liver contributes to protein metabolism. It is responsible for the hydrolysis (called deaminization) of amino acids and the conversion of certain types of amino acids to other needed amino acids.
7. It synthesizes heparin, an anticoagulant.
8. It synthesizes the proteins prothrombin and thrombin, which are needed for clotting when a person experiences a cut or other traumatic injury.
9. When proteins are broken down into amino acids, the amino acids are taken up by the mitochondria in the cells and synthesized into ATP. The process produces the toxic waste substance, ammonia. The liver cells are responsible for converting the ammonia to the harmless substance urea, which is excreted by the kidneys in the urine.
10. The liver is responsible for the metabolism of anesthetic drugs and gases. The anesthesia provider must be aware of the physiological status of the liver in order to make decisions related to the types of drugs given to the patient and the amount. For example, if a patient has cirrhosis, the ability of the liver to metabolize anesthetic gases and drugs is impaired, meaning the substances will remain in the body much longer as compared to a patient who has a healthy liver. The anesthesia provider will have to make adjustments to account for the patient's condition.
11. The hepatocytes form and secrete bile.

BOX 15-4

Liver Excisional Biopsy

The indications for a wedge resection include trauma to a small section of the liver, cysts, or tumors. Wedge resection is the removal of a small piece or section of the liver that is in the shape of a pie wedge. The incision employed by the surgeon is determined by the area of the liver to be excised. Most often a subcostal approach or midline approach is used. The patient is placed in a supine position. As with any procedure involving the liver, hemorrhage will be a concern; therefore, the surgical technologist must make sure to have enough suture, small vascular clamps, and chemical hemostatic agents. After the incision has been made and the liver exposed, the first step of the procedure involves placing sutures approximately 2 inches above the edge of the lesion. Using the knife and suction electrocautery, the lesion is removed with at least 1 inch of healthy tissue to ensure that all of the lesion or any migrating cells from the lesion are removed. The specimen is sent to the pathologist to confirm that all of the lesion has been excised. After hemostasis has been achieved, the previously placed sutures are tied to approximate the wound.

Bile is yellowish-green in color and contains cholesterol, bile pigments, bile salts, and a small amount of electrolytes. Bile salts are the most abundant and are the only substance in bile that have a digestive function. The only function of the cholesterol is in the production of bile salts. The hepatocytes release cholesterol to produce bile salts, and consequently in the process the cholesterol is released into the bile. Bilirubin is the primary bile pigment, which is produced from the breakdown of hemoglobin from erythrocytes. It is a normal component of bile; however, an excessive production of the pigment produces the condition known as jaundice, which is characterized by the yellowish color of the skin, sclerae of the eyes, and mucous membranes.

Healing of the Liver

As previously mentioned, the liver is highly vascular. When surgery is performed, the vessels, especially the arteries, must be ligated (the process of using a suture strand with or without a needle to tie off a blood vessel) as surgery progresses. Additional difficulty with controlling hemorrhage is encountered when the liver has sustained a traumatic injury or wound. Occasionally, due to the severity of the trauma and inability to control the hemorrhage, a wedge resection, lobectomy, or segmentectomy is performed in the area of the injury.

The liver tissue is exceptionally **friable**, since the organ, as compared to other body organs, has little connective tissue. Sutures are placed widely apart with little tension and not deep in the tissue. The suture of choice is absorbable with a relatively short absorption rate, since the liver tissue tends to heal quickly, and in the absence of hemorrhage, small-size sutures can be used. Other methods of hemostasis must be available to control bleeding. The raw surface of the liver can also be repaired by using an absorbable mesh that is sutured in place or by placing a piece of omentum over the area of the wound and tacking it in place with sutures.

GALLBLADDER

The **gallbladder** is a pear-shaped sac located in a fossa on the inferior surface of the right lobe of the liver above the transverse colon (Figures 15-12 and 15-13). It is approximately 8–9 cm long and can store about 50

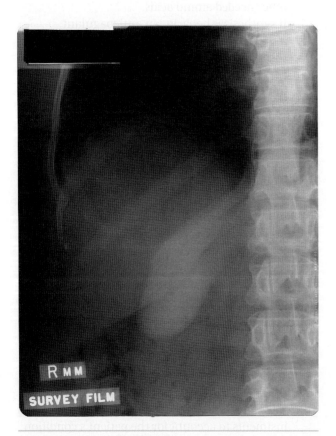

FIGURE 15-12 Gallbladder

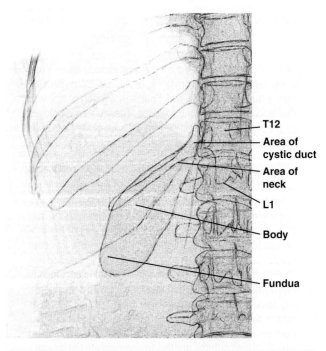

T12

Area of cystic duct

Area of neck

L1

Body

Fundua

FIGURE 15-13 Gallbladder

mL of bile. The organ is divided into a fundus, body, and neck. The neck is attached to the liver by loose connective tissue. Enlargement of the neck of the gallbladder due to the collection of a stone or stones forms a pouch called **Hartmann's pouch**. The fundus is rounded and lies anterior to and extends slightly past the edge of the liver. It is the portion of the gallbladder that can be palpated during a physical examination. The body is attached to the inferior surface of the liver and lies near the superior portion of the duodenum.

The gallbladder is held in position by peritoneum, which is continuous with the liver. During a cholecystectomy, surgical removal of the gallbladder, the surgeon must meticulously dissect the peritoneum to free up the gallbladder. The **cystic artery** and **cystic duct** are important anatomic structures associated with the gallbladder. The cystic duct exits the gallbladder and joins the common hepatic duct, which exits the liver to form the common bile duct (CBD). During surgery the surgeon must identify the cystic artery and duct. The surgeon will use an imaginary anatomic landmark called the **triangle of Calot** to locate the cystic artery. The boundaries of the triangle are the cystic duct, common hepatic duct, and inferior border to the liver, and the cystic artery is often located within the triangle.

The cystic duct is usually 1–8 cm in length, and the circumference will vary from 4–12 mm. The mucosal layer of the cystic duct has several folds that appear as a spiral valve, called the valves of Heister, which aid in controlling the flow of bile into and out of the gallbladder (Caruthers & Price, 2001). The CBD will vary in length from 6–20 cm, and the circumference is approximately 10 mm in diameter. The mucosal layer is continuous with the cystic duct. The distal portion of the CBD travels behind the superior border of the head of the pancreas and passes through the parenchyma of the pancreas to join with the duct of Wirsung to form the ampulla of Vater.

It is important for the surgical team to remember the anatomic variations that can occur with the ampulla of Vater and duct of Wirsung. In approximately 10%–15% of the population, the ampulla and duct will be separately attached to the duodenum and therefore have separate openings. In addition, the openings can occur at any point along the duodenum.

The gallbladder has four coats: serous, subserosal, muscular, and mucosa. The serous coat derives from the peritoneum; it completely invests the fundus but covers only the inferior surface of the body and neck. The subserosal layer is composed of connective and adipose tissue. The muscular layer is a thin, strong layer that covers the entire gallbladder. It is composed

BOX 15-5
Laparoscopic Cholecystectomy

Cholecystectomy, removal of the gallbladder, is performed primarily due to the presence of gallstones that have caused cholecystitis, but is occasionally necessary due to a malignancy or presence of polyps. The patient will often experience severe pain that radiates to the front of the abdomen, right side, and back. The gallbladder can be removed through the laparoscope and is the standard procedure. The patient is placed in the supine position. A small incision is made at the umbilicus to allow the insertion of the Veress needle through which carbon dioxide is pumped to distend the abdominal cavity. The needle is removed and a trocar is placed; a laparoscope is inserted through the trocar. Three other small incisions are made and trocars are placed through which the special laparoscopic instruments can be inserted to retract, dissect, and remove the gallbladder. The gallbladder is grasped at the fundus and pulled upward; the cystic artery and duct are identified. At this time, if indicated, a cholangiogram will be performed to confirm if stones are present or not present in the common bile duct. A small incision is made in the cystic duct, and a small catheter is inserted into the duct toward the common bile duct.

Dye is injected through the catheter into the common bile duct. X-rays are taken and will show if stones are present in the CBD. If present, the stones are removed from the CBD. Once the cholangiogram has been completed, the cystic artery and duct are ligated with clips. The gallbladder is dissected from its attachment to the liver using a special laparoscopic instrument in which the tip is shaped like a hook, and it is connected to electrocautery to achieve hemostasis while cutting. Electrocautery, also called the bovie machine, is an electrical unit that sends electric current to the laparoscopic instrument, heating the tip so as to cauterize or close bleeding vessels with the use of heat, or in this case, to dissect tissue. Once the gallbladder is dissected free, it is placed in a bag to prevent the contents from spilling and removed through the umbilical trocar. The four small incisions, each ranging in length from 1 to $1\frac{1}{2}$ inches, are closed with suture.

of smooth muscle fibers that interlace and run in all directions. The mucosa is the inner layer that is connected to the fibrous coat. It is yellowish-brown with mucosal folds, similar to the rugae of the stomach, which allows the gallbladder to extend when bile enters.

The blood is supplied to the gallbladder by the cystic artery, right hepatic artery, and superior portion of the pancreaticoduodenal artery. The veins that drain the upper biliary tree and gallbladder flow into the liver. The veins that drain the inferior biliary tree and portion of the gallbladder flow into the portal vein. The lymphatics follow the pathway of the venous system collecting at the lymph nodes around the cystic duct, then join the pancreatic lymphatics and travel to the lymph nodes of the porta hepatis.

The nerve innervation is as follows:

1. Parasympathetic innervation: derived from the myenteric and submucosal plexuses.
2. Sympathetic innervation: derived from the splanchnic nerve and hepatic plexus.
3. The nerves have both sensory and motor functions and communicate with the right phrenic nerves.

The functions of the gallbladder are to serve as a storage area for bile until it is needed for digestive purposes in the small intestine, concentrate the bile during storage by reabsorbing water, and release the bile for entrance into the duodenum when stimulated by the hormone cholecystokinin, which originates from the small intestine. The common bile duct attaches to the duodenum. The bile enters the

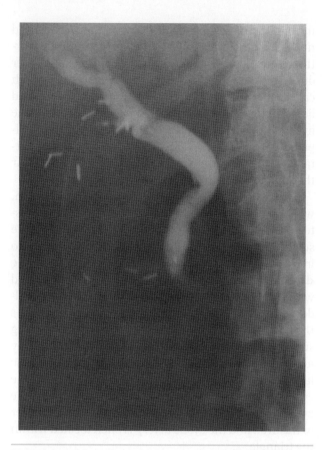

FIGURE 15-15   Operative cholangiogram with stones

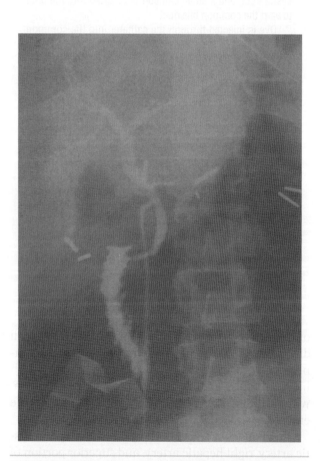

FIGURE 15-14   Normal operative cholangiogram

duodenum through the ampulla of Vater. The opening of the ampulla is controlled by the sphincter of Oddi, which is formed of a thick coat of longitudinal and circular muscle to control the flow of bile into the duodenum. When the sphincter is contracted, the bile flows back into the gallbladder and vice versa when the sphincter is open.

As previously mentioned, the bile becomes concentrated as the inner lining of the gallbladder reabsorbs water and electrolytes. One consequence of this physiological action is that the cholesterol will separate from the bile and form gallstones (Figures 15-14 and 15-15). The gallstones can block the flow of bile from the gallbladder into the CBD, leading to possible cholecystitis and pain in the upper right quadrant that radiates to the back. In addition, because the bile is static, it serves as an excellent medium for the growth of bacteria, which could lead to a serious infection of the gallbladder and biliary tree. An anatomic feature of the gallstone condition to be considered by the surgical team is that the cystic duct will appear on x-ray to exit the gallbladder on the left side rather than at the apex of the organ.

Cholecystokinin is released by the mucosa of the small intestine in response to the presence of proteins and fats in the intestine. The hormone travels in the bloodstream to the gallbladder, causing it to contract to push bile into the CBD. The peristalsis of the duodenum causes the sphincter of Oddi to relax and the bile to enter the duodenum.

Healing of the Biliary Tract

The cystic and common bile ducts heal quickly. For example, as long as stones are not present in the gallbladder or they can be treated with extracorporeal shock-wave lithotripsy, a surgeon may perform a CBD exploration to remove stones that are in the duct. The duct will be closed with small-diameter absorbable suture. Because the biliary ducts and gallbladder are prone to crystal formation, suture can precipitate the formation of stones. The use of absorbable suture to close the tissue for healing helps to avoid the formation of stones. The healing of the ducts is primarily by reepithelization and fibrous protein synthesis, which occurs rapidly.

SMALL INTESTINE

The processes of digestion and absorption occur primarily in the **small intestine** (Figure 15-16). The small intestine begins at the pyloric sphincter and ends at the beginning of the colon, taking a twisting and tortuous course and filling much of the space in the abdominal cavity. The small intestine is divided into three sections: duodenum, jejunum, and ileum. Overall it is approximately 5–7 m in length and the diameter of the lumen is 3–6 cm.

The blood supply to the small intestine is complex and requires several branches of the superior mesenteric artery (Caruthers & Price, 2001). The arterial blood supply to the duodenum is from the right gastric and gastroepiploic, supraduodenal and superior and inferior pancreaticoduodenal branches of the gastroduodenal and hepatic arteries. Venous drainage is to the splenic, portal, and superior mesenteric veins. The jejunum and ileum are supplied by the jejunal and ileal arteries, which are branches of the superior mesenteric artery. The venous drainage is to the superior mesenteric vein.

The nerve supply to the small intestine is from the celiac plexus, thoracic splanchnic, and vagus nerves. The nerves stimulate or inhibit peristalsis and sphincter reaction, and stimulate the small intestine to release digestive secretions. Lymph drainage is

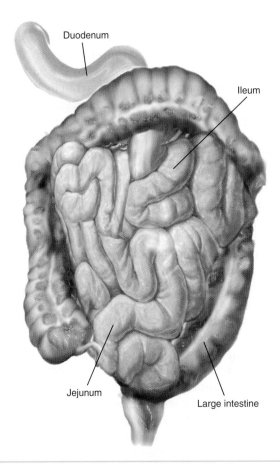

FIGURE 15-16   The small intestine

from the muscularis and mucosa and drains into the mesentery.

The duodenum is approximately 30 cm in length and has no mesentery. It is subdivided into four sections. The first portion, approximately 5 cm long, is called the duodenal cap and is continuous from the pylorus. There are two unique features of the cap. First, it contains longitudinal mucosal folds as compared to the rest of the small intestine, which has transverse mucosal folds. Second, it is covered with peritoneum, whereas the rest of the duodenum is not covered. The peritoneum forms the hepatoduodenal ligament within which is located the hepatic artery, portal vein, and CBD. The cap is the area where peptic ulcers most often occur.

The second portion is approximately 12 cm long and is located retroperitoneally, descending slightly to the right of the midline from the first to the third lumbar vertebrae and is situated close to the medial border of the pancreas. The second portion is where the transverse mucosal folds begin. The third portion is approximately 15 cm in length, located retroperitoneally, and travels in a horizontal fashion at the level of the third lumbar vertebra. It travels over the inferior vena cava and abdominal aorta. The last portion of the duodenum travels upward, forward, and to the left of the aorta below the level of the pancreas. The end of the fourth portion is marked by the **ligament of Treitz**, which indicates the beginning of the jejunum. The ligament of Treitz is an important surgical landmark for surgeons performing abdominal surgery, in particular when trauma or pathological conditions have obscured the normal anatomy.

The jejunum is approximately 8 feet in length and lies in the left upper portion of the abdominal cavity. The jejunum can be distinguished from the ileum because the diameter of the lumen is greater and its wall is thicker. The ileum is about 12 feet in length, located in the right abdomen and pelvis, and is distinguished from the jejunum by its smaller diameter and is more vascular. It connects to the cecum of the colon at the **ileocecal valve**. The layers of the small intestine are from the outside to the inside serosa, muscular, submucosa, and mucosa. The serosa is derived from the peritoneum. The muscular has two layers of fibers, longitudinal and circular. The submucosa connects the muscular layer with the mucosal layer. The mucosa is a thick, highly vascular layer.

As previously mentioned, the small intestine is the organ that carries out the major portion of digestion. Three structures aid in increasing the absorptive sur-

---

BOX 15-7

Bowel Technique During Surgery

The small intestine and colon are reservoirs for bacteria. The bacteria that live in the GI tract are known as opportunistic bacteria. They are actually needed for necessary functions within the bowel, but given the opportunity can cause an infection. One type of well-known resident bacteria of the bowel is *Escherichia coli*. When bowel surgery is performed, the surgerical team must be very careful not to allow the contents of the open bowel to spill into the abdominal cavity. If this occurs, there is a good chance the patient will experience a postoperative infection due to the opportunistic bacteria that were allowed to enter the cavity. Precautions the surgical technologist takes to prevent infection are called bowel technique. The bowel instruments that have come into contact with the open bowel will not be used on any other portion of the body; for instance, they will not be used for closure of the surgical wound. Even though the open end of the bowel is clamped with an instrument, it should be held upward and not downward to prevent spillage of bowel contents. After the bowel has been closed, the surgical team, at the minimum, should change their sterile gloves; occasionally the team will also change their sterile gowns. By strictly following the principles of bowel technique and aseptic technique, the chances of the patient acquiring a postoperative infection are greatly reduced.

BOX 15-6

Small-Bowel Resection

Removal of a portion of the small bowel is more frequently performed during the course of another primary procedure such as partial gastrectomy, or treatment of tumors of nearby organs or diverticulitis. Occasionally resection is performed for tumors, mesenteric infarctions, or other pathologies. This discussion will concentrate on the removal of a portion of the small bowel due to a tumor. The surgeon will make a midline incision over the area of bowel to be removed. The portion of the bowel to be excised is mobilized from its attachments to the posterior abdominal wall. The mesentery is divided and vascular structures are ligated as well. Two clamps are placed over the small bowel approximately 10 cm proximal to the tumor and two other clamps are placed 10 cm distal. The knife is used to excise the portion of the small intestine to be removed by cutting between the two clamps on each end. The two ends of the small intestine are brought together and a two-layer anastomosis is achieved using suture.

---

face area of the small intestine; the plicae circulares, villi, and microvilli (Figure 15-17). The inner lining of the small intestine contains numerous folds of mucosa that are circular in shape called plicae circulares. They are more numerous and better developed in the distal portion of the duodenum and proximal portion of the jejunum.

Also throughout the inner lining are thousands of minute projections called **villi**. These vastly increase the surface area of the epithelium for absorption of nutrients by projecting into the lumen of the small intestine so as to make contact with digestive contents. They are most numerous in the duodenum and proximal portion of the jejunum. Each villus is approximately 0.5 to 1 mm in length and is composed of the following:

1. Outer layer of simple columnar epithelium.
2. One venule to transport nutrients.
3. One arteriole to pick up nutrients.
4. A lymphatic capillary called a **lacteal** to pick up fats.

into the mucous membrane of the small intestine called intestinal glands or crypts of Lieberkühn. The simple epithelial lining of the glands is continuous with the villus. The glands secrete a watery-like fluid that has a neutral pH and contains no digestive enzymes. However, the villi absorb the fluid to aid in the transport of digestive products into the villi.

Two other important secreting structures are goblet cells and Brunner's glands, also called duodenal glands and mucus-secreting glands. The goblet cells are located in the simple columnar epithelium throughout the small intestine and Brunner's glands are located in the submucosa of the duodenum and proximal portion of the jejunum. Both of these structures secrete large quantities of alkaline mucus, which protects the inner walls of the small intestine from being destroyed by the enzymes and acids found in the chyme.

The other secretions of the intestine come from the epithelial cells in the mucosal membrane of the microvilli, which secrete various enzymes responsible for breaking down the food particles before absorption can take place. The following are the enzymes and their action:

1. Lipase: Breaks down fat molecules into glycerol and fatty acids
2. Enterokinase: Changes trypsinogen to trypsin
3. Peptidase: Splits peptides into amino acids
4. Sucrase, maltase, lactase: Breaks down the disaccharides (double sugars) sucrose, lactose, and maltose into monosaccharides (simple sugars)

Brunner's glands are stimulated to secrete mucus by mechanical stimulation of the stomach and small intestine, and by the presence of acidic irritants such as gastric juice. Goblet cells and crypts of Lieberkühn are stimulated by contact with chyme. The other small-intestine secretions such as the enzymes are released due to the nerve plexuses being activated by distention of the small-intestine wall. This activation stimulates the parasympathetic response that activates the release of the small-intestine secretions.

Just like the stomach, the small intestine moves the digested food forward by peristalsis. Parasympathetic impulses stimulate peristalsis and sympathetic impulses inhibit them. Peristalsis is stimulated by food entering the stomach and chyme entering the duodenum. If the small intestine becomes overdistended, the peristaltic waves can be very strong, quickly propelling the food through the small intestine. When this occurs, the water, electrolytes, and nutrients that are usually absorbed are not and the result is diarrhea.

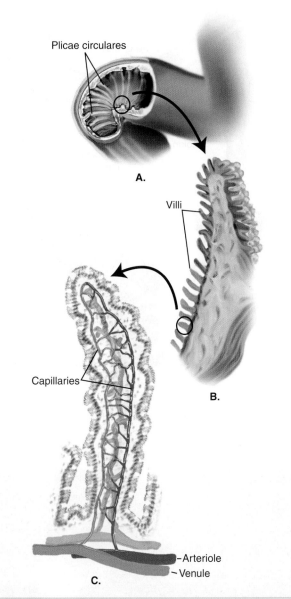

FIGURE 15-17   Structures of absorption in the small intestine: (A) plicae circulares; (B) villi; and (C) capillaries

5. On the surface of the epithelium are fine extensions called microvilli, which give a villus a brush border that further increases the absorption ability of the small intestine.

The nutrients pass through the simple epithelial cells and then pass through the endothelial cells of the capillary walls. Within the lacteal, the nutrients enter the blood and lymphatic circulatory systems to be delivered to the cells of the body. The activity of the villi are stimulated or inhibited by nerve fibers.

Finally, there are the tubular pouches located between the bases of each villi and extending downward

The ileocecal valve is normally contracted to prevent contents from the ileum from entering the colon, but also to prevent the contents of the colon from reflux into the ileum. However, the peristalsis stimulates the valve to relax and allow contents of the small intestine to enter the cecum. The valve is composed of two valvular folds of mucous membrane that project into the colon with a narrow aperture. The valve is approximately 15 cm diagonal to the ligament of Treitz, and this area is important when evaluating a patient for bowel obstruction.

Healing of the Small Intestine

The small intestine heals rapidly, usually achieving preoperative tissue strength in approximately two to three weeks. Probably because of a better blood supply, the digestive contents are more liquified, the muscular layer is stronger and better developed, and there is a lower bacterial count, surgical wounds of the small intestine tend to heal predictably and with fewer complications as compared to the colon.

The most frequent complication of healing is obstruction, usually due to the technique of anastomosis, which is the surgical rejoining of bowel segments following the removal of a section of bowel wherein the two ends need to be rejoined, in which the diameter of the lumen has been decreased. This can occur when the inverted closure technique is utilized and the cuff of tissue protrudes into the lumen causing the obstruction. Absorbable suture is most often used, although nonabsorbable suture is occasionally used in the serosal-to-serosal layer closure.

COLON AND RECTUM

The **colon** is approximately 1 m to $1\frac{1}{2}$ m in length and the diameter ranges from 2–8 cm. The colon begins at the right side of the abdominal cavity traveling upward and across to the left, then downward to end at the opening of the anus. It is divided into seven portions: cecum, ascending colon, transverse colon, descending colon, sigmoid colon, rectum, and anal canal (Figures 15-18, 15-19, and 15-20). The colon has four coats: serosa, muscular, submucosa, and mucosa. The mucosal layer is different from that of the small intestine, since it contains more goblet cells and does not have villi. The submucosa contains a complex network of veins, arteries, lymph vessels, and nerve plexus of Meissner. The muscular layer consists of a series of circular rings.

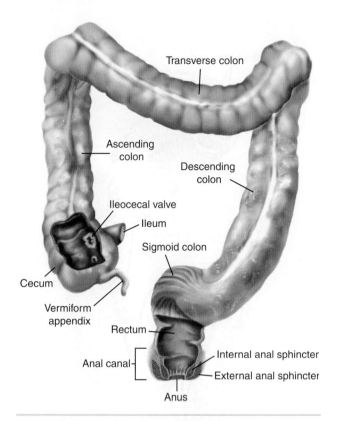

FIGURE 15-18 **The large intestine**

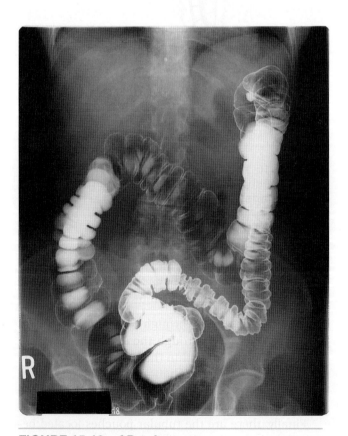

FIGURE 15-19 **AP colon**

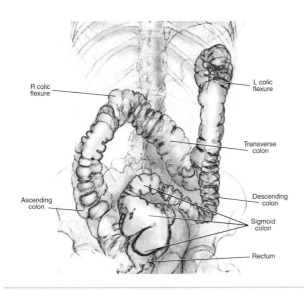

R colic
flexure

L colic
flexure

Transverse
colon

Ascending
colon

Descending
colon

Sigmoid
colon

Rectum

FIGURE 15-20 AP colon

A distinguishing feature of the colon is a series of pouches called **haustrae**. The layer of longitudinal muscle fibers are separated into the three bands called tenia coli that extend the entire length of the colon. The longitudinal tension of the bands on the wall of the colon creates the series of haustrae.

The primary functions of the colon are the absorption of water and electrolytes to condense the feces in preparation for expulsion, production of vitamin K by the bacteria within the organ, and expulsion of the feces; therefore, the colon basically has no digestive functions. However, throughout the mucous mem-

brane lining of the colon are many tubular glands composed of goblet cells that secrete mucus, the only secretion of the organ. Chyme and parasympathetic impulses stimulate the production of the mucus. The mucus is important for the following reasons:

1. It lubricates the inner wall to protect the intestinal tissue from the abrasive materials passing through.
2. It is alkaline, so it controls the pH level of the digestive content, which can be acidic due to the bacterial activity.
3. It aids in holding the pieces of fecal matter together

The blood supply to the cecum, ascending colon, and right portion of the transverse colon is from the ileocolic, right, and middle colic branches of the superior mesenteric artery. The left portion of the transverse colon, descending colon, sigmoid colon, and rectum are supplied by the sigmoid, superior left colic, and superior rectal branches of the inferior mesenteric artery. The veins have the same names as the arteries. The mesentery contains several lymph nodes and the lymphatic drainage of the colon is next to the arterial blood supply. The lymph fluid from the nodes drains into the cysterna chyli near the aorta.

The nerve supply is sympathetic and parasympathetic. The innervation is from the following plexuses:

1. Superior hypogastric
2. Inferior hypogastric
3. Celiac
4. Intermesenteric
5. Superior mesenteric

In addition, nerve fibers from the vagus nerve, splanchnic, and third and fourth sacral nerves innervate the colon.

The **cecum** is the first portion of the colon located in the lower right quadrant. It is about 7 cm in length and wider than most of the other sections of the colon. The cecum is very mobile, since it has no mesenteric attachment and is held in position by the peritoneum. At the superior portion of the cecum is the location of the ileocecal valve and indicates the joining of the ileum to the colon. Attached to the cecum is the vermiform **appendix**. The appendix is a short blind tube, about 7–15 cm in length when not inflamed. It is attached to the cecum by a fold of peritoneum called the mesoappendix, which contains the appendiceal artery. There is no known function of the appendix, but at one time during the evolution of the human species it may have functioned in the some capacity in the digestive system. It often becomes

BOX 15-8

Colonoscopy

Colonoscopy is a diagnostic procedure performed to confirm a diagnosis such as a tumor or diverticulitis, but tissue and fluid samples can be obtained through the colonoscope with the use of specialized endoscopic surgical instrumentation. Colonoscopy involves viewing the colon from the rectum to the cecum. If more of the colon needs to be examined, a sigmoidoscopy is performed using a flexible sigmoidscope. The patient is placed either on their side (lateral position) or jackknife (patient lies facedown on a table, which is flexed in the middle to raise the buttocks). The tip of the endoscope is inserted through the anus and advanced by the surgeon. As the endoscope is being withdrawn, the surgeon is examining the bowel. As mentioned, instruments such as biopsy forceps, cytology brush, or irrigating tube can be used to obtain specimens.

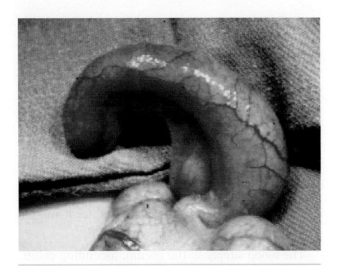

Figure 15-21 Appendicitis (Courtesy of The Division of Pediatric Surgery, Brown Medical School, Providence, RI)

inflamed and infected, in particular when feces become impacted within the tube requiring an appendectomy to be performed (Figure 15-21). The appendix often is difficult for the surgeon to remove, since it is frequently situated upward and inward behind the cecum, known as **retrocecal**. The mesoappendix must be dissected during the course of surgery to free up the appendix prior to removal.

The **ascending colon** is approximately 15–20 cm in length, beginning at the ileocecal valve, traveling upward along the right side of the abdominal cavity, and ending at the hepatic flexure. It is held in place by peritoneum to the posterior abdominal wall and a fold of peritoneum that extends downward for the hepatorenal ligament supports the hepatic flexure.

The **transverse colon** is the longest portion at 40–50 cm and the most mobile section of the colon. It begins at the hepatic flexure, travels across the top of the abdominal cavity in a slight upward curve, and ends at the splenic flexure. It is attached to the undersurface of the diaphragm by the phrenocolic ligament, which is also responsible for providing support to the spleen, thereby pulling the transverse colon slightly upward to create the splenic flexure. A portion of the peritoneum called the transverse mesocolon attaches the posterior side of the transverse colon to the spine. The hepatic flexure is at such an extreme angle that the end of the transverse colon often overlaps the anterior portion of the descending colon making it difficult to examine abdominal x-rays (Caruthers & Price, 2001). It is important for the surgical team to know the various flexures and ligaments that serve as important anatomic landmarks during abdominal surgery.

The **descending colon** is about 25–30 cm in length, beginning at the splenic flexure, traveling downward along the left lateral abdominal cavity toward the pelvic cavity. Only about two thirds of the anterior surface of the descending colon is covered with peritoneum and other support comes from being directly attached to the posterior abdominal wall.

The **sigmoid colon** varies considerably in length and is held in place by a fold of peritoneum called the iliac mesocolon. The name sigmoid comes from the S shape, aiding in identification, in addition to the easily identified epiploic appendices that are filled with fat located on the serosal layer (Caruthers & Price, 2001). The sigmoid flexure is the narrowest part of the colon. The sigmoid commences at the end of the descending colon, approximately at the margin of the crest of the ilium, and terminates at the rectum. The sigmoid is the most frequent site of colon cancer and **volvulus**.

The **rectum** is approximately 10–15 cm long (Figures 15-22 and 15-23). The rectum descends in an anteroposterior curve called the sacral flexure, passing into the pelvic cavity to join the anal canal. It is situated anterior to the sacrum and coccyx. A key

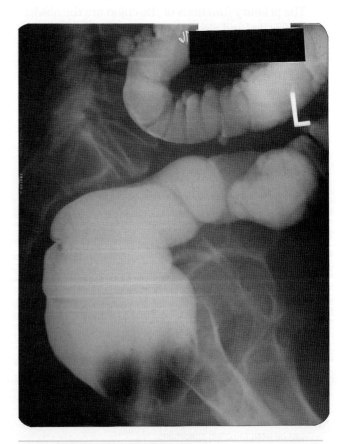

FIGURE 15-22 Lateral rectum

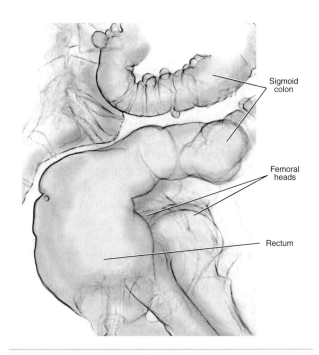

Sigmoid colon

Femoral heads

Rectum

FIGURE 15-23   Lateral rectum

identifying feature of the rectum is that the tenia organization of the longitudinal coat, which is found throughout the colon, now changes to a continuous layer of muscle that envelops the rectum.

The last 2–4 cm of the colon is the **anal canal** and opens to the exterior of the body through the **anus**. Two sphincter muscles are located around the anus, the internal sphincter composed of involuntary smooth muscle, which is supported by the levator ani muscles, and the external sphincter composed of voluntary skeletal muscle. Within the lining of the anal canal, the mucous-secreting columnar epithelium changes to stratified squamous epithelium. The mucous membrane of the anal canal is arranged into several longitudinal folds called anal columns that contain arteries and veins. The anal valves are situated just above the anus and just superior to these valves are the **anal sinuses**, which can become compacted with fecal matter, leading to the formation of abscesses.

The three mechanical movements of the colon are peristalsis, haustral churning, and mass peristalsis. The peristaltic waves of the colon, as compared to the small intestine, are different in that they do not occur as frequently. The peristaltic waves produce mass peristalsis, which is a strong peristaltic wave that begins in the transverse colon and vigorously pushes the intestinal contents forward into the rectum.

When the chyme has been in the colon for approximately two to eight hours, it has become a semisolid mass due to the absorption of water and electrolytes, and is known as feces. Feces are composed primarily of water, but also contain inorganic salts, mucus, electrolytes, and bacteria, in particular, *E. coli,* a normal inhabitant of the intestine that feeds on undigested materials. The odor of feces is from products of bacterial action, including phenol, ammonia, and hydrogen sulfide gas, which produces the "rotten egg" odor. Undigested materials are also found in the feces, such as fiber from eating vegetables and fruits.

The mass peristalsis pushes the feces into the rectum and initiates the defecation reflex. As the feces fill the rectum, its walls distend, stimulating pressure-sensitive receptors also located in the rectal wall and sending an impulse to the nervous system to begin the reflex action. This also stimulates other reactions:

1. Peristaltic waves occur in the descending colon.
2. The internal sphincter relaxes involuntarily.
3. The abdominal muscles contract.
4. The external sphincter is relaxed.

When all of this has taken place the individual can defecate, the act of forcing the feces from the rectum through the anus to the outside of the body. A person can also voluntarily contract the external sphincter, since it is composed of skeletal muscle, to inhibit defecation.

Healing of the Colon and Rectum

The knowledge of the tissue layers of the colon and rectum is highly important during surgery. Many surgeons prefer to use a double-layer closure of the colon. For example, when an end-to-end anastomosis is being performed, many surgeons will use a continuous 3-0 absorbable suture for the mucosa-to-mucosa portion of the anastomosis. The intestine is everted to facilitate the placement of the sutures on the back wall of the intestine, and 3-0 silk interrupted suture is often used for the closure of the serosa. Silk suture is also used when a colostomy is performed. A colostomy is when an opening is created in the skin and an opening in the colon is sutured to the skin opening. The colostomy can be temporary or permanent. The colon heals at about the same rate as the stomach.

The rectum is slow healing. The lower portion is posterior to the pelvic peritoneum and therefore has no serosa. Absorbable suture is used for an anastomosis and the muscle layer is included due to the absence of the serosa. The surgeon also takes care when tying the sutures to avoid cutting through the tissues.

BASIC NUTRITION INFORMATION

The cells and tissues of the body rely on the food that is ingested by a person in order to carry out their daily duties to maintain homeostasis. The food should be nutritious and the individual should have a well-balanced diet. In order for proper cell functioning to take place, the intake of the following nutrients is important:

- water
- carbohydrates
- proteins
- minerals
- lipids
- vitamins

Water is one of the most important components to maintaining life. In humans it comprises approximately 50%–65% of the total body weight. Water must be replaced on a daily basis due to loss through respiration, evaporation, and excretion by sweating. Many diseases can also deplete the body of water, in particular those that involve vomiting. Important functions of water include:

1. It aids in controlling normal body temperature by evaporation from the surface of the skin.
2. It acts as a solvent during biochemical reactions within the body.
3. Within the blood and lymph vessels, it contributes to the fluid level to aid in transporting material to the cells of the body.

Carbohydrates include monosaccharides, disaccharides, and polysaccharides. Monosaccharides are carbohydrates that are small enough molecules to be transported through the cell wall and into the cell for use as energy. The other carbohydrates must be broken down into smaller molecules in order to be used by the body.

Carbohydrates are the primary source of energy. Excess carbohydrates are stored as reserve energy in the form of fat in adipose tissue. Nutrition experts recommend that 50%– 60% of the daily intake of calories be carbohydrates. **Calorie** is defined as the amount of heat required to raise the temperature of 1 gram of water by 1°C. The calorie content of any type of food is measured by the amount of heat that is released when the food is burned. One thousand calories is equal to a kilocalorie. The average adult requires approximately 1,500 to 3,000 kilocalories per day; the number depends on the person's weight, age, sex, and amount of physical activity.

Proteins are synthesized within the cytoplasm of the cell from amino acid molecules and contain an amino group. Proteins have many functions in the body; two of the most important are that they are critical to the growth and repair of various types of body tissue and that they are enzymes that stimulate or inhibit chemical reactions within the body.

Not all amino acids can be synthesized by the body; those that can't be made by the body are called essential amino acids. Proteins that contain all of the essential amino acids are called complete proteins; meat, milk, and eggs are some of the foods that contain these complete proteins. Proteins that do not contain all of the essential amino acids are called incomplete proteins; vegetables are just one example of food that contains incomplete proteins.

The human body cannot store excess amino acids. The leftover amino acids are broken down by the liver and excreted in the urine as a nitrogenous waste product called **urea**. Because protein synthesis cannot take place with any of the amino acids missing, it is important that a source of complete protein be ingested with the diet. Nutrition experts recommend the daily intake of protein calories should be no more than 15%–20%.

Minerals are a chemical element obtained from the food humans eat. They are important for normal human growth and maintenance. Some of the more important minerals include iron, sodium, phosphorus, calcium, and potassium.

The term *trace elements* indicates that these elements are needed in only small amounts in the body. Examples of trace elements include zinc, iodine, cobalt, selenium, fluorine, copper, and manganese. Minerals and trace elements, as mentioned, are sufficiently present in the diet of the average human in the United States and do not usually require supplementation except in the cases of disease, old age, or pregnancy. Refer to Table 15-1 for a summary of the essential minerals and trace elements.

Lipids are composed of fatty acids combined with an alcohol. There are two groups of lipids: simple lipids, which include fats and oils, and compound lipids, which include phospholipids and glycolipids. This section of the discussion concentrates on fats and oils (simple lipids).

As previously mentioned, fats are a source of energy, but excess fats are stored in the fat cells of the body in adipose tissue and represent stored energy. Fats are an essential part of the diet. Stored fat is a source of energy during times of emergency such as a debilitating sickness whereby an individual has a deficient caloric intake. Other important functions include:

1. Fats aid in the formation of bile.
2. They aid in the formation of some steroid hormones.

TABLE 15-1 Summary of Essential Minerals and Trace Elements Needed for Health

MINERAL	FOOD SOURCES	FUNCTION	DEFICIENCY DISEASES
Calcium	Milk, cheese, dark green vegetables, dried legumes, sardines, shellfish	Bone and tooth formation Blood clotting Nerve transmission	Stunted growth Rickets Osteoporosis Convulsions
Chlorine	Common table salt, seafood, milk, meat, eggs	Formation of gastric juices Acid–base balance	Muscle cramps Mental apathy Poor appetite
Chromium	Fats, vegetable oils, meats, clams, whole-grain cereals	Involved in energy and glucose metabolism	Increased ability to metabolize glucose
Copper	Drinking water, liver, shellfish, whole grains, cherries, legumes, kidney, poultry, oysters, nuts, chocolate	Constituent of enzymes Involved with iron transport	Anemia
Fluorine	Drinking water, tea, coffee, seafood, rice, spinach, onions, lettuce	Maintenance of bone and tooth structure	Higher frequency of tooth decay
Iodine	Marine fish and shellfish, dairy products, many vegetables, iodized salt	Constituent of thyroid hormones	Goiter (enlarged thyroid)
Iron	Liver, lean meats, legumes, whole grains, dark green vegetables, eggs, dark molasses, shrimp, oysters	Constituent of hemoglobin Involved in energy metabolism	Iron-deficiency anemia
Magnesium	Whole grains, green leafy vegetables, nuts, meats, milk, legumes	Involved in energy conversions and enzyme function	Growth failure Behavioral disturbances Weakness Spasms
Phosphorus	Milk, cheese, meat, fish, poultry, whole grains, legumes, nuts	Bone and tooth formation Acid–base balance Involved in energy metabolism	Weakness Demineralization of bone
Potassium	Meats, milk, fruits, legumes, vegetables	Acid–base balance Body water balance Nerve transmission	Muscular weakness Paralysis
Selenium	Fish, poultry, meats, grains, milk, vegetables (depending on amount in soil)	Necessary for vitamin E function	Anemia Deficiency is rare
Sodium	Common table salt, seafood, most other foods except fruit	Acid–base balance Body water balance Nerve transmission	Muscle cramps Mental apathy
Sulfur	Meat, fish, poultry, eggs, milk, cheese, legumes, nuts	Constituent of certain tissue proteins	Related to deficiencies of sulfur-containing amino acids
Zinc	Milk, liver, shellfish, herring, wheat bran	Involved many enzyme systems Necessary for vitamin A metabolism	Growth failure Lack of sexual maturity Impaired wound healing Poor appetite

3. Fats contain fat-soluble vitamins that are important to the diet.
4. They are one of several components of the cell membrane.

It is recommended that the total daily intake of fat should not exceed 25%–30% of the daily caloric intake.

Cholesterol is a type of fat that is ingested with foods such as eggs, meat, and cheese. Much of the information pertaining to cholesterol seems to be negative; however, it is an essential component of the diet as long as foods high in cholesterol are not eaten in excess. Cholesterol is important in the manufacturing of body cells and synthesizing of certain hormones. But because cholesterol is not digested, it is important

TABLE 15-2   Summary of Major Vitamins Needed in the Human Diet

VITAMIN	FOOD SOURCES	FUNCTION	DEFICIENCY DISEASES
A (Fat soluble)	Butter, fortified margarine, green and yellow vegetables, milk, eggs, liver	Night vision Healthy skin Proper growth and repair of body tissues	Night blindness Dry skin Slow growth Poor gums and teeth
B_1 (Thiamine) (Water soluble)	Chicken, fish, meat, eggs, enriched bread, whole-grain cereals	Promotes normal appetite and digestion Needed by nervous system	Loss of appetite Nervous disorders Fatigue Severe deficiency causes beriberi
B_2 (Riboflavin) (Water soluble)	Cheese, eggs, fish, meat, liver, milk, cereals, enriched bread	Needed in cellular respiration	Eye problems Sores on skin and lips General fatigue
B_3 (Niacin) (water soluble)	Eggs, fish, liver, meat, milk, potatoes, enriched bread	Needed for normal metabolism Growth Proper skin health	Indigestion Diarrhea Headaches Mental disturbances Skin disorders
B_{12} (Cyanocobalamin) (Water soluble)	Milk, liver, brain, beef, egg yolk, clams, oysters, sardines, salmon	Red blood cell synthesis Nucleic acid synthesis Nerve cell maintenance	Pernicious anemia Nerve cell malfunction
Folic Acid (Water soluble)	Liver, yeast, green vegetables, peanuts, mushrooms, beef, veal, egg yolk	Nucleic acid synthesis Needed for normal metabolism and growth	Anemia Growth retardation
C (Ascorbic acid) (Water soluble)	Citrus fruits, cabbage, green vegetables, tomatoes, potatoes	Needed for maintenance of normal bones, gums, teeth, and blood vessels	Weak bones Sore and bleeding gums Poor teeth Bleeding in skin Painful joints Severe deficiency results in scurvy
D (Fat soluble)	Beef, butter, eggs, milk	Needed for normal bone and teeth development Controls calcium and phosphorus metabolism	Poor bone and teeth structure Soft bones Rickets
E (Tocopherol) (Fat soluble)	Margarine, nuts, leafy vegetables, vegetable oils, whole wheat	Used in cell respiration Protects red blood cells from destruction Acts as an antioxidant	Anemia in premature infants No known deficiency in adults
K (Fat soluble)	Synthesized by colon bacteria Green leafy vegetables, cereal	Essential for normal blood clotting	Slow blood clotting

to maintain a normal level of cholesterol. An important substance in relation to cholesterol is **triglycerides**—fats and oils. Excess calories are converted into triglycerides, which are stored as adipose tissue.

Cholesterol and triglycerides are transported through the blood cells by a special protein called **lipoprotein**. There are three kinds of lipoprotein:

1. High-density lipoprotein (HDL)
2. Low-density lipoprotein (LDL)
3. Very low-density lipoprotein (VLDL)

LDL is known as the "bad" lipoprotein, since it carries fats to the cells, and HDL is "good" lipoprotein because it removes excess cholesterol from the cells to be transported back to the liver for elimination by the body. **Atherosclerosis** is caused by the buildup of cholesterol inside an artery. If more cholesterol is ingested and carried by LDL to the cells than can be removed by HDL, atherosclerosis results. The recommended level of blood cholesterol for individuals age 40 and older is less than 200 mg/dl.

Vitamins are coenzymes that are necessary for growth and maintaining homeostasis. The majority of action by enzymes is dependent on the presence of vitamins. Vitamins must be obtained from the diet; if vitamins are not present in the diet in sufficient quantity, the individual must take a vitamin supplement. A deficiency in a certain type of vitamin results in a specific disease or disorder of the body; for example, a deficiency of vitamin D results in rickets and resulting bone deformities if not treated. There are two types of vitamins: fat-soluble vitamins, which are stored by the body and include A, D, E, and K, and water-soluble vitamins, which are excreted by the body when in excess and include B_1, B_2, B_3, B_6, B_{12}, vitamin C, folic acid, biotin, and pantothenic acid. Table 15-2 provides a summary of the major vitamins needed by humans.

The baseline caloric needs of a person are determined by calculating the basal metabolic rate (BMR). It is the measure of the total energy used by the body to maintain homeostasis. BMR is estimated as follows:

Females: $661 + (4.38 \times$ weight in lbs.) $+ (4.33 \times$ height in inches) $- (4.7 \times$ age) $=$ BMR
Males: $67 + (6.24 \times$ weight in lbs.) $+ (12.7 \times$ height in inches) $- (6.9 \times$ age) $=$ BMR

Now estimate the total number of calories the body requires by multiplying the BMR by one of the following categories:

1. 1.2 for an inactive person
2. 1.3 for a moderately active person (exercises three times per week)
3. 1.7 for a very active person (exercises more than three times per week, but not seven days a week)
4. 1.9 for an extremely active person (runs, swims, bikes every day)

When the metabolic rate is lower than the intake of calories, the excess calories are stored as fat and the person's weight increases. If metabolic rate equals intake of calories, the body weight is maintained. If the metabolic rate exceeds the intake of calories, the person loses weight.

BOX 15-9

Exploratory Laparotomy

An exploratory laparotomy is an incision through the abdominal wall into the cavity for the purpose of exploration, diagnosis, and possible treatment. If a surgeon cannot make a definitive diagnosis of a patient's condition, an exploratory laparotomy is often performed. The patient will be placed in a supine position and the surgeon will usually make an incision from the xiphoid process, around the umbilicus and to the level of the pubis. The surgeon will use the knife and scissors to incise through the tissue layers of the abdomen, and electrocautery to control bleeding. The tissues are incised in order from outside to inside skin, subcuticular tissue, subcutaneous fat, abdominal muscle, fascia, and the peritoneum. Once inside the abdominal cavity large retractors are placed to hold open the surgical wound edges and the surgeon explores the interior to determine if any pathol-

ogy exists. If the surgeon discovers a pathology such as a tumor, bowel obstruction, or infection, she or he will perform the necessary procedure to correct the disorder. During the course of the surgery large sponges will be used for various purposes such as to aid in holding an organ, soak up blood and body fluids, and wall off organs in order to better visualize other portions of the cavity. The sponges are removed before the tissue layers of the cavity are closed with suture. An important factor for the surgical technologist to remember is that when preparing for an exploratory laparotomy any type of abdominal procedure could eventually be performed based on the intraoperative diagnosis. The surgical technologist must have available the proper surgical instrumentation, supplies, and equipment that are specific to the organ to be operated upon.

Case Study 2

A 43-year-old man visits his physician and presents the following clinical and physiological symptoms particularly after eating:

- Chronic heartburn
- Dysphagia
- Nausea/vomiting
- Increased gastric acidity
- Regurgitation
- Epigastric pain
- Decreased gastric emptying
- Decreased lower esophageal sphincter (LES) pressure

Based on these symptoms answer the following questions:

1. What disease is the patient most likely experiencing and what anatomy does it involve?

2. What complications can occur due to the disease?

3. What diagnostic tests are performed to confirm the disease and LES?

4. What are the nonsurgical treatments?

5. What is the primary surgical treatment?

CHAPTER SUMMARY

- The process of digestion involves chemical and mechanical functions that break down food into small substances that can be used by the cells of the body.

- The functions of the digestive system are ingesting food, the mechanical and chemical breakdown of food, the breakdown and absorption of complex nutrient molecules into simple organic molecules, and the formation and elimination of feces.

- The general order of the tunics or coats from innermost layer to outside is tunica, mucosa, tunica submucosa, tunica muscularis, and serosa.

- There are two types of peritoneum: parietal peritoneum and visceral peritoneum.

- The mesentery is an extension of the peritoneum that attaches the small intestine and colon to the posterior abdominal wall.

- The folds of peritoneum, called mesocolon, serve to connect portions of the colon to the posterior abdominal wall.

- There are eight primary anatomic landmarks of the abdomen that serve as reference points for abdominal incisions and muscular attachments.

- The four muscles encountered during surgery of the abdomen are the external oblique muscle, internal oblique muscle, transverse abdominis, and rectus abdominis.

- A special type of tendon that connects the transverse abdominis and both obliques is the aponeurosis.

- The oral cavity is responsible for the first portion of the digestive process by breaking down food through the process of mastication and mixing it with saliva.

- The cheeks form the lateral sides of the mouth and are continuous with the lips.

- The four primary muscles of the cheek are the buccinator, zygomatic, masseter, and platysma.

- The tongue is a muscular structure composed of skeletal muscle, connected to the floor of the mouth by the lingual frenulum. The tongue contains the taste buds.

- The hard and soft palates form the roof of the mouth. Connected in the posterior part of the soft palate is the uvula.

- The teeth are embedded in the mandible and maxillary bones. The human has two sets of teeth: deciduous and permanent.

- Each tooth is composed of three portions: crown, root, and neck.

- The root of the tooth has two layers: periodontal ligament and cementum.

- The majority of the mass of the tooth is composed of dentin, which encloses the pulp cavity containing the blood vessels and nerve that supply the tooth.

- Enamel forms the outer layer of the crown and is the hardest substance in the body.

- The primary supply of saliva is from the salivary glands.

- Saliva moistens the food particles, brings the particles together into a food bolus, and chemically begins the breakdown of carbohydrates.

- There are two types of cells in the salivary glands: mucous and serous cells. Serous cells produce the digestive enzyme called amylase.

- The sympathetic nerve impulses stimulate the glands to secrete mucus; the parasympathetic nerve impulses stimulate the release of watery fluid.

- There are three pairs of salivary glands: parotid, submandibular, and sublingual.

- The excretory duct of the parotid is Steno's duct; the submandibular excretory duct is Wharton's duct; and the sublingual excretory duct is Rivini-ani ducts.

- The pharnyx is the only structure of the body that serves as part of the digestive and respiratory tracts.

- The pharynx is divided into the nasopharynx, oropharynx, and laryngopharynx.

- The pharynx is continuous with the esophagus and has three coats: mucous, muscular, and fibrous.

- The role of the pharynx is to begin the process of deglutition.

- The muscles of the pharynx are skeletal muscles so the individual can voluntarily begin deglutition.

- The esophagus is a long tube that provides a passageway for food to the stomach. It begins at the laryngopharynx and ends at the cardiac sphincter, traveling through an opening in the diaphragm called the esophageal hiatus.

- Peristalsis of the smooth muscle layer of the esophagus pushes the food bolus to the stomach.

- The esophagus has three coats: muscular, submucosa, and mucosa.

- At the point where the esophagus joins the stomach, a layer of circular muscle fibers form the lower esophageal sphincter (LES).

- The esophagus lacks a serosal layer and is slow healing.

- The stomach is the primary organ of digestion, responsible for carrying out the process of chymification.

- The superior border is called the lesser curvature and hanging from it is the lesser omentum.

- The inferior border of the stomach is called the greater curvature and hanging from it is the greater omentum.

- The gastrophrenic ligament aids in holding the stomach in its anatomic position.

- The stomach is divided into the cardiac, fundus, body, and pyloric regions.

- The stomach is connected to the duodenum via the pyloric sphincter.

- The gastric glands of the stomach contain three kinds of secretory cells: goblet cells, chief cells also called peptic cells, and parietal cells also called oxyntic cells.

- Pepsin, converted from pepsinogen, is responsible for beginning the digestion of proteins.

- The three layers of the muscularis coat are: inner oblique, middle circular, and outer longitudinal.

- There are three stages of gastric secretion: cephalic, gastric, and intestinal.

- The action of the vagus nerve is important to understand, since it affects the release of gastric juice.

- The stomach usually heals quickly when an infection is not present.

- It is the only organ of the body that performs endocrine and exocrine functions.

- It is divided into the head, body, and tail.

- The acinar cells perform the exocrine function by secreting pancreatic juice.

- The pancreatic juice travels through the duct of Wirsung to enter the duodenum.

- The pancreatic juice breaks down fats, proteins, carbohydrates, and nucleic acids.

- The duct of Wirsung joins the common bile duct (CBD) to enter the duodenum through the ampulla of Vater. The opening of the ampulla is called the sphincter of Oddi. Sometimes a second separate duct will exist called the duct of Santorini.

- The parasympathetic impulses and the hormone cholecystokinin stimulate the pancreas to release the pancreatic juice.

- The liver is the second largest organ of the body.

- It is covered by a fibrous and serous coat, and a thin coat of connective tissue called Glisson's capsule.

- It is divided into two lobes, right and left, by the falciform ligament.

- An important surgical landmark is the porta hepatis where the right and left lobes meet, and blood vessels and ducts enter or exit the liver.

- The coronary ligament aids in anchoring the liver to the diaphragm.

- The cells of the liver are called hepatocytes and form the hepatic lobules. They are responsible for the production of bile.

- A bile canal exits each lobule and they join to form the right and left hepatic ducts that exit the liver and join to the form the common hepatic duct, which joins with the cystic duct of the gallbladder to form the CBD.

- The liver is highly vascular. The vessels are the hepatic artery, portal vein, and hepatic vein.

- Kupffer cells within the liver remove bacteria by the process of phagocytosis.

- The liver has many functions including metabolizing carbohydrate, storing of iron and vitamins, contributing to protein metabolism, synthesizing heparin, metabolizing anesthetic drugs and gases, and forming and secreting bile.

- Bile is a yellowish-green thick liquid; the active digestive substance in bile is the bile salts.

- The gallbladder is located in a fossa on the inferior surface of the right lobe of the liver.

- It is divided into the fundus, body, and neck.

- When stones collect at the neck they form a pouch called Hartmann's pouch.

- The cystic duct exits the gallbladder to join the common hepatic duct to form the common bile duct.

- The anatomic landmark called the triangle of Calot is used to locate the cystic artery.

- The gallbladder has four coats: serous, subserosal, muscular, and mucosal.

- The blood supply to the gallbladder is the cystic artery, right hepatic artery, and superior portion of the pancreaticoduodenal artery.

- The cystic duct has the dual purpose of transporting bile to and from the gallbladder.

- The functions of the gallbladder are to store bile, concentrate the bile by absorption of water, and release the bile for entrance into the duodenum when stimulated by the hormone cholecystokinin.

- A pathological condition that can occur is cholesterol separating from the bile within the gallbladder and forming gallstones.

- The processes of digestion and absorption occur primarily in the small intestine, which is divided into three sections: duodenum, jejunum, and ileum.

- The arterial blood supply is complex and requires several branches from the superior mesenteric artery.

- The end of the duodenum is marked by the ligament of Treitz, which indicates the beginning of the jejunum.

- The layers of the small intestine from outside to the inside are the serosa, muscular, submucosa, and mucosa.

- The ileum connects to the cecum of the colon at the ileocecal valve.

- Three structures aid in increasing the absorptive surface of the small intestine: plicae circulares, villi, and microvilli.

- Thousands of minute villi are located throughout the inner lining of the small intestine. They absorb the nutrients that come into contact with the projections.

- Located at the base of each villi are the intestinal glands, also called the crypts of Lieberkühn, which secrete digestive enzymes. Two other important secreting structures are goblet cells and Brunner's glands, which secrete alkaline mucus.

- The digestive process is called chymification and the digested contents in the small intestine are called chyme.

- The colon is divided into four portions: cecum, colon, rectum, and anal canal.

- The colon has four coats: serosa, muscular, submucosa, and mucosa.

- The colon is divided into three sections: ascending colon, transverse colon, and descending colon.

- The primary functions of the colon are absorption of water and electrolytes, production of vitamin K by the resident bacteria, and expulsion of feces.

- The ileocecal valve is the opening from the ileum into the cecum.

- The appendix is a closed-end tube that extends from the cecum and has no known function.

- The hepatic flexure is where the ascending colon angles to the left to begin the transverse colon and is an important anatomic landmark.

- The splenic flexure is where the transverse colon curves beneath the spleen and marks the beginning of the descending colon and is an important anatomic landmark.

- The name sigmoid colon comes from its S shape.

- The last portion of the colon is the anal canal, which opens to the exterior through the anus.

- The anal canal is arranged into a series of longitudinal folds called anal columns.

- The three movements of the colon are peristalsis, haustral churning, and mass peristalsis.

- When the chyme has condensed it is now known as feces.

- Water comprises approximately 50%–65% of the total body weight and is one of the most important components for maintaining life.

- Carbohydrates are the primary source of energy.

- Calorie is the amount of heat required to raise the temperature of 1 gram of water by 1°C. The average adult requires 1,500 to 3,000 kilocalories per day.

- Proteins are important in the growth and repair of body tissue and are enzymes.

- Essential amino acids are those that can't be made by the body; proteins that contain all of the essential amino acids are called complete proteins. Incomplete proteins do not contain all of the essential amino acids.

- Excess amino acids are excreted in the form of urea.

- Minerals are obtained from food. They are important for growth and maintenance of the body.

- Trace elements are present in food.

- Simple lipids include fats and oils. Fat is a source of energy.

- Cholesterol is a type of fat that is essential in the manufacturing of body cells and synthesis of certain hormones.

- Excess calories are converted into triglycerides and stored as adipose tissue.

- LDL is the "bad" lipoprotein and HDL is the "good" lipoprotein.

- Vitamins are coenzymes that are necessary for maintaining homeostasis.

- The BMR is used to determine the baseline caloric needs of an individual.

CRITICAL THINKING QUESTIONS

1. Describe the functions of the mesentery.
2. Explain why the facial nerve must be preserved when performing surgery in the area of the mouth.
3. Explain why there is a high incidence of failure of esophageal anastomosis.
4. Describe the three layers of the muscularis coat of the stomach and how they relate to the esophagus.
5. Describe the bile duct system of the liver and gallbladder.

REFERENCES

Acute peritonitis (2003). Retrieved July 24, 2003, from http://surgery.4t.com/56.2.htm

Association of Surgical Technologists. (2003). *Surgical technology for the surgical technologist: A positive care approach* (2nd ed.). Clifton Park, NY: Thomson Delmar Learning.

Bosscha, K., van Vroonhoven, T. J. M. V., & van der Werken, C. (1999). Surgical management of severe secondary peritonitis. *British Journal of Surgery, 86,* 1371–1377.

Shier, D., Butler, J., & Lewis, R. (2002). *Hole's human anatomy & physiology* (9th ed.). New York: McGraw-Hill.

16

URINARY SYSTEM

CHAPTER OBJECTIVES

After completing the study of this chapter, you should be able to:

1. List the organs of the urinary system and their functions.
2. Describe the location and structures of a kidney.
3. Name the functions of the kidney.
4. Describe the blood supply to the kidney.
5. Describe a nephron to include major parts.
6. Describe how a nephron functions.
7. Explain glomerular filtrate including how it is formed and its composition.
8. Explain the roles of tubular absorption and tubular secretion in the formation of urine.
9. Describe the anatomic structure of the ureter, bladder, and urethra.
10. Explain how micturition occurs and how it can be controlled.

KEY TERMS

acidosis	detrusor muscle	hematuria	renal corpuscles
aldosterone	dysuria	hypospadias	renal fascia
alkalosis	epispadias	internal urethral sphincter	renal pyramids
antidiuretic hormone (ADH)	erythropoietin	intracellular fluid (ICF)	renal tubule
atrial natriuretic hormone (ANH)	external urethral sphincter	juxtaglomerular apparatus	stress incontinence
	extracellular fluid (ECF)	ketoacidosis	tubular reabsorption
Bowman's capsule	filtration	kidney	ureters
calciferol	Gerota's fascia	meatus	urethra
calculi	glomerular filtration	osmosis	urinary bladder
calyces	glomerular filtration rate (GFR)	podocytes	urinary tract infection (UTI)
collecting tubule	glomerulus	renal columns	vesical trigone

Case Study 1

A male patient is admitted to the emergency department complaining of extreme pain to the left flank that radiates to the back and upper abdomen. He informs the physician that earlier in the week he experienced hematuria and dysuria. The physician orders a urinalysis and kidney-ureter-bladder (KUB) x-ray. The urinalysis is negative for pyuria, but is positive for hematuria. The KUB confirms the diagnosis.

1. Define the words hematuria, dysuria, and pyuria.

2. What did the KUB and physical signs and symptoms most likely confirm?

3. Why are individuals who are prone to the formation of renal calculi told by a physician to limit their intake of calcium-containing foods?

4. What are the two reasons for the cause of the pain due to renal calculi?

5. If the patient cannot eliminate the stone(s) through urination, what other methods may have to be employed in order to remove them?

INTRODUCTION

The urinary system consists of two kidneys located on each side of the body, two ureters that exit each kidney and connect to the urinary bladder, which collects urine, and the urethra through which urine exits the body (Figure 16-1). The formation of urine by the kidneys is important to eliminate the body's waste products, which are toxic to the body. The tubules in the kidneys resorb substances that are needed by the body such as amino acids, glucose, and various ions, and, most important, water. After the useful substances have been resorbed, the toxic substances are voided in the urine. The process of urine formation, therefore, is highly important to homeostasis in that it maintains the normal composition, pH level, and volume of blood and extracellular fluids.

KIDNEYS

Each **kidney** is located in the lower thoracic and upper lumbar areas on each side of the vertebral column and is referred to as being in a retroperitoneal position. It is a reddish-brown-colored organ that is shaped like a kidney bean. The left kidney is larger than the right; the right kidney is situated slightly lower than the left. The size of a kidney is 10–12 cm in length, 5–6 cm in width, and 3 cm thick. Lying on the medial side of the kidney is the psoas muscle, on the lateral side are the transverse abdominal muscles, and the quadratus lumborum muscles lie posteriorly.

In relation to the abdominal organs, the right and left kidney are situated as follows:

1. Right kidney: The medial border is situated posterior to the second portion of the duodenum. The superior portion of the kidney is in contact with the right lobe of the liver. The inferior portion lies lateral to the right flexure of the colon and part of the jejunum.

2. Left kidney: The pancreas lies across the hilum (Junge, 2004). The superior portion rests against the stomach and spleen. The left flexure of the colon is situated laterally and a portion of the jejunum medially.

Each kidney is surrounded by a layer of fibrous dense connective tissue referred to as the capsule. The kidneys rest in a concave bed of adipose tissue that acts as a cushion referred to as **Gerota's fascia** or **renal fascia**, which aids in supporting and holding the kidneys in place.

On the medial side of a kidney is the hilum where the renal artery enters the kidney and the renal vein and ureter exit. The renal artery is a branch from the abdominal aorta and the renal vein carries deoxygenated blood back to the inferior vena cava.

Structure

The kidney is divided into three sections: the outer, middle, and inner. The renal cortex contains the **renal corpuscles** and renal tubules, which are parts of the nephron. The renal cortex is recognized by its

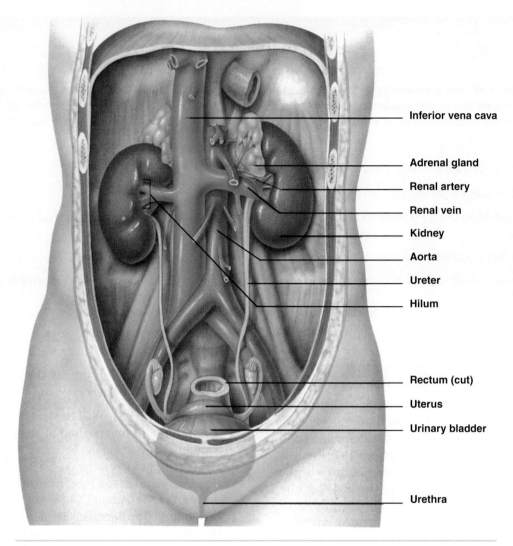

FIGURE 16-1 Organs of the urinary system

Inferior vena cava

Adrenal gland

Renal artery

Renal vein

Kidney

Aorta

Ureter

Hilum

Rectum (cut)

Uterus

Urinary bladder

Urethra

granular appearance when a transverse section of the kidney is viewed (Figure 16-2).

The renal medulla also contains parts of the nephron called the loop of Henle and **collecting tubules**. The renal medulla is distinguished from the renal cortex by its striated appearance and is composed of wedge-shaped structures called **renal pyramids**. The pyramidal shape of each renal pyramid contributes to dividing the kidney into several lobes, making the kidney multilobar. Individual lobes of the kidney are delineated by the **renal columns**. Renal columns are extensions of cortical substance from the renal cortex into the medulla. The columns are located on the lateral margins of individual lobes, referred to as interlobar cortical tissue, and aid in recognizing each lobe of the kidney. A branch of the renal artery, the interlobar artery, travels across each renal column; more detailed information concerning

the interlobar arteries is provided later in the chapter. Therefore a lobe consists of the renal pyramid and the renal columns. The superior portion of each renal pyramid tapers to form 8–12 renal papillae. The papillae enter the 4–13 minor calyces in the renal pelvis.

The renal pelvis is actually an area of the kidney located at the hilum that indicates where the ureter enters the kidney and expands into funnel-shaped structures called the **calyces** (singular, **calyx**), which surround the papillae of the renal pyramids. There are two calyces, the aforementioned minor calyces and the major calyces. The minor calyces empty into two or three major calyces. The major calyces drain the superior, middle, and inferior sections of the kidney into the common renal pelvis. The calyces serve as the collection point of urine; the urine flows from the renal papillae into the calyces and continues into the ureter.

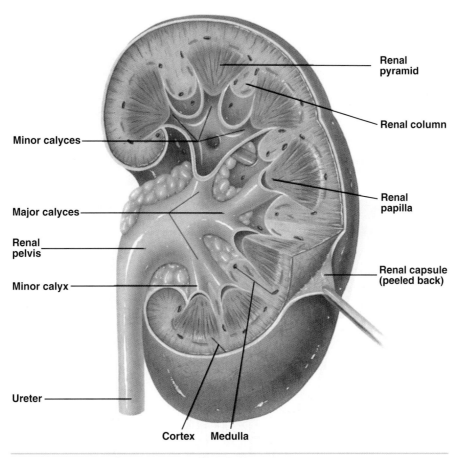

FIGURE 16-2   The internal anatomy of a kidney

Nephron

The nephron is a very small structure but is the structure of the kidney that does all of the work. Each kidney contains approximately 1 million nephrons and it is here that urine is formed. A nephron is composed of two parts: the renal corpuscle and the renal tubule. Each of these two portions is further subdivided (Figure 16-3).

Renal Corpuscle

The renal corpuscle consists of the **glomerulus** and **Bowman's capsule**, which lie in the cortex of the kidney. The glomerulus is actually a network of capillary vessels that is a division of an afferent arteriole and empties into an efferent arteriole. Bowman's capsule is a double-layered cup that is an extension of the end of a renal tubule and it surrounds the glomerulus. The outer layer of Bowman's capsule is the parietal layer and the inner is a visceral layer (Junge, 2004). A small space exits between the two layers and contains renal filtrate, which is the fluid formed in the glomerulus that eventually becomes urine. The parietal layer contains a type of epithelial cells called

podocytes (Junge, 2004). Branches extend from the podocytes that attach to the glomerular capillaries. The branches and the spaces between them form one of the several filtering devices of the kidney through which substances and materials must pass before entering Bowman's capsule.

Renal Tubule

The second portion of a nephron is the **renal tubule**, which is a continuation of Bowman's capsule. The renal tubule is subdivided into the following:

1. Proximal convoluted tubule: located in the renal cortex
2. Loop of Henle: located in the renal medulla
3. Distal convoluted tubule: located in the renal cortex

Distal convoluted tubules from groups of nephrons empty into a collecting tubule and several of the collecting tubules join to form a papillary duct that transfers the urine into a calyx. Peritubular capillaries surround each part of the renal tubule; the capillaries are a division of the efferent arteriole.

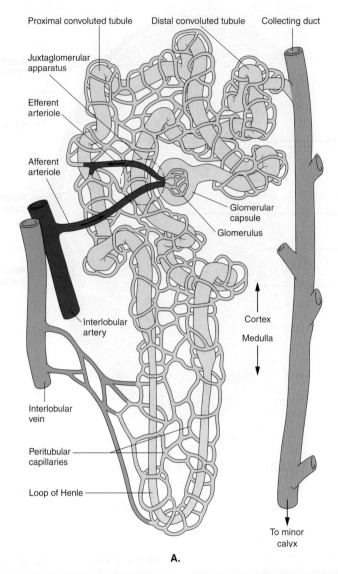

Proximal convoluted tubule

Distal convoluted tubule

Collecting duct

Juxtaglomerular apparatus

Efferent arteriole

Afferent arteriole

Glomerular capsule

Glomerulus

Interlobular artery

Cortex

Medulla

Interlobular vein

Peritubular capillaries

Loop of Henle

To minor calyx

A.

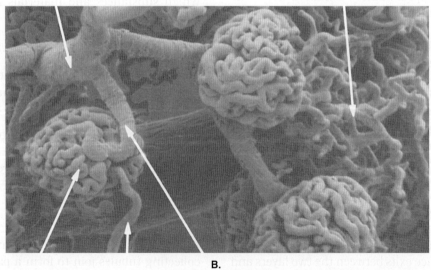

B.

FIGURE 16-3 (A) The anatomy of a nephron, the functional unit of a kidney. (B) A scanning electron micrograph of glomerular capillaries

In the cortex at the origin of the distal convoluted tubule, the tubule travels between the afferent and efferent arterioles and makes contact with them. At the point of contact, the epithelial cells in the wall of the tubule are vertical and densely packed and form a structure called the macula densa. Next to the afferent arteriole near its attachment to the glomerulus are large smooth muscle cells called juxtaglomerular cells. The juxtaglomerular cells and macula densa together comprise the **juxtaglomerular apparatus**, which is important in the regulation of the secretion of renin. This regulation is discussed in more detail later in the chapter.

To facilitate full understanding of the nephron's anatomic complexity, the following is a review of its structure:

1. The renal corpuscle and proximal convoluted tubule are located in the renal cortex.
2. The proximal convoluted tubule continues its course downward into the renal medulla and is now referred to as the descending portion of the loop of Henle.
3. Within the deep portion of the medulla the descending portion forms a U-turn and begins traveling upward back to the cortex; this is called the ascending portion of the loop of Henle.
4. The ascending loop reenters the cortex and the tubule becomes twisted to form the distal convoluted tubule.
5. The distal convoluted tubule straightens to travel through the cortex slightly downward to join a collecting tubule.
6. The collecting tubule travels downward through the medulla and opens into a papilla.

Blood, Nerve, and Lymphatic Supply to the Kidneys

The blood supply is described in two parts: flow of blood through the kidney and the arterial and venous blood supply to the kidney itself.

Blood Flow Through the Kidney

The flow of blood through the kidney is one of the most important aspects of the formation of urine and maintenance of homeostasis in the body. As previously mentioned, the blood from the abdominal aorta enters the branch called the renal artery. The renal artery enters the kidney through the hilum and divides into several branches called the interlobar arteries that pass between the renal pyramids and across the renal columns. At the junction between the

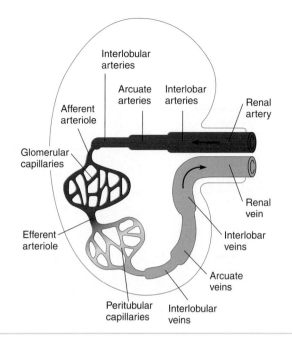

FIGURE 16-4   Blood flow through the kidney

medulla and cortex, the interlobar arteries divide to form incomplete arteries in the shape of arches called the arcuate arteries, which eventually give rise to interlobular arteries. The last branches of the interlobular arteries are the afferent arterioles that lead to the nephrons (Figure 16-4). The flow of blood through the kidney and nephron is as follows:
Renal artery → interlobar artery → arcuate artery → interlobular artery → afferent arteriole → glomerular capillary → efferent arteriole → peritubular capillary → interlobular vein → arcuate vein → interlobar vein → renal vein → inferior vena cava.

Blood Supply to the Kidneys

The renal arteries branch off the abdominal aorta at the level of the second lumbar vertebra and travel in a transverse route to the kidney. The arteries travel anterior to the crura of the diaphragm and the psoas muscle (Junge, 2004). The right renal artery passes posterior to the inferior vena cava, head of the pancreas, and duodenum (Junge, 2004). The left renal artery is posterior to the left renal vein, splenic vein, and pancreas. Branches from the renal arteries called the ureteric branches supply the ureter.

The renal veins lie anterior to the arteries. The left renal vein is anterior to the aorta and posterior to the superior mesenteric artery and empties into the inferior vena cava. Along the route to the inferior vena cava the left adrenal and left testicular or ovarian veins empty into the left renal vein (Figure 16-5).

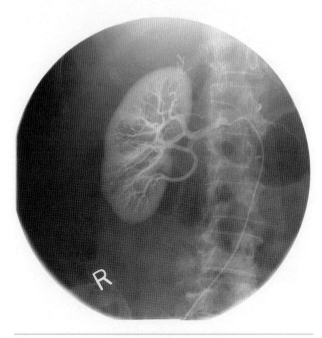

FIGURE 16-5   Renal arteriography

Lymphatic and Nerve Supply

The lymphatic vessels form three plexuses. One plexus is located within the parenchyma of the kidney, the second is located just underneath the capsule of the kidney, and the third is located in the perirenal fat. The lymph vessels of the plexuses from the kidney and capsule join at the hilum and follow the course of the renal vein to empty into the lumbar lymph nodes. The perirenal fat plexus drains directly into the lumbar lymph nodes.

The afferent nerve innervation to the kidney arises from the renal plexus. The efferent innervation consists of autonomic, vasomotor nerves (Junge, 2004).

Urine Formation

The exchange of fluids occurs in the two sets of capillaries: glomeruli and peritubular capillaries. Remember, capillaries are only one cell thick and so are conducive to the efficient process of fluid exchange. The exchange at these two sites of capillaries in the kidneys results in the formation of urine.

Urine formation occurs in three steps: glomerular filtration within the renal corpuscles, tubular reabsorption, and tubular secretion within the renal tubules.

Glomerular Filtration

Glomerular filtration involves plasma, waste products, and small protein particles being forced out of

the glomeruli by blood pressure and into Bowman's capsule to form the liquid called renal filtrate. The blood pressure in the glomeruli is much higher than that found in other capillaries. The pressure in Bowman's capsule is low and, remember, the inner layer is permeable. Therefore, about 25% of the blood that enters the kidney and flows through the glomeruli becomes renal filtrate. The erythrocytes, leukocytes, and large proteins are too large to exit the glomeruli and remain in the circulatory system.

The amount of urine formed by the kidneys in one minute is measured by the **glomerular filtration rate (GFR)**. The average amount that is formed is 125 ml per minute. GFR is affected if the blood flow through the kidney changes. If the blood flow increases, the GFR increases and the amount of urine formed increases. The opposite occurs when the blood flow decreases.

Tubular Reabsorption

Tubular reabsorption occurs between the renal tubules and peritubular capillaries. The majority of renal filtrate does not become urine; approximately 99% of the renal filtrate is reabsorbed into the blood flow in the peritubular capillaries. Therefore, only 1% of the renal filtrate enters the renal pelvis to eventually be excreted as urine. The reabsorption and secretion of renal filtrate occur primarily in the proximal convoluted tubules. The distal convoluted tubules and collecting tubules contribute to the reabsorption of water. The reabsorption of water is affected by hormones, which are discussed later.

There are four processes of reabsorption:

- Active transport: The cells that make up the renal tubule use ATP to transfer needed substances such as vitamins and glucose from the renal filtrate to the blood. The reabsorption rate of these substances is affected by the level in the renal filtrate. For example, a normal blood glucose level indicates that the renal filtrate level of glucose is also normal. Therefore, all of the glucose will be reabsorbed by the tubules and the urine will not contain any glucose. However, if the blood glucose level is high, the amount of glucose in the renal filtrate will also be above normal. Therefore, the glucose will not be reabsorbed by the tubules and will be present in the urine.

  Another important example of active transport is the reabsorption of calcium ions. The reabsorption of the ions is increased by the secretion of parathyroid hormone (PTH). The parathyroid glands secrete PTH when the blood calcium level is low. The reabsorption process of the kidneys is one mechanism in which the body is able to raise the blood calcium level back to normal.

- Passive transport: The negative ions reenter the circulating blood after positive ions are reabsorbed. The principle that applies here is that unlike charges, positive–negative, attract.
- Pinocytosis: Some proteins are too large to be reabsorbed through the process of active transport. Therefore, the protein particles are absorbed by the process of pinocytosis by the proximal convoluted tubules. This is comparable to phagocytosis of bacterial cells. The cell membrane of the tubules indents and folds around the protein to pull within the lumen. Normal urine will not contain any proteins; they are all reabsorbed through the process of pinocytosis.
- **Osmosis**: Osmosis involves the reabsorption of water, which is affected by the action of hormones. Water is reabsorbed along with minerals.

Hormones and the Reabsorption of Water

The three hormones that are important in influencing the reabsorption of water are **aldosterone**, **atrial natriuretic hormone (ANH)**, and **antidiuretic hormone (ADH)**. Aldosterone is secreted by the adrenal gland that rests on the superior portion of the kidney. Aldosterone is secreted when the blood potassium level is above normal, blood sodium level is below normal, or the blood pressure decreases. Aldosterone stimulates the reabsorption of sodium ions, which in turn causes water to be reabsorbed from the renal filtrate back to the circulating blood. This aids homeostasis by maintaining a normal circulating blood volume and blood pressure. The adrenal gland is stimulated to release aldosterone by the renin–angiotensin mechanism, which is described later.

ANH is the antagonist to aldosterone. It is secreted by the atria of the heart. When the atrial walls expand due to high blood pressure or an increase in blood volume, ANH is released to decrease the reabsorption of sodium ions from the renal filtrate into the circulating blood. Consequently, the sodium ions remain in the renal filtrate, including water, and are excreted in the urine. The elimination of the sodium and water from the body lowers the blood pressure and blood volume.

ADH is secreted by the posterior pituitary gland when the water level in the body is too low. ADH causes the distal convoluted tubules and collecting tubules to increase their reabsorption of water from the renal filtrate. The water level rises and this aids in maintaining normal blood volume and blood pressure. The urine that is excreted is more concentrated, but still essential to eliminating the waste products of the body.

Once the water level within the body returns to normal, the posterior pituitary is no longer stimulated to secrete ADH and less water is reabsorbed. The urine returns to being dilute due to the presence of water.

Maintenance of the pH Level

The kidneys are the primary organ for maintaining the normal blood pH level and normal level of tissue fluid. If the blood and body fluids are too acidic, the kidneys increase the secretion of hydrogen ions into the renal filtrate and cause an increase of bicarbonate ions into the blood. This aids in increasing the pH level back to normal. When the blood and body fluids are too alkaline, an opposite reaction occurs. The kidneys cause the hydrogen ions to be returned to the circulating blood and the bicarbonate ions are excreted in the urine. This lowers the pH level back to normal. Later in the chapter the acid–base balance and electrolytes will be discussed in more detail.

Additional Functions of the Kidneys

The additional functions of the kidneys include secretion of renin, conversion of vitamin D, and production of erythropoietin. When the blood pressure decreases, the juxtaglomerular cells located in the walls of the afferent arterioles are stimulated to secrete the enzyme renin. The secretion of renin is the first step in the renin–angiotensin mechanism, the end product of which is angiotensin II, which causes vasoconstriction and stimulates the increase in the secretion of aldosterone. Aldosterone and angiotensin II both increase the blood pressure. The steps of the renin–angiotensin mechanism are as follows:

1. Renin is secreted by the kidneys in reaction to an abnormal decrease in the blood pressure.
2. Renin causes angiotensinogen, a plasma protein synthesized by the liver, to break apart to form angiotensin I.
3. An enzyme secreted by the lung tissue causes angiotensin I to be converted to angiotensin II.
4. Angiotensin II stimulates vasoconstriction and the release of aldosterone by the adrenal cortex of the adrenal gland.

The maintenance of homeostasis relies on a normal blood pressure. For example, when a person experiences severe hemorrhage after a traumatic accident, the blood pressure will suddenly and drastically decrease. To compensate, the kidneys respond by decreasing filtration, which in turn causes a decrease in urinary output, and the renin–angiotensin mechanism is stimulated to form angiotensin II. This is one way the body attempts to ensure that cardiac output and blood pressure remain normal.

The kidneys are responsible for converting vitamin D to **calciferol**. Calciferol increases the absorption of calcium and phosphate in the small intestine. Kidneys produce the hormone **erythropoietin**. The hormone is secreted when a person experiences hypoxia. Erythropoietin acts on the red bone marrow to increase the rate of erythrocyte production. The increase in erythrocytes will increase the oxygen-carrying level of the blood, thereby resolving the hypoxic state.

URETERS, URINARY BLADDER, AND URETHRA

The ureters, urinary bladder, and urethra allow urine to travel from the kidneys to be excreted to the outside of the body (Figures 16-6 and 16-7).

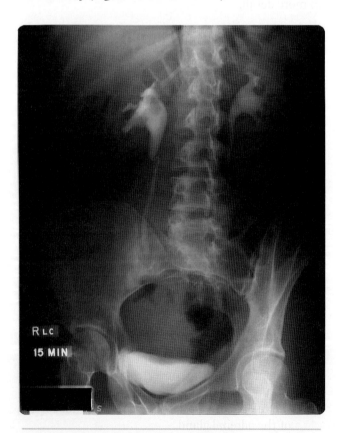

FIGURE 16-6   Posterior IVU oblique

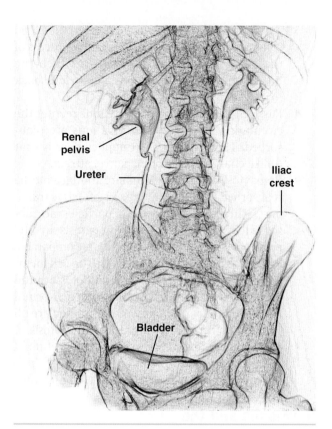

FIGURE 16-7   Posterior IVU oblique

Ureters

The **ureters** conduct urine from the kidney to the bladder. The position of the ureters is retroperitoneal. The course of the ureter is divided into an abdominal course and a pelvic course. The ureters travel downward on the psoas muscles and eventually cross the bifurcation of the common iliac arteries where it becomes the pelvic course. The average length of a ureter is 25 cm. The ureters terminate on the right and left posterolateral walls of the urinary bladder, approximately 3 cm apart. The ureter exits from the hilum of the kidney and travels the abdominal course in extraperitoneal connective tissue. The blood supply to the abdominal course is branches of the renal and testicular or ovarian arteries. The veins follow the course of the arteries. Innervation is from the renal and testicular or ovarian plexuses.

The pelvic course travels downward on the side of the pelvic wall. The course curves anteromedially (Junge, 2004). The blood supply to the pelvic course is branches of the superior and inferior vesical artery. The veins follow the course of the arteries.

Ureters have no submucosa in their walls. The inner portion of the wall is mucosa and external to this layer is a thick coat of smooth muscle. Peristaltic contractions of the smooth muscle push the urine

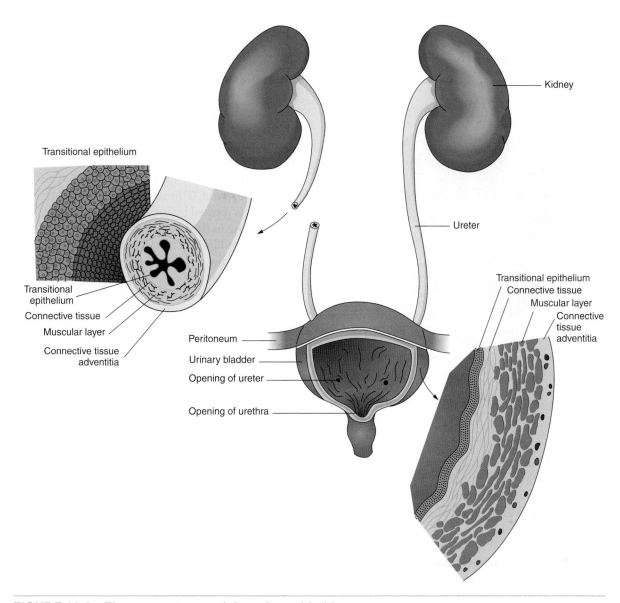

Transitional epithelium

Kidney

Ureter

Transitional epithelium
Connective tissue
Muscular layer
Connective tissue adventitia

Transitional epithelium
Connective tissue
Muscular layer
Connective tissue adventitia

Peritoneum

Urinary bladder

Opening of ureter

Opening of urethra

FIGURE 16-8   The two ureters and the urinary bladder

downward to the bladder. To prevent the reflux of urine, as the bladder fills with urine and expands, the opening of the ureters into the bladder compresses. In addition, rugae of the bladder mucosa cover the orifices of the ureters to aid in reflux when the bladder is full (Cormack, 2001). The outer coat of the ureter, the adventitia, consists of fibroelastic connective tissue (Cormack, 2001) (Figure 16-8).

Urinary Bladder

The **urinary bladder** is a hollow, but muscular, organ located in the anterior of the pelvis (Figure 16-9). The bladder lies posterior to the symphysis pubis—the walls of the pelvis lie on each side—and anterior to the rec-

tovesical septum. In males, the bladder is located superior to the prostate gland, and in females, inferior to the uterus. The location of the bladder is important to the surgeon for two reasons:

1. In the male, prostate tumors can be removed by performing the surgical procedure called suprapubic prostatectomy, which involves an incision into the bladder to expose the prostate and tumor.
2. When performing a vaginal hysterectomy, removal of the uterus through the vaginal canal and opening, the surgeon must be careful not to place sutures through the bladder while closing the vaginal cuff, the area where the vagina was attached to the cervix and uterus.

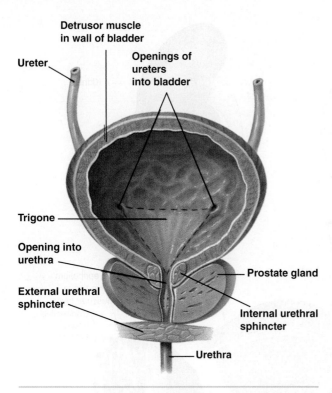

Detrusor muscle
in wall of bladder

Ureter

Openings of
ureters
into bladder

Trigone

Opening into
urethra

External urethral
sphincter

Prostate gland

Internal urethral
sphincter

Urethra

FIGURE 16-9 **The anatomy of the urinary bladder**

In males, the bladder is attached to the superior portion of the prostate gland. In females, it rests on the pelvic diaphragm. Also, in males, the puboprostatic ligament originates at the neck of the bladder and attaches to the parietal fascia on the posterior of the pubis and superior fascia of the pelvic diaphragm (Junge, 2004). This attaches and stabilizes the inferior portion of the bladder. Additional stabilization is achieved by the attachment of the median umbilical ligament to the connective tissue of the umbilicus.

The bladder serves as the collecting point of urine and contracts to eliminate the urine through the urethra. The muscular coat of the bladder consists of three layers of smooth muscle. The inner mucosal lining of the bladder consists of transitional epithelium, which allows the bladder to expand as it fills with urine. When the bladder is empty the mucosa forms folds called rugae, much like the rugae within the stomach. In actuality, the bladder is never completely empty, since there is always a small residual amount of urine left inside. This prevents the walls of the bladder from rubbing against each other and causing irritation of the mucosal tissues. However, a minor complication can occur called "runner's bladder," named for long-distance runners. In addition to avoiding dehydration, long-distance runners are recommended to drink sufficient fluids to ensure

that there is a small amount of urine in the bladder to keep the walls from rubbing against each other. If the bladder is empty, the excessive rubbing action due to the impact of running will irritate the mucosal tissue, causing slight bleeding, and the urine will contain blood. Additionally, this can lead to a bladder infection.

The **vesical trigone** of the urinary bladder is an important anatomic landmark. It is located on the floor of the bladder and contains no rugae, and so does not expand. The vesical trigone is a triangular area that is formed by the two openings of the ureters and opening to the urethra.

The outer fibroelastic adventitial layer is covered by peritoneum on the superior portion of the bladder (Cormack, 2001). The inner smooth muscle layer that surrounds the bladder is the **detrusor muscle**. When the muscle contracts, it pushes on the bladder to force the urine through the urethra. The muscle forms the **internal urethral sphincter** around the opening of the urethra at the neck region of the bladder, which is an involuntary sphincter (Cormack, 2001). Refer to Figure 16-9.

The arterial blood supply to the bladder is from the superior and inferior vesical arteries, branches of the anterior branch of the internal iliac artery. The veins form a plexus within the endopelvic areolar tissue that surrounds the neck of the bladder (Junge, 2004). The veins empty into the internal iliac vein.

Innervation of the bladder occurs from the vesical plexus, which contains sympathetic and parasympathetic fibers. The nerves supply the bladder and lower portion of the ureters. The parasympathetic fibers stimulate the contraction of the detrusor muscle to cause the urination reflex.

Urethra

The **urethra** transports urine from the bladder, through the penis (in the male), and to the outside of the body. Surrounding the urethral meatus is a voluntary sphincter composed of skeletal muscle fibers called the **external urethral sphincter** (Cormack, 2001).

The male urethra is approximately 20 cm in length. It is divided into the prostatic urethra, membranous urethra, and spongy urethra. It extends through the prostate gland and penis, and ends in the urethral **meatus** at the tip of the penis. The male urethra serves the dual function of transporting urine and semen.

The prostatic urethra travels through the prostate gland and is 3–4 cm in length. Ducts from reproductive organs join the prostatic urethra. The membranous urethra is approximately 2 cm in length. It begins just distal to the prostate gland and travels through the urogenital diaphragm. The spongy urethra is about 15 cm in length. It passes through the corpus spongiosum of the penis and the erectile tissue surrounds it. The bulbourethral glands enter the spongy urethra. It terminates at the urethral meatus.

The female urethra is approximately 4 cm long and travels anterior to the lower portion of the vagina. The urethra is in strict contact with the anterior wall of the vagina by a layer of fibrous connective tissue (Cormack, 2001). It is a straight tube as compared to the male urethra, in which the membranous section can assume a tortuous course.

The urethral opening of the female urethra is just superior to the vaginal opening. The shortness and location of the urethral opening, including the straightness of the tube, contribute to why females acquire **urinary tract infections (UTIs)** more often than males. Females are instructed to clean themselves after a bowel movement by using a posterior swiping motion away from the vaginal opening to keep the bacteria from spreading to the vaginal and urethral openings. The arterial supply is from the inferior vesical and vaginal branches of the internal iliac artery.

HEALING OF THE URINARY TRACT

The closure of tissues in the urinary tract must be correctly performed to avoid incomplete closure in order to prevent the leakage of urine. Just as with the biliary tract, nonabsorbable sutures can induce the formation of urinary calculi, and so are not used (Figure 16-10). Absorbable sutures are the suture of choice.

The tissues of the urinary tract tend to heal rapidly. The transitional epithelium quickly migrate and cover the denuded surfaces (Ethicon, 2002). A distinguishing characteristic of the transitional epithelium is that it undergoes mitosis and cell division unlike other epithelium. Healing of specific urinary system structures is discussed in the following sections.

Kidney

Due to the capsule that surrounds the kidney, the repair of wounds is not as difficult as compared to the liver, spleen, or pancreas, and healing usually occurs with fewer complications. However, most injuries to the kidney are due to blunt or penetrating trauma that

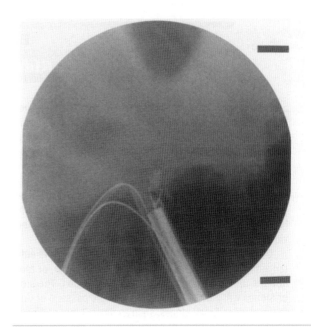

FIGURE 16-10 Percutaneous stone removal

causes jagged-edge fractures of the tissue. These types of injuries are often not reparable by suturing. Simple, uncomplicated injuries are usually treated nonsurgically and healing occurs by fibrous protein synthesis (Peacock, 1984). A scar may occur, which can affect a few of the nephrons, but it is not a complication.

If the kidney must be operated upon, it is most often because the diagnostic evaluation reveals that a major portion of the organ or vessels have been compromised due to injury. The diagnosis is achieved by performing arteriography or pyelography. Surgery will involve either excision of the injured portion of the kidney—as long as the blood supply and good portion of the urinary collecting systems can be preserved—or nephrectomy. The occasional clean laceration is repaired by suturing the capsule (Peacock, 1984). Postoperative complications when the kidney injury is approximated with suture include subcapsular hematoma, perirenal abscess, and hemorrhage. The risk of developing complications is lessened when suction drainage of the retroperitoneal region is utilized.

As mentioned, heminephrectomy is preferred to treat blunt trauma and fractures that do not require a nephrectomy. The intraoperative complications after a portion of the kidney has been excised are control of hemorrhage and wound closure. Hemorrhage is managed by compression such as with the capsule tissue, if enough is left after the heminephrectomy, free grafts of fascia, or peritoneum, and use of a hemostatic agent such as Avitene.

BOX 16-1

Kidney Stones

Stones, or **calculi**, are small and can form in one or both kidneys. The stones are solid due to their composition, which is primarily calcium. Calcium stones occur in approximately 75% of instances of patients with kidney stones. The exact reasons for the formation of stones is not known; however, because the stones are composed of calcium, diet is most likely the leading factor. Changes in diet that lower the ingestion of calcium often prevent recurrences of calcium stones. However, urinary calculi recur in approximately 50% of individuals who have been affected.

One of two actions will occur with stones: they will either remain in the kidney, most often in the renal pelvis, or move into the ureter where they often become lodged. The stone or stones will partially or totally block the passage of urine to the bladder. Small stones, such as those 3 mm or smaller, have a high probability of passing through the ureter to the bladder and being excreted to the outside of the body with the urine. However, this can be very painful and so the individual may be prescribed analgesic and anti-inflammatory drugs.

Calculi can cause the following symptoms:

1. **dysuria**
2. urinary frequency
3. pain in the side in which the stones are located, referred to as flank pain
4. **hematuria**
5. urinary tract infection

The location of the stone(s) can be confirmed by x-ray, ultrasound, CT scan, and intravenous urography. Stones that do not spontaneously pass through the urinary tract must be removed. The options for the removal of stones include:

1. Extracorporeal shock wave lithotripsy (ESWL): a noninvasive method of breaking up the calculi so the smaller fragments will spontaneously pass to the outside of the body with the urine. A patient is placed in the supine position in a special chair and the exact locations of the stone(s) are found with the use of fluoroscopy. The patient is given analgesic drugs in order to relax and reduce the discomfort during the procedure. Shock waves, generated by an electrical discharge, travel to the area of the stones to break them apart.

2. Percutaneous lithotomy: the stone(s) are removed with the use of a scope, special instrumentation, and a small flank incision.

3. Transurethral removal of the stone(s): a flexible ureteroscope can be inserted through the urethra and ureter. Special instruments are used to remove the stone(s).

4. Surgery: stones that are lodged in the renal pelvis or ureter that can't be removed through other methods must be surgically removed. The patient is placed on the unaffected side on the OR table, a flank incision is utilized, and the renal pelvis is entered; or a small incision is made in the ureter to facilitate the removal of the stone(s).

BOX 16-2

Nephrectomy

A nephrectomy is the surgical removal of the entire kidney. A subtotal nephrectomy may be performed in which the upper or superior portion of the kidney is removed. A simple nephrectomy is removal of just the kidney and a radical nephrectomy is removal of the kidney, adrenal gland, perirenal fat, upper ureter, and Gerota's fascia en bloc (meaning removed all together). A simple nephrectomy is performed for malignancies, benign tumors, or chronic obstructive disorders that have not been resolved through other nonsurgical or surgical means. The following is a brief description of a simple nephrectomy.

The patient is positioned on his or her side (lateral position) with the operative site exposed. A flank incision is made just inferior to the 12th rib. The incision is extended through the muscle layers down to Gerota's fascia, which is opened. The perirenal fat and adrenal gland are dissected from the kidney and the kidney is freed up from any tissue attachments.

The ureter is identified, hemostatic clamps are placed on it, a knife is used to divide the ureter, and strands of suture material called ties are used to tie shut the ends of the ureter. Next the renal artery and vein are identified. The renal artery is clamped first, and then the vein. Three strands of strong nonabsorbable ties are placed on the renal artery; two strands are tied as close to the aorta as possible and the third approximately 1 cm from the aorta. The ties are placed in similar fashion on the renal vein; however, they are placed in relation to the vena cava. The renal artery and vein are now divided with the knife between the ties. All remaining attachments to Gerota's fascia are dissected from the kidney and it is now removed. The renal fossa is thoroughly irrigated with saline solution and all bleeding controlled. The wound is closed in layers and the skin layer is closed with staples. Postoperative complications include hemorrhage and infection.

Ureter

Most injuries of the ureter are due to surgical errors, and complications during the healing process are serious and difficult to treat. Surgeons are aware of one of the most important factors in preserving the function of the ureter: it lies on a cushion of retroperitoneal fat (Peacock, 1984). To maintain the downward flow of urine, the slight movement of the ureter on the cushion must be preserved. Healing of the ureter that causes it to be attached to an immovable anatomic structure such as the spine or fascia will decrease peristalsis and inhibit the flow of urine to the bladder (Peacock, 1984). The retroperitoneal fat should be preserved and confirmation must be made that the ureter is in place on the cushion.

Bladder

Surgical incisions and traumatic wounds that are approximated with suture heal by collagen synthesis, which continues until the original strength of the bladder tissue is attained. In approximately 14 days, bladder wounds will have regained 100% of the strength of the remainder of the bladder wall (Peacock, 1984). Collagen synthesis takes place for about seven days and then decreases. Between 30 and 70 days the tensile strength of the wound is almost 100%, and by the 70th day, healing is complete.

However, the actual incision or wound itself heals by fibrous scar formation, which does not have the same strength to resist rupture as compared to normal bladder tissue. As compared to the small intestine and colon, a scar indicates an area of least resistance to increased intraluminal pressure and, if a rupture occurs in a bladder previously operated on, the rupture will most likely happen at the area of healing (Peacock, 1984).

Bladder incisions should be closed with absorbable suture, since suture material can be a nidus for the formation of stones. One of the most frequently used suture material is plain catgut.

Recall that mucosa lines the inner surface of the bladder. Mucosal tissue defects heal by rapid epithelization. The regeneration has been observed in cases in which epithelium must be excised for surgical treatment of bladder cancer. The rapid regeneration of epithelium is due to the migration of epithelial cells and undamaged epithelial cells that undergo mitosis. However, studies have shown that a complication related to the healing process is the high incidence of some ureteral reflux of urine. This may mean that the bladder does not return to complete normal function-

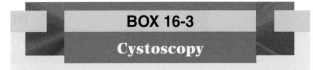

BOX 16-3

Cystoscopy

A cystoscopy involves the insertion of an endoscope called a cystoscope through the urethra and into the bladder to visualize the inside for diagnostic purposes; and some procedures, such as bladder tissue biopsy, resection and removal of a bladder tumor, and the removal of stones too large to pass through the urethra, can then be performed.

The patient is placed in the lithotomy position on a special type of OR table called a cystoscopy table. The patient may receive general anesthesia or, more commonly, spinal anesthesia, in which a drug is injected into the region of the spine that numbs the spinal nerves so the patient has no feeling from the waist down. If necessary, the urethra is dilated with a type of surgical instrument called Van Buren urethral sounds; the diameter of the instrument is round in shape, which facilitates the insertion of the cystoscope to avoid damage to the urethral tissue. As the surgeon advances the cystoscope, the urethra is visualized for any abnormalities, and then the scope enters the bladder.

Through an irrigation port in the cystoscope, the bladder is filled with irrigation fluid. The surgeon inspects the bladder in order to diagnose any pathology. He or she may want to take a bladder tissue biopsy. Special instruments such as a flexible endoscopic biopsy punch can be advanced through another port and a small amount of tissue is removed under direct visualization with the use of the cystoscope. Upon conclusion of the procedure the cystoscope is removed, the bladder thoroughly irrigated, and an indwelling urinary catheter may be inserted for a short period after the surgery.

ing after the process of reepithelization has been completed (Peacock, 1984).

Urethra

The healing of the urethra will be discussed in two parts: posterior urethra and anterior urethra. The posterior urethra heals by epithelization. If the urethra is completely dissected transversely by trauma, the goal, obviously, is to preserve as much length of the urethra as possible and surgically realign the two ends. The short-term use of an indwelling catheter aids in establishing the correct course of healing by reepithelization (Peacock, 1984). A postoperative complication can be excessive fibrous protein synthesis in the tissue surrounding the urethra, causing a chronic stricture that will eventually require treatment such as incision of the area of stricture or dilation.

BOX 16-4

Urinary Catheterization

The bladder is often drained of urine by catheterization, the introduction of a flexible tube called a urinary catheter through the urethra into the bladder. This is a sterile procedure in which strict aseptic technique must be followed to avoid the patient acquiring a UTI. In addition, this is considered an invasive procedure, since the catheter is being placed internally in the body, and so a surgeon's order is required. There are two types of urinary catheters: straight and indwelling. If the patient is undergoing a short surgical procedure, but the bladder still requires drainage, a straight catheter called a Robinson catheter is inserted, the urine is allowed to drain, and the catheter is removed. An indwelling catheter is inserted and remains in place until removal at the appropriate time postoperatively. The most popular type of indwelling catheter is called a Foley catheter. The following information pertains to the insertion of a Foley catheter.

The Foley catheter does the following:

1. It decompresses the bladder to prevent injury to the bladder during abdominal or pelvic surgical procedures, improves visualization of the operative site during abdominal or pelvic procedures, and aids in the postoperative healing of urinary tract structures.

2. It drains urine from the bladder to prevent overfilling during long surgical procedures, obtains a urine specimen from the urinary bag for urinalysis, and monitors the perioperative urinary output to aid in assessing kidney function and fluid balance. The output is periodically documented throughout the surgical procedure in the patient's operating room record.

3. The Foley catheter has openings in which irrigation fluids can be injected to irrigate the bladder.

Foley catheters are available in a variety of sizes. The diameter of the catheter is measured in what is called French size. The smallest size is 8 French for pediatric patients up to the largest, 30 French. For pediatric patients, 8 French through 12 French are commonly used; 14 French and 16 French are commonly used for adults. Near the tip of the catheter is a balloon, which is inflated with sterile water to keep the catheter in place. Sterile water is used to inflate the balloon rather than sterile saline, since the saline can break down the latex composition of the catheter. Typically, in the adult, it is a 5-cc balloon, however, 10 cc's of water are required to inflate the balloon to compensate for the fluid that remains in the inflation portion of the tube.

Catheterization of the surgical patient is usually performed after the patient has been given spinal or general anesthesia to alleviate any pain or discomfort the patient could feel. The female patient must be placed in the "frog-leg" position to facilitate access to the urethral opening. The required supplies include sterile gloves, sterile drape, KY lubricant, antiseptic cleansing solution, cotton balls, forceps, 10-cc syringe prefilled with water, specimen cup, and Foley catheter with drainage tubing and bag attached. Typically, most operating rooms have sterile urinary catheterization trays available with all of the needed supplies and the trays are commercially purchased.

The following are the general steps for placing a Foley catheter in a female patient, since that is the more difficult procedure to perform:

1. The patient is placed in the frog-leg position.

2. Create enough space between the legs to place and open the catheter tray without contaminating any of the contents.

3. Don the sterile gloves using the open-glove technique.

4. Attache the syringe to the appropriate port on the catheter.

5. Open the packet of KY lubricant and empty it into a corner of the tray. Open the packet of antiseptic cleansing solution and pour the solution over the sponges within the container.

6. Place the sterile drape under the buttocks of the patient and place the opening of the drape over the vulva.

7. Use the nondominant hand to retract the labia and expose the urethral meatus. From this point on, this hand cannot be used to touch any sterile supplies and is left in place retracting the labia.

8. Using the forceps, use the dominant hand to pick up a sponge soaked in the antiseptic solution. Using a wiping motion anterior to posterior from the clitoris toward the anus, clean the labial fold and urethral meatus. This is performed three to four times with a new sponge each time.

9. Grasp the end of the catheter with the dominant hand, ensure that the tip is lubricated with the KY lubricant, and slowly insert the catheter through the urethral meatus. If by accident the tip is inserted into the vaginal opening, the catheter is then considered contaminated and a new Foley catheter will need to be obtained.

10. For adult females, the catheter is inserted approximately 2 inches.

11. IMPORTANT: The flow of urine through the catheter tubing and into the urinary bag *must* be confirmed before the balloon is inflated. If urine flow is not confirmed, this could be an indication that the catheter has not been fully inserted and is not within the bladder. Premature inflation of the balloon could cause severe damage to the urethra. If the catheter has been deemed to be inserted quite a distance, the nondominant hand can be used to externally push on the area of the bladder right above the pubic region to force the flow of urine and confirm catheter placement.

12. Once the catheter has been inserted, use the nondominant hand to hold the catheter in place and the dominant hand to inject the sterile water in the syringe to inflate the balloon. Gently pull the catheter to feel resistance and disconnect the syringe from the catheter.

13. Tape the catheter tube to the patient's leg and place the urinary bag below the level of the urinary catheter to prevent the reflux of urine through the urethra and back into the bladder.

Traumatic wounds and congenital defects affect the anterior urethra. Most often traumatic wounds involve blunt or sharp injuries, and lacerations. Two of the more frequent congenital defects are **hypospadias** and **epispadias.** Traumatic wounds heal by reepithelization with very little fibrous protein synthesis (Peacock, 1984). Postoperatively, the repair of traumatic wounds is rarely complicated by stenosis. Congenital defects heal by fibrous protein synthesis. Postoperative complications include wound contraction during the healing process and formation of a fistula.

URINE

The urination reflex and the physical and chemical characteristics of urine will be discussed in the following section. The discussion will also include normal lab values of urine and laboratory findings that indicate an abnormality.

Micturition

Two terms that also refer to the act of urinating are micturition and voiding. The urination reflex is voluntary, since it is a spinal cord reflex. The bladder can hold approximately 800 ml of urine. However, the urination reflex is stimulated when the volume reaches 200–300 ml. The stretching of the detrusor muscle is the stimulus for the urination reflex.

When the urine volume stretches the detrusor muscle, sensory impulses are generated that travel to the sacral portion of the spinal cord. Motor impulses return along parasympathetic nerve pathways to the detrusor muscle, stimulating it to contract. At the same time the muscle is stimulated, the internal urethral sphincter involuntarily relaxes. When an individual urinates, the external urethral sphincter is voluntarily relaxed and the urine flows from the bladder into the urethra and out of the body, thereby emptying the bladder.

Some individuals, due to age, congenital defects, disease or disorders, or, for females, having one or more children, experience urinary incontinence. Many females are affected by a type of incontinence referred to as **stress incontinence**, meaning when the bladder area and muscles are stressed, such as by sitting, laughing, or exercise, urine leaks from the bladder. The condition results from a change in the base of the bladder and distortion of the urethrovesical angle caused by childbirth or because of aging. Surgery is performed to restore both the base of the bladder and the urethrovesical angle back to

their normal position by elevating the base of the bladder.

Physical and Chemical Aspects of Urine

The composition of urine, both physical and chemical, is useful in determining many urinary system, adrenal gland, and systemic conditions of the body, as well as confirming the health of the individual as related to the normal functioning of the kidneys. Urinalysis (UA) is the laboratory analysis of urine that aids in diagnosing pathologies such as urinary tract infection (UTI), diabetes mellitus, eclampsia, tumors, and many other kinds of diseases.

The following summarizes some of the more important normal and abnormal values and constituents of urine:

1. Volume: In a 24-hour period, the normal adult output of urine is approximately 1,200–1,500 ml (Burke, 1980). Factors that can increase the output include fluid intake, diabetes mellitus and insipidus, and certain types of tumors. Excessive consumption of alcohol increases the output, since alcohol inhibits the secretion of ADH and less water is reabsorbed by the kidneys. Dehydration is one contributor to the morning-after hangover. Factors that can decrease the output include dehydration, renal failure, and intestinal disorders and diseases. Dehydration can be caused by excessive sweating due to exercise and loss of fluid such as through diarrhea.

2. Color: The normal color of urine is referred to as being straw- or amber-colored. The more concentrated the urine, meaning there is not much water in the urine, the darker the color.

3. pH: The pH range is 4.5–8.0 (Kee, Paulanka, & Purnell, 2004). Diet has the greatest effect on the pH level. A vegetarian diet will tend to make the urine alkaline, whereas a high-protein diet will make the urine acidic.

4. Specific gravity: The normal range is 1.005–1.030 (Kee et al., 2004). Specific gravity is the measure of the dissolved materials in the urine. A level of 1.000 means that a liquid or solution has no solutes present. The higher the specific gravity number the more dissolved materials are present. Specific gravity provides an indication of the concentrating performance of the kidneys. For example, if a person has been exercising and water has been lost through sweat, less urine will be produced and it will be more concentrated, and will thus have

a higher specific gravity. But this still indicates that the kidneys are doing their job of excreting waste products with the water that is available. A decrease in the specific gravity could indicate diabetes insipidus or nephritis (Burke, 1980).

5. Composition: Urine consists of approximately 95% water and 5% waste products and salts.
6. Aldosterone: Normal value 6–25 μg/24 hours (Kee et al., 2004). An abnormal decrease can indicate eclampsia or Addison's disease.
7. Amylase: Normal value 4–37 U/L/2 hours (Kee et al., 2004). An abnormal increase in the value could indicate the presence of a perforated duodenal ulcer, stone(s) in the common bile duct, or cancer of the pancreas (Burke, 1980).
8. Bilirubin and bile: Should not be present in the urine. Their presence can indicate hepatitis or jaundice.
9. Calcium: Normal value 100–250 mg/24 hours (Kee et al., 2004). An abnormal decrease occurs in the presence of tetany.
10. Ketone bodies (acetone): These should not be present in the urine (Kee et al., 2004). Their presence can be an indicator of eclampsia, starvation, or diabetes mellitus (Burke, 1980).
11. Uric acid: Normal value 250–500 mg/24 hours (Kee et al., 2004). An abnormal increase can be an indicator of eclampsia, liver disorders, and leukemia. An abnormal decrease can be an indicator of an approaching attack of gout (Burke, 1980).
12. Glucose: This should not be present in the urine (Kee et al., 2004). Its presence is an indicator for diabetes mellitus.
13. Casts: These should be present in only a very small amount if at all in the urine. Their presence is an indicator for eclampsia, pyelonephritis, and glomerulonephritis.

WATER–ELECTROLYTE AND ACID–BASE BALANCE

The primary fluid component of the human body is water; approximately 60%–70% of the total body weight is water. Within the body fluids are the positive and negative ions called electrolytes. A primary function of the some of the electrolytes is maintaining the normal pH level in the body fluids. The following sections of this chapter will discuss the water–electrolyte balance and physiology of the acid–base balance.

BOX 16-5

Blood Urea Nitrogen (BUN)

Urea is the chief nitrogenous constituent of urine. Urea forms in the liver and is an end product of protein metabolism. It travels through the circulatory system and is eventually filtered by the kidney to be excreted in urine. Laboratory measurements of the BUN are determined by taking a blood sample from the patient. The measurements are a strong indicator of the excretory function of kidney and metabolic function of the liver. The normal adult value is 3.6–7.1 mm/L; in children the normal value is 5–18 mg/dl (deciliter). The value of 100 mg/dl or higher indicates a serious dysfunction of the kidney(s).

BOX 16-6

Hemodialysis

Hemodialysis is a procedure used to remove excess fluids, waste products, and impurities from the circulating blood. It is indicated for patients who have renal failure or other toxic conditions such as diabetic nephropathy. The patient's blood is passed through the dialysis machine for filtration and diffusion and returned to the circulatory system.

The first step in the process is the insertion of a dual-lumen catheter, usually in the forearm of the nondominant upper extremity, which serves as the access port. The vessels of choice for insertion of the lumens of the catheter are the cephalic vein and the radial artery. Two dialysis cannulas are connected to the catheter. One cannula is the outflow and the other is the inflow, thus the reason for using a dual-lumen catheter. The patient's blood is pumped from the body to the dialysis machine and back to the body. The incoming blood passes over a semipermeable membrane, much like the filter system found in the kidney. As the blood passes over the membrane, excess fluid, waste products, and impurities are filtered into a liquid substance called dialysate, while the necessary blood components such as proteins and blood cells that cannot pass through the membrane are returned to the body. The dialysate is disposed of at the end of the procedure.

The frequency of treatments depends on the type of pathology that is causing the patient to undergo dialysis. However, generally the individual must have dialysis treatment three times per week and the procedure lasts two to four hours each time.

Compartments

Approximately 60% of the water is inside the cells of the body, and is referred to as **intracellular fluid (ICF)**. The other portion of the water is called **extracellular fluid (ECF)** and includes plasma, tissue fluid, synovial fluid, serous fluid, aqueous fluid, and cerebrospinal fluid.

Water is always moving from one compartment of the body to another by the processes of **filtration** and osmosis. For example, the blood vessels of the body are one type of compartment and the water inside the vessels is called plasma. The process of filtration in the capillaries forces some of the plasma into the extracellular tissue spaces, which is another compartment, and now the water is referred to as tissue fluid. The tissue fluid will then enter cells, a third compartment, by osmosis and is now intracellular fluid. Lymph capillaries represent another compartment in which tissue fluid enters and is then called lymph fluid.

Osmosis is an important component for maintaining the water–electrolyte homeostasis. Osmosis is the diffusion of water that most often occurs through the semipermeable cell membranes. Water moves through the membranes from an area of greater concentration to an area of lesser concentration. This movement is affected by the level of electrolytes that are present in the water compartments. Consequently, when the water balance is normal in the water compartments, the electrolytes are also balanced.

Nervous System and Hormonal Control

The majority of the water that humans take in is derived from drinking liquids. Other sources of water include foods that are eaten and metabolic water, which is the by-product of cellular respiration. The normal intake of water in the adult is approximately 2.5–3.0 L per day.

The output of water is primarily through urine of which approximately 1,500 ml are produced per day. Additional water is lost through sweat, water vapor that is contained in exhaled air, and the feces. The total output of water is equal to the intake, 2.5–3.0 L per day. Obviously, individuals who perform strenuous exercise on a frequent basis must replace the fluids by drinking more water.

The hypothalamus is the portion of the brain that is involved in the body's balance of water. The hypothalamus contains osmoreceptors that detect the differing levels of osmolarity in the body fluids. Osmolarity refers to the concentration of dissolved substances in the body fluids. For example, dehydration increases the osmolarity of the blood, thereby making the blood a more concentrated liquid. Therefore, when dehydrated we are thirsty, which produces the desire to drink water to relieve the symptoms such as dry mouth and throat. The water is absorbed by the stomach and small intestine and the osmolarity of the blood is decreased, causing the blood to be more dilute and the symptoms of thirst disappear.

The hypothalamus is also involved in the water balance because of its production of ADH, which is then stored in the posterior pituitary gland. When dehydrated, the hypothalamus stimulates the secretion of ADH from the posterior pituitary gland. ADH stimulates the tubules in the kidneys to increase the reabsorption of water, which is returned to the circulatory system, and urine output is decreased.

The adrenal cortex secretes the hormone aldosterone, which aids in regulating water output. Aldosterone causes an increase in the reabsorption of sodium ions from the kidney tubules and by doing so, water from the renal filtrate naturally follows the ions back to the circulatory system.

Several situations contribute to the loss of water, including the following:

- Excessive abnormal diaphoresis: examples include individuals who are sick with AIDS, flu, malaria, or other infectious diseases.
- Hemorrhage: due to trauma or disease.
- Diarrhea: due to disease.
- Vomiting: due to disease.
- Extensive burns of the body: The two major complications of burns are infection and loss of body fluid.
- Fever: Due to disease or illness such as appendicitis.

These types of situations must be immediately addressed by health care providers, in particular emergency department personnel and the surgical team. The balance of body fluids and maintenance of electrolytes are essential to homeostasis. For example, a burn victim will require the quick administration of large amounts of fluid through intravenous administration, and the fluid must contain needed electrolytes. Even the patient with appendicitis will require some fluid replacement due to the presence of fever, which causes the loss of body fluids.

Electrolytes

Electrolytes are chemicals that dissolve in water and are either positive or negative ions. Positive ions are called cations and negative ions are called anions. Electrolytes aid in the osmolarity of body fluids and osmosis of water between water compartments. The primary electrolytes, with their chemical symbol, are as follows:

- Sodium (Na^+)
- Potassium (K^+)
- Calcium (Ca^{+2})
- Chloride (Cl^-)
- Phosphate (HPO_4^{-2})
- Bicarbonate (HCO_3^-)
- Magnesium (Mg^{+2})
- Sulfate (SO_4^{-2})

The electrolytes that are absorbed through the consumption of food and beverages enter the bloodstream to become a component of the body fluids. The levels of many of the electrolytes are controlled by hormones. As previously mentioned, aldosterone increases the reabsorption of Na^+ ions, but also increases the excretion of K^+ ions by the kidneys. Therefore, the blood level of sodium is increased and the potassium level is decreased. ANH is responsible for increasing the excretion of Na^+ ions by the kidneys to decrease the blood level of sodium. PTH and calcitonin regulate the circulatory levels of calcium and phosphate. Calcitonin stimulates calcium and phosphate to be removed from the blood to be used in the formation of bone matrix. PTH increases reabsorption of calcium and phosphate from bones to increase their circulatory levels.

Electrolytes are also removed from the body through sweat, urine, and feces. Urine contains electrolytes such as Na^+ that are not reabsorbed by the kidney tubules due to the size of the ion particles. Na^+ and Cl^- ions are the primary electrolytes that are found in sweat.

Acid–Base Balance

Homeostasis of the acid–base balance is maintained by the three buffer systems in respirations, kidneys, and body fluids. Buffer systems prevent abnormal changes in the pH levels of the body by chemical reactions. Each buffer system contains a weak acid and base that react with strong acids or bases to change the strong substances into substances that do not affect the body's pH. The buffer systems maintain blood and tissue fluid pH level at 7.35 to 7.45 and intracellular fluid pH level at 6.8 to 7.0. The three buffer systems are the bicarbonate buffer system, protein buffer system, and phosphate buffer system.

Bicarbonate Buffer System

The bicarbonate buffer system consists of carbonic acid (H_2CO_3), a weak acid, and sodium bicarbonate ($NaHCO_3$), a weak base. The bicarbonate buffer system is important in maintaining the normal pH in the tissue fluids and blood. During the processes of metabolism the blood and tissue fluids have a tendency to become acidic. Consequently, sodium bicarbonate is needed more than carbonic acid.

For example, if the pH level changes due to the blood becoming more acidic, the following chemical reaction occurs in the body:

$$HCl \text{ (strong acid)} + NaHCO_3 \rightarrow NaCl + H_2CO_3 \text{ (weak acid)}$$

The HCl reacted with the sodium bicarbonate to produce NaCl (salt), which does not affect the pH level, and also a weak acid has been produced, which does not affect the pH level.

If the pH changes and becomes more basic, the following chemical reaction occurs in the body:

$$NaOH \text{ (strong base)} + H_2CO_3 \rightarrow H_2O + NaHCO_3 \text{ (weak base)}$$

The NaOH reacted with the carbonic acid to produce H_2O (water) and a weak base, neither of which has an effect on the pH level.

Protein Buffer System

As the name suggests, the protein buffer system is composed of proteins that are made up of amino acids. The amino acids contain a carboxyl group (COOH) and amino group (NH_2), and either group can work as acids or bases. The protein buffer system is important to maintaining the normal pH level in the intracellular fluids.

The carboxyl group can act as an acid due to donating a hydrogen ion (H^+) to the ICF to act against the increase in the alkaline level of the fluid. The chemical reaction is as follows:

$$\begin{array}{ccc} & H & & H \\ & | & & | \\ NH_2-C-COOH & \rightarrow & NH_2-C-COO^- + H^+ \\ & | & & | \\ & R & & R \end{array}$$

The amino group can act as a base due to picking up an excess hydrogen ion from the intracellular fluid to act against an increase in acidity. The chemical reaction is as follows:

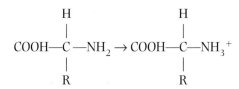

The buffer systems are effective, but short acting due to the limited number of molecules within the body fluids. Therefore, to counteract a pathologic condition, such as **acidosis** or **alkalosis**, the buffer systems are supported by respiratory and renal mechanisms.

Phosphate Buffer System

The phosphate buffer system consists of sodium dihydrogen phosphate (NaH_2PO_4), a weak acid, and sodium monohydrogen phosphate (Na_2HPO_4), a weak base. The phosphate buffer system aids in the regulation of the pH level of the blood by the kidneys. The kidney tubules remove excess hydrogen ions by synthesizing NaH_2PO_4, which is then excreted in the urine. The Na^+ ions and bicarbonate ions that are retained are returned to the bloodstream in the peritubular capillaries.

If a strong acid affects the pH level, the following chemical reaction takes place:

$$HCl \text{ (strong acid)} + Na_2HPO_4 \rightarrow NaCl$$
$$+ NaH_2PO_4 \text{ (weak acid)}$$

The HCl reacted with the sodium monohydrogen phosphate to produce salt, which does not effect the pH level, and a weak acid, which has very little effect on the pH level.

If a strong base affects the pH level the following chemical reaction takes place:

$$NaOH \text{ (strong base)} + NaH_2PO_4 \rightarrow H_2O$$
$$+ Na_2HPO_4 \text{ (weak base)}$$

In this instance, NaOH reacted with sodium dihydrogen phosphate to synthesize water, which has no effect on the pH level, and a weak base, which has very little effect on the pH level.

Respiratory Mechanism

The respiratory system contributes to the homeostasis of the body's pH level by regulating the level of CO_2 in body fluids. Thus, the respiratory system can help to return the pH to normal levels when an imbalance is created by various factors within the body; these changes are referred to as metabolic acidosis or b.

Causes of metabolic acidosis include diabetes mellitus, severe vomiting, severe diarrhea, and kidney disease. The pH decreases when an excess of H^+ ions is within the body fluids. This stimulates the respiratory center in the medulla to increase the rate of breathing so an increase of CO_2 is exhaled by the individual and the level of H^+ ions decreases. The end result is an increase of the pH back to the normal range.

Causes of metabolic alkalosis include vomiting or overuse of antacid medicines. In this instance, as the pH level of the body fluids increases, the individual breathes slower, thus decreasing the amount of CO_2 that is exhaled. The CO_2 helps to increase the synthesis of H^+ ions, lowering the pH back to normal range.

Renal Mechanism

The renal mechanism is the strongest and most effective buffer for countering pH changes. It does not react as quickly, sometimes taking several hours to days to be functional, but is effective much longer than is the respiratory mechanism. The kidneys aid in regulating the pH of the ECF by excreting or reabsorbing H^+ ions and by excreting or reabsorbing Na^+ ions and HCO_3^- ions. The following is an example of the respiratory and renal mechanisms at work:

1. The patient has diabetes mellitus that has not been controlled by medication.
2. **Ketoacidosis** is now occurring.
3. As the level of acidic ketones continues to increase, the ECF buffer systems are exhausted.
4. Now the respiratory mechanism begins by increasing the respiratory rate in order for the level of exhaled CO_2 to increase and cause a decrease in H^+ ion level. However, the respiratory mechanism eventually becomes exhausted.
5. But this has allowed the renal mechanism to become fully functional and effective. The kidneys are now working to keep the pH level normal. However, the kidneys can do only so much; the ketoacidosis requires medical intervention to correct the condition or death will most likely occur.

IMPLICATIONS FOR THE SURGICAL TECHNOLOGIST

Surgical procedures of the urinary system range from the simple such as diagnostic cystoscopy to the very complicated including nephrectomy and renal transplant. Having in-depth knowledge of and understanding the anatomy and physiology of the urinary system are highly important for the following reasons:

1. The name of the surgical procedure provides the number one indication of what organ(s) of the urinary system will be operated upon. The surgical technologist must know the surgical position in which to place the patient, the type of incision that will be made, surgical supplies, equipment and instrumentation that the surgeon will use, drains specific to urinary system surgery, dressings, and immediate postoperative care.

2. Many urinary system procedures require the identification of the ureters in order to prevent damage to them during the surgical procedure. Knowing the approximate anatomic location of the ureters allows the surgical technologist to aid the surgeon in their identification. Additionally, often dyes are injected into the kidney or through the openings in the bladder so x-rays can be taken that allow visualization of the ureters. The surgical technologist must be ready to assist the surgeon in the insertion of the cystoscope and other instrumentation in order to perform these procedures.

3. Surgical technologists are trained to insert catheters through the urethra into the bladder to facilitate the drainage of urine. The surgical technologist must be able to distinguish the opening of the urethra in the female as opposed to other nearby structures such as the vaginal opening. In the male, because of the length of the urethra, it can occasionally be difficult to insert the catheter, and manipulative measures are taken in order to straighten out the urethra and put the catheter in place.

4. The choice of suture material and size is determined by the urinary organs that will be operated on. Obviously, the suture used for the ureter will be very small in diameter, whereas the suture material used on the bladder will be larger in diameter. Additionally, the surgical technologist must remember that the suture material should be absorbable, since it can be a nidus for stone formation in the bladder.

5. As previously mentioned, the name of the surgical procedure aids in indicating the patients surgical position. Some positions, such as prone, can place pressure on the ureters and prevent the flow of urine from the kidneys to the bladder. Proper positioning of the patient with the use of positioning devices is essential to prevent this mishap. The surgical technologist can be another set of eyes to help in monitoring the flow of urine during surgery, the color of the urine, and whether blood is present in the urine.

As the preceding examples indicate, the surgical technologist is a key member of the surgical team whose knowledge of the complicated urinary tract system is valuable to good patient outcomes in surgery.

Case Study 2

A physician examines an infant who has been experiencing hematuria, pyuria, dysuria, and occasionally anuria. When touched on the right side of the body, the infant cries and exhibits signs of pain. The mother also reports bouts of vomiting. The physician orders an ultrasound and urography, which confirm a congenital stricture (stenosis) of the right ureter and hydronephrosis.

1. What are the two most common sites for a ureteral stricture?

2. Define hydronephrosis.

3. Define anuria.

4. What is a urography?

5. How is the stricture treated?

CHAPTER SUMMARY

- The urinary system consists of: two kidneys, two ureters, a urinary bladder, and a urethra.

- The formation of urine is important to aid in the elimination of wastes from the body that are toxic.

- Substances that are needed are absorbed by the tubules to be returned to the body.

- Urine formation aids in homeostasis by maintaining the normal composition, pH level, and volume of blood and extracellular fluids.

- Each kidney is located in a retroperitoneal position, is reddish brown in color, and is shaped like a kidney bean.

- The kidney is surrounded by a capsule. It rests in a bed of adipose tissue called Gerota's fascia.

- The hilum is located on the medial side; the renal artery enters and the renal vein exits at this area of the kidney. The renal artery is a branch of the abdominal aorta and the renal vein travels back to the inferior vena cava.

- The kidney is divided into three sections: the renal cortex, renal medulla, and renal pelvis. The renal cortex contains the renal corpuscles and convoluted tubules.

- The renal medulla contains the loop of Henle and collecting tubules. It is composed of renal pyramids, which divide the kidney into lobes. Individual lobes are identified by the renal columns.

- The lobes consist of a renal pyramid and renal column.

- The upper portion of each renal pyramid tapers to form renal papillae, which enter minor calyces in the renal pelvis.

- The renal pelvis indicates where the ureter enters the kidney and the pelvis expands into funnel-shaped structures called calyces.

- The calyces surround the papillae of the renal pyramids. There are two calyces: minor and major calyces. The minor calyces drain into the major calyces. The calyces serve as the collection point of urine.

- The nephron is the working structure of each kidney. It is composed of two parts: the renal corpuscle and renal tubule.

- The renal corpuscle consists of the glomerulus and Bowman's capsule.

- The glomerulus is a network of capillary vessels that are a division of the afferent arteriole and efferent arteriole.

- Bowman's capsule is a double-layered cup that is an extension of the end of a renal tubule and it surrounds the glomerulus. Bowman's capsule consists of two layers with a space between and podocytes that branch to the glomerulus. This forms one of several filtering devices of the kidney.

- The second portion of a nephron is the renal tubule that is a continuation of Bowman's capsule. It is subdivided into three parts: the proximal convoluted tubule, the loop of Henle, and the distal convoluted tubule.

- Distial convoluted tubules empty into a collecting tubule. Several collecting tubules join to form a papillary duct that transfers the urine to a calyx. Peritubular capillaries surround each part of the renal tubule.

- The juxtaglomerular apparatus is composed of juxtaglomerular cells and the macula densa.

- Blood flow through the kidney begins with the renal artery. After entering through the hilum, it divides into several branches called interlobar arteries. The interlobar arteries divide to form incomplete arteries called arcuate arteries that give rise to the interlobular arteries. The last branch of the interlobular arteries are the afferent arterioles, which travel to the nephrons.

- The renal arteries branch from the abdominal aorta at the level of the second lumbar vertebra and travel in a transverse route to the kidney. Branches from the renal arteries called the ureteric branches supply the ureter.

- The renal veins lie anterior to the arteries. As the left vein travels to the inferior vena cava, the left adrenal and left testicular or ovarian veins empty into it.

- There are three lymphatic vessel plexuses: one located within the parenchyma of the kidney, the second located underneath the capsule of the kidney, and the third located in the perirenal fat.

- Afferent nerve innervation arises from the renal plexus. The efferent innervation consists of autonomic, vasomotor nerves.

- Urine formation is in three steps: glomerular filtration, tubular reabsorption, and tubular secretion.

- Glomerular filtration involves plasma, waste products, and small protein particles forced from the glomeruli by blood pressure and into Bowman's capsule to form renal filtrate.

- The glomerular filtration rate (GFR) is the measurement of the amount of urine formed by the kidneys in one minute. The average amount that is formed in 125 ml per minute.

- Tubular reabsorption occurs between the renal tubules and peritubular capillaries. The majority of renal filtrate does not become urine; it is reabsorbed into the bloodstream in the peritubular capillaries. The reabsorption and secretion of renal filtrate occur primarily in the proximal convoluted tubules.

- There are four processes of tubular reabsorption: active transport, passive transport, pinocytosis, and osmosis.

- Three hormones that influence the absorption of water are: aldosterone, atrial natriuretic hormone (ANH), and antidiuretic hormone (ADH).

- Aldosterone is secreted by the adrenal gland. It stimulates the reabsorption of sodium ions, which causes water to be reabsorbed from the renal filtrate back to the circulating blood.

- ANH is the antagonist to aldosterone. It is secreted by the atria of the heart. ANH is released to decrease the reabsorption of sodium ions from the renal filtrate into the circulating blood. Thus, the sodium ions remain in the renal filtrate, including water, and are excreted in the urine to aid in lowering the blood pressure and blood volume.

- ADH is secreted by the posterior pituitary gland when the water level in the body is low. ADH stimulates the distal convoluted tubules and collecting tubules to increase the reabsorption of water from the renal filtrate.

- The kidneys are the primary organ responsible for maintaining the normal blood pH level and normal level of tissue fluid. If blood and body fluids are acidic, the kidneys stimulate the secretion of hydrogen ions into the renal filtrate and cause an increase of bicarbonate ions into the blood. When blood is too alkaline, the kidneys cause the hydrogen ions to be returned to the circulating blood and bicarbonate ions are excreted in the urine.

- Additional functions of the kidney include secretion of renin, conversion of vitamin D, and production of erythropoietin.

- When the blood pressure decreases, the juxtaglomerular cells are stimulated to secrete renin, the first step in the renin–angiotensin mechanism, the end product of which is angiotensin II, which causes vasoconstriction and stimulates the increase in the secretion of aldosterone. Together aldosterone and angiotensin II increase the blood pressure.

- The kidneys convert vitamin D to calciferol, which increases the absorption of calcium and phosphate in the small intestine.

- The kidneys produce erythropoietin, which is secreted when a person is hypoxic.

- All three structures have the overall responsibility of allowing urine to travel from the kidneys to be excreted to the outside of the body.

- The ureters allow urine to flow from the kidneys to the bladder. They are positioned retroperitoneally. The course of the ureter is divided into an abdominal course and pelvic course. The ureters terminate on the right and left posterolateral walls of the urinary bladder.

- The blood supply to the ureters is from branches of the renal and testicular or ovarian arteries, and branches of the superior and inferior vesical arteries. The veins follow the course of the arteries. Innervation is from the renal and testicular or ovarian plexuses.

- The inner portion of the ureteral wall is mucosa and overlying this is a smooth muscle layer. Peristaltic contractions of the smooth muscle push the urine downward to the bladder.

- The urinary bladder is a hollow, muscular organ located anterior to the pelvis, posterior to the symphysis pubis, and anterior to the rectovesical septum. In males it is superior to the prostate gland; in females, it is superior to the uterus.

- The anatomic location of the bladder is important to the surgeon for two reasons: first, in the male, prostate tumors can be removed, which involves an incision in the bladder to expose the prostate and tumor; second, when performing a vaginal hysterectomy the surgeon must be careful not to place sutures through the bladder wall.

- The bladder serves as the collecting point and reservoir for urine, and contracts to eliminate the urine through the urethra.

- The bladder consists of three layers of smooth muscle. The inner mucosal lining consists of transitional epithelium, which allows the bladder to expand when filling with urine. When empty, the mucosa forms folds called rugae.

- The vesical trigone is an important anatomic landmark within the bladder. It is located on the floor of the bladder and contains no rugae; therefore, it does not expand. It is formed by the two openings of the ureters and opening to the urethra.

- The inner smooth muscle layer of the bladder is the detrusor muscle. The muscle contracts to push on the bladder, thus forcing out the urine through the urethra. The muscle forms the internal urethral sphincter around the opening of the urethra at the neck region of the bladder, an involuntary sphincter.

- The arterial blood supply to the bladder is from the superior and inferior vesical arteries, branches of the anterior branch of the internal iliac artery. The veins form a plexus within the endopelvic areolar tissue that surrounds the bladder neck. The veins empty into the internal iliac vein.

- Innervation of the bladder is from the vesical plexus, which contains sympathetic and parasympathetic fibers. The parasympathetic fibers stimulate the contraction of the detrusor muscle.

- The urethra transports urine from the bladder to the outside of the body.

- The urethral meatus is surrounded by a voluntary sphincter composed of skeletal muscle fibers called the external urethral sphincter.

- The male urethra is divided into the prostatic urethra, membranous urethra, and spongy urethra. The male urethra serves the dual function of transporting urine and semen.

- The female urethra is much shorter and travels anterior to the lower portion of the vagina; it is connected to the anterior wall of the vagina by a layer of connective tissue.

- The female urethral opening is just superior to the vaginal opening. The short length, location of the urethral opening, and straightness of the tube contribute to the higher frequency with which urinary tract infections (UTI) occur in females relative to males.

- The blood supply to the female urethra is from the inferior vesical and vaginal branches of the internal iliac artery.

- Closure of urinary tract tissues must be complete to prevent leakage of urine.

- Absorbable sutures are used, since nonabsorbable sutures induce the formation of urinary calculi.

- The majority of the tissues of the urinary tract tend to heal rapidly. Unlike other types of epithelium, the transitional epithelium undergoes mitosis and cell division.

- Most injuries sustained by the kidney are due to blunt or penetrating trauma that causes jagged-edge wounds of the tissue, which are usually not repairable with suture.

- Diagnosis of the kidney is performed through an arteriography or pyelography, which help to determine if an operation must be performed.

- Surgery of the kidney will be either excision of the injured portion or a nephrectomy. Occasionally a clean laceration can be repaired by suturing the capsule.

- Postoperative complications of kidney surgery include subcapsular hematoma, hemorrhage, and perirenal abscess.

- Heminephrectomy is performed to treat blunt trauma and fractures. Hemorrhage is the primary intraoperative complication.

- Most injuries sustained by a ureter are due to surgical errors.

- One of the most important factors that contributes to the healing of the ureter and preserving its function is retaining the cushion of retroperitoneal fat on which it lies.

- Healing of the ureter that causes it to be attached to an immobile anatomic structure will decrease peristalsis, thereby inhibiting the flow of urine.

- Incisions and traumatic wounds of the bladder that are approximated with suture heal by collagen synthesis. In 14 days, bladder wounds regain 100% of their original strength.

- The actual incision or wound heals by fibrous scar formation, which does not have the same strength as the rest of the bladder tissue.

- Bladder incisions are closed with absorbable suture material, usually plain catgut.

- Mucosal tissue defects heal by rapid epithelization. However, a complication of the healing process is the high incidence of some ureteral reflux of urine.

- The posterior urethra heals by epithelization. Postoperative complication of healing is excessive fibrous protein synthesis in the tissue surrounding the urethra, causing a chronic stricture that will require treatment.

- The anterior urethra is usually injured by traumatic wounds or congenital defects.

- Traumatic wounds of the anterior urethra heal by reepithelization. Congenital defects heal by fibrous protein synthesis, and often postoperatively wound contraction and formation of a fistula occur.

- Micturition and voiding refer to the act of urinating.

- The urination reflex is voluntary, since it is a spinal cord reflex.

- The bladder can hold approximately 800 ml of urine. The urination reflex is stimulated when the volume is at 200–300 ml. The stretching of the detrusor muscle is the stimulus for the urination reflex.

- The urinary reflex pathway is as follows: the detrusor muscle is stretched by urine volume → sensory impulses travel to the sacral portion of the spinal cord → motor impulses return to the detrusor muscle stimulating it to contract → internal urethral sphincter involuntarily relaxes → external urethral sphincter is voluntarily relaxed → urine flows from bladder through urethra to the outside of the body.

- Many females are affected by stress incontinence, most often because of a change in the base of the bladder and distortion of the urethrovesical angle caused by childbirth or due to aging. Surgery is performed to correct the condition.

- The composition of urine is used as a gauge to confirm the health of the individual as related to normal functioning of the kidneys and other systems of the body.

- Urinalysis (UA) is a laboratory analysis of urine.

- The normal adult output of urine in a 24-hour period is 1,200–1,500 ml.

- The normal color of urine is referred to as being straw- or amber-colored. The more concentrated the urine, the more yellow the color.

- The pH range is 4.7–8.0. Diet has the greatest effect on the pH level.

- The normal range of the specific gravity is 1.010–1.020. Specific gravity is the measure of the dissolved substances in the urine, and provides an indication of the concentrating performance of the kidneys.

- Urine consists of 95% water and 5% waste products and salts.

- Approximately 60%–70% of the total body weight is water.

- Within the body fluids are the electrolytes, a primary function of which is maintaining the normal pH level in the body fluids.

- Sixty percent of the water is intracellular fluid (ICF). The other portion is extracellular fluid (ECF).

- Water moves from one compartment of the body to another by either filtration or osmosis.

- Osmosis is the diffusion of water through the semipermeable cell membranes. Water moves through the membranes from an area of greater concentration to an area of lesser concentration. When the water balance is normal, the electrolyte balance is normal.

- The majority of water intake of humans is derived from drinking liquids.

- The output of water is primarily through urine. The total output of water equals the intake.

- The hypothalamus contains osmoreceptors, which detect differing levels of osmolarity in the body fluids. Osmolarity is the concentration of dissolved substances in the body fluids. The hypothalamus aids in maintaining the body's balance of water.

- The hypothalamus also produces antidiuretic hormone (ADH), which is then stored in the posterior pituitary gland. When dehydrated ADH is secreted, it stimulates the tubules in the kidneys to increase the reabsorption of water to be returned to the circulatory system.

- The adrenal cortex secretes aldosterone to aid in regulating water output. Aldosterone causes an increase in the reabsorption of sodium ions from the kidney tubules, and water follows the ions back to the circulatory system.

- Emergency situations that contribute to the loss of water and body fluids must be immediately treated by the emergency department personnel and surgery team. Maintaining the normal level of water and body fluids, including electrolytes, is essential to homeostasis.

- Electrolytes are either positive ions called cations or negative ions called anions. Electrolytes contribute to the osmolarity of body fluids and affect the osmosis of water in the water compartments.

- Electrolytes are absorbed through the consumption of food and beverages and enter the bloodstream to become a component of the body fluids.

- The levels of many of the electrolytes are controlled by hormones such as aldosterone, atrial natriuretic hormone, and parathyroid hormone.

- Electrolytes are removed by the body through sweat, urine, and feces.

- The acid–base balance is maintained by buffer systems that prevent abnormal changes in the pH levels of the body through chemical reactions.

- The bicarbonate buffer system consists of carbonic acid, a weak acid, and sodium bicarbonate, a weak base. The system maintains the normal pH in the tissue fluids and blood.

- The protein buffer system consists of proteins that are made up of amino acids. The amino acids contain a carboxyl group and amino group, and either group can work as an acid or base. The system maintains the normal pH in the intracellular fluids.

- The phosphate buffer system consists of sodium dihydrogen phosphate, a weak acid, and sodium monohydrogen phosphate, a weak base. The system aids in the regulation of the pH of the blood by the kidneys.

- The buffer systems are effective, but short acting, and, therefore, cannot counteract a chronic condition such as acidosis or alkalosis for a very long time.

- The respiratory system contributes to maintaining a normal pH level by regulating the level of CO_2 in body fluids.

- During episodes of metabolic acidosis the pH decreases, which stimulates the respiratory center in the medulla to increase the rate of breathing in order to increase the amount of CO_2 that is exhaled.

- During episodes of metabolic alkalosis the individual breathes slower to decrease the amount of CO_2 that is exhaled.

- The renal mechanism is the strongest and most effective buffer to counter changes in the pH level. It can take several hours to days to become fully functional, but lasts much longer than the respiratory mechanism.

- The renal mechanism works by excreting or reabsorbing H^+ ions and by excreting or reabsorbing Na^+ ions and HCO_3^- ions.

- The surgical technologist must have in-depth knowledge of the anatomy and physiology of the urinary system in order to know proper patient surgical positions; types of incisions utilized in urinary tract surgery; surgical supplies, equipment, and instrumentation that will be used; and drains and dressings.

- Knowing the location of the ureters will provide the surgical technologist with the ability to aid the surgeon in identifying their location.

- The surgical technologist must know the location of the urethral opening in the female in order to place catheters. In the male, due to the length of the urethra and its tortuous course through the membranous portion, it can be difficult to insert a catheter, and the surgical technologist must know the manipulative techniques in order to place the catheter in position without harming the patient.

- Knowing the urinary organs and type of tissue aids in the choice of suture material and size.

Additionally, the surgical technologist must remember that absorbable suture is the suture of choice to prevent the formation of stones.

- Often the patient must be placed in difficult surgical positions to facilitate surgery on the organs of the urinary system. These positions can place pressure on the ureters and prevent the flow of urine from the kidneys to the bladder. Proper positioning and use of positioning devices is essential to the protection of the patient.

- The surgical technologist can serve as another set of eyes to help in monitoring the flow of urine during any type of lengthy surgery, including the color of the urine and the amount excreted during a set period of time.

CRITICAL THINKING QUESTIONS

1. A urinalysis on a patient indicates the presence of glucose in the urine. What does this most likely indicate for the patient?
2. When a nephrectomy is performed, what artery and vein must be cut and tied closed with suture material to free up the kidney?
3. A patient's spinal cord is injured during a car accident but recovers. However, the patient is diagnosed with an atonic or flaccid bladder. What has happened to the patient? What anatomic structures are involved?
4. Based on your knowledge of the anatomic position of the kidney, what surgical patient position is often utilized when operating on the kidney?
5. If the blood flow decreases through the kidney, what happens to the GFR?

REFERENCES

Burke, S. R. (1980). *The composition and functions of body fluids* (3rd ed.). St. Louis: C. V. Mosby.

Cormack, D. H. (2001). *Essential histology* (2nd ed.). Philadelphia: Lippincott Williams & Wilkins.

Ethicon Products Worldwide. (2002). *Wound closure manual.* Somerville, NJ: Ethicon, Inc.

Junge, T. (2004). Genitourinary surgery. Association of surgical technologists, *Surgical technology for the surgical technologist: A positive care approach* (pp. 731–790). Clifton Park, NY: Thomson Delmar Learning.

Kee, J. L., Paulanka, B. J., & Purnell, L. D. (2004). *Handbook of fluid, electrolytes, and acid-based imbalances* (2nd ed.). Clifton Park, NY: Thomson Delmar Learning.

Peacock, E. E. (1984). *Wound repair* (3rd ed.). Philadelphia: W. B. Saunders.

17

REPRODUCTIVE SYSTEM

CHAPTER OBJECTIVES

After completing the study of this chapter, you should be able to:

1. List the functions of the male and female reproductive systems.
2. List the components of the male reproductive system and describe each of their functions.
3. Describe the process of meiosis.
4. Describe the process of spermatogenesis.
5. Describe the pathway of sperm cells from the beginning point within the body to the outside of the body.
6. List the hormones that play an important role in the male reproductive system and development of male secondary sex characteristics and their functions.
7. List the components of the female reproductive system and describe each of their functions.
8. Describe the process of oogenesis.
9. List the hormones that play an important role in the female reproductive system and development of female secondary characteristics and their functions.
10. List and describe the steps of the menstrual cycle.
11. Describe the changes the female body undergoes during pregnancy and the role of hormones.
12. Describe the process of cleavage.
13. State the origination of the primary germ layers and the structures produced.
14. Describe the anatomic structure and functions of the placenta.
15. Describe each stage of fetal development.
16. Trace the flow of blood in the fetal circulatory system.
17. List and describe the immediate anatomic changes that occur in a newborn.
18. Define genes and chromosomes.
19. Define genome.

CHAPTER OUTLINE (*continued*)

Mammary Glands
    Breast Development
    Production of Milk
    Blood and Nerve Supplies of the Breasts
    Healing of Breast Tissue
Genetics
    Genetic Traits
    The Y & X of the Whole Gene Situation
    Gene Therapy

CHAPTER OBJECTIVES (*continued*)

20. State the difference between the two types of chromosomes.
21. Explain alleles.
22. Describe the various modes of inheritance.
23. Explain how genetic traits are transmitted through the sex chromosomes.
24. Describe how abnormalities in the chromosome number can affect the health or condition of an individual.
25. Describe gene therapy.

KEY TERMS

alleles	ejaculatory duct	lactiferous duct	puberty
androgens	embryo	Leydig cells	seroma
autosomes	estrogens	marsupialization	somatic cells
Bartholin's glands	fimbriae	menopause	spermatic cord
chorion	genes	ovarian follicles	spermatids
chorionic villi	genome	placenta	spermatogonia
chromosomes	genotype	primordial follicles	spermatozoa
circumcision	glans penis	progesterone	tubal pregnancy
crossover	infundibulum	prolactin	vulva
ductus venosus vessel	karyotype		

Case Study 1

A pregnant woman in the 35th week of gestation is rushed into the emergency department with the following signs and symptoms: severe, agonizing uterine pain that radiates to the abdomen; tender uterus; signs of fetal distress; and onset of shock. An IV with a large-bore catheter is immediately started for the rapid infusion of lactated Ringer's solution. A blood sample is drawn for type-and-crossmatch and, as soon as possible, the infusion of blood is started. The woman is stabilized; however, signs of fetal distress continue and the surgeon decides that a cesarean section must be performed.

1. Based on the signs and symptoms, what is most likely happening to the patient and describe the pathology?

2. Why is the rapid infusion of fluids and possible blood transfusion necessary?

3. What are some of the causes of the pathology that is identified in the answer to Question 1?

4. When the newborn is delivered by cesarean section, what should the pediatric team in the OR be ready to immediately treat?

INTRODUCTION

The organs of the male and female reproductive systems are formed as such in order to perform the specialized functions of producing sperm cells and eggs, and transporting these sex cells. In addition, organs such as the ovaries in the female and the testes in the male produce hormones that initiate the development of secondary sex characteristics and support pregnancy.

In the male, as mentioned, the reproductive system is focused on the production and maintenance of the sex cells, called sperm cells, and the transport of these cells to the outside of the body and then into the female reproductive tract. The primary organs of

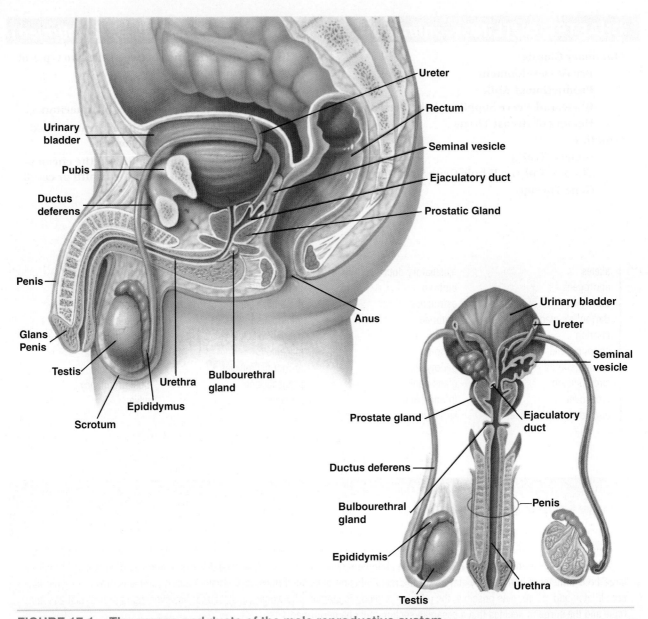

FIGURE 17-1 The organs and ducts of the male reproductive system

the system are the testes. The generic term gonads is used to refer to the testes in the male and the ovaries in the female. Within the testes, the spermatozoa are formed; they also produce the male sex hormones. The other reproductive structures, which support the functions of the testes, are located internally and externally (Figure 17-1). These will be discussed later.

TESTES

The testes (singular, testis), also called testicles, are ovoid structures approximately 3–4 cm in diameter, 4–5 cm in length, and 2 cm thick. They are contained

in an external saclike structure called the scrotum and held in place by the **spermatic cord**. The scrotal septum separates the scrotum in halves with a testis in each half. Each half contains the same set of anatomic structures.

Testicular Descent

In the fetus, the testes form in an area that is posterior to the parietal peritoneum next to where the kidneys are forming. Approximately two months prior to birth, the testes descend through the inguinal canal and into the scrotum. The male hormone testosterone, which is produced and secreted by the testes, stimulates the descent of the testes. Attached to each testicle is a thick cord called the gubernaculum, which travels through the inguinal canal and is attached to the outside of the scrotal skin. As the testicle descends, the gubernaculum serves as a guide, allowing the testicle to travel downward through the inguinal canal of the abdomen and enter the scrotum. Attached to each testicle is a developing vas deferens, nerves, and blood vessels, which will eventually be a part of the spermatic cord that replaces the gubernaculum.

If one or both testicles fail to descend from the abdominal cavity, the condition is referred to as unilateral or bilateral cryptorchidism. If the condition is not surgically treated, the cells that produce sperm will die and eventually the tissue of the testis itself will deteriorate. Because the body temperature is high in the abdominal region, when the testis remains there, most often in the inguinal canal, damage to the testis occurs. If both testicles are affected, infertility results. The testes are located in the external scrotal sac precisely because the temperature is a few degrees cooler there as compared to the rest of the body. Surgical treatment for cryptorchidism involves incision of the scrotal sac and inguinal canal to "pull" the testis into place within the scrotum and surgically fix the testis in place with the use of suture. The procedure is called an orchiopexy.

Anatomic Structure of the Testicle

The tunica vaginalis is an invaginated serous sac that covers the majority of the testis, epididymis, and lower part of the spermatic cord. However, it does not cover the posterior of the testis where the nerves and blood vessels enter. The thick external connective tissue covering of the testis is called the tunica albuginea. At the posterior border, the tunica albuginea forms the mass called the mediastinum testis. Extending from the mediastinum testis are thin layers of connective tissue called the septa, which travel inward into the testis and subdivide it into lobules. Between the septa and within each lobule are a large number of convoluted seminiferous tubules that are coiled; each testis contains approximately 800 of the convoluted seminiferous tubules. The convoluted seminiferous tubules join to form the straight seminiferous tubules, which travel in a posterior direction and unite to form a network of channels called the rete testis (Shier, Butler, & Lewis, 2002). The channels of the rete testis unite to form approximately 15 efferent ducts, which travel through the tunica albuginea and open into the single duct on the coiled tube called

the epididymis. The epididymis rests on the superolateral outer surface of the testis.

The seminiferous tubules are lined by stratified epithelium that contains the spermatogenic cells that eventually become spermatozoa. Another set of cells called cells of Leydig are located in the interstitial spaces between the tubules. The cells of Leydig produce and secrete male sex hormones. Refer to Figure 17-2 for an illustration of the anatomy of a testis.

Blood and Nerve Supply of the Testis

The testicular arteries branch from the abdominal aorta just inferior to the renal arteries. The vessels are long and small in diameter. They descend in an oblique fashion in the retroperitoneal space. The arteries eventually cross over the psoas muscles, ureters, and external iliac arteries and enter the deep inguinal rings. During their descent, branches from the testicular arteries supply the ureter. The testicular artery exits from the spermatic cord to form several branches to supply the testis. Some of the branches travel next to the vas deferens to supply the epididymis. The testicular vein travels next to the testicular artery on the lateral side.

The nerve supply consists of the testicular plexus, which contains parasympathetic fibers from the vagal system and sympathetic neurons from the 10th thoracic spinal cord segment.

SPERMATOGENESIS

Spermatogenesis is a broad term that refers to the whole process that ends in the production of **spermatozoa** (Figure 17-3). In the male embryo, the endoderm layer of the yolk sac gives rise to primordial germ cells that migrate to the developing testes where they lodge in the embryonic seminiferous tubules. It is here that the primordial cells differentiate into diploid (2n) **spermatogonia**, which remain inactive until puberty when they become active. With the onset of puberty, the spermatogonia begin to produce primary spermatocytes that eventually complete the first division of maturation. The secondary spermatocytes that are produced from this first division immediately undergo a second maturation division, thus producing the haploid (n) **spermatids**, which transform into spermatozoa. The following section goes into detail as related to this brief introduction to spermatogenesis.

Contained in the epithelium of the seminiferous tubules are the spermatogenic cells and Sertoli cells. The Sertoli cells are columnar cells that extend through the wall to the lumen of the seminiferous

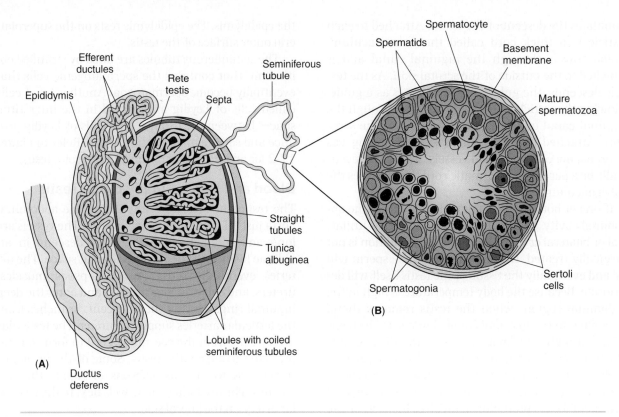

Labels (A): Epididymis, Efferent ductules, Rete testis, Septa, Seminiferous tubule, Straight tubules, Tunica albuginea, Lobules with coiled seminiferous tubules, Ductus deferens

Labels (B): Spermatocyte, Spermatids, Basement membrane, Mature spermatozoa, Sertoli cells, Spermatogonia

FIGURE 17-2   The anatomy of a testis

tubule. Processes extend from the cells between the spermatogenic cells. The functions of the Sertoli cells include:

1. Produce and secrete testicular fluid, which enters the lumen of the seminiferous tubules.
2. Transport nutrients from capillaries to support and nourish the spermatogenic cells.
3. Transport newly formed spermatozoa to the seminiferous tubule lumen.
4. Phagocytose surplus spermatic cytoplasm that is not required for the formation of spermatozoa.

As previously mentioned, in the male embryo the primordial cells are undifferentiated and eventually differentiate into the cells called spermatogonia. Each spermatogonia contains the normal number of 46 chromosomes in its nucleus. With the onset of puberty, the spermatogonia give rise to primary spermatocytes by mitosis. As the level of testosterone secretion increases, the primary spermatocytes reproduce by the cell division called meiosis.

Meiosis consists of two divisions that occur successively, called meiosis I and meiosis II. Just before meiosis I begins, each homologous chromosome is replicated to create two DNA strands, referred to as chromatids, attached to each other at a central region

called the centromere. Meiosis I involves the division of these homologous chromosome pairs, resulting in half the number of chromosomes. This reduced number is referred to as a haploid. The cells that undergo meiosis II are referred to as being haploid, since they contain one member of each homologous pair. The chromatids are separated during the second division, meiosis II, but are not replicated prior to division and as a result, haploid cells are produced. Post–meiosis II, each chromatid is now a separate and independent chromosome.

Meiosis I is a continuous process involving many, many cells, as illustrated in Figure 17-4. However, to better understand this process of division, the steps of meiosis are described in more detail:

1. Prophase I: The chromosomes shorten within the nucleus and become visible. While this is occurring, the nucleoli disappear and the nuclear membrane also temporarily disappears. The microtubules begin to form the spindle fibers. The homologous chromosomes form pairs in a process called synapsis; one member of this pair comes from the mother and the other comes from the father. During synapsis the chromatids of homologous chromosomes make contact, break apart, and form new chromatids, which contain new genetic information. This process

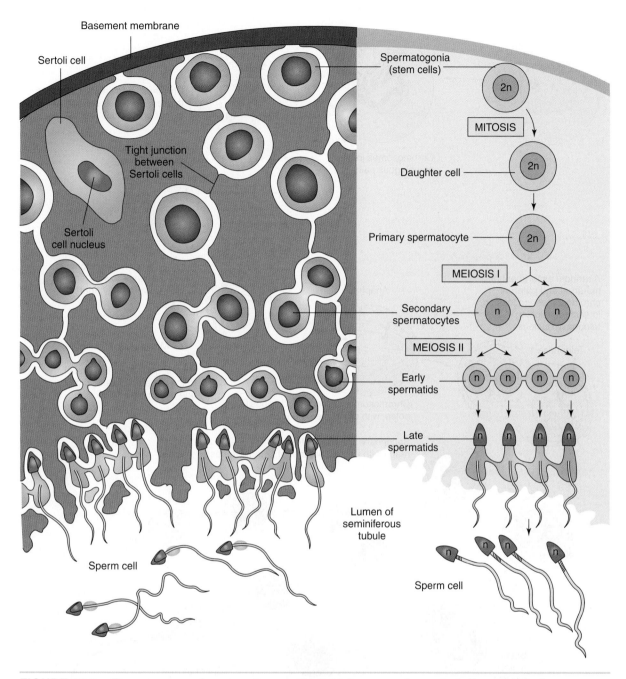

Basement membrane

Sertoli cell

Tight junction between Sertoli cells

Sertoli cell nucleus

Spermatogonia (stem cells)

MITOSIS

Daughter cell

Primary spermatocyte

MEIOSIS I

Secondary spermatocytes

MEIOSIS II

Early spermatids

Late spermatids

Lumen of seminiferous tubule

Sperm cell

Sperm cell

FIGURE 17-3   The process of spermatogenesis, which occurs in a seminiferous tubule

of **crossover** between homologous chromosomes creates chromatids that contain genetic information from both parents.

2. Metaphase I: The chromosomes now line up halfway between the spindle fiber poles attached to spindle fibers on the outside of their centromeres. Each pair of chromosomes consists of four chromatids.

3. Anaphase I: The homologous chromosome pairs separate, and each replicated chromosome trav-

els to the pole of the spindle fiber. This ensures that each new cell will receive only one replicated chromosome of the original pair of homologous chromosomes, thus cutting the number of chromosomes in half.

4. Telophase I: The cell divides in two. A nuclear membrane re-forms around the chromosomes in each new cell, the nucleoli reappear, and the spindle fibers disappear to allow the microtubules to reform. Meiosis II will now begin.

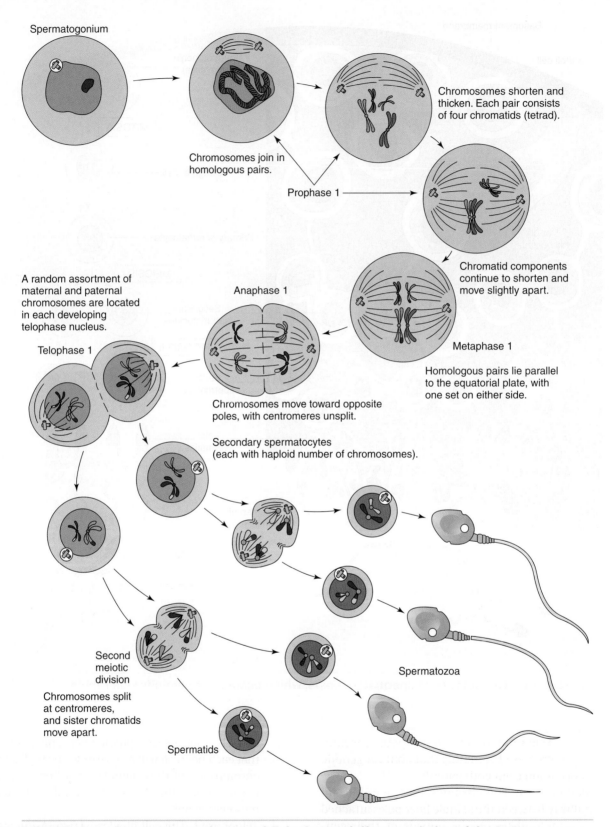

Spermatogonium

Chromosomes join in homologous pairs.

Prophase 1

Chromosomes shorten and thicken. Each pair consists of four chromatids (tetrad).

Chromatid components continue to shorten and move slightly apart.

Metaphase 1

Homologous pairs lie parallel to the equatorial plate, with one set on either side.

Anaphase 1

Chromosomes move toward opposite poles, with centromeres unsplit.

A random assortment of maternal and paternal chromosomes are located in each developing telophase nucleus.

Telophase 1

Secondary spermatocytes (each with haploid number of chromosomes).

Second meiotic division

Chromosomes split at centromeres, and sister chromatids move apart.

Spermatids

Spermatozoa

FIGURE 17-4 **Spermatogenesis occurring in the seminiferous tubules of the testes**

The steps of meiosis II are:

1. Prophase II: The replicated chromosomes gather and line up halfway between the poles of the spindles that develop.
2. Metaphase II: The chromosomes attach to the spindle fibers.
3. Anaphase II: The chromatids are freed up due to the separation of the centromeres and they travel to the spindle fiber poles. The chromatids are now referred to as chromosomes.
4. Telophase II: The two cells that were formed during meiosis I now divide to form two cells, thereby producing four gametes. In the male, the gametes will undergo maturation into four sperm cells. In the female, three of the cells of meiosis develop into polar bodies that have no function and soon degenerate, but one cell will develop into an egg.

During the process of spermatogenesis the primary spermatocytes divide into two secondary spermatocytes. The secondary spermatocytes then divide to form two spermatids, which eventually mature into sperm cells. As previously mentioned, the process of meiosis decreases the number of chromosomes in each sperm cell by one half. Therefore, after each primary spermatocyte has completed meiosis, there will be four sperm cells with 23 chromosomes each in the cellular nucleus. Therefore, when a sperm cell and egg join during fertilization, since the number of chromosomes has been halved, the embryo will have a normal set of 23 chromosome pairs or 46 chromosomes.

Remember, the spermatogonia are responsible for producing primary spermatocytes. As spermatogenesis occurs, the spermatogonia that are in advanced stages of development travel upward to the lumen of the seminiferous tubule. Spermatogenesis is a continual process in the male starting with the onset of puberty. The sperm cells that develop from this process collect in the lumen of the seminiferous tubule, then travel through the rete testis to the epididymis where they are stored and mature, ready to fertilize an egg.

Sperm Cell Structure

The sperm cell, which is shaped like a tadpole, is approximately 0.06 mm long. It consists of three parts: head, round body, and long, round tail. The head is oval-shaped and consists primarily of a nucleus, which contains the 23 chromosomes. The rounded tip of the head is called the acrosome; it contains various enzymes, hyaluronidase being one of the primary enzymes. Hyaluronidase is released to help create an opening in the egg of the female to allow the sperm cell to penetrate it (Shier et al., 2002). Refer to Figure 17-5 for an illustration of the structures of a sperm and ovum.

The rounded body contains a number of mitochondria, which provide ATP for the back-and-forth movement of the tail that propels the sperm forward. The tail, or flagellum, is composed of microtubules, which are enclosed in the cell membrane that extends from the head of the sperm cell.

INTERNAL MALE REPRODUCTIVE ORGANS

The internal male reproductive organs include the epididymis, vas deferens, ejaculatory ducts, seminal vesicles, prostate gland, bulbourethral glands, and urethra.

Epididymis

The epididymis is a long, coiled tube that is connected internally to each testis, and serves as a storage reservoir for spermatozoa. As the spermatozoa travel along the duct, they mature and acquire the ability to fertilize an egg: their movement occurs via peristaltic contractions of the epididymis duct. The duct exits from the superior end of the testis, descends along the posterior surface of the testis, and curves upward to eventually become the vas deferens. The covering of the duct is a continuation of the tunica albuginea, a visceral layer of tunica vaginalis, and just external to the basement membrane of the epididymis is a circular layer of smooth muscle that increases with thickness as the epididymis duct travels toward the vas deferens. The inner wall of the epididymis is lined by pseudostratified columnar epithelium that contains nonmotile cilia called stereocilia (Shier et al., 2002). The epithelium secretes glycogen and other nutritive substances that help to maintain the viability and maturation of the spermatozoa, and are a primary site of fluid resorption.

Vas Deferens and Ejaculatory Ducts

The vas deferens, also called ductus deferens, is a muscular tube that is approximately 40 cm in length. Its

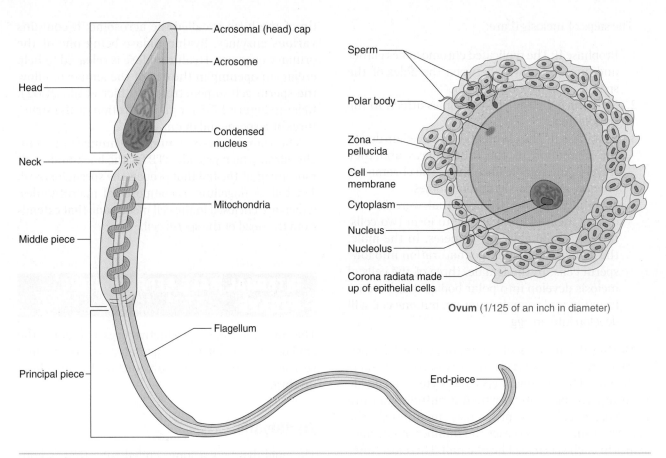

FIGURE 17-5 **Structures of the human sperm and ovum**

inner wall is also lined with pseudostratified columnar epithelium that contains nonmotile cilia (stereocilia). The layers of the wall of the vas deferens are, from outside to inside: adventitia, outer longitudinal muscle layer, middle circular muscle layer, inner longitudinal muscle layer, and epithelium lined with cilia. It begins at the proximal end of the epididymis, traveling in a superior direction along the medial side of the testis to eventually become one of the structures contained in the spermatic cord. Each vas deferens travels through the inguinal canal as part of the spermatic cord, enters the abdominal cavity exterior to the parietal peritoneal layer, goes in front of the ureter extending backward, and ends behind the urinary bladder (Shier et al., 2002).

Near its distal end, the vas deferens widens into an area called the ampulla. The tube then narrows again to unite with the duct of the seminal vesicle just superior to the prostate gland; together these two ducts form the **ejaculatory duct**. The ejaculatory duct passes through the prostate gland to eventually become the urethra.

Seminal Vesicles

Each seminal vesicle is a sac approximately 5–6 cm in length that is attached to the vas deferens by an external adventitial coat of connective tissue located near the base of the urinary bladder. The walls of the seminal vesicle are composed of smooth muscle with an inner circular layer and outer longitudinal layer. The lining of the inner wall of the seminal vesicle is glandular and secretes a mild alkaline fluid. The purpose of the fluid is to help regulate the pH level of the fluid portion, called **semen**, that contains the sperm cells as it travels through the vas deferens and into the urethra. The secretion of the seminal vesicle also contains fructose, a simple sugar that the sperm cells use for energy, and prostaglandins, which stimulate muscular contractions in the female reproductive tract that help the sperm cells move forward to reach the egg. When emission occurs, the smooth muscle layer contracts and the stored contents of the seminal vesicles flow into the ejaculatory ducts; this increases the amount of fluid traveling from the vas deferens to the urethra. The secretory activity of the seminal vesicles is dependent on an adequate amount of the hormone testosterone. The important male and female hormones are discussed in more detail later in the chapter.

Prostate Gland

The prostate gland is somewhat round and approximately 4 cm wide. It surrounds the proximal portion of the urethra, referred to as the prostatic urethra, where it emerges from the bladder. The prostate gland consists of tubular glands that are arranged around the prostatic urethra. The tubular glands have openings into the prostatic urethra. Refer to Box 17-1, which briefly describes enlargement of the prostate gland and the surgical procedure called transurethral resection of the prostate (TURP).

The prostate produces and secretes a thin, slightly acidic milky fluid that contains enzymes and other

---

BOX 17-1

Transurethral Resection of the Prostate

Prostatectomy is the surgical removal of all or part of the prostate. The procedure can be accomplished transurethrally, referred to as a transurethral resection of the prostate (TURP), or may have to be performed as an open procedure. The approach will be determined primarily by the patient's pathological condition. Removal of a cancerous prostate usually requires an open procedure, whereas the patient with BPH (benign prostatic hypertrophy) is most often treated transurethrally. A patient with an enlarged prostate, whether cancerous or due to BPH, has a constricted urethra. Because of the constriction, the patient feels a frequent urgency to urinate, although the amount of urine expelled each time is a very small volume; this urgency to urinate can also cause him to awaken several times during the night. The patient is also prone to frequent bladder infections. By removing a portion of the prostate, the constriction of the urethra is removed and, upon recovery, the patient is able to urinate in a normal fashion.

TURP is a procedure that is typically performed in the cystoscopy operating room, since the room contains a special cysto operating table, which is conducive to performing these type of procedures. Also, the specialty equipment and supplies for performing genitourinary procedures can be kept in the room.

The patient is anesthetized regionally (preferred) or generally, then placed in a lithotomy position, preppeder and draped. The surgeon may place an O'Connor shield to allow for trans-rectal digital manipulation of the prostate during the procedure without fecal contamination. The O'Connor shield is a disposable sterile item that is placed over the anus and allows the surgeon to examine the prostatic urethra digitally through the rectum during the surgical procedure without contaminating the sterile field.

If necessary, the urethra is dilated or a meatotomy is performed. A preliminary cystoscopy may be performed to visualize the urethra, bladder, and prostate gland so as to become oriented to the position of the gland and its size. Following removal of the cystoscope, the lubricated resectoscope is inserted. The resectoscope is a special instrument specifically used for the resection of the prostate. A scope is inserted into the instrument so the surgeon can see the prostate and the tissue to be removed. The resectoscope is plugged into the electrocautery, the tip of which has a half-loop that is used to cut (resect) or "scoop away" the prostate tissue. The prostate tissue enters the bladder, which is kept dilated by the continuous infusion of irrigating fluid. The resection requires multiple strokes or passes with the loop electrode. The surgeon will intermittently remove tissue fragments with the Ellik evacuator, which has a rubber bulb and container. The surgeon connects the Ellik evacuator to the irrigation tubing and compresses the rubber bulb; as the bulb decompresses, prostate tissue is removed. The surgical technologist must save the tissue as a surgical specimen. Total removal of all tissue fragments is necessary. The bladder, prostatic fossa, and urethra are inspected for debris, and any blood vessels that were not cauterized with the loop electrode will be coagulated with a blade or ball-style electrode prior to final removal of the instrument.

A large Foley catheter (22–24 Fr) with a 30-ml balloon is inserted, and the balloon is inflated with water. The catheter may be manually irrigated to assess hemostasis. Initially the irrigation fluid and postoperative urine that flows from the irrigation tube will be slightly reddish in color due to some bleeding. However, this should subside in 12–24 hours; if bright red, this coloration could indicate arterial bleeding, in which case the surgeon may have to perform a cystoscopy to assess what is occurring. Traction may be applied to the Foley by taping the external portion to the patient's inner thigh. The maneuver applies moderate pressure to the operative site and helps to reduce bleeding. The number one complication during the surgical procedure and postoperatively is hemorrhage.

The amount of time required for a TURP is directly related to the size of the prostate gland and can range from 30 minutes to 3 hours.

The patient remains hospitalized for several days until the urine draining from the catheter is clear, the catheter is removed, and the patient is able to void satisfactorily. Normal activity, including sexual relations, can be resumed in four to six weeks.

substances. Contractions force stored prostatic fluid from the gland, which contributes to the semen. The fluid aids in the mobility of the sperm and, in addition, even though the fluid is slightly acidic, it helps to neutralize the highly acidic secretions of the vagina, thereby protecting the sperm when they enter the female reproductive system.

Lying between the tubular glands are dense fibroelastic connective tissue and smooth muscle, which provides firmness to the gland (Cormack, 2001). The prostatic fluid is released into the urethra when the smooth muscles and prostatic capsule contract. At the same time, the fluid in the vas deferens and seminal vesicles also enters the urethra to increase the volume of the semen.

Bulbourethral Glands

The bulbourethral glands, also called Cowper's glands, are located just inferior to the prostate gland and on each side of the membranous urethra. They are small structures, only about 1 cm in diameter, with openings into the urethra. They are also composed of tubular glands that are lined with epithelium. The epithelial lining secretes a viscous fluid that is released in response to sexual stimulation, which aids in slightly lubricating the penis prior to insertion into the vagina of the female.

Urethra

The male urethra serves the dual function of transporting urine and semen. It is divided into three sections. The prostatic urethra, the most proximal portion, is lined with transitional epithelium and, as it transitions to the membranous urethra, the cells become stratified columnar epithelium. As previously mentioned, the prostatic urethra is so named because the prostate gland surrounds this portion of the urethra. Because the prostate is so close to where the urethra emerges from the bladder, prostatic enlargement can occlude the urethral opening of the bladder and the urethra itself. Prostatic enlargement is common in middle-aged and older men. The condition can be benign, referred to as benign prostatic hypertrophy (BPH), or caused by prostatic gland cancer. The male will experience difficulty with urinating and also experience urinary urgency, the need to frequently urinate since the bladder cannot be fully emptied. In addition, this can lead to frequent bladder infections if left untreated. When the male has cancer, the prostate and tumor will be removed regardless of the size of the prostate gland. However, only in instances of severe obstruction due to BPH will the male undergo surgery to remove a portion or most of the prostate, which will restore normal urination function.

The next section of the urethra is the membranous urethra, which travels through the urogenital diaphragm. The last portion, which is also the longest, is the spongy or penile urethra, which begins where the urethra enters the corpus spongiosum of the penis and ends at the urethral orifice.

EXTERNAL MALE REPRODUCTIVE ORGANS

The external male reproductive organs are the scrotum, testes and the penis.

Scrotum

The scrotum, also referred to as the scrotal sac, is a wrinkled pouch located on the exterior of the male body posterior to the penis. The layers of the scrotum are as follows: skin, the dartos tunic, which is subdivided into the dartos muscle and Colles' fascia (Agur, 1991). When exposed to colder temperatures, the dartos muscle is responsible for contracting in order to bring the testes closer to the body where they can absorb heat and preserve the viability of the sperm. When exposed to warm temperatures, the dartos muscle fibers relax to allow the scrotum to hang loosely and prevent overheating of the testes, which would kill the sperm.

A septum divides the scrotum into halves, each of which contains a testicle. Each half of the scrotum is lined by a serous membrane that covers the anterior and sides of the testis and the epididymis, which helps to reduce friction as the structures move within the scrotal sac.

Penis

The penis contains the erectile tissue and urethra to convey urine and semen to the outside of the body. The erectile tissue allows the male to attain an erection to facilitate insertion of the penis into the vagina during sexual intercourse.

The erectile tissue is arranged in three cylindrical-shaped bodies called the cavernous bodies, which are surrounded and held together by elastic connective tissue that is covered by the skin layer. Each cavernous body is surrounded by a tough fibrous sheath called the tunica albuginea. The interior of each cavernous body is filled with vascular spaces that are lined by endothelium and separated by smooth muscle. On the dorsal side of the penis, the paired corpora cavernosa are located and on the ventral side is the single corpus spongiosum. The corpus spongiosum surrounds the urethra and extends to the end of the penis which enlarges to form the **glans penis**. The urethral opening is situated near the tip of the glans penis and along with the rest of the penis contains sensory receptors for sexual stimulation. The penile skin is able to move freely over the underlying structures of the penis and extends over the glans penis as a loose fold of skin called the prepuce or foreskin. This is the skin that is removed during the surgical procedure referred to as **circumcision**.

At the base of the penis the cavernous bodies separate. The corpora cavernosa travel laterally in the perineum and attach to the inferior surface of the pubic arch by connective tissue (Shier, et al., 2002). This area of separation is called the crura of the penis. The corpus spongiosum enlarges around the urethra to form a round bulb of the penis and is attached to the perineal membranes. Superior to the crura is the triangular suspensory ligament of the penis, which is attached to the pubic symphysis region and blends with the deep fascia of the penis (Agur, 1991).

Erection and Ejaculation

An erection occurs in the following manner:

1. Parasympathetic nerve impulses generated from the sacrum of the spinal cord cause the release of nitric oxide, a vasodilator that causes the arteries that supply the penis to dilate and increase blood flow to the erectile tissues (Shier et al., 2002).
2. The pressure of the arterial blood entering the vascular spaces of the erectile tissues squeezes the penile veins, thus inhibiting the flow of venous blood out of the penis.
3. The blood accumulates in the erectile tissues; the penis becomes engorged, swells, and elongates, producing an erection.
4. The ending response is an orgasm in which emission and ejaculation occur.

Emission is when the sperm cells travel from the testes and the secretions from the seminal vesicles and prostate gland empty into the urethra to mix and form semen. It is stimulated by sympathetic nerve impulses that generate from the spinal cord and cause peristaltic contractions in the smooth muscles located in the walls of the ejaculatory ducts, testicular ducts, epididymis, and vas deferens.

As the semen enters and fills the urethra, sensory impulses travel to the sacrum of the spinal cord. In re-

action, the motor impulses are transmitted from the spinal cord to the skeletal muscles at the base of the cavernous bodies, causing them to contract in a rhythmic fashion. The contractions increase the pressure within the erectile tissues to force the semen through the urethra and urethral orifice to the outside of the body. The fluid is secreted by the bulbourethral glands, then the prostate gland, and finally the seminal vesicles—a process is referred to as ejaculation.

Within moments after ejaculation, sympathetic impulses cause the arteries that supply the erectile tissues to constrict, inhibiting the flow of blood into the penis. The smooth muscles in between the vascular spaces contract and the penile veins begin transporting the blood from the spaces. The penis eventually returns to its original flaccid state and it may be a few minutes before the male can sustain another erection.

Blood and Nerve Supply

The blood supply to the penis includes the following:

1. Dorsal artery
2. Deep artery of the penis
3. Accessory artery to the bulb
4. Artery to the bulb
5. Dorsal vein
6. Superficial dorsal vein
7. Deep dorsal vein

The nerve supply is derived from the pudendal nerve and hypogastric plexus. The pudendal nerve is one of the branches of the pudendal plexus and divides into five branches, which supply the genitalia and pelvic region. One branch of the nerve is the dorsal nerve of the penis (Agur, 1991). The hypogastric plexus is located in the pelvic region near the termination of the aorta and beginning of the common iliac artery.

MALE HORMONES

The hormones secreted by the testes, anterior pituitary gland, and hypothalamus affect the male reproductive functions such as sperm cell production and initiate and maintain the secondary sex characteristics.

Androgens

Androgens are the male sex hormones, the majority of which are produced by the testicular interstitial cells, called **Leydig cells**. Testosterone is the hormone produced in the greatest quantity. When produced by the interstitial cells, it is secreted into the circulatory system and attaches to plasma proteins.

The hormone then travels to specific organs to combine with the receptor molecules within the nuclei of the organs' target cells. However, before testosterone can stimulate the cells of these organs, which include the external reproductive organs, prostate gland, and seminal vesicles, it is converted to the androgen called dihydrotestosterone (Shier et al., 2002).

Testosterone is first secreted in the fetus and for a short period after childbirth, but the secretion completely stops during childhood. Approximately between the ages of 12 and 15, the male enters **puberty** and testosterone production begins and dramatically increases. Postpuberty, testosterone continues to be produced throughout life, however, in smaller quantities as an adult.

Within the fetus, the embryonic testicular cells produce testosterone starting at approximately the eighth week of development. The hormone stimulates the body to form the male reproductive organs. Much later in fetal development testosterone is responsible for the descent of the testes into the scrotal sac.

During puberty, testosterone causes the following to occur:

1. Development of primary sex characteristics: enlargement of the testes and other reproductive organs
2. Development of secondary sex characteristics
   a. Growth of body hair
   b. Change in voice in which the pitch lowers
   c. Enlargement of the larynx or what is commonly referred to as the development of the Adam's apple
   d. Thickening of the skin of the body
   e. Increase in muscular growth
   f. Shoulders broaden and waist narrows
   g. Bones thicken
3. Increase in the rate of cellular metabolism, which explains the increased appetite of the teenager
4. Increase in the production of erythrocytes by stimulating the release of erythropoietin

Hormones of the Hypothalamus and Anterior Pituitary Gland

The hypothalamus secretes a hormone called gonadotropin-releasing hormone (GnRH). It enters the circulatory system and travels to the anterior pituitary gland. The anterior pituitary gland is stimulated to release the gonadotropin hormone called luteinizing hormone (LH), which in males is referred to as interstitial cell–stimulating hormone (ICSH) and

follicle-stimulating hormone (FSH). ICSH aids in the development of the Leydig cells in the testes. FSH stimulates the sustentacular cells located in the seminiferous tubules to multiply and mature. Together FSH and testosterone cause the sustentacular cells to stimulate the spermatogenic cells to go through the process of spermatogenesis, leading to the end result of the development of sperm cells. The secretion of FSH is also controlled by the sustentacular cells that secrete the hormone inhibin, which inhibits the anterior pituitary gland by a negative-feedback mechanism.

Testosterone is also regulated by a negative-feedback mechanism. As the level of testosterone increases in the circulatory system, the action of the hypothalamus is inhibited, thereby decreasing the level of GnRH and stimulation of the anterior pituitary gland. The level of secretion of ICSH by the anterior pituitary gland decreases in response and accordingly the level of testosterone secreted by the Leydig cells decreases.

As the level of testosterone continues to lower in the circulatory system, the hypothalamus becomes less inhibited and begins to release GnRH, stimulating the release of ICSH by the anterior pituitary gland once again. The increased secretion of ICSH causes Leydig cells to secrete more testosterone and the level increases in the circulatory system. This back-and-forth process continues in the body in order to maintain a constant level of testosterone.

INTERNAL FEMALE REPRODUCTIVE ORGANS

The female reproductive organs are responsible for producing eggs, transporting the eggs to the region where fertilization will occur, protecting the fertilized eggs, and providing an environment where it will remain viable and develop into a fetus, providing the means for birth to take place, and producing the female sex hormones (Figures 17-6 and 17-7).

Ovaries

The ovaries are a pair of almond-shaped organs that are approximately 3 cm long, 2 cm wide, and .5–1 cm in thick (Figure 17-8). They are located on each side of the superior portion of the uterus in a slight depression called the ovarian fossa, which helps to keep the ovaries in normal anatomic position.

Three other ligaments also keep the ovary in place: the broad ligament, ovarian ligament, and suspensory ligament. The broad ligament is aptly named, since it is a large, broad fold of peritoneum that

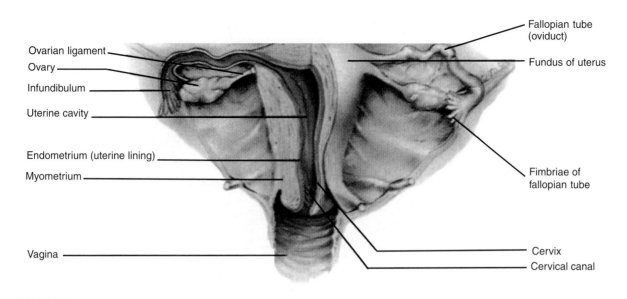

FIGURE 17-6 Structures of the female reproductive system

attaches to each side of the uterus, the cervix, and down to the level of the beginning of the vagina, superiorly and posteriorly to the fallopian tubes and ovary. A small fold of peritoneum that is cylindrical in shape and contains the ovarian blood vessels and nerves is the suspensory ligament, which holds a distal portion of the fallopian tube in place and the ovary. A cylindrical fold of the broad ligament called the ovarian ligament is attached to the medial end of the ovary, also helps to keep the ovary in position.

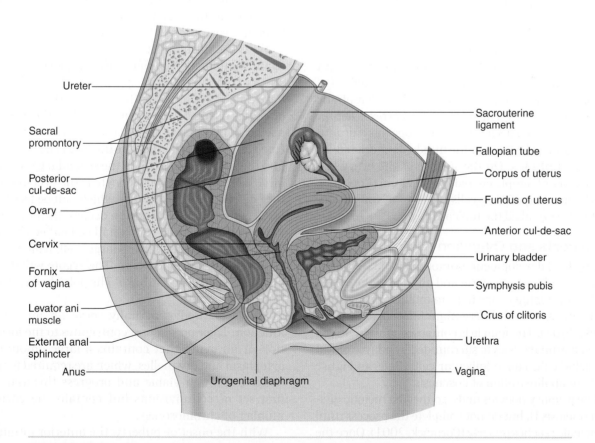

FIGURE 17-7 Structures of the female reproductive system

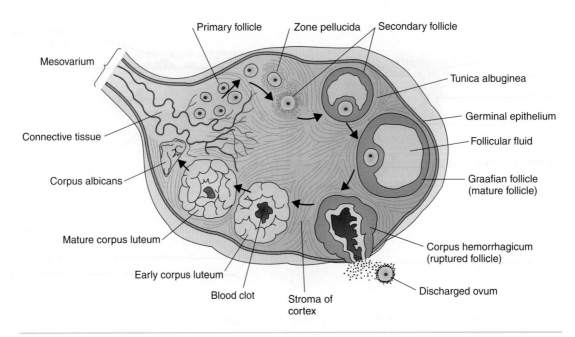

FIGURE 17-8 **A microscopic view of an individual ovary and its internal anatomy**

During fetal life, the ovaries start out as a mass of tissue posterior to the peritoneum next to the developing kidneys. Once the ovaries have progressed somewhat in development and separated into two distinct structures, they descend to an area inferior to the pelvic brim and become attached to the lateral pelvic wall as their final destination.

The ovary consists of two layers, the outer cortex and the inner medulla. The medulla is composed of connective tissue that contains blood and lymphatic vessels, and nerves. The tissue of the cortex is denser and when viewed under the microscope has a granular appearance because of the hundreds of cells called **ovarian follicles**. On the surface of the ovary is a single layer of simple cuboidal epithelium (Cormack, 2001). Just below these cells is a layer of tough connective tissue called the tunica albuginea.

Oogenesis and Ovulation

During fetal development, primordial germ cells arise from the yolk sac endoderm and migrate to the cortex of the developing ovary to form millions of **primordial follicles**, and differentiate into oogonia (Cormack, 2001). The follicle is composed of a single cell called a primary oocyte surrounded by a layer of flat epithelial cells called follicular cells. Refer to Figure 17-9 for an illustration of oogenesis.

The primary oocytes undergo the first meiotic division (meiosis I), but do not complete the process until the female reaches puberty (Cormack, 2001). Once the primordial follicles form, no new ones will develop. The number of oocytes will decrease due to degeneration. Of the millions of follicles originally developed, approximately 1 million are present at birth, but when puberty occurs only about 500,000 are present. Of the 500,000, around 350,000–400,000 will be released from the ovary prior to the onset of menopause.

With the onset of puberty, primary oocytes are again stimulated to complete the processes of meiosis. As compared to the sperm cells, the eggs will have 23 chromosomes in their nuclei. The formation of eggs is referred to as oogenesis. When the primary oocyte divides the cytoplasm is unevenly distributed. One cell is called the **first polar body**, a small cell, and the second cell is called the secondary oocyte, a large cell. The secondary oocyte is the precursor to the egg cell, called an ovum, which can be fertilized by a sperm cell. If fertilization occurs, the oocyte divides and produces a very small cell called the second polar body and a second larger cell, which is the fertilized egg called a zygote. The zygote will divide and develop into an **embryo**. The polar bodies eventually degenerate.

The polar bodies actually serve an important function. Their production contributes to the formation of an ovum that contains a large amount of cytoplasm and organelles, which are required for the ovum to remain viable and progress through the first set of cell divisions but contain the correct number of chromosomes.

With the onset of puberty, the anterior pituitary gland secretes FSH, which stimulates the ovaries to

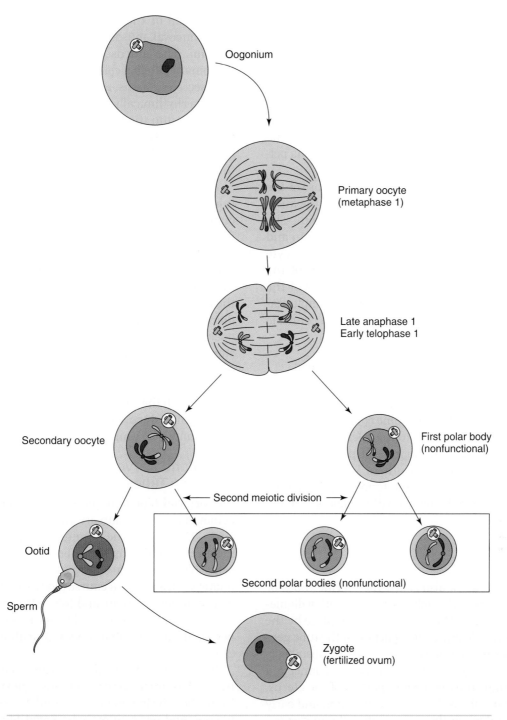

FIGURE 17-9   Oogenesis in the ovary

increase in size. Occurring at the same time, some of the primordial follicles mature. Within the follicles, the oocytes become larger and the follicular cells divide by mitosis to form a stratified epithelium that consists of granulosa cells. A layer composed of glycoprotein called the zona pellucida separates the oocyte from the granulosa cells; now the structure is referred to as a primary follicle (Shier et al., 2002).

The ovarian cells outside the follicle develop into a layer of connective tissue cells called thecal cells (Shier et al., 2002). The follicular cells continue to multiply and when approximately 10 to 12 layers of cells have formed, fluid-filled spaces appear between the layers. The spaces join to form the cavity called the antrum, and the oocyte is now shoved against one side of the follicle, now called a secondary follicle.

It takes approximately 10 to 14 days for a follicle to mature. A mature follicle is called a Graafian follicle. Due to the fluid in the antrum, the follicle is identifiable by the bulge it creates on the surface of the ovary. The secondary oocyte inside the Graafian follicle is large and circular in shape and is surrounded by a layer of zona pellucida that is attached to a second layer of follicular cells called corona radiata. Processes from the cells of the corona radiata travel through the zona pellucida to transport nutrients to the oocyte.

The process of ovulation refers to the release of the oocyte from the follicle. LH is secreted from the anterior pituitary gland, stimulating ovulation. The Graafian follicle swells in size and the walls thin and weaken. Eventually the wall ruptures and the oocyte and cytoplasm are released from the surface of the ovary. The oocyte travels toward the opening of the fallopian tube for possible fertilization and implantation in the uterus. If fertilization does not occur, the oocyte degenerates.

Blood and Nerve Supply of the Ovaries

The arterial blood supply to the ovaries is from the ovarian arteries that branch off the abdominal aorta. The ovarian veins follow the same course as the arteries; however, they empty into the inferior vena cava. The lymphatic vessels drain into the pelvic and lumboaortic lymph nodes (Caruthers & Allen, 2004). Innervation of the ovaries is autonomic, parasympathetic, and postganglionic sympathetic fibers from the ovarian plexus.

Fallopian Tubes

The fallopian tubes, also called the uterine tubes or oviducts, are approximately 10 cm long with a diameter of about .5 cm. The tubes are held in place by the broad ligament. The proximal portion of the tube gently curves to its opening near the ovary; the distal portion travels slightly posterior to the uterus, connecting to and opening into the superior portion of the uterus. The fallopian tube is the site of fertilization and early cleavage, and when the zygote enters the uterus approximately five days later it has reached the blastocyst stage of development (Cormack, 2001).

The proximal opening of the tube expands and is funnel-shaped; it is called the **infundibulum**. On the edges of the infundibulum are a number of extensions called **fimbriae**. The infundibulum does not come into contact with the ovary; however, it often has one fimbria longer than the others that extends and connects to the ovary, called the ovarian fimbria (Shier et al., 2002).

The wall of the fallopian tube has three layers: inner mucosal, muscular, and outer covering of peritoneum. The mucosal layer is lined with simple columnar epithelial cells that are ciliated. The epithelium secretes mucus, and together with the fimbriae, the cilia rhythmically beat toward the uterus to draw the ovum into the tube. Once inside, the ciliary action and peristaltic contractions of the muscular layer of the fallopian tube propel the ovum through the tube.

A pathology that can occur within the fallopian tube is referred to as a **tubal pregnancy**, which occurs when the fertilized ovum remains in the fallopian tube and the embryo begins developing. Due to the small diameter of the tube, it does not take long before the developing embryo bursts through the tube's wall. This constitutes a dire emergency due to the amount of internal hemorrhaging that can take place. The woman will be immediately taken to the operating room for emergency surgery. In most instances, the fallopian tube cannot be surgically repaired, but the section that has been injured will be removed to control the bleeding. However, this does not diminish the woman's chances of becoming pregnant again, since she still has another intact and functioning ovary and fallopian tube.

Blood and Nerve Supply of the Fallopian Tubes

The arterial blood supply to the fallopian tubes is achieved by the ovarian arteries that branch from the aorta. They join at the termination point of the uterine arteries and enter at the border of the ovary. The veins follow the same course as the arteries. The lymphatic vessels follow a course along the superior edge of the broad ligament and join with the lymphatic vessels from the uterus and ovary to empty into the periaortic and lumbar nodes (Caruthers & Allen, 2004).

Innervation of the fallopian tubes is from fibers of the 10th thoracic to second lumbar plexuses, branch from the uterine nerves, second to fourth sacral nerves, and parasympathetic vagal fibers from the ovarian plexus (Caruthers & Allen, 2004).

Uterus

The uterus is a hollow, pear-shaped, muscular organ in which the fertilized ovum is implanted and the embryo develops. The primary purpose of the uterus is to sustain and protect the development of the embryo.

The broad ligament is the primary structure that keeps the uterus in anatomic position. The broad

BOX 17-2

Hysterectomy

A hysterectomy is the surgical removal of the uterus. However, often the fallopian tubes and ovaries are excised with the uterus. The medical term for the surgical procedure in which all structures are removed is *total abdominal hysterectomy–bilateral salpingo/oophorectomy* (TAH-BSO) or *total vaginal hysterectomy–bilateral salpingo/oophorectomy* (TVH-BSO). The medical term for fallopian tube is *salpingo* and the medical term for ovary is *oophor;* the suffix *-ectomy* means surgical removal of. The procedure is performed either through an abdominal incision or vaginally. Increasingly, the procedure is performed laparoscopically; this involves the excision of the structures through the vagina, but with the use of instruments and a laparoscope placed through small abdominal incisions—the procedure is called laparoscopic assisted vaginal hysterectomy (LAVH).

The following is a brief overview of an abdominal TAH-BSO. The skin incision is most often vertical, extending from just below the umbilicus to just above the pubis. A large retractor that stays open on its own due to ratchets, referred to as a self-retaining retractor, is used to expose the uterus, fallopian tubes, and ovaries. Large clamps called Heaney clamps are placed across the broad, round, and ovarian ligaments. The round ligaments are cut with scissors and suture is placed to ligate the ligaments. Next, the peritoneum that is continuous over the bladder and uterus is divided with scissors. The ureters can now be seen and identified to ensure they are protected and not injured during the procedure.

The bladder is bluntly dissected from the uterus. Blunt dissection refers to the use of the fingers or an instrument called a sponge forceps to dissect tissue. The opposite of blunt dissection is sharp dissection, meaning a knife blade or scissors is used.

The uterus and associated structures are now totally freed up by completing the dissection of the ligaments. The cardinal ligament and broad ligament are clamped with a large surgical instrument called a Heaney clamp, cut with scissors called curved Mayo scissors, and tied with a suture in order to free up the uterus, fallopian tubes, and ovaries for removal. Two Heaney clamps are placed across the ligaments and closed tightly. Next, the surgeon uses the curved Mayo scissors to cut the tissue between the two clamps and then places a suture to tie off the tissue; this process is referred to as clamp, cut, tie, and is repeatedly performed until the ligaments are no longer attached to the uterus.

The removal of the uterus leaves an opening to the vagina called the vaginal cuff. This is closed with suture; suture is also used to close the peritoneum over the cuff. The surgeon can now close the abdomen in layers with suture.

ligament extends laterally from the uterus to the pelvic walls and floor, thus covering the top of the pelvic cavity. Two other ligaments aid in positioning the uterus: the round ligament and cardinal ligament. The round ligament is a fold of peritoneum that extends from the anterior surface of the uterus through the inguinal canal and to the labium majus. It is homologous to the spermatic cord in the male. The cardinal ligament is located within the inferior portion of the broad ligament on each side of the uterus and represents a continuation of the broad ligament. During a **hysterectomy**, the surgical removal of the uterus, these are the ligaments that are cut to free the uterus for removal.

The uterus is situated medially toward the anterior region of the pelvic cavity, superior to the vagina and slightly anterior to the bladder. It is divided into three sections:

1. Fundus: The rounded upper portion of the uterus where the fallopian tubes are attached. This is the part of the uterus that is slightly anterior to the bladder; the peritoneum is continuous from the bladder over the uterus at this area.

2. Body: The next two thirds of the uterus is the body, which is broad at the superior portion and begins to narrow posteriorly as it leads into the third section of the uterus.

3. Cervix: The last portion of the uterus is the narrow cervical region that ends in the opening called the cervical orifice, which serves as the opening of the uterus into the vagina. The orifice is the opening that dilates when a pregnant female is in labor in preparation for the delivery of the fetus; this is discussed in more detail later in the chapter.

The wall of the uterus is composed of three layers of tissue:

1. Endometrium: The endometrium is the inner mucosal layer, which is lined by columnar epithelium and contains many tubular glands. Some females are affected by a condition called endometriosis, which is the abnormal implantation and growth of endometrial tissue outside of its normal anatomic position. The endometrium will grow primarily on the outside of the uterus, creating fibroids. This is a

benign condition; however, the fibroids can become large enough to cause pain, discomfort, abnormal bleeding, and dysmenorrhea. At this point, the female will most likely undergo a hysterectomy.

2. Myometrium: The myometrium is the second muscular layer, which is composed of smooth muscle fibers in varying patterns including circular and longitudinal. The fibers are interlaced with connective tissue. The myometrium is the muscular layer that contracts during labor to propel the fetus into the vaginal canal.

3. Perimetrium: The perimetrium is the outer serosal layer that covers the uterus and some of the cervix.

Blood and Nerve Supply of the Uterus

The arterial blood supply to the uterus is from the two uterine arteries that branch from the paired internal iliac arteries. The veins are large and travel adjacent to the arteries. The lymphatics travel through the utero-ovarian pedicle and terminate in the pelvic and lumbar glands (Caruthers & Allen, 2004). The size of the lymphatic vessels dramatically increases during pregnancy.

The uterus is innervated by the following nerves:

1. Ovarian plexus
2. Hypogastric plexus
3. First lumbar spinal segment
4. Third and fourth sacral nerves
5. 12th thoracic spinal segment

Vagina

The vagina is a fibromuscular tube approximately 8–9 cm long, extending from the cervix to its opening to the outside of the body. It has three functions:

1. The erect penis is inserted into the vagina during sexual intercourse.
2. During menstruation, the secretions from the uterus flow through the vagina to the outside of the body.
3. It serves as the birth canal during labor.

The vagina is posterior to the ureters and urinary bladder, but anterior to the rectum. Just superior to the vaginal orifice is the urethral orifice. The superior portion of the vagina is separated the rectum by a thin layer of tissue called Douglas' cul-de-sac or rectouterine pouch; the pouch is formed by the broad ligament. A rectovaginal fistula is a pathology that can occur in which a small abnormal passageway develops through this thin layer of tissue causing an opening between the rectum and vagina. Fecal material can then enter the vagina and cause chronic infections. The fistula requires surgery to close the opening.

In the area in which the vagina and cervix meet are recesses called fornices (singular, fornix). The wall of the vagina at this point is also thin, allowing a physician to palpate the abdominal organs by inserting one to two fingers into the vagina during a physical examination.

Females who have not had sexual intercourse or inserted a tampon during the menstrual cycle will often have a thin mucous membrane of skin and fibrous tissue called the hymen covering the vaginal introitus (introitus is another term for orifice or opening). When the hymen is penetrated, the tissue will recede and small "tags" of tissue will remain.

The wall of the vagina consists of three layers:

1. Mucosal layer: The mucosal layer is the inner layer, which consists of stratified squamous epithelium and forms rugae. The layer does not contain mucous glands. The mucus found on the mucosal wall of the vagina actually is secreted by the glands of the cervix and Bartholin's glands located next to the vaginal introitus; the mucus serves as lubrication to facilitate the insertion of the penis during sexual intercourse.
2. Muscular layer: The muscular layer is the middle layer, which consists of smooth muscle fibers arranged in circular and longitudinal patterns.
3. Fibrous layer: The fibrous layer is the outer layer, which is composed of dense connective tissue; intertwined among the tissue are elastic fibers. The fibrous layer serves as the point of attachment of the vagina to the surrounding organs.

EXTERNAL FEMALE REPRODUCTIVE ORGANS

The external organs are the labia majora and labia minora, clitoris, and Bartholin's glands (Figure 17-10). Collectively, these structures make up what is referred to as the **vulva**.

Labia Majora and Labia Minora

The labia majora are longitudinal folds of tissue located on each side of the vaginal introitus. They are homologous to the scrotum of the male, composed of adipose tissue and a layer of smooth muscle covered

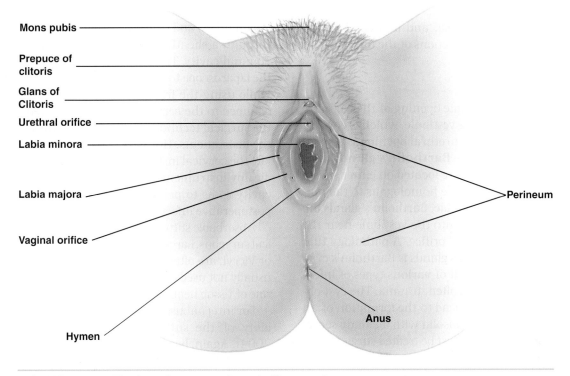

Mons pubis

Prepuce of clitoris

Glans of Clitoris

Urethral orifice

Labia minora

Labia majora

Vaginal orifice

Hymen

Perineum

Anus

FIGURE 17-10 The female external genitalia or vulva

by skin. The outer portion of the labia majora is covered by pubic hair and contains sweat glands and sebaceous glands. The inner side is smooth and hairless. The anterior ends of the labia majora come together to form a small elevated, rounded area called the mons pubis, which contains adipose tissue. The posterior ends taper and merge together just superior to the perineal area.

The labia minora are situated just inside the labia majora forming small longitudinal folds that extend along the same length. They are composed of connective tissue and are highly vascular. The anterior ends merge with the labia majora to form the clitoral hood and the posterior ends merge with the labia majora.

Clitoris

The clitoris is a small region of highly sensitive tissue that projects at the anterior end of the vulva between the ends of the labia minora. Exteriorly, it is approximately 1–2 cm long, but a portion of it is imbedded into the tissue. The clitoris is homologous to the penis and the structure is similar. It consists of two columns of erectile tissue called the corpora cavernosa; a septum of connective tissue divides the two columns. At the root of the clitoris, the corpora cavernosa form the crura, which attaches to the pubic arch (Shier et

al., 2002). The end of the clitoris is formed by erectile tissue and supplied with many sensory nerve fibers. During sexual intercourse the clitoris becomes erect and the stimulation of it contributes to the sensation known as an orgasm.

A ritual mutilation practiced in many countries of the world is known as clitoridectomy, the excising of all or part of the clitoris and sometimes part of the labia. The reasons for this ancient practice are complex; however, a primary reason is the male desire to control female sexuality. Unfortunately, it is performed on young females, using crude instruments without any type of anesthesia and with no regard for protecting against infection. In the United States, the practice is banned by federal law.

Nerve Supply of the Clitoris

A large nerve plexus is the pudendal nerve plexus; the pudendal nerve is a branch that arises from the second, third, and fourth sacral nerves. The pudendal nerve divides into branches that innervate the genital structures and pelvic region. Three of the main branches are inferior rectal nerve, perineal nerve, and dorsal nerve of the clitoris or penis.

During labor a pudendal block can be performed to ease the pain of contractions. An anesthetic agent is injected transvaginally and the pudendal nerves are anesthetized, thereby anesthetizing the perineum, vulva, clitoris, labia majora, and perirectal region with no effect on the contractions of the uterus.

Bartholin's Glands

Surrounding the immediate opening of the vagina is an area referred to as the vestibule, which is covered by the labia minora. The urethral opening is also located in the vestibule. The **Bartholin's glands** (also called vestibular glands) are located on either side of the vaginal orifice. They are homologous to the bulbourethral glands of the male. Bartholin's glands are actually ducts that open into the vestibule near the lateral sides of the vaginal orifice. A pathology that can occur with Bartholin's glands is Bartholin's cyst, which can form as a result of various types of infections of the area or, most often, trauma. The cyst obstructs the duct and can lead to the formation of an abscess. The cysts are semisolid with a cloudy secretion. Most often the cyst must be treated surgically, by performing an incision and drainage. However, if the cyst is in advanced stages and infection is present, **marsupialization** must be performed, in which the closed cavity is converted into an open cavity to allow healing to occur.

HEALING OF THE FEMALE GENITAL TRACT

The external female structures and the area within the vagina are considered contaminated areas when performing surgery, which can present a challenge to the surgery team in terms of preventing a postoperative infection. Another challenge is the small amount of space for the surgeon to work in when performing a vaginal procedure, such as a vaginal hysterectomy. What has helped the efforts of the surgeon is the use of the laparoscope. Laparoscopic surgical techniques as well as the instrumentation have improved through the years; this improvement has broadened the use of the laparoscope. Two other important factors can present a challenge to the surgeon: (a) highly vascular tissues of the pelvis and vagina and (b) highly muscular tissues such as the uterus.

As previously mentioned, the vaginal canal is considered a contaminated area. The surgical technologist must keep this in mind when a surgical procedure calls for instruments that are placed within both the vagina and the abdominal cavity. For example, during an abdominal laparoscopic procedure instruments are placed within the vaginal canal and clamped onto the cervix to facilitate manipulation of the uterus, fallopian tubes, and ovaries. The laparoscope is inserted through a sheath that has been placed into the abdominal cavity. The surgeon is able to look through the laparoscope to view the internal female structures while using the free hand to move the instruments clamped to the cervix, or the surgeon requests that the surgical technologist manipulate the cervix with the instruments. However, the hand used to manipulate the cervical instruments must not be used to handle any instruments to be used within the abdominal cavity so as to prevent contamination and possible postoperative infection.

Absorbable sutures are the preference of gynecological surgeons. Larger-sized sutures, such as #1 chromic or Vicryl, are often used to close the abdomen, but are usually not used on the reproductive organs due to the rate of tissue healing and incisional stresses.

For internal use in the pelvis and vagina, the pliability of the sutures is very important (Ethicon, 2004). Again, because of the limited amount of space in which to work within the vagina, a suture that has excellent handling characteristics and pliability is required in order to place the suture and efficiently tie knots that will hold. Vicryl suture is one of the most popular types used; the sizes often used are 0 to 2-0. Vicryl suture is excellent for use on the highly vascular tissues of the pelvis and vagina, as well as the muscular structures. It is also a suture of choice for repair of an episiotomy.

FEMALE HORMONES

The anterior pituitary gland, hypothalamus, and ovaries secrete the female hormones that are responsible for the development and maintenance of the female secondary sex characteristics, female reproductive cycle, and eggs.

At about 10 years of age, the hypothalamus starts secreting gonadotropin-releasing hormone (GnRH), which stimulates the anterior pituitary gland to release the gonadotropins follicle-stimulating hormone (FSH) and luteinizing hormone (LH). These are two of the primary hormones that play a role in the production of female sex hormones and controlling oocyte maturation.

The female sex hormones are secreted by the placenta during pregnancy, as well as by the ovaries and adrenal gland cortices. There are two categories of hormones: **estrogens** and **progesterone**. The most plentiful estrogen hormone is estradiol (Shier et al., 2002).

In the nonpregnant female, the ovaries are the primary source of estrogens. When the female enters puberty, the anterior pituitary gland stimulates the ovaries to secrete the estrogens. Estrogens cause the female reproductive organs such as the vagina, uterus, fallopian tubes, and ovaries to enlarge. The estrogens also stimulate the development of the female secondary sex characteristics. Estrogens affect the female secondary sex characteristics as follows:

1. Breast development including the ductile system
2. Increase in the amount of adipose tissue in the subcutaneous layer, particularly in the breasts, buttocks, and thighs

The ovaries are also the primary source of progesterone in the nonpregnant female. Progesterone affects the cycles of the uterus and the mammary glands, and aids in regulating the secretion of gonadotropins from the anterior pituitary gland.

Other changes as related to the female secondary sex characteristics; for instance, the growth of pubic hair and axillary hair, are caused by the male sex hormone, androgen. However, due to the small amount of androgen in the female, skeletal development is affected, resulting in narrow shoulders and broad hips.

MENSTRUAL CYCLE

The menstrual cycle begins in approximately the 12th to 13th year of life in a female (Figure 17-11). The first menstrual cycle a female experiences, referred to as menarche, is when the female reproductive organs have reached maturity and are affected by the hormones of the body. GnRH is secreted by the hypothalamus, which stimulates the anterior pituitary gland to release FSH and LH. FSH stimulates the ovarian follicles to mature. The granulosa cells within the follicle produce estrogens and a small amount of progesterone.

The estrogen stimulates the development of the female secondary sex characteristics. The estrogens will continue to be secreted during each menstrual cycle in order to maintain the characteristics.

The start of the menstrual flow indicates the end of the menstrual cycle and the beginning of a new one. Consequently, the progesterone and estrogens level are low, thus stimulating the anterior pituitary gland and hypothalamus to begin secreting FSH and LH to increase their levels and stimulate a new follicle to mature. The follicle will secrete estrogens, the uterine lining is repaired after the discontinuation of the menstrual flow, and the endometrial layer thickens again.

MENOPAUSE

Women will continue to have menstrual cycles until approximately their late 40s or early 50s. The cycles will become irregular until eventually the female enters menopause and the cycles completely stop. Menopause begins due to the few remaining follicles that can respond to the gonadotropins. The follicles will not mature, which means ovulation does not occur, causing the level of estrogens to significantly decrease.

The reduced level of estrogens has an effect on the female secondary sex characteristics. The breasts, fallopian tubes, uterus, and vagina may decrease in size. A serious side effect is osteoporosis, the abnormal loss of bone density, which can cause pain, in particular in the lower back, loss of stature whereby some individuals have a stooped posture, and a proneness to pathological fractures. Often, a fracture of the hip joint or femur must be repaired surgically in individuals with osteoporosis who fall, and who otherwise would not have stained a fracture.

Many women going through menopause are afflicted by the discomfort of "hot flashes," which are vasomotor symptoms and include heat on the forehead, face, neck, and upper body that lasts for a short period of time. Often the hot flash is accompanied by sweating and chills. To help with the symptoms of menopause and to combat osteoporosis, some women are treated with estrogen replacement therapy (ERT), which usually consists of an estrogen transdermal patch or pill. However, ERT carries the risk of development of endometrial cancer, and so women on ERT must be sure to have regular checkups.

PREGNANCY AND BIRTH

Pregnancy is the result of fertilization, the union of a sperm cell with an egg cell. The oocyte released during ovulation survives approximately 12 to 24 hours. However, the sperm cells can live up to 72 hours inside the female reproductive tract. Therefore, sexual intercourse must occur 72 hours prior to ovulation or within 24 hours following ovulation for fertilization to occur. Fertilization takes place in the fallopian tube.

Fertilization

When a sperm cell reaches the oocyte, it penetrates the follicular cells that are attached to the corona radiata, the surface of the oocyte, and attach to the zona

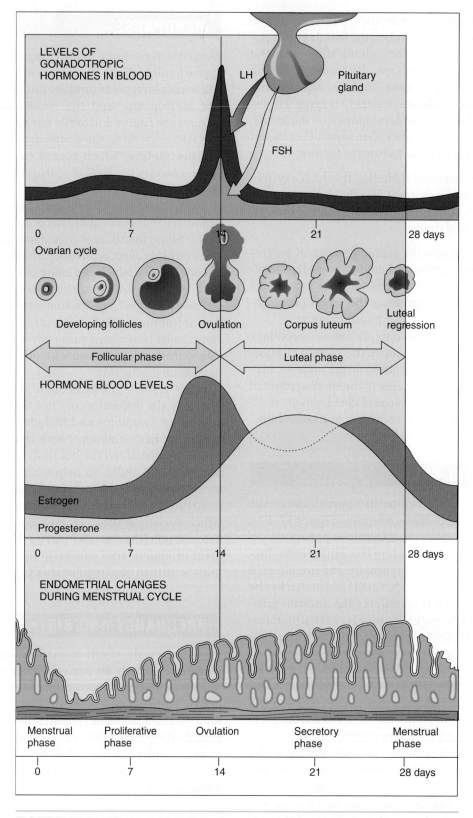

FIGURE 17-11 The menstrual cycle

TABLE 17-1   Coinciding Phases of the Menstrual Cycle

FOLLICULAR PHASE: FIRST 14 DAYS	PROLIFERATIVE PHASE: FIRST 14 DAYS
Anterior pituitary gland secretes FSH and LH.	Increase in level of estrogens causes the endometrial layer of the uterus to thicken, and the uterine lining also changes.
FSH stimulates the ovarian follicle to mature.	The level of progesterone also increases.
The granulosa cells within the follicle that encircle the oocyte and connect it to the inner wall loosen. This causes follicular fluid to accumulate.	
During follicular maturation, estrogen secreted by it inhibits the release of LH from the anterior pituitary gland. The estrogens also cause the anterior pituitary gland to be receptive to the GnRH that is released in doses from the hypothalamus approximately 60–90 minutes apart.	

OVULATION: 14TH DAY	
The anterior pituitary gland responds to the GnRH and LH. The LH causes the follicular wall to rupture, allowing the oocyte and follicular fluid to escape from the ovary.	

LUTEAL PHASE: 15TH TO THE 28TH DAY	SECRETORY PHASE: 15TH TO THE 28TH DAY
The space left by the rupture of the oocyte fills with blood. Additionally, granulosa and thecal cells stimulated by LH form the corpus luteum. The corpus luteum is yellow.	Progesterone secreted by the corpus luteum causes the endometrium to increase in vascularity and become more glandular.
The corpus luteum secretes a large amount of progesterone and estrogens.	Progesterone causes the uterine glands to increase their secretion of glycogen and lipids. This results in the endometrial layer containing more nutrients in preparation for embryo development.
The increased levels of estrogens and progesterone inhibit the additional release of FSH and LH from the anterior pituitary gland. This prevents the development of other follicles while the corpus luteum is active.	
If the oocyte is not fertilized by a sperm cell, the corpus luteum degenerates starting at approximately the 24th day of the cycle and is now referred to as a corpus albicans, a white fibrous scar (Cormack, 2001).	
Because the corpus luteum no longer functions, the levels of estrogens and progesterone rapidly decreases. This causes the blood vessels in the endometrium to constrict.	

	MENSTRUATION: BEGINS ON 28TH DAY OF CYCLE
	The constriction of the blood vessels in the endometrium reduces the supply of oxygen and nutrients to the tissue layer. The endometrial tissues slough off.
	At the same time of tissue sloughing, blood is released from the capillaries that have been damaged, creating a flow of blood and dead cells that passes through the vaginal orifice to the outside of the body, referred to as the menstrual flow.

pellucida, which encircles the cell membrane of the oocyte. The head of the sperm cell, called the acrosome, releases an enzyme that helps the sperm to penetrate the zona pellucida. Once penetration occurs, the cell membrane of the sperm cell and the oocyte join and the sperm movement discontinues. The tail of the sperm cell breaks off. When this happens, the cell membrane of the oocyte becomes unresponsive to the other sperm cells (Shier et al., 2002). The joining of the two membranes causes cortical granules that are located just underneath the oocyte cell membrane to release an enzyme that hardens the zona pellucida, thus forming a protective shell around the fertilized oocyte and preventing other sperm cells to penetrate.

The nucleus of the sperm enters the cytoplasm of the oocyte. The oocyte then divides to form a large cell and a smaller polar body that is eventually expelled. This is the process of oocyte meiosis and occurs only after the oocyte is fertilized. The nuclei of the sperm and oocyte can now unite and the chromosomes become mixed together, thereby completing the process of fertilization.

The chromosomal product of fertilization is 46 chromosomes, since the sperm cell contained 23 and the oocyte contained 23. The human cell is now referred to as a zygote.

Approximately 24 to 30 hours after fertilization, the zygote divides by mitosis and the result is two cells. These cells keep dividing by mitosis and, while this is occurring, the cell mass moves through the fallopian tube to the uterine cavity. At this point, the zygote is referred to as a blastocyst. The blastocyst, on approximately the eighth day after fertilization, becomes implanted in the uterine wall.

Prenatal Growth

Obviously, humans grow and age, which is a continuous process involving various stages of life. These stages are placed under two primary periods of growth: prenatal growth and postnatal growth. This section of the chapter will discuss prenatal growth; postnatal growth is discussed later. Prenatal growth is divided into three stages: cleavage, embryonic, and fetal.

Cleavage Stage

As previously mentioned, the union of an egg and sperm results in a zygote that eventually undergoes mitosis to form two new cells. These cells keep dividing at a fast rate; thus, the new cells do not have time to grow, resulting in smaller and smaller cells. This process of division is called cleavage and the cells are called blastomeres. The group of cells produced by cleavage is referred to as a cleavage embryo.

The cleavage embryo travels through the fallopian tube to the uterus, taking approximately three to four days. During its travel to the uterus the ball of cells solidifies and is now called a morula, consisting of about 20 cells (Shier et al., 2002). Once inside the uterine cavity, the morula does not become immediately stationary and is free for approximately three days. The cell division continues, but the zona pellucida of the

original oocyte disintegrates and the morula is now called a blastocyst. It is at this stage that the ball of cells implants in the endometrium of the uterus.

The cells of the blastocyst arrange themselves into two groups. One group is an inner mass of cells that will form the embryo. The other, outer cell group makes up the trophoblast, which will develop into structures such as the placenta. The trophoblast secretes the hormone HCG, which sustains the corpus luteum and prevents the immune system of the pregnant female from rejecting the blastocyst. HCG also stimulates the placenta to synthesize other hormones.

Embryonic Stage

The embryonic stage occurs in the second week through eighth week of pregnancy. The primary developments during this stage include the formation of the placenta; body structures such as the fingers, toes, and so on, begin to be recognizable, and the internal organs develop.

During the second week the amniotic cavity develops and is located between the inner cell mass and the trophoblast that is attached to the endometrium. The inner cell mass becomes flat and is now called the embryonic disk. The disk is composed of three layers—the outer ectoderm, middle mesoderm, and inner endoderm—collectively called the primary germ layers. Another important anatomic structure also develops—the stalk that attaches the embryo to the placenta.

All of the internal organs of the body form from the primary germ layers. The cells of the ectoderm form the organs of the nervous system, contribute to the formation of the sensory organs; the epidermis, and glands of the skin, hair, nails; and form the linings of the mouth and anal canal. The cells of the mesoderm form muscle tissue of all types, bone tissue and marrow, blood and blood vessels, lymphatic vessels, internal reproductive organs, and connective tissues of all types. The cells of the endoderm form the respiratory tract, urethra, urinary bladder, and epithelial lining of the intestines.

A second layer of cells develops and lines the trophoblast, and together the cells and trophoblast form the **chorion**. Thin projections push outward from the trophoblast and embed into the endometrium. The projections are called **chorionic villi** and are fully developed by the fourth week of pregnancy. Refer to Figure 17-12, which shows an illustration of the germ layers, chorionic vili, and other structures.

By the fourth week of pregnancy, the embryonic disk develops from being a flat structure to being

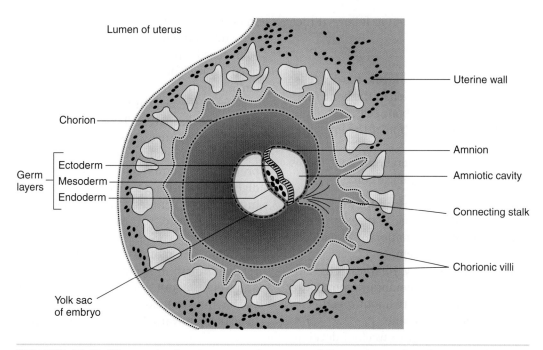

FIGURE 17-12 **The early developmental stages of the embryo showing germ layers, chorionic villi, and other structures**

somewhat elongated in shape. By the end of the fourth week, the heart is beating and the head as well as the beginning of what will be the arms and legs can be distinguished.

Rapid development occurs during the fifth to seventh weeks. The head grows, becoming more rounded, and the face becomes more human as the eyes, nose, and mouth can be distinguished. The arms and legs develop further, with toes and fingers appearing. By the end of the seventh week, all of the primary internal organs have developed and continue to grow.

Beginning in the ninth week of development the **placenta** forms from the chorion. As the embryo enlarges, only a certain portion of the chorion remains attached to the endometrial layer. The area of attachment is what becomes the placenta. A membrane that is part of the placenta is the placental membrane. The membrane consists of epithelium of the chorionic villus and endothelium of a capillary. It serves to separate the embryonic blood within the capillary of a chorionic villus from the maternal blood. It is through this membrane that various substances such as nutrients and oxygen move from the maternal blood to the embryo's blood, and waste products and carbon dioxide move from the embryo's blood into the maternal blood. The placenta is divided into two parts: the embryonic part is composed of the chorion and chorionic villi and the maternal portion arises from the region of the endometrium underneath the implantation site.

During placental formation, the amnion develops, surrounding the embryo. The amnion is membrane that begins to appear during the second week of development. It is attached to the embryonic disk, and amniotic fluid fills up the space between the membrane and embryonic disk.

As the embryo enlarges, the amnion contributes to the development of tissues, in particular the connecting stalk that attaches the embryo to the chorion and placenta. Eventually the connecting stalk is converted into the umbilical cord.

The umbilical cord is the lifeline of the fetus. It is approximately $1-1\frac{1}{2}$ cm in diameter and 60 cm in length. Its starting point is at the abdomen of the embryo and it attaches to the placenta. Within the cord are two umbilical arteries and one umbilical vein responsible for the transport of blood to and from the embryo. The fetal circulation will be discussed in detail later in the chapter.

The amniotic fluid keeps the placenta from collapsing around the embryo, providing an environment much like being constantly underwater in which the embryo can easily grow and remain suspended. The amniotic fluid also serves as a cushion to protect the embryo from the movements of the mother's body.

Two other important structures develop during the embryonic stage, the yolk sac and allantois. The yolk sac develops during the second week of pregnancy and attaches to the embryonic disk. The yolk sac contributes to embryo development as follows (Shier et al., 2002):

1. It forms blood cells.
2. It forms cells that later develop into the sex cells.
3. It forms the stem cells located in the bone marrow that later develop into bone cells.
4. It contributes to the formation of the intestinal tract.
5. A portion of the yolk sac membrane contributes to the formation of the umbilical cord.

The allantois develops during the third week. It is a tube that extends from the yolk sac to the connecting stalk. Its functions include formation of blood cells and the umbilical arteries and vein.

The amniotic cavity, obviously, enlarges as the embryo grows. Soon the amnion membrane comes into contact with the chorion. The two join together to form the amniochorionic membrane.

At the conclusion of the eighth week of development, the embryo is becoming an identifiable human. The embryo weighs approximately 5–8 grams and is about 30–35 mm long. It still has a long way to go as far as development, but it has made it through the most critical developmental stage and is now entering the fetal stage.

Fetal Stage

The fetal stage starts at the ninth week of development and ends at birth. During this stage the fetus grows rapidly and the body proportions become normal. During the third month the body of the fetus becomes taller while the growth of the head slows down in order to become proportioned to the body. The ossification of the bones begins and the external reproductive organs can be seen.

During the fourth month the body grows to approximately 20–25 cm in length and weighs about 175 grams. The fetus develops hair, nails, and nipples while the bones continue to ossify. Starting in the fifth month growth slows. The limbs of the body achieve their maximum length. The mother will start to feel the fetus move and the movement, as time goes on, will become more frequent. More hair will grow on the scalp and a fine hair called lanugo grows on the skin of the body. The fetus now weighs about 500 grams and is about 30–35 cm in length. The fetus is more or less forced into the fetal position due to lack of room, but is still in a buttocks-first presentation.

In the sixth month, the fetus develops eyelashes and eyebrows. In addition, the skin at this point is still very wrinkled. In the seventh month, the skin smooths out due to the accumulation of a fat layer in the subcutaneous tissue. The eyelids, which have been fused shut since the third month, are able to open again. The fetus is now approximately 40–45 cm in length.

During the last three months, the final trimester, the brain cells mature. The rest of the internal organs grow and mature. However, the respiratory and digestive systems mature last, which explains why premature infants have difficulty breathing and digesting, requiring temporary assistance in breathing such as a ventilator and placement of a feeding tube. The testes of the male descend into the scrotum.

About nine months after conception, the fetus is ready for birth. It is now about 50–55 cm in length and weighs about 2.5–3.5 kg. The fetus prepares for the birthing process by turning where it is positioned head down toward the cervix and vaginal canal.

Fetal Circulation

The fetus relies on the mother to supply its oxygen and nutrients, and transport away the waste products. The mother brings the oxygen and nutrients to the fetus by route of the maternal blood supply via the umbilical arteries and vein; the substances diffuse through the placental membrane.

In fetal circulation, the roles of the arteries and vein are reversed; in this instance, the umbilical vein transports oxygenated blood and nutrients from the placenta to the fetus. After the vein enters the body of the fetus, it travels next to the anterior abdominal wall up to the liver. Approximately 50% of the blood enters the liver and the other half enters the **ductus venosus vessel**, which bypasses the liver (Shier et al., 2002).

The ductus venosus travels superiorly to connect to the inferior vena cava. The oxygenated blood mixes with deoxygenated blood and the mixture travels into the right atrium. It must be remembered that the lungs of the fetus do not function, so the blood has to also bypass them. When the blood enters the right atrium, a good portion is shunted into the left atrium, through an opening in the atrial septum called the foramen ovale. A valve in the left atrium called the septum primum opens and closes to prevent regurgitation of the blood from the left to the right atria (Shier et al., 2002).

A small portion of blood in the right atrium travels into the right ventricle and exits into the pulmonary trunk. Even though the lungs are not yet functioning, the tissue needs to be sustained; the small amount of blood that travels to the lungs is enough to keep them viable.

Most of the blood that enters the pulmonary trunk bypasses the lungs and enters the ductus arteriosus vessel. The ductus arteriosus connects the pulmonary trunk to the descending aorta. The result of this connection is that the blood with a low oxygen level, which returns to the heart via the superior vena cava, bypasses the lungs, and so does not enter the area of the aorta that sends out branches to the brain and heart.

The blood with a high level of oxygen that entered the left atrium mixes with deoxygenated blood that is returning from the pulmonary veins. The mixture travels into the left ventricle and is pumped into the aorta. This mixture then travels through the coronary arteries to sustain the myocardium of the heart and through the carotid arteries to enrich the brain tissue.

The blood in the descending aorta is a mixture of oxygenated and deoxygenated blood. Some of the blood exits into the branches from the aorta that lead to the lower part of the fetal body. The other portion of blood exits into the umbilical arteries, which go to the placenta for reoxygenation.

Hormones and Pregnancy

To prevent spontaneous abortion of the blastocyst a layer of tissue, called the trophoblast, forms a wall that functions in the implantation of the blastocyst in the uterine wall and supplies nutrients to the embryo. Additionally, the trophoblast cells secrete the hormone HCG, which surrounds the embryo to help prevent spontaneous abortion. HCG also aids in maintaining the corpus luteum so it can continue secreting estrogens and progesterone. The level of HCG secretion is high for about two months and then decreases significantly by the fourth month. By the end of the first trimester, the placenta now secretes sufficient levels of estrogens and progesterone to maintain the uterine wall. The placental progesterone along with another hormone called relaxin, which is secreted from the corpus luteum, inhibits the myometrium of the uterus to suppress uterine contractions until labor begins. Relaxin also loosens the ligaments that hold the symphysis pubis and sacroiliac joints together (Shier et al., 2002). This helps the fetus pass through the vaginal canal during birth.

The placenta secretes placental lactogen, a hormone that stimulates the mammary glands in preparation for milk secretion. Other important hormones include aldosterone and parathyroid hormone. Aldosterone is secreted from the adrenal cortex and encourages renal reabsorption of sodium, which causes fluid retention (Shier et al., 2002). Parathyroid hormone is secreted by the parathyroid glands and helps to maintain a high circulating level of calcium in the blood of the mother. The fetal demand for calcium is very high, so if the mother does not maintain an adequate amount in her circulation, it can lead to hypocalcemia.

Body Changes and Physiology

Obviously, as the fetus grows in size the uterus enlarges. However, in situations where surgery on a pregnant woman cannot be avoided, the surgeon must be aware of how the size of the uterus has now temporarily displaced some of the abdominal organs. The uterus itself now extends in a superior direction, causing the intestines and stomach to be pushed upward. The uterus also presses against the bladder; this pressure causes frequent urination. Also, because of the pressure on the intestines and stomach, large meals will often make a pregnant woman uncomfortable and can lead to frequent bouts with heartburn.

In many pregnant women, a dark longitudinal line called the linea nigra will appear on the abdomen at about the 24th week of pregnancy, extending from the symphysis pubis to a few inches above the umbilicus. Another development, which can be permanent, are lineae albicantes, or what are commonly called stretch marks. The lines appear white or grayish in color, and usually occur on the abdomen, buttocks, breasts, and thighs, and are caused by the stretching of the skin. The application of skin lotion containing vitamin E to the affected areas is recommended to either prevent the stretch marks or, after a period of time, help to eliminate some of them. However, the efficacy of this treatment is unknown at this time.

The pregnant woman's cardiac output, urine production, and breathing rate all increase to compensate for the growth of the fetus. The fetus places a large demand on the body of the woman. As the placenta enlarges, it requires more blood and as the fetus enlarges, it requires more oxygen and produces waste that must be eliminated.

To compensate for these increased demands, the pregnant woman must increase her intake of food to ensure the ingestion of an adequate amount of nutrients. In order to stay healthy, the mother must remember she is now eating for two individuals, herself and the fetus.

Labor

The average length of a pregnancy is approximately nine months and the pregnacy ends with labor and birth. Two factors contribute to the beginning of labor:

1. The level of progesterone, which serves to suppress the uterine contractions, decreases as time progresses during pregnancy.
2. The uterine and vaginal tissues stretch.

Labor begins when the cervix dilates and ends when the placenta is delivered. The myometrial layer of the uterus begins contracting in order to dilate the cervix and push the fetus into the birth canal. The contractions begin superiorly and travel down the uterus to force the fetus and placenta forward. To aid the effort, a powerful hormone called oxytocin is released from the posterior pituitary gland, which stimulates the muscle in order to sustain contractions. For woman who are in labor for a long period of time, the production of oxytocin and muscle contractions will eventually start to decrease. Therefore, the obstetrician may order that the woman receive by IV doses of the commercial preparation of oxytocin called pitocin to aid in sustaining the contractions. Also, women who are overdue for delivering their baby may be given pitocin to kick-start the labor process.

Normally the fetus is positioned head downward. As the fetus moves forward its head stretches the cervix, resulting in a positive feedback system that induces stronger contractions and the release of more oxytocin. During later stages of labor, the abdominal wall muscles are stimulated to contract due to the positive feedback system. These muscles, along with the myometrium of the uterus, aid in moving the fetus through the cervix and vagina to the outside of the body. As the infant passes through the birth canal, it can stretch the perineum (the area between the vaginal opening and the anus), in the process tearing it. To prevent this mishap, the obstetrician will perform an episiotomy, which involves the following:

1. Local anesthetic is injected into the perineal area to numb the sensory nerves.
2. Using scissors, the surgeon makes a cut along the midline of the perineum from the vestibule to approximately 1 cm above the anus.
3. Once the infant is born and the placenta delivered, the obstetrician will suture the incision to allow for normal healing to take place.

Almost immediately after the birth of the infant, the contractions of the uterus cause the expulsion of the placenta. Some bleeding occurs after the expulsion, since the capillaries are damaged in the process of the placenta separating from the uterine wall. However, the action of oxytocin aids in keeping the bleeding to a minimum, since the contraction of the uterus compresses the bleeding vessels. When a woman has to undergo a cesarean section, pitocin is immediately administered by IV to stimulate contractions of the uterus and to minimize the bleeding.

During the weeks after childbirth, the uterus shrinks back to normal size. The endometrium sloughs off through the vagina and the mother may pass a bloody discharge for a short period of time. However, eventually the tissue lining of the uterus returns to normal and resembles that of a nonpregnant female.

Postnatal Growth

Postnatal growth is the longest period of life, starting at birth and ending with death. The period of postnatal growth that will be discussed in this section is the neonatal period.

Neonatal Period

The neonatal period begins at birth and ends at the fourth week of life. The first few minutes after birth are some of the most critical for the baby. Everything the mother was doing for the fetus the baby must now take over, including breathing, digesting, and maintaining proper body temperature. Of these, the most important immediately after exiting the birth canal is breathing: bringing in oxygen and getting rid of carbon dioxide.

The first breath will hopefully be a strong one in order to expand the lungs. Up to this point the lungs have been collapsed and the surface tension can hold them together. However, to combat the surface tension the fetus has been producing and secreting surfactant, which decreases the surface tension and explains why the obstetrician wants to get the baby to start crying very hard immediately after delivery, this brings in lots of oxygen and eliminates the carbon dioxide.

During pregnancy, the mother provides the nutrients needed by the fetus. However, the newborn is now reliant on external sources of nutrients. The mother does not produce milk for approximately two to four days after giving birth, but does produce colostrum, which contains maternal antibodies and is rich in nutrients. Also, the newborn's digestive system is not immediately ready to be able to digest milk, but can handle the colostrum.

Some of the most important changes to the infant's body occur with the circulatory system. When

BOX 17-3

Anesthesia of the Pregnant Female

The pain caused by labor and delivery of the infant results from two factors: (a) visceral pain caused by the dilation of the cervix during uterine contractions, and (b) somatic pain due to the stretching of the perineum and vagina as the fetus travels through the vaginal canal. The visceral pain radiates to the lower abdomen and lower back. Somatic pain is primarily conducted from the pudendal nerve to the sacral nerve roots.

When a woman in labor is given any type of medication, in particular for pain, the vital signs of the mother and fetus must be closely monitored. In addition, an IV must be in place in order to keep the mother hydrated or in case the rapid administration of drugs is required.

Pain relief is provided to the mother in labor through the administration of systemic medication, inhalation agents, and regional anesthetic agents. Only systemic medication and regional anesthetic agents are discussed here. Systemic medications are administered through the IV. The most popular class of drugs administered is opioids. They are given in the first stage of labor. Meperidine was the drug of choice, but has been replaced by fentanyl or butorphanol. Frequent small doses are given IV, since the actions of the drugs can be better predicted.

The term regional anesthesia refers to numbing an area or region of the body by injecting a local anesthetic drug that blocks the nerve impulses of the sensory nerves. The techniques of regional anesthesia that are in use for the woman in labor are injection into the perineum, the pudendal nerve block, and the epidural block. The pudendal nerve block is performed prior to delivery in a transvaginal fashion, meaning the long needle is placed through the opening of the vagina into the vaginal canal and into the tissues surrounding the nerve to inject the local anesthetic. The somatic pain is eliminated and allows for the episiotomy to be performed, including the repair. This block does not have any maternal or fetal side effects.

The standard for vaginal delivery is the continuous lumbar epidural analgesia. It eliminates the pain due to labor and delivery, usually with no effect on the mother or fetus. The epidural block is administered during labor, usually when the cervix is dilated to 5–6 cm. A catheter is inserted in the lumbar region and left in place. The anesthetic agent is injected through the catheter into the tissues just superior to the dura mater of the spinal cord, and the agent is then absorbed into the cerebrospinal fluid. The visceral pain from the cervix and uterus is blocked. Anesthesia is maintained by the ability to repeat injections through the catheter. The block provides a pain-free second stage of labor and allows for the episiotomy to be performed and repaired.

Anesthesia for cesarean section (C-section) is spinal, epidural, or general anesthesia. The incidence of C-sections in the United States has increased over the past two decades. C-sections are performed as a scheduled, urgent, or emergency procedure. Urgent C-sections are most often due to failure to progress when the mother is in labor. Emergency C-sections are due to fetal compromise such as a prolapsed umbilical cord or a cord that is wrapped around the baby, or maternal hemorrhage. Emergency C-sections must be performed quickly in order to save the baby and mother.

Regional anesthesia, spinal or epidural, is preferred for C-section since, it usually does not affect the infant or mother. Additionally, the mother can remain awake in order to share the birth experience with their significant other. Regional anesthetic techniques can take time to perform; therefore, they are optimal for scheduled and urgent C-sections, but not best for emergency C-sections because of the time factor.

General anesthesia is the technique of choice for emergency C-sections. A minimal depth of general anesthesia is sufficient; however, this technique still presents complications to the mother and, in particular, the infant. General anesthesia will affect the infant since the mother is still breathing for the baby and the agent can enter into the infant's body systems. Therefore, the anesthetic agent is not delivered until just before the surgeon is ready to make the skin incision. The provider of the anesthesia will perform the technique of rapid induction to quickly put the mother to sleep, and the surgical team will work rapidly to have the baby delivered in five to eight minutes or less. Just prior to being administered the anesthetic agent, the mother will breathe 100% oxygen via a mask to increase both her and the infant's blood oxygen level so as to keep the effects of the anesthetic gas to a minimum. Anesthetic gases of choice include halothane, isoflurane, and enflurane with or without nitrous oxide.

Surgery of any type, a C-section, is highly avoided for the pregnant female. Again, the risks to the mother and fetus are greatly increased when the mother must undergo surgery. There have been instances where surgery is urgent, such as for the removal of a tumor, but surgery is delayed due to the risks to the mother and fetus. If surgery must be performed, obviously regional anesthesia is the technique of choice depending on the type of surgery to be performed. However, if the mother is involved in a traumatic accident and surgery cannot be avoided, general anesthesia will most likely be required. In these instances, the life of the mother takes precedence over the life of the fetus. If scheduled surgery is unavoidable, every effort is taken to preserve the life of the fetus. One last note: if general anesthesia must be utilized, halothane must not be used. Halothane causes profound uterine relaxation and could cause the mother to abort the fetus.

BOX 17-4

Cesarean Section

The following is a brief description of a C-section performed as a scheduled procedure. The classic C-section incision is the Pfannenstiel incision, which is a transverse incision made just above the symphysis pubis following what is referred to as the pubic line, a natural skin-increase line. The skin incision is carried down to the fascia, which is opened with large scissors called Mayo scissors. The fascia is separated from the rectus abdominus muscle by using the fingers (blunt dissection) toward the umbilicus and then toward the symphysis pubis. Using scissors that have thinner blades, called Metzenbaum scissors, the surgeon is incises and opens the peritoneum. A retractor called the bladder blade is placed to retract the bladder away from the uterus. A transverse incision is made in the uterus; the surgical technologist should have the suction tube immediately avaliable to suction away the amniotic fluid once the incision is made. The surgical technologist now pushes the abdominal area while the surgeon manipulates the infant and removes it from the uterus.

Things move very quickly now. Immediately the surgeon uses a small bulb syringe to suction the mouth and nares of the infant while the surgical technologist places two clamps over the umbilical cord. Another type of large scissors, called bandage scissors, are used to cut the cord and the neonate is given to the pediatrician. The clamp nearest the cut end of the umbilical cord is removed and a blood sample called cord blood sample is taken for analysis by the laboratory. The surgeon confirms two umbilical arteries and one vein.

The anesthesia person gives IV pitocin to prevent hemorrhaging from the uterus. The placenta with cord is delivered from the uterus and placed in a large round basin, which is then passed off from the surgical technologist to the circulating person, since this is a surgical specimen to be sent to the pathology department. The uterus is delivered through the surgical wound and the interior cleaned with sponges. The closure of the uterus is in two layers using size 0 absorbable suture. Once closed, the uterus is placed back into anatomic position and the abdomen is closed in layers.

blood pressure in the right atrium decreases. With the expansion of the lungs due to the infant's first breaths of air, the previous low level of blood flow through the pulmonary trunk is eliminated and a normal level of blood flow through the left atrium via the pulmonary veins is established, thereby increasing the blood pressure in the left atrium (Shier et al., 2002).

As pressure decreases in the right atrium and increases in the left atrium, the septum primum valve located on the left side of the atrial septum covers the opening of the opening foramen. Eventually the valve tissue joins the tissue of the septum.

Most important, the ductus arteriosus closes immediately after birth to prevent the continued bypass of the lungs. The blood now follows a normal course of travel to and from the lungs.

MAMMARY GLANDS

The mammary glands are specialized structures of the female that produce and secrete milk for the feeding of the infant. Female breasts are considered by many in society as one of the defining sexual characteristics of a female (Figure 17-13).

The mammary glands are situated within the adipose tissue of the breasts. Twothirds of the breast lies anterior to the pectoralis major muscle and is also attached to the muscle. The second muscle layer is the pectoralis minor muscle which lies a top the ribs. The remaining onethird of the breast lies anterior to the

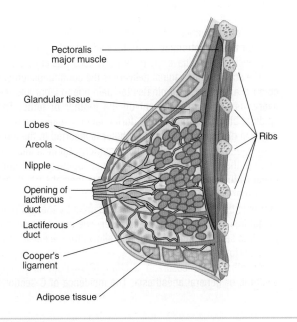

FIGURE 17-13 Sagittal section of the female breast

the infant is delivered the umbilical arteries constrict, which closes them. Until the umbilical cord is clamped and cut, blood continues to travel through the umbilical vein from the placenta to the newborn; this contributes somewhat to the blood volume level of the newborn.

The foramen ovale closes due to changes in blood pressure in the right and left atria. When the umbilical cord is cut, obviously blood flow through the umbilical vein to the inferior vena cava stops; consequently, the

serratus anterior muscle. The breasts extend from the second to the sixth ribs and from the sternum to the axillae. In the majority of women, there is a portion of the lateral quadrant of the breast that is elongated and enters the axilla. This is called the tail of Spence; it enters the deep fascia of the medial axillary region and is the only breast tissue located beneath the deep fascia (Skandalakis, Skandalakis, & Skandalakis, 2000). At the tip of each breast is the nipple , approximately in the center, at the about the level of the fourth intercostal space. Surrounding the nipple is a pigmented area of skin called the **areola**.

A mammary gland consists of approximately 15 irregularly shaped lobes. Each lobe contains an alveolar gland and a **lactiferous duct**, which travels to the nipple and has an opening to the outside of the body. Separating each lobe are adipose and connective tissues, which support the mammary glands and the breast. A type of connective tissue, the suspensory ligaments of Cooper, extends from the dermis of the breast to the fascial layer to also help support the breast. The ligaments form a network of strong connective tissue fibers that pass between the lobes of the breast tissue and connect the dermis of the skin with the deep layer of the superficial fascia.

Breast Development

In the female, the hormones secreted by the ovaries stimulate the development of the breasts during puberty. The alveolar glands and lactiferous glands enlarge while adipose tissue is deposited, thereby enlarging the breasts. Males have the same tissue structure in the chest region; however, obviously the breasts normally don't develop like the female. In certain instances, males who are going through puberty can experience an abnormal enlargement of one or both breasts called gynecomastia. The condition is often due to a hormonal imbalance and is usually temporary and nonmalignant. But if the condition

---

BOX 17-5

Surgical Anatomy of a Mastectomy

The following is a description of the surgical anatomy as related to the surgical procedure called a modified radical mastectomy, the surgical removal of a breast. Rather than provide a brief description of the procedure, the information will be more relevant to the general breast anatomy that has already been discussed and provide additional details.

Position the patient on the operating room table in the supine position. An important anatomic landmark as related to the modified radical mastectomy is the triangular bed. The superior portion of the triangle is marked by the axillary vein, or what some surgeons refer to as "big blue" when performing the surgery; the vein must be identified, protected from injury, and preserved. The lateral side of the triangle is marked by the medial border of the latissimus dorsi muscle and the medial side of the triangle is the retracted margin of the pectoralis major and minor muscles (Skandalakis et al., 2000). The floor of the triangle is formed by the subscapularis and serratus anterior muscles. This is the area in which the surgeon must have excellent dissection.

After the breast is removed, the continuing dissection must include the following:

1. Excise the remaining pectoralis major fascia at the axillary border.
2. Remove the remaining fascia of the pectoralis minor.
3. Dissect axillary fat and, in particular, axillary lymph nodes from the thoracic wall.
4. Remove some of the fascia from the subscapularis, latissimus dorsi, and serratus anterior muscles.

The surgeon must be aware of the following nerves; they must be identified and preserved to prevent subsequent postoperative complications and deformities:

1. Thoracodorsal nerve: innervates the latissimus dorsi muscle. It is located at the medial border of the latissimus dorsi. Once found, it should be marked with what is called a vessel loop, a colored $\frac{1}{8}$-inch strip of silicone that is ideal for the retraction of delicate structures such as nerves and blood vessels. White–or yellow–colored loops are used for nerves.
2. Medial anterior thoracic nerve: located lateral to the pectoralis minor muscle.
3. Lateral anterior thoracic nerve: innervates the pectoralis major muscle at the clavicular and sternal regions. It is located at the medial edge of the pectoralis minor muscle. Injury to either of these anterior thoracic nerves will result in atrophy of the pectoralis major and minor muscles.
4. Long thoracic nerve: innervates the serratus anterior muscle and lies on the surface of the muscle. The anatomic landmark for identifying the nerve is where the axillary vein travels over the second rib. Damage to this nerve can result in a condition referred to as winged scapula, in which there is an abnormal protuberance of the scapula due to paralysis of the serratus anterior muscle.
5. Subscapular nerve: located near the subscapular artery and vein.

persists, it can be surgically corrected for cosmetic and psychological reasons.

Production of Milk

During pregnancy, the estrogens and progesterone secreted by the placenta stimulate the increased development of the mammary glands. Estrogens stimulate the lactiferous ducts to enlarge and branch, and an increased amount of adipose tissue is deposited. Progesterone stimulates further development of the alveolar glands. Due to this enlargement of the ducts, the deposition of adipose tissue, and production of milk, the breasts will grow larger in size.

In approximately the fifth to sixth week of pregnancy, the anterior pituitary gland secretes the hormone **prolactin**. Although prolactin is released throughout pregnancy, the secretion of milk does not start until after delivery because the progesterone secreted by the placenta inhibits milk production, and, lactogen, also secreted by the placenta, inhibits the prolactin.

This all changes after delivery of the infant and placenta and the levels of hormones decrease, thus removing the inhibition of the action of prolactin. Milk is not secreted immediately after birth. For approximately a week, the mammary glands produce colostrum, a thin, watery cloudy fluid. Providing the infant the colostrum is highly important; the colostrum contains maternal antibodies that are passed onto the infant, and it is rich in proteins. The antibodies are temporary, but provide protection to the infant.

In order for milk to flow through the ducts to the mammary glands, specialized cells contract called myoepithelial cells that surround the alveolar glands. When the nipple and areola are mechanically stimulated, such as when an infant is nursing, the sensory receptors in the breast AQ7 to the hypothalamus. The hypothalamus sends a signal to the posterior pituitary gland to release a small amount of oxytocin. The oxytocin enters the circulatory system, travels to the breasts, and stimulates the myoepithelial cells to contract. The mother can literally feel the milk enter the breasts when the infant suckles, a process referred to as let down. If the mother is nursing the infant on a regular schedule, let down may occur minutes before nursing begins. In addition, there is a strong connection between the hormones and the mind. Often when a nursing mother hears another baby cry, the milk may start to flow.

If the mother discontinues breast feeding the infant or mechanically removing milk such as with a breast pump, the hypothalamus will inhibit the secretion of prolactin and, within five to seven days, the mammary glands will no longer be able to produce milk.

Blood and Nerve Supplies of the Breasts

The arterial blood supply to the breasts is derived from the thoracic branches of the axillary artery (Gray, 1991). The primary branches are the internal thoracic, intercostal, and lateral mammary arteries. The following is a more detailed description of the arterial supply:

1. Internal thoracic artery: branch of the subclavian artery.
2. Three branches of the axillary artery: (a) supreme thoracic, (b) pectoral branch of the thoracoacromial, and (c) lateral thoracic arteries (Skandalakis et al., 2000).
3. Intercostal arteries: lateral portion of the breast is supplied by the third, fourth, and fifth intercostal arteries.

The veins follow an anastomotic circle around the nipple called the circulus venosus. The blood travels from this central region of the breast to the circumference and empties into the axillary and internal mammary veins (Gray, 1991). Additionally, the axillary, internal thoracic, and third to fifth intercostal veins drain the mammary gland; they follow the course of the arteries. The lymphatic system of the breast is highly important due to its role in breast cancer. The lymphatics travel along the lower border of the pectoralis major muscle to the axillary glands (Gray, 1991). This cutaneous lymphatic network is located on the anterolateral thoracic wall and connects with the abdomen inferiorly and the neck superiorly. The mammary cutaneous lymphatic network is a part of this system (Caruthers & Allen, 2004).

The nerves of the breast are derived from the anterior and lateral cutaneous branches from the anterior thorax. The majority of the anterior and medial mammary branches is derived from the anterior branches of the lateral cutaneous intercostal nerves. The skin of the superior portion of the breast is innervated by branches of the supraclavicular nerves (Caruthers & Allen, 2004).

Healing of Breast Tissue

The breast tissue as previously described is primarily composed of adipose tissue. Adipose tissue is a friable, loose type of tissue and is conducive to forming spaces during the healing process. However, some surgeons will not approximate the breast tissue, reasoning that the **seroma** will eventually form fibrous tissue to fill the defect (Skandalakis et al., 2000). On the other hand, there are surgeons who will place sutures to close the defect and approximate the tissue edges using 2-0 or 3-0 Vicryl suture. The sutures are placed without tension so as not to tear the tissue and are widely spaced.

With surgical procedures, such as a lumpectomy, in which a larger incision is made and a larger amount of tissue is removed, one or two drains must be placed to avoid a hematoma. A hematoma is the buildup of blood and fluid in a dead space in a wound. The result is the separation of the wound edges beneath the skin, delaying healing and increasing the chance of a postoperative wound infection. The drains prevent dead space from forming by allowing the evacuation of air and fluids from the wound. In addition, a pressure dressing helps to prevent dead space.

GENETICS

The following section is an overview of genetics, the area of science that studies the genes, chromosomes, and gene therapy. Individuals inherit certain characteristics determined by genes, such as baldness, from their parents, who inherit genes from their parents, and so forth. The genetic information is transferred by **genes**, which are made up of DNA. Genes are found on the structures called **chromosomes**. The transmission of genetic traits occurs when the egg is fertilized by the sperm and meiosis takes place.

The DNA in human cells makes up what is referred to as the **genome**. In the cells of the human body, the genes are located on 23 chromosome pairs (total of 46 chromosomes). These cells are called **somatic cells**, since they are the nonsex cells, and they are referred to as being diploid, since the cells have a pair of chromosomes (Shier et al., 2002). Beacuse the egg and sperm each have 23 chromosomes, they are referred to as **haploid**.

The 23 chromosomes are often placed on a chart called a **karyotype** to be viewed (Figure 17-14). The first 22 pairs are referred to as **autosomes** and are lined up according to size on the karyotype. These chromosomes do not carry the X and Y genes that determine sex. The last pair of chromosomes, pair #23, contains the X and Y genes, and is therefore referred to as the sex chromosomes.

On each chromosome are thousands of genes. Since there are pairs of chromosomes, it makes sense that there are two copies of genes and each one is located at the same position on the chromosome pairs. But, it must be remembered that genes are made up of sequences of nucleotides that can occur in various forms called **alleles** (Shier et al., 2002). If an individual has two identical alleles, they are said to be homozygous for that particular gene. But if the individual has two different alleles, they are said to be heterozygous. The genetic makeup of a person's genome forms their **genotype**. The appearance of a person or a specific health condition that develops due to the way genes are expressed is called the phenotype. An allele that produces an unusual phenotype is termed mutant.

Dominant and recessive inheritance is determined by alleles, which thus determine the phenotypes. An allele the expression of which is stronger than that of another is called a dominant allele; the allele the expression is with the weaker is called a recessive allele. Dominant alleles are indicated by using a capital letter. A gene that is responsible for causing a disease or genetic disorder can be dominant or recessive. The gene can also be autosomal, carried on a nonsex chromosome, or carried on the X or Y chromosome, where it is referred to as being X-linked or Y-linked.

Knowing this information, geneticists can use the Punnet square or pedigree diagram to explain inheritance. The Punnet square is used to present the probability of specific genotypes occurring in the offspring of a family. The mother's alleles for a particular gene are listed on top of a box divided into four squares; the father's alleles are listed on the left side of the box. Placed within each square is the combination of alleles that can occur at fertilization.

The pedigree diagram shows the genotypes and phenotypes. Females are represented by circles and males by squares. These are then shaded-in to represent a female or male as having a trait or condition; when the square or circle is half-shaded it means the person is a carrier. Roman numerals are used to indicate generations.

Genetic Traits

Most inherited chromosomal disorders are monogenic, meaning a single gene is responsible for the disorder and is influenced to a very small degree by the environment. However, most often several genes contribute toward the phenotype of an individual and the degree of expression of the genes varies greatly. Traits that are determined by multiple genes are called polygenic, examples of which are eye and skin color.

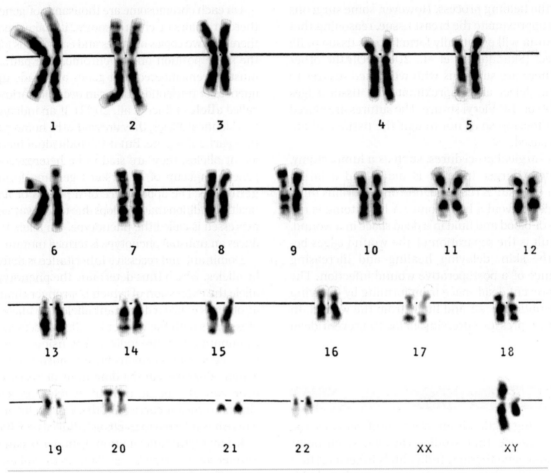

FIGURE 17-14 Karyotype of human from a male somatic cell. A karyotype is the arrangement of chromosome pairs according to shape and size

Eye color is a good example of how multiple genes form a single trait. The iris of the eye becomes darker when the amount of melanin produced in the iris increases. Individuals with blue eyes have just enough melanin to produce the color. Two genes with two alleles each interact to produce the eye colors—light blue to green, light brown to dark brown, and black. If each dominant allele contributes pigment and there are a larger number of dominant alleles, then the eye will be darker in color. For example, let's say that eye color is controlled by dominant genes E and F, but each is in two alleles that form E and e and F and f. The lightest color of the eye would then be eeff and the darkest would be EEFF. Many combinations can be formed from the two genes to account for the various colors of the eye.

Traits that are determined by one or more genes and are also influenced by the environment are called complex traits. An example of a complex trait is height, which is also polygenic. The environment affects height in that an individual needs to have a good diet and nutrition in order to reach the height that is determined by the genes.

The Y & X of the Whole Gene Situation

Sex is determined when fertilization takes place. Oocytes have a single X chromosome and the sperm cell has either a Y or an X chromosome; therefore, it is the male who determines the sex of the infant. Obviously, Y chromosomes are male and X chromosomes are female. The somatic cells in a male will have a Y and an X chromosome and in females two X chromosomes.

It was not until 1990 that the gene responsible for determining that a fetus would be male was discovered, referred to as the SRY gene (Shier et al., 2002). The SRY gene encodes a type of protein called transcription factor, which inhibits the formation of female anatomic structures, but gears the other genes of the body to develop male structures. Females do not have the SRY gene, since they do not have a Y chromosome, and so female development in the fetus will occur.

A sex-limited trait influences an anatomic structure or function of the body that is seen only in males or only in females. The gene is either autosomal or X-linked. An example is the beard growth in males. Females do not grow a beard due to the lack of hormones that influence the growth. However, the sons can receive the genes for beard growth from their mother.

Sex-influenced inheritance refers to an allele that is dominant within one sex but recessive in the other. Just as with a sex-limited trait, the gene is either autosomal or X-linked. The difference as to which sex contains the dominant allele accounts for hormonal differences between males and females. A well-known example of sex-influenced inheritance is male-pattern baldness. The gene for hair growth has two alleles; one allele is the cause of male-pattern baldness and the other allows for a head full of hair. The male-pattern baldness allele is dominant in males and recessive in females, which provides the explanation for why more males than females are bald.

Gene Therapy

Gene therapy is used to treat disorders and diseases and represents another important scientific step forward in the fight against difficult and life-threatening pathologies. Gene therapy is used to alter, stop the functioning of, or enhance the functions of a gene or genes. There are two types of gene therapy: germline gene therapy and somatic gene therapy. Nonheritable gene therapy targets affected cells of the body, so the changes cannot be passed on to the next generation. Germline gene therapy involves inducing genetic changes in an egg, sperm, or fertilized egg, and every cell in the individual will also then be changed. The change is repeated in the gametes of the individual, thereby the changes are passed on to the next generation. Germline gene therapy is highly controversial and is considered an unethical practice that will never be performed on humans.

The following specific examples of gene therapy are provided to show of how the research in gene therapy is being applied. The liver is one of the primary organs being focused on for gene therapy due to its multitude of functions. If a small percentage of the liver cells could be influenced by gene therapy, the effects could be dramatic. Another primary target is the lungs, because a gene could be placed in an aerosol, which, once inhaled, can go directly to the cells lining the inner wall of the lung. The cells could absorb the gene and produce a needed protein to aid in treating an inherited disease or illness. The endothelium lines the inner wall of blood vessels and is another target of gene therapy. Gene therapy may produce a method by which the endothelium is induced to secrete a substance that would directly enter the circulatory system. For example, the endothelium could possibly be stimulated to secrete insulin to aid in the treatment of diabetes mellitus.

IMPLICATIONS FOR THE SURGICAL TECHNOLOGIST

As noted in previous chapters, the primary reason for knowing and understanding the anatomy and physiology of the human body is to be able to better assist during surgical procedures. This also applies to understanding the anatomy and physiology of the reproductive system. However, the reproductive system of either males or females it does not involve just one or two organs, but several organs; each of which has a separate functions that contribute to the whole. For example, the cardiovascular system, however complicated it, still involves only one organ: the heart and its supporting cast of vessels. The reproductive system of the female involves the ovaries, fallopian tubes, uterus, cervix, vagina, external structures, and supportive internal structures, which include the bony pelvis, muscles, ligaments, arteries, veins, nerves, and the breasts. Whenever a female undergoes gynecologic or breast surgery, several anatomic structures have to be taken into account. Remember Box 17-5, which discusses modified radical mastectomy and the number of nerve structures and vessels that must be preserved. Another example is a traumatic bony pelvic injury, which is most likely going to involve several key internal reproductive structures. Key things for the surgical technologist to do to be effective when assisting the surgeon during gynecologic and breast procedures include the following:

1. Know the anatomy in detail in order to better assist during laparoscopic procedures. As previously mentioned, the surgical technologist may have to manipulate the uterus with the use of surgical instruments placed through the vaginal canal and clamped onto the cervix in order for the surgeon to better visualize the internal structures.
2. Be able to help the surgeon to identify nerves and other vessels during a modified radical mastectomy.
3. Be able to apply knowledge of suture and what type and size the surgeon may want according to the tissue involved.
4. Know the male anatomical structures, and, in particular, the groin region in order to anticipate the needs of the surgeon, such as during an inguinal herniorrhaphy or TURP.

5. Have the experience and ability to efficiently and quickly assist the surgeon during traumatic procedures such as a STAT cesarean section or repair of a pelvic injury. Trauma surgery requires much experience and the ability to think independently while working with the surgery team, which requires excellent knowledge of the anatomy and physiology of the body

The last issue as always is aseptic technique. This can never be overemphasized. A lay person would never have a clue that the vaginal canal is considered a contaminated area. However, through didactic studies and surgical rotation, the surgical technologist learns the methods by which to ensure that she or he does not violate the rules of aseptic technique when a procedure involves the vagina and possibly the abdominal cavity.

Case Study 2

A 10-year-old male patient is brought into the emergency department with extreme pain in the scrotum. The physical examination reveals a tender scrotum with significant swelling. Ultrasonography reveals a left-sided testicular torsion. The patient is immediately taken to surgery.

1. Why is ultrasonography necessary to confirm testicular torsion? Define testicular torsion.

2. If not immediately treated, what can occur?

3. What is the name of the surgical procedure that will be performed and its definition?

4. When performing the surgical procedure, what anatomic portion of the testis is involved and what anatomic portion of the scrotum is involved?

CHAPTER SUMMARY

- The testes are the primary sex organs in males and produce sperm cells and male sex hormones. The overies are the primary sex organs in females and produce eggs and female sex hormones.

- The tunica vaginalis covers the testis, epididymis, and the lower portion of the spermatic cord. The external connective tissue covering is called the tunica albuginea.

- On the posterior border, the tunica albuginea forms the mediastinum testis. Extending from the mediastinum testis is the septa, which extends inward into the testis and subdivide it into lobules. Between the lobules are the coiled seminferous tubules. The coiled tubules join and form the straight tubules that unite to form the rete testis. The rete testis unites to form ducts, which travel through the tunica albuginea and eventually form the single duct called the epididymis, which rests on the outer surface of the testis.

- The seminiferous tubules are lined by stratified epithelium that contains the spermatogenic cells. The cells of Leydig are located between the tubules and secrete male sex hormones.

- Spermatogenesis refers to the process of producing spermatozoa.

- In the embryo, the endoderm layer produces primordial germ cells that migrate to the developing testes where they lodge in the seminiferous tubules to differentiate into spermatogonia.

- With the onset of puberty, the spermatogonia form primary spermatocytes by mitosis. The primary spermatocytes reproduce by meiosis. Meiosis consists of two divisions: meiosis I and meiosis II. Meiosis I involves the following steps: prophase I, metaphase I, anaphase I, and telophase I. Meiosis II involves the following steps: prophase II, metaphase II, anaphase II, and telophase II.

- During this process of development, the primary spermatocytes divide into two secondary spermatocytes, which divide to form two spermatids each.

The result is four spermatids that mature into sperm cells with 23 chromosomes in the cellular nucleus. The sperm cells collect in the seminiferous tubule and travel to the epididymis where they mature and are stored.

- The sperm cell consists of the head, round body, and tail. The tip of the head is called the acrosome and contains enzymes. The body contains mitochondria to produce ATP for energy used for the movement of the tail.

- The epididymis is a coiled tube that is connected to each testis. Spermatozoa are stored in the epididymis. It exits the superior end of the testis and eventually becomes the vas deferens. It is lined by epithelium, which secretes nutritive substances that aid in maintaining the viability of the spermatozoa.

- The vas deferens begins at the proximal end of the epididymis and eventually becomes one of the structures in the spermatic cord. The vas deferens unites with the duct of the seminal vesicle to form the ejaculatory duct. The ejaculatory duct passes through the prostate gland to become the urethra.

- Each seminal vesicle is a saclike structure that is attached to the vas deferens. The seminal vesicle secretes an alkaline fluid that regulates the pH level of semen. The secretion also contains fructose, which the sperm cells use for energy, and prostaglandins, which stimulate muscular contractions in the female reproductive tract. The activity of the seminal vesicle is affected by testosterone.

- The prostate gland surrounds the proximal portion of the urethra. It secretes an acidic fluid that contain enzymes. The fluid aids in the mobility of the sperm. Contractions force the fluid from the prostate gland into the urethra to contribute to the fluid from the vas deferens and seminal vesicles.

- Cowper's glands are located on each side of the membranous urethra. They have openings into the urethra and secrete a viscous fluid that aids in lubricating the erect penis prior to insertion into the vagina.

- The male urethra serves the dual function of transporting urine and semen. The three sections of the urethra are: prostatic urethra, membranous urethra, and spongy urethra. Two pathologies that can occur involving the prostate gland are benign prostatic hypertrophy or cancer of the prostate gland. Enlargement of the gland causes constriction of the urethra making it difficult to urinate. Often surgery to remove some of the prostate gland is the only option.

- The scrotum is a pouch that contains the testicles. The layers of the scrotum are the skin and dartos tunic, which is subdivided into the dartos muscle and Colles' fascia. During colder temperatures the dartos muscle contracts to bring the testicles closer to the body and relaxes in warmer temperatures. A septum divides the scrotum into two halves.

- The penis contains the urethra and erectile tissue to convey urine and semen to the outside of the body. The erectile tissue is arranged into cylindrical-shaped bodies called cavernous bodies. The cavernous bodies are surrounded by the tunica albuginea. The paired corpora cavernosa are located on the dorsal side of the penis, and, on the ventral side is the corpus spongiosum, which surrounds the urethra and extends to the end of the penis to form the glans penis. The penile skin is freely movable and forms an extension over the glans penis called the prepuce or foreskin, which is often removed by performing a circumcision.

- At the base of the penis, the cavernous bodies separate at an area called the crura. The corpora cavernosa attach to the inferior surface of the pubic arch. The corpus spongiosum attaches to the perineal membranes. Superior to the crura the suspensory ligament attaches to the pubic symphysis.

- Refer to text for a complete description of the physiology of an erection.

- Emission is when the sperm cells travel from the testes and semen is formed. Emission is stimulated by sympathetic nerve impulses.

- Ejaculation is the forcing of the semen through the urethra and urethral orifice caused by nerve impulses that affect the various internal reproductive organs. After ejaculation the sympathetic impulses cause the arteries that supply blood to the erectile tissues to constrict, the smooth muscles contract, and the penile veins transport blood away from the penis causing it to become flaccid.

- Refer to the text for a list of blood vessels that supply the penis.

- The nerve supply to the penis is the pudendal nerve and hypogastric plexus. A branch of the pudendal nerve is the dorsal nerve of the penis.

- The term androgens refers to the male sex hormones.

- Leydig cells produce the majority of androgens and are located in the testes. Testosterone is the hormone produced in the largest quantity.

- Testosterone is secreted into the circulatory system and then travels to specific organs to combine with receptor molecules within the nuclei of the cells of the target organ. Before testosterone can be used by the cells, it is converted to dihydrotestosterone.

- When a male enters puberty the production of testosterone begins and rapidly increases. It is produced throughout life, however, in small quantities as an adult.

- During fetal life small amounts of testosterone stimulate the development of the male reproductive organs and cause the testes to descend into the scrotal sac. Soon after birth the secretion stops until puberty.

- During puberty, testosterone causes the development of primary sex characteristics and secondary sex characteristics, increases the rate of metabolism, and increases the production rate of erythrocytes.

- The hypothalamus secretes gonadotropin-releasing hormone into the circulatory system and travels to the anterior pituitary gland. The anterior pituitary gland is then stimulated to release interstitial cell–stimulating hormone (ICSH) and follicle-stimulating hormone (FSH). ICSH aids the development of Leydig cells. FSH stimulates the sustentacular cells to multiply and mature in the seminiferous tubules. FSH and testosterone cause the sustentacular cells to stimulate the spermatogenic cells to go through spermatogenesis.

- Testosterone is controlled by a negative-feedback mechanism that involves GnRH and ICSH.

- The ovaries are almond-shaped organs that are located on each side of the uterus in the ovarian fossa.

- The broad ligament, ovarian ligament, and suspensory ligament also keep the ovary in place. The broad ligament is a large fold of peritoneum that attaches to each side of the uterus and, cervix, and down to the beginning of the vagina.

- The suspensory ligament, cylindrical in shape, is a small fold of peritoneum that contains the ovarian blood vessels and nerves. It holds the distal portion of the fallopian tube and ovary in place.

- The ovarian ligament is a fold of the broad ligament attached to the medial end of the ovary to aid in holding it in place.

- During fetal life the ovaries are a mass of tissue developing next to the kidneys. They eventually descend and attach to the lateral pelvic wall.

- The layers of the ovary are the outer cortex and inner medulla. The cortex contains the cells called ovarian follicles. The surface layer of the ovary is the tunica albuginea.

- During fetal life primordial germ cells from the yolk sac endoderm migrate to the ovarian cortex to form primordial follicles that eventually differentiate into oogonia. The follicle is a single cell called a primary oocyte.

- The primary oocyte undergoes meiosis I. When a female enters puberty the primary oocytes complete the process of meiosis. The primary oocyte divides; one cell is the first polar body and the other is the secondary oocyte, which is the precursor to an ovum.

- If fertilization occurs, the oocyte divides into a second polar body and a zygote. The zygote develops into an embryo.

- During puberty, FSH stimulates the ovaries to increase in size. The primordial follicles mature and divide by mitosis to form an epithelium that is composed of granulosa cells. The glycoprotein zona pellucida separates the oocytes from the granulosa cells and this is now called a primary follicle.

- The ovarian cells outside the follicle form thecal cells.

- The follicular cells multiply, and fluid-filled spaces appear between the layers of cells. The spaces form the antrum cavity and the follicle is now called a secondary follicle.

- A mature follicle is called a Graafian follicle. It takes 10–14 days for a follicle to mature. The follicle now causes a bulge on the surface of the ovary. The secondary oocyte inside the Graafian follicle is attached to the follicular cells called corona radiata. Processes from the corona radiata transport nutrients to the oocyte.

- Ovulation is the release of the oocyte from the follicle. LH stimulates ovulation. The oocyte, upon release, travels to the opening of the fallopian tube for possible fertilization.

- The arterial blood supply to the ovaries is from the ovarian arteries, branches of the abdominal aorta. The ovarian veins follow the course of the arteries and empty into the inferior vena cava. The lymphatic vessels drain into the pelvic and lumboaortic lymph nodes. Innervation is from autonomic, parasympathetic, and postganglionic sympathetic fibers from the ovarian plexus.

- The fallopian tubes are held in place by the broad ligament. They connect to the superior portion of the uterus. Fertilization takes place in the fallopian tube.

- The opening of the tube is called the infundibulum and on the edges are the fimbriae. A fimbriae longer than the others extends and connects to the ovary and is called the ovarian fimbria.

- The three layers of the fallopian tube are inner mucosal, muscular, and outer peritoneum.

- The fimbriae beat rhythmically toward the uterus to draw the ovum into the tube. The mucosal layer is lined with cilia, which also beat rhythmically and along with peristaltic contractions of the muscular layer propel the ovum through the tube.

- A pathologic condition that can occur is a tubal pregnancy in which the fertilized ovum remains in the fallopian tube and develops. Soon it is too big for the lumen of the tube and bursts through the wall of the tube. This is an emergency situation due to hemorrhaging, and the female must undergo immediate surgery.

- The arterial blood supply to the fallopian tube is by the ovarian arteries. The veins follow the same course as the arteries. The lymphatic vessels join with the lymphatic vessels of the uterus and ovary and empty into the periaortic and lumbar nodes.

- Innervation of the fallopian tubes is from fibers of the 10th thoracic to 2nd lumbar plexuses, branch of the uterine nerves, 2nd to 4th sacral nerves, and parasympathetic vagal fibers from the ovarian plexus.

- The uterus is a hollow organ that sustains and protects the embryo. It is kept in place by the broad ligament, round ligament, and cardinal ligament. The round ligament is homologous to the spermatic cord in the male.

- The uterus is divided into the fundus, body, and cervix. The cervix is the last portion and ends in the cervical orifice.

- The wall of the uterus consists of the endometrium, myometrium, and perimetrium.

- The arterial blood supply to the uterus comprises the two uterine arteries, and the veins are adjacent to the arteries. The lymphatics travel through the utero-ovarian pedicle and terminate in the pelvic and lumbar glands. Refer to the text for the nerve supply.

- The vagina is a muscular tube that extends from the cervix to the outside of the body. It serves as the opening for the erect penis during sexual intercourse, for menstrual secretions flow through the vagina to the outside of the body, and as the birth canal.

- The vagina is posterior to the ureters and urinary bladder, but anterior to the rectum. The superior portion of the vagina is separated by the Douglas' cul-de-sac.

- The fornices are the area where the vagina and cervix meet.

- The hymen is a thin membrane of skin that covers the vaginal introitus and remains intact until either sexual intercourse or a tampon is inserted into the vagina.

- The layers of the vagina consist of the mucosal, muscular, and fibrous.

- The labia majora are longitudinal folds of tissue located on each side of the vaginal opening. They are homologous to the scrotum of the male. The anterior ends form the mons pubis.

- The labia minora are located just inside the labia majora. They are highly vascular. The anterior ends merge to form the clitoral hood.

- The clitoris is a small projectile of highly sensitive tissue that is homologous to the penis, and the anatomic structure is similar. The end of the clitoris is formed by erectile tissue and is supplied with sensory nerve fibers.

- The nerve supply to the clitoris is from the pudendal nerve, which divides into branches, one of which is the dorsal nerve that innervates the clitoris. During labor the pudendal nerve is anesthetized with a local anesthetic drug to relieve the pain from contractions.

- Bartholin's glands are located on either side of the vaginal orifice. They are homologous to the bulbourethral glands of the male. Ducts from the glands open into the vestibule. A pathology that can occur is Bartholin's cyst, which often has to be surgically removed.

- The external female structures and vaginal canal are considered contaminated areas. Therefore, when surgery is performed in this area, the surgery team must be aware of preventing postoperative infections by utilizing good aseptic technique. Three other important factors to consider:

  1. When performing vaginal surgery there is not much room for the surgeon within the vaginal canal.

  2. The tissues of the pelvis and vagina are highly vascular.

  3. The uterus and other structures consist of muscular tissues.

- Absorbable suture is the suture material of choice. The pliability of the sutures is an important characteristic. Vicryl suture is one of the most popular types used in sizes 0 to 2-0.

- At the onset of puberty the hypothalamus secretes GnRH, which stimulates the anterior pituitary gland to secrete FSH and LH. FSH and LH are the two primary hormones.

- The female sex hormones are secreted by the placenta during pregnancy, ovaries, and adrenal gland cortices. The two categories of hormones are estrogens and progesterone.

- In nonpregnant females, the ovaries are the main source of estrogens. Estrogens cause the internal reproductive organs to enlarge and stimulate the development of the female secondary sex characteristics.

- The ovaries are also the main source of progesterone. Progesterone affects the cycles of the uterus and the mammary glands, and aids in regulating the secretion of gonadotropins.

- Small amounts of androgen cause the growth of pubic hair and axillary hair.

- The menstrual cycle begins in about the 12th year of life in the female. The first menstrual cycle is called menarche.

- Refer to the text for the phases of the menstrual cycle.

- Females go through menstrual cycles until their late 40s or early 50s. The cycles become irregular and the female will then enter menopause during which the cycles discontinue.

- Menopause begins due to the few number of follicles that respond to the gonadotropins. The level of estrogen decreases because the follicles do not mature.

- The reduced level of estrogens affects the female secondary sex characteristics and has other effects, one of which is loss of bone density, which can result in osteoporosis.

- Many women who go through menopause are afflicted with hot flashes. To help with this, some women are treated with estrogen replacement therapy.

- Sexual intercourse must occur 72 hours prior to ovulation or within 24 hours following ovulation for fertilization to occur.

- The sperm cells penetrate the follicular cells and the acrosome releases an enzyme that helps the sperm penetrate the zona pellucida. Once inside, the sperm cell and the oocyte join.

- The nucleus of the sperm cell enters the cytoplasm of the oocyte and the oocyte then divides to form a large cell and smaller polar body. The nuclei of both cells unite and the chromosomes mix together, completing the fertilization process. The cell is now called a zygote.

- The zygote divides by mitosis and keeps dividing while the cell mass moves through the fallopian tube to the uterus. Now the zygote is called a blastocyst. Eight days after fertilization the blastocyst implants into the uterine wall.

- Prenatal growth is divided into three stages: cleavage, embryonic, and fetal.

- The rapid process of cell division of the zygote is called cleavage and the individual cells in the cell mass blastomeres. The group of cells produced by cleavage is called a cleavage embryo.

- While traveling to the uterus, the mass of cells solidifies and is now called a morula. When inside the uterus the morula does not immediately implant. When the zona pellucida disappears the morula is called a blastocyst, which implants in the wall of the uterus.

- The blastocyst consists of two groups of cells: the inner mass, which will form the embryo, and the trophoblast.

- The embryonic stage occurs during the second week through eighth week of pregnancy.

- The amniotic cavity develops during the second week. The inner cell mass flattens and is called the embryonic disk. The disk is composed of three layers called the primary germ layers and all of the internal organs develop from this layer.

- A second layer of cells develops and with the trophoblast forms the chorion. Chorionic villi extend from the chorion into the endometrium of the uterus.

- At the fourth week of pregnancy, the embryonic disk starts becoming elongated and humanlike features begin to develop.

- At the ninth week of pregnancy, the placenta forms from the chorion, including the development of the placental membrane. The membrane separates the embryonic blood from the maternal blood. Also substances such as nutrients and oxygen travel through the membrane from the maternal blood to the embryo's blood, and waste products and carbon dioxide travel from the embryo's blood to the maternal blood. The placenta is divided into the embryonic portion and the maternal portion.

- Amnion develops during placental formation. Amniotic fluid fills the space between the amnion membrane and the embryonic disk; the fluid keeps the placenta from collapsing and serves as a cushion to protect the embryo. The amnion contributes to the growth of the umbilical cord.

- The umbilical cord is the lifeline of the fetus. It begins at the abdomen of the embryo and attaches to the placenta. Two arteries and one vein are located within the cord.

- The yolk sac develops during the second week of pregnancy and is attached to the embryonic disk. Refer to the text for the contributions of the yolk sac to the development of the embryo.

- The allantois develops during the third week of pregnancy. It is a tube extending from the yolk sac to the connecting stalk. It contributes to the formation of blood cells and the umbilical arteries and vein.

- As the amnion increases in size, it comes into contact with the chorion to form the amniochorionic membrane.

- The fetal stage begins at the ninth week of pregnancy and ends with birth of the fetus.

- Third month: body of fetus grows longer and head growth slows; ossification of bones begins; external reproductive organs are visible.

- Fourth month: hair, nails, and nipples develop; bones continue to ossify.

- Fifth month: limbs achieve maximum length; fetal movement increases; hair on scalp grows.

- Sixth month: eyelashes and eyebrows develop.

- Seventh month: skin smoothes out; eyelids are open.

- During the last trimester the brain cells mature; internal organs mature; testes descend into scrotum. At the ninth month, the fetus prepares for birth by turning to a head-down position toward the cervix and vagina.

- In fetal circulation, the umbilical vein transports oxygenated blood to the fetus. Fifty percent enters the liver; the other half enters the ductus venosus vessel.

- The oxygenated blood mixes with deoxygenated blood and travels into the right atrium. The blood is shunted into the left atrium through the foramen ovale.

- A small portion of the blood in the right atrium travels to the right ventricle and into the pulmonary trunk to maintain the viability of the nonfunctioning lungs.

- The majority of blood that enters the pulmonary trunk enters the ductus arteriosus vessel. The vessel connects the pulmonary trunk to the descending aorta. This results in blood with low oxygen level bypassing the lungs and does not enter the branches of the aorta that supply the brain and heart.

- The highly oxygenated blood mixes with deoxygenated blood and travels into the left ventricle and is pumped into the aorta. This mixture travels to the coronary and carotid arteries.

- The mixture of blood in the descending aorta exits into branches from the aorta that travel to the lower portion of the fetal body. The other portion of blood travels through the umbilical arteries to the placenta for reoxygenation.

- The trophoblast also secretes HCG, which aids in preventing spontaneous abortion and maintains the corpus luteum.

- The corpus luteum secretes estrogens and progesterone ,but by the end of the first trimester the level of secretion greatly declines. The placenta now secretes enough estrogen and progesterone.

- The placental progesterone with relaxin secreted from the corpus luteum inhibits the myometrium to suppress uterine contractions. Relaxin also loosens the ligaments of the symphysis pubis and sacroiliac joints to aid the passage of the fetus during birth.

- Placental lactogen stimulates the mammary glands to prepare for milk secretion.

- Aldosterone causes fluid retention.

- Parathyroid hormone helps maintain a high circulating level of calcium in the mother.

- With the growth in the size of the fetus, the uterus is much larger and extends in a superior direction. This displaces the abdominal organs in a superior direction. The uterus presses against the urinary bladder, causing the mother to have to frequently urinate.

- At about the 24th week of pregnancy, the linea nigra appears. Also lineae albicantes can develop.

- The mother's cardiac output, urine production, and breathing rate increase during pregnancy.

- Labor begins when the cervix dilates and ends when the placenta is delivered. The myometrial layer of the uterus contracts to dilate the cervix and push the fetus into the birth canal. Oxytocin is released to stimulate the muscles to sustain contractions. Pitocin is a commercial preparation of oxytocin.

- As the fetus moves forward and stretches the cervical opening, it induces stronger contractions and the release of more oxytocin. The abdominal wall muscles also contract to aid in the forward movement of the fetus.

- To prevent tearing of the perineum during birth, the obstetrician will perform an episiotomy.

- Right after birth of the infant, the placenta is also delivered. The action of oxytocin aids in decreasing the bleeding from the uterus due to the contractions of the muscles, which constrict the blood vessels.

- The postnatal growth is the longest period of life. The neonatal period begins at birth and ends at the fourth week of life.

- Immediately after birth the infant must now breathe, digest, and maintain all other body functions that the mother used to take care of for the fetus. The most important immediate function is breathing and expanding the lungs for the first time.

- The colostrum produced by the mother prior to milk production contains maternal antibodies and is rich in nutrients.

- Upon birth the foramen ovale closes. When the umbilical cord is cut, blood flow through the umbilical vein to the inferior vena cava stops and the blood pressure in the right atrium lowers. A normal level of blood flow through the left atrium through the pulmonary veins is established and the blood pressure increases in the left atrium.

- The septum primum valve covers the foramen ovale opening and eventually fuses with the tissue of the septum.

- The ductus arteriosis closes immediately after birth to prevent the continued bypass of the lungs. Failure to close results in patent ductus arteriosus, which must be surgically treated.

- The mammary glands produce and secrete milk. They are located in the adipose tissue of the breasts.

- The breasts lie anterior to and are attached to the pectoralis major muscle and serratus anterior muscle. They extend from the second to the sixth ribs and sternum to axillae. At the tip of each breast is the nipple surrounded by the areola.

- An elongated portion enters the deep fascia of the medial axillary region called the tail of Spence.

- Fifteen irregularly shaped lobes make up the mammary gland. Each lobe contains an alveolar gland and lactiferous duct, which opens to the outside of the body via the nipple. The lobes are separated by adipose and connective tissue; the connective tissue is called the suspensory ligaments of Cooper.

- Ovarian hormones stimulate breast development during puberty. Alveolar glands and lactiferous ducts enlarge, whereas adipose tissue is deposited.

- Gynecomastia is the abnormal enlargement of the male breasts and usually occurs during puberty.

- During pregnancy, estrogens and progesterone stimulate the increased development of the mammary glands. Prolactin is released throughout pregnancy, but is inactive until the infant is delivered and the inhibiting actions of progesterone and lactogen are no longer present.

- When the nipple and areola are stimulated, such as by a nursing infant, sensory receptors travel to the hypothalamus. The hypothalamus signals the posterior pituitary gland to release a small amount of oxytocin, which travels to the breasts and causes the myoepithelial cells that surround the areola to contract. The milk now enters the breasts and exits at the nipple.

- When breastfeeding is discontinued, the hypothalamus will inhibit the secretion of prolactin and within a few days the mammary glands will no longer produce milk.

- The arterial blood is supplied to the breasts by the internal thoracic, intercostal, and lateral mammary arteries. The veins follow the course of the arteries and are the axillary, internal thoracic, and third to fifth intercostals. The lymphatics travel along the inferior border of the pectoralis major muscle to the axillary glands. The lymphatic network is located on the anterolateral thoracic wall. The mammary cutaneous lymphatic network is part of this system.

- The nerves to the breasts are derived from the anterior and lateral cutaneous branches of the anterior thorax. The anterior and medial mammary branches are from anterior branches of the lateral cutaneous intercostal nerves. The skin of the breast is innervated by branches of the supraclavicular nerves.

- The breast tissue is largely adipose tissue that is friable and conducive to forming spaces when healing. Some surgeons will approximate the breast tissue and others do not. If the tissue is approximated, the sutures are placed without tension and widely spaced; 2-0 and 3-0 Vicryl is often used.

- For larger excisions, drains are placed to avoid the formation of a hematoma.

- Genetics is the study of genes, chromosomes, and gene therapy. Genetic information is transferred by genes that are made up of DNA. Genes are located on the chromosomes.

- The genome is the DNA makeup in the human cells.

- The nonsex cells are called somatic cells; they contain 23 chromosome pairs and are referred to as diploid.

- The egg and sperm each have 23 chromosomes so they are referred to as haploid.

- Chromosomes are placed on a karyotype to be viewed. The autosomes are the first 22 pairs and do not carry the X and Y genes. Pair #23 comprises sex chromosomes and contains the X and Y genes.

- Genes consist of sequences of nucleotides that occur in various forms called alleles. Homozygous is an individual with two identical alleles for a particular gene. Two different alleles is referred to as heterozygous. The genetic makeup of a person's genome is called their genotype. Phenotype refers to the way genes are expressed. An allele that produces an unusual phenotype is called a mutant.

- Dominant and recessive inheritance is determined by alleles. An allele with a strong expression is called a dominant allele; the weaker allele is called a recessive allele.

- Geneticists use the Punnet square or pedigree diagram to explain inheritance.

- A monogenic chromosomal disorder means a single gene is responsible for the disorder and is hardly influenced by the environment.

- Traits determined by multiple genes is called polygenic. Eye and skin color are examples of polygenic traits.

- Traits determined by one or more genes but also influenced by the environment are called complex traits.

- Oocytes have a single X chromosome and the sperm cell has either an X or a Y; therefore, the male determines the sex of the infant. Y chromosomes are male and X chromosomes are female. Somatic cells in males will have an X and a Y chromosome, females will have two X chromosomes.

- The gene responsible for determining if a fetus will be male is the SRY gene. Females don't have the SRY gene, since they don't have the Y chromosome.

- A sex-limited trait influences the development of characteristics in males and females. Beard growth in males is an example of a sex-limited trait.

- Sex-influenced inheritance is a dominant allele in one sex, but recessive in the other sex. Male pattern baldness is an example.

- Gene therapy is used to treat disorders and diseases. It is used to alter, stop the functioning of, or enhance the functions of genes. There are two types of gene therapy: germline gene therapy and somatic gene therapy.

- Targeted organs of gene therapy include the liver, lungs, and endothelial lining of the inner wall of blood vessels.

- Several organs are involved in the male and female reproductive systems as opposed to other body systems, which may involve only one organ. Whenever surgery is performed that involves the male or female reproductive system, several anatomic structures will need to be considered.

- Knowing the anatomy in detail to better assist during laparoscopic procedures is important for the surgical technologist.

- The ability to identify nerves and other vessels during a modified radical mastectomy is important for the surgical technologist.

- Due to the various types of tissues encountered during reproductive surgery, the surgical technologist must be able to apply his or her knowledge of suture.

- The surgical technologist must be able to quickly and efficiently assist the surgeon during traumatic procedures. Often trauma victims, in particular females, will have several internal reproductive organs that are injured.

- The practice of strict aseptic technique is critical, especially since the vagina and external female reproductive structures are considered contaminated areas.

CRITICAL THINKING QUESTIONS

1. In many high-caliber women athletes, abnormal menstrual cycles are common including amenorrhea. What hormonal abnormalities can occur?

2. When a woman is being treated with estrogen replacement therapy, what other factors can increase the risk of endometrial cancer in combination with the ERT?

3. What vessels are located in the umbilical cord?

4. How does the action of oxytocin aid in decreasing bleeding from the uterus after the infant is delivered?

5. In which male reproductive structure are the sperm cells stored and mature?

REFERENCES

Agur, A. M. R. (1991). *Grant's atlas of anatomy* (9th ed.). Baltimore: Williams & Wilkins.

Cormack, D. H. (2001). *Essential histology* (2nd ed.). Philadelphia: Lippincott Williams & Wilkins.

Ethicon. (2004). *Ethicon wound closure manual*. Somerville, NJ: Ethicon, Inc.

Gray, H. (1991). *Anatomy, descriptive and surgical*. St. Louis: Mosby-Year Book.

Shier, D., Butler, J., & Lewis, R. (2002). *Hole's human anatomy & physiology* (9th ed.). Boston: McGraw-Hill.

Skandalakis, J. E., Skandalakis, P. N., & Skandalakis, L. J. (2000). *Surgical anatomy and technique* (2nd ed.). New York: Springer-Verlag.

18

ENDOCRINE SYSTEM

CHAPTER OBJECTIVES

After completing the study of this chapter, you should be able to:

1. Describe the difference between endocrine and exocrine glands.
2. Explain the effects of steroids on human cells.
3. Discuss how hormone secretion is regulated by negative feedback mechanisms.
4. List the endocrine glands and the hormones each secretes.
5. Describe how hormonal secretions are regulated.
6. Describe the role of the nervous system in the secretion of hormones.

KEY TERMS

chief cells	islets of Langerhans	thymic hormones	vasopressin (antidiuretic
chromaffin cells	parafollicular cells (C cells)	(thymosins)	hormone or ADH)
hypophysioportal circulation	pinealocytes	thyroglobulin	

Case Study 1

A patient is transported to the post-anesthesia care unit (PACU) following a thyroidectomy. Within a few minutes the patient experiences severe convulsions, twitching of the muscles, extreme flexion of the wrist and ankle joints, and stridor. The patient is immediately administered calcium gluconate through the IV to increase the circulating level of calcium. Anticonvulsant drugs are administered and the patient is intubated to maintain an open airway. Answer the following questions based on this scenario:

1. Based on the signs and symptoms, what is occurring with this patient?

2. What has caused this condition to occur?

3. What therapy will the patient be required to maintain for the rest of their life?

INTRODUCTION

The endocrine system consists of organs called endocrine glands that secrete hormones within the body (hence the use of the prefix *endo-*, which means within). The hormones travel through the circulatory system to the target cells. These glands are opposite of the exocrine glands, which have been discussed in other chapters (Figure 18-1). A prime example of an exocrine gland (the prefix *exo-* means outside or outward) is the skin, which contains sweat glands that secrete sweat to the skin's surface.

Hormones regulate internal metabolic processes of the body. They aid in controlling chemical reactions, help control blood pressure, and regulate water and electrolyte balance. In addition, they are important in the processes of reproduction and growth as evidenced by the discussion of the hormones secreted by the ovaries and testes in the previous chapter. This chapter will focus on the following endocrine glands: pituitary gland, thyroid gland, parathyroid glands, adrenal glands, pancreas, and thymus.

STEROID HORMONES

Depending on their chemical structure, hormones are classified as either steroids, which the body synthesizes from cholesterol, or proteins, amines, and peptides, or glycoproteins, which the body synthesizes from amino acids. Hormones are specific to the cells on which they act. The hormone receptor site or binding site is a protein or glycoprotein molecule that is specific for a particular hormone. The hormone acts on the cell by connecting to the binding site of the receptor cell.

Remember that a large portion of the cell membrane consists of lipids. Steroid hormones are soluble; therefore, the hormone can penetrate the cell membrane and enter the cell in easy fashion (Shier, Butler, & Lewis, 2002). Inside the cell, steroid hormones combine with protein receptors; this combination binds inside the cell nucleus to activate specific genes on the DNA. The genes are transcribed into messenger RNA, which enters the cellular cytoplasm to activate the synthesis of specific proteins (Shier et al., 2002). The proteins are responsible for causing the cellular processes that bring about the specific change in the metabolic process within the body.

NONSTEROID HORMONES

A protein, peptide, or amine is referred to as a nonsteroid hormone. The mechanism of these hormones is more involved as compared to steroidal hormones. The nonsteroid hormone combines with a protein receptor molecule on the cell membrane of the target cell. The receptor molecule has two sites: the activity site and the binding site; the hormone connects with the binding site. This binding causes biochemical changes in the cellular components of the receptor cell, such as changing the function of certain enzymes. The hormone that causes these changes is referred to as the first messenger. The cellular biochemicals that cause the changes in response to the hormone are called second messengers.

The most common second messenger that hormones use is cyclic adenosine monophosphate (cAMP). The following are the steps of the mechanism:

1. Hormone binds with the receptor in the cell.
2. G protein is activated, which stimulates the enzyme adenylate cyclase.

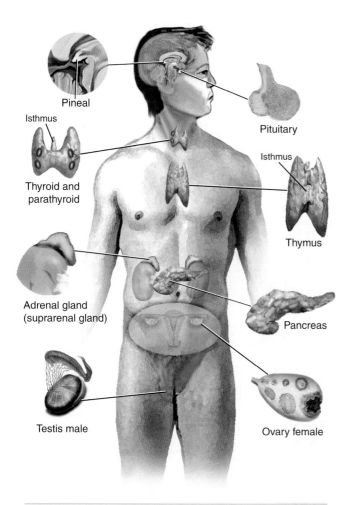

FIGURE 18-1 Locations of the endocrine glands

Pineal

Isthmus

Pituitary

Thyroid and parathyroid

Isthmus

Thymus

Adrenal gland (suprarenal gland)

Pancreas

Testis male

Ovary female

3. Adenylate cyclase causes the removal of phosphates from ATP thus forming cAMP.
4. Cyclic AMP stimulates the enzymes called protein kinases, which cause the transfer phosphate from ATP to protein substrate molecules; this converts the protein substrate molecules from being inactive to being active.
5. The active protein substrate molecules are responsible for causing changes in the intracellular processes.
6. The enzyme phosphodiesterase inactivates cAMP. Therefore, the action of cAMP is very short. Since the enzyme destroys the cAMP, the target cell is reliant on the continual secretion of the hormone in order to sustain a prolonged action.

Examples of hormones that rely on cAMP are thyroid-stimulating hormone (TSH), adrenocorticotropic hormone (ACTH), and follicle-stimulating hormone (FSH) from the hypothalamus; antidiuretic hormone (ADH) from the posterior pituitary gland; luteinizing hormone (LH) from the anterior pituitary gland; parathyroid hormone (PTH) from the parathyroid glands; and calcitonin from the thyroid gland.

NEGATIVE FEEDBACK SYSTEM

The secretion of hormones is precisely controlled by the body in order to avoid disorders that can have devastating effects on the body. Methods of control include the following:

1. Nervous system: directly stimulates a few glands. For example, the adrenal medulla is stimulated by preganglionic sympathetic nerve impulses, which cause the release of the hormones norepinephrine and epinephrine.
2. Hypothalamus: controls the release of hormones from the anterior pituitary gland.
3. Glandular responses: glands that secrete hormones or inhibit the secretion of a hormone due to homeostatic changes within the body. This is a continuing give-and-take system that is constantly in motion. The classic example, which will be discussed in further detail later in the chapter, is the blood glucose level. The pancreas secretes the hormone insulin in response to an increase in the glucose level and as soon as the level decreases, the gland secretes the hormone glucagon.

The insulin–glucagon example is also an example of a negative feedback system, the common method used by the body to maintain hormonal homeostasis. An endocrine gland senses when a hormone has reached its optimum level within the body and decreases the secretion of the hormone; this is the negative portion of the feedback system. As the level of the hormone decreases, the gland senses the decrease and the secretion of the hormone increases again.

PITUITARY GLAND

The pituitary gland, also called the hypophysis, is a small gland located in a fossa of the sphenoid bone called the sella turcica at the base of the brain (Figure 18-2). It is reddish-gray in color and highly vascular. The gland is attached to the hypothalamus by a small length of tissue called the pituitary stalk. The entire gland is surrounded by a dura-derived fibrous capsule (Cormack, 2001).

The pituitary gland consists of two lobes that are separated by a narrow region of fibrous lamina

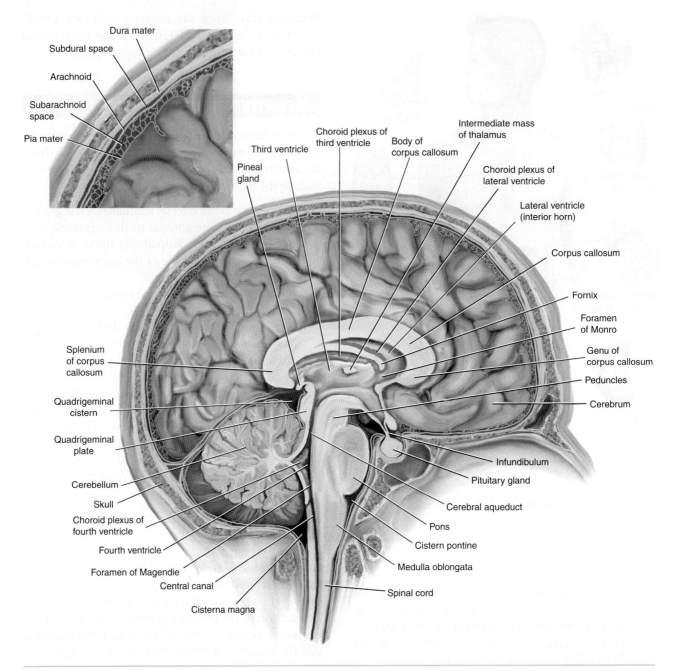

FIGURE 18-2 **The pituitary gland in relation to the brain**

called the pars intermedia. The two lobes are the anterior pituitary lobe, or adenohypophysis, and posterior pituitary lobe, which is also called the neurohypophysis or pars nervosa. The anterior lobe is the larger of the two; posteriorly it is slightly concave and it is there in which the posterior lobe rests (Gray, 1991). The posterior lobe is rounder and darker than the anterior lobe. The anterior lobe secretes the following hormones: TSH, ACTH, growth hormone (GH), prolactin (PRL), and LH (Figure 18-3). The posterior lobe does not synthesize any hormones; it is the neural component of the pituitary, since it is composed of nervous tissue. However, oxytocin (OT) and ADH are secreted by neurosecretory cells, the axons of which are located within the posterior lobe.

The portal system is an interesting anatomical arrangement for the transfer of the hormones from

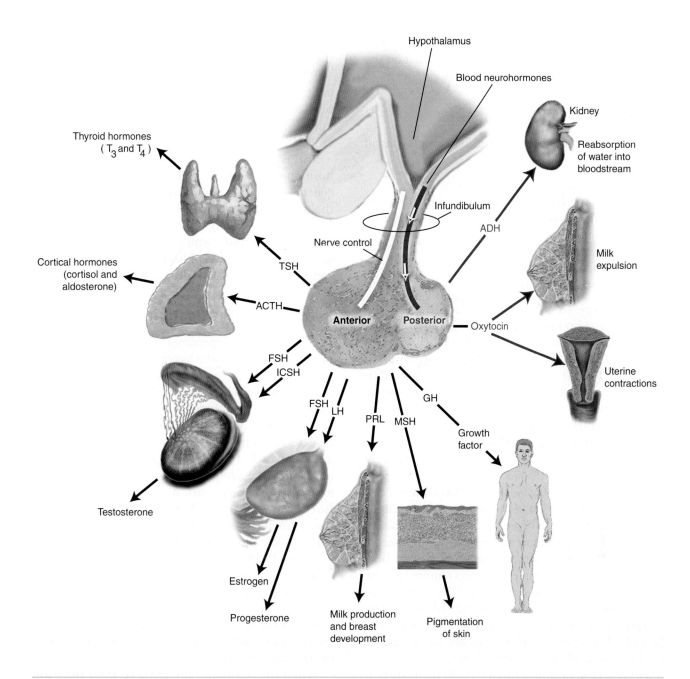

FIGURE 18-3   The pituitary gland and its hormonal secretion

the hypothalamus to the anterior lobe. Since the hypothalamus releases hormones that travel directly to the anterior lobe, a method of transfer is required and this is accomplished by a portal system of capillaries. A portal system is the arrangement of blood vessels in which the blood exits one tissue and travels directly to another tissue before the blood returns to the heart. A plexus of capillaries interconnected by portal vessels (portal venules and veins) exits the hypothalamus, travels through the pituitary stalk, and forms a capillary plexus within the anterior lobe (Cormack, 2001). Venous blood passes down the portal vessels to the capillary plexus in the anterior lobe forming what is referred to as the **hypophysioportal circulation** (Cormack, 2001). Consequently, the hormones secreted by the hypothalamus are transferred directly to the anterior lobe.

The neurosecretory regions of the hypothalamus contain neurosecretory cells, which secrete the peptide hormones from the terminal portion of the axon. When the hormones reach the pituitary, they stimulate the anterior lobe to secrete hormones that act on the other endocrine glands to secrete their hormones.

Hormones of the Anterior Lobe

The anterior lobe contains the following types of secretory cells:

1. Corticotrophs: secrete ACTH
2. Gonadotrophs: Secrete FSH and LH (however, remember that in males, LH is called interstitial cell–stimulating hormone [ICSH])
3. Somatotrophs: secrete GH
4. Mammatrophs: secrete PRL
5. Thyrotrophs: secrete TSH

Refer to Figure 18-4 for an illustration of the hypothalamus and how it interacts with the anterior lobe of the pituitary gland.

ACTH is a peptide that controls the secretion of hormones from the cortex of the adrenal glands. In response to a decrease in the circulating level of adrenal cortical hormones, the hypothalamus releases corticotrophin-releasing hormone, which has some effect on causing the release of ACTH.

FSH and LH are glycoproteins and are collectively referred to as gonadotropins, since they affect the gonads. FSH is responsible for the growth of the follicles that contain the oocyte in the ovaries. It also stimulates the secretion of estrogen by the follicular cells. In males, FSH stimulates spermatogenesis at the onset of puberty. LH stimulates the secretion of the sex hormones in females and males. It is also required for the oocyte to be released from an ovary. The hypothalamus controls the release of the gonadotropins by secreting gonadotropin-releasing hormone when puberty begins. Thus, gonadotropins are not present in the circulation of infants and children.

GH is a protein that stimulates cells to divide at a faster rate, decreases the use of carbohydrates by the cells, and increases the use of fats by the cells. It also increases the rate of protein synthesis. The hypothalamus secretes two substances that control the secretion of GH; however, they are not released at the same time but rather alternatively, since they have opposite effects. One substance is growth hormone–releasing hormone (GHRH), which stimulates the secretion of GH, and the other is somatostatin, which inhibits the secretion.

Nutrition also effects the secretion of GH. When the blood glucose and protein levels are low, additional GH is released; but when the levels rise, GH secretion decreases. This process indicates that the hypothalamus is provided feedback as to the level of these substances and secretes GHRH in response.

PRL is a protein that stimulates the production of milk in the mammary glands. The hypothalamus regulates PRL secretion by secreting prolactin release–inhibiting hormone, which decreases the secretion of PRL.

TSH is a glycoprotein that controls the secretion of hormones from the thyroid gland. A pathology associated with an excess of TSH levels is goiter. The hypothalamus regulates the secretion of TSH by secreting thyrotropin-releasing hormone (TRH). The circulating level of thyroid hormones also regulates the level of TSH. When the level of hormones increases, the secretions of TSH and TRH decrease and vice versa.

Hormones of the Posterior Lobe

The posterior lobe represents an extension of the unmyelinated axons of the hypothalamus and also contains a network of capillaries. The axons are from the neurosecretory neurons the cell bodies of which are located in the hypothalamus; therefore, the cells are not neurotransmitters but secretory bodies. The neurosecretory cell bodies synthesize two peptide hormones, which travel to the posterior lobe to be released by the axon terminals. The two peptide hormones are **vasopressin**, also called **antidiuretic hormone (ADH)**, and oxytocin. The hormones travel down the axons from the hypothalamic cells, through the pituitary stalk, and into the posterior lobe. The hormones are stored in the vesicles at the end of the axons and are released in response to nerve impulses from the hypothalamus by the process of exocytosis (Cormack, 2001). Refer to Figure 18-5 for an illustration of the relationship between the hypothalamus and the posterior lobe of the pituitary gland.

When the hormones are released from the axon terminals, they pass into capillaries that are situated near the terminals. The posterior lobe also contains a specialized type of glial cells called pituicytes; their function is not fully understood, but it is thought that they support the neurophysiological function of the lobe in some manner.

ADH causes a decrease in the level of urine formation by acting on the kidneys to decrease the volume of water they excrete. The net effect is a decrease in urination and an increase in the level of circulating body fluids. ADH also contracts the smooth muscle layer in blood vessels, thereby acting as a vasoconstrictor that aids in raising the blood pressure. In

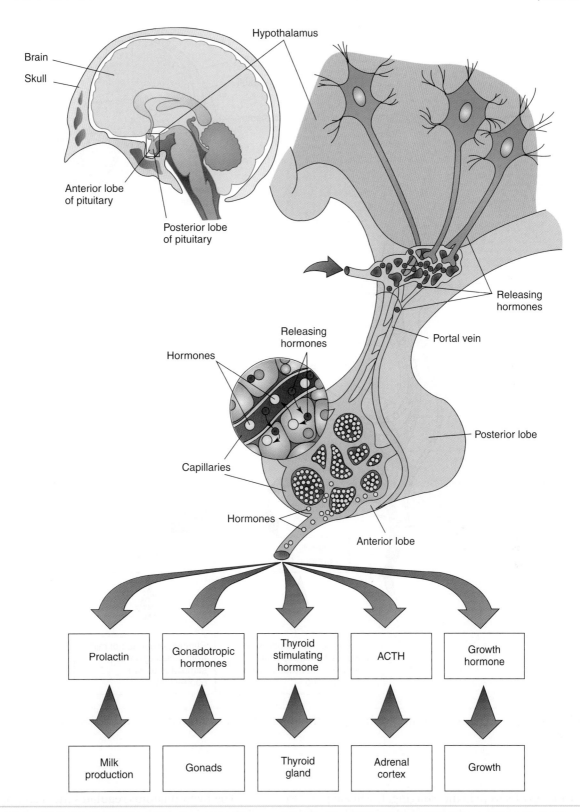

FIGURE 18-4   The relationship of the hypothalamus of the brain with the anterior lobe of the pituitary gland

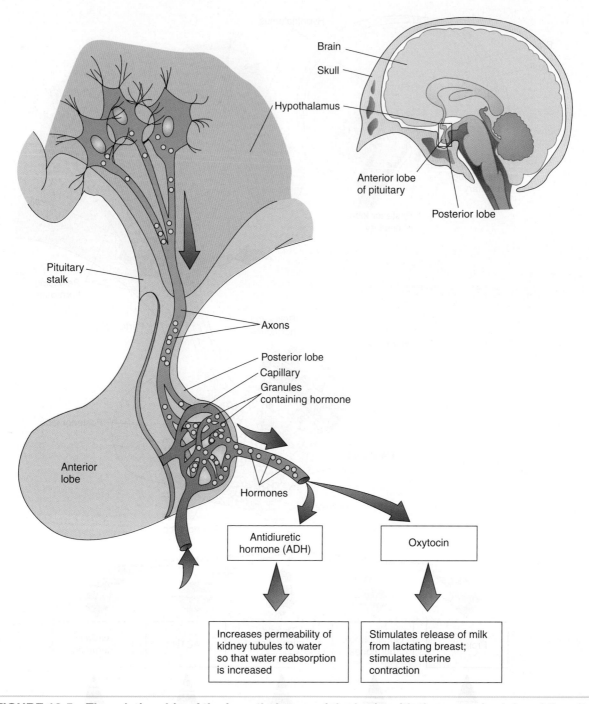

FIGURE 18-5 **The relationship of the hypothalamus of the brain with the posterior lobe of the pituitary gland**

instances of severe hemorrhaging, the blood pressure drops in response to the loss of blood and body fluids. The secretion of ADH increases in an attempt to normalize the blood pressure. Commercial drugs called vasopressors are available that perform the same vasoconstriction actions as ADH; two of these drugs are vasopressin and metaraminol.

The hypothalamus regulates the secretion of ADH. Let's use blood volume as an example. An increase in the blood and body fluid volumes stretches the walls of the vessels. Nerve receptors in the walls of the vessels send signals to the hypothalamus, which reacts by inhibiting the release of ADH. But if severe hemorrhage occurs and the blood and body fluid volumes are decreasing, the hypothalamus receives fewer signals, since the vessel walls are no longer stretched. Therefore, ADH secretion increases, causing the blood vessels to constrict and the kidneys to reduce the volume of water that is excreted, which also aids in keeping the body fluid volume normal.

Oxytocin has three roles:

1. It initiates the contractions of the uterus to begin labor in a pregnant female.
2. It causes contractions of the myometrium in the uterus after the infant is born to aid in constricting the blood vessels and expelling the placenta.
3. It is important in relation to breast feeding.

Due to the stretching of the uterine tissues by the fully developed fetus, nerve impulses travel to the hypothalamus. The hypothalamus then sends impulses to the posterior lobe to secrete oxytocin, which stimulates the uterus to begin the process of labor through contractions. Refer to Figure 18-6 for an illustration outlining the hormones of the posterior lobe and structures in which they act.

Once the female has delivered the infant, additional oxytocin is secreted, which has two important effects:

1. It causes the uterus to contract in order to expel the placenta.
2. It causes the smooth muscle layer of the uterus to contract, which constricts the small blood vessels in the uterus that have been damaged by labor and decreases the bleeding.

In the breasts, oxytocin causes the contraction of myoepithelial cells surrounding the lactiferous ducts. This forces the milk through the ducts and to the outside of the body. When the infant begins to suckle, nerve impulses travel to the hypothalamus of the mother. The hypothalamus then signals the posterior lobe to secrete oxytocin, which causes the milk to be released.

THYROID GLAND

The thyroid gland consists of two lobes situated on each side of the trachea, just inferior to the larynx, connected in the middle by a thin longitudinal band of tissue called the isthmus (Figure 18-7). The isthmus connects the lower third of the two lobes and is approximately $\frac{1}{2}$ inch in width, covering the second and third rings of the trachea (Gray, 1991). Occasionally during surgery, the surgical team will discover that the isthmus is absent, but this does not present any physiological difficulties to the patient. Additionally, a

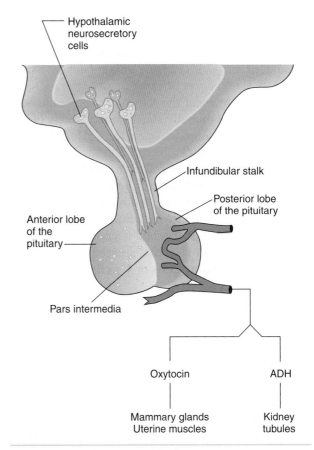

FIGURE 18-6   Pituitary gland

third lobe called the pyramid, a thin tissue layer that ascends as high as the hyoid bone, may or may not be present.

The thyroid gland extends from the level of the fifth cervical vertebra to the first thoracic vertebra. The

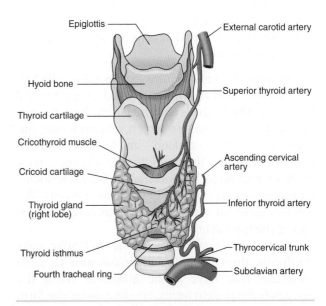

FIGURE 18-7   Thyroid gland

gland is contained in a capsule of connective tissue that is the true capsule of the thyroid. Outside the true capsule is a layer of fascia referred to as the false capsule or surgical capsule (Skandalakis, Skandalakis, & Skandalakis, 2000).

The parenchyma of the gland consists of spherical structures called thyroid follicles and the cavity of the follicle is lined by simple cuboidal thyroid follicular epithelial cells (Cormack, 2001). The thyroid follicles contain the glycoprotein called **thyroglobulin.** The thyroglobulin combines with iodine to be stored within the follicles in an iodinated form. Subsequently, the iodinated thyroglobulin is always available for the synthesizing and secretion of thyroid hormone. The other cells that secrete hormones are called **parafollicular cells** or **C cells** (the *C* stands for calcitonin).

Hormones of the Thyroid Gland

Three hormones are synthesized by the thyroid gland: thyroxine, triiodothyronine, and calcitonin. Thyroxine, also referred to as T_4, since it has four atoms of iodine, and triiodothyronine, also referred to as T_3, since it has three atoms of iodine, are produced by the follicular cells. The levels of the hormones are controlled by TSH secreted by the anterior lobe of the pituitary gland. These two hormones are responsible for regulating the metabolism of proteins, carbohydrates, and lipids. The specific actions of both hormones include the following:

1. Increase the rate of protein synthesis.
2. Aid in the breakdown of lipids.
3. Essential to the development and maturation of the nervous system.
4. Increase the rate that cells release energy from carbohydrates.

The follicular cells require iodides (also called iodine salts) in order to synthesize triiodothyronine and thyroxine. The iodine is obtained from the diet—primarily from table salt to which sodium iodide has been added and from seafood—and absorbed from the small intestine into the circulating blood to be carried to the thyroid gland. The mechanism called the iodine pump transfers the iodides to the follicular cells. The iodides combined with tyrosine, an amino acid, synthesize the thyroid hormones.

As previously mentioned, the follicular cells synthesize thyroglobulin, which contains tyrosine molecules that have iodine attached. While the thyroglobulin protein forms, tyrosine molecules form bonds that create thyroid molecules. The follicular cells take up the tyrosine molecules of the thyroglob-

ulin and break down the protein, thereby releasing the thyroid hormones into the circulatory system. Within the blood, the thyroid hormones attach to proteins called alpha globulins to be transported to the target cells of the body. Thyroxine is more abundant than triiodothyronine in the bloodstream, but triiodothyronine is much more potent.

The parafollicular cells are located throughout the thyroid gland; the cells are round with a central nucleus. The cells contain secretory granules that contain the polypeptide hormone calcitonin, which explains the other name, C cells.

Calcitonin is important in the control of the calcium level and phosphate ion concentration in the circulation. Calcitonin is responsible for lowering the concentrations of circulating calcium and phosphate ions by decreasing the rate in which the two substances disperse from the bones, in particular the long bones of the body, by inhibiting the action of osteoclasts. Simultaneously, calcitonin increases the rate of calcium and phosphate ion deposition in the bone matrix by stimulating the action of osteoblasts. Calcitonin also increases the level of calcium and phosphate ions that are excreted by the kidneys in the urine.

As mentioned above, the primary target cell of calcitonin is the osteoclast. The hormone secreted by the parathyroid glands, PTH (discussed in the next section), is an antagonist to calcitonin. It causes the ruffled borders of the osteoclasts to enlarge and increase their resorption of bone matrix. Calcitonin also performs an antagonistic action by decreasing the size and number of ruffled borders, thereby inhibiting the amount of calcium that is released due to resorption of the bone matrix. Calcitonin also reduces the number of osteoclasts.

The secretion of calcitonin is stimulated by a high level of circulating calcium ions, usually after an individual eats and the calcium ions are absorbed from the food. When the calcium level is greater than normal, the parafollicular cells are stimulated to release calcitonin by exocytosis. Calcitonin prevents an elevation of the circulating calcium ions for a long period after eating.

Strap Muscles

An important group of muscles as related to the thyroid gland are called the strap muscles, since they resemble thin straps or belts. The strap muscles are the sternohyoid, sternothyroid, and omohyoid. These muscles must be retracted when a thyroidectomy is being performed, but care is taken, since important structures such as the common carotid artery and nerves are situated in relation to the anatomic position of the muscles.

The first muscle actually encountered is the platysma. The platysma is a broad, thin muscle situated on each side of the neck located immediately beneath the skin. It arises from the fascial covering of the superior portion of the pectoralis major muscle, extends upward crossing the anterior length of the clavicle, and continues medially along side the neck to insert on the whole length of the inferior border of the mandible. It covers the external jugular vein and is innervated by a branch of the facial nerve; it serves to draw down the lower lip and corners of the mouth (Gray, 1991).

The sternohyoid is a narrow, ribbonlike band of muscle that arises from the inner portion of the clavicle and upper portion of the sternum. It extends upward and inward and inserts on the lower border of the hyoid bone. The sternothyroid is situated immediately posterior to the sternohyoid, but is a shorter muscle. It arises from the posterior surface of the upper portion of the sternum, inferior to the origin of the sternohyoid and inserts on the side of the thyroid cartilage. The omohyoid arises from the superior border of the scapula, travels upward in an oblique fashion along the side of the neck next to the lateral border of the sternohyoid, and inserts on the posterior border of the hyoid bone, lateral to the insertion of the sternohyoid (Gray, 1991). The omohyoid consists of two muscular sections joined by a central tendon.

Blood Supply

The arterial blood supply is from the superior and inferior thyroid arteries, and the thyroid ima artery. The superior thyroid artery is the first branch from the external carotid artery near the bifurcation of the common carotid artery. It travels in an anterior direction to the superior pole of the thyroid gland. At the superior pole, the artery divides into the anterior and posterior thyroid arteries.

The inferior thyroid artery branches from the thyrocervical trunk of the subclavian artery. It travels upward behind the carotid artery and jugular vein. It then divides into two or more branches to supply the inferior pole of the thyroid gland. The inferior thyroid artery crosses the recurrent laryngeal nerve at the point where the nerve is ascending and the artery is dividing.

The thyroid ima artery branches from one of the following: brachiocephalic artery, aortic arch, or right common carotid artery (Skandalakis et al., 2000). It supplies the lower region of the isthmus and travels downward lying on the anterior surface of the trachea, making it an important artery to remember when a tracheostomy is performed.

The venous drainage consists of a plexus of vessels that are within the parenchyma of the gland and on the surface. The plexus is drained by three veins:

1. Superior thyroid vein, which travels next to the superior thyroid artery and joins the internal jugular vein
2. Middle thyroid vein, which lies on the lateral surface of the gland and joins the internal jugular vein
3. Inferior thyroid vein, the largest of the three, which travels downward from the inferior lobe of the gland and joins the right and left brachiocephalic veins

Laryngeal Nerves

The laryngeal nerves that must be preserved during surgery are the right and left recurrent laryngeal nerves and the superior laryngeal nerve. The course of the right recurrent laryngeal nerve is as follows:

1. The nerve arises from the vagus nerve and travels across the right subclavian artery.
2. It loops around the subclavian artery going from anterior to posterior.
3. It ascends within the tracheoesophageal groove.
4. It travels posterior to the right lobe of the thyroid gland and enters the larynx.

The left recurrent laryngeal nerve loops under the aorta, but the remainder of its course is the same as that of the right recurrent laryngeal nerve. Both nerves cross the inferior thyroid arteries (Skandalakis et. al., 2000).

The superior laryngeal nerve travels inferiorly and medial to the carotid artery, and at one point parallels the course of the superior thyroid artery. At the level of the hyoid bone, it divides into the internal laryngeal branch, which is a sensory nerve, and the external laryngeal branch, which is a motor nerve. The external laryngeal branch innervates the cricothyroid muscle.

The results of injury to the recurrent laryngeal nerve and external laryngeal branch of the superior laryngeal nerve include hoarseness, loss of voice, and inability to cough. The injury can be temporary or permanent. If permanent, the voice may improve, but the airway may narrow necessitating a tracheostomy. Therefore, it is highly important for the surgeon to identify these nerves when performing surgery in the neck region, such as a thyroidectomy, in order to isolate and preserve them.

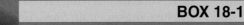

BOX 18-1

Thyroidectomy

A thyroidectomy is performed primarily for two reasons: cancer of the gland or hyperthyroidism. Before surgery is performed to treat hyperthyroidism, medications that block the effects of TSH or radioiodide ablation of the thyroid tissue are first tried. If these treatments fail, surgery will be performed.

The patient will be placed supine on the OR table, but a rolled towel will be placed posteriorly at the base of the neck to slightly hyperextend the neck to expose the operative area. The surgeon will make a transverse incision over the thyroid following the lines of the skin called Langer lines, a location chosen because it aids in healing, since the skin naturally comes together in this area and for cosmetic reasons, since the scar will be less noticeable.

The skin incision is carried through the subcutaneous tissue and the platysma muscle is bluntly divided. Retractors are placed to retract the developed skin flaps in superior and inferior directions. The strap muscles are bluntly divided and the thyroid gland is now exposed. The thyroid ima artery is

identified; two clamps are placed on the artery, the artery is divided between the two clamps, and the two ends of the artery are ligated with suture ties.

Additional vessels are clamped, ligated, and divided. At this point, the surgeon will identify the following so as to preserve them from injury: the parathyroid glands, recurrent laryngeal nerve, superior laryngeal nerve, and inferior thyroid artery. The parathyroid glands are freed from the thyroid tissue, but their vascular supply is preserved.

Branches from the inferior thyroid artery are clamped, divided, and ligated. The superior portion of the thyroid lobes is freed from the trachea and the surgeon will work her or his way downward, freeing up the rest of the lobes and carefully dissecting the tissue away from the trachea.

Once the thyroid gland is removed, the surgeon checks for bleeding, gently irrigates the wound, and closes it in layers. The strap muscles do not require suturing, since they were opened in the direction of their fibers, which will naturally rejoin.

PARATHYROID GLANDS

There are four parathyroid glands located on the posterior border of the thyroid gland, internal to the thyroid fascial sheath (Cormack, 1991). One pair is located superiorly and the other pair inferiorly (Figure 18-8). The glands are small, spherical structures that are yellowish-brown in color, making them very hard to distinguish from the thyroid gland tissue. They are covered by a thin layer of connective tissue, and the parenchyma consists of packed secretory cells interspersed with a network of capillaries.

Parathyroid Hormone

The parathyroid glands secrete the protein hormone PTH. There are two types of parenchymal cells within the parathyroid glands: chief cells and oxyphil cells. The **chief cells** secrete PTH; they are small, round cells with a centrally located spherical nucleus (Cormack, 1991). PTH is an antagonist to calcitonin; it increases the circulating level of calcium ions and decreases the circulating level of phosphate ions. As mentioned in Chapter 6, two of the main components of the bone matrix are calcium phosphate and calcium carbonate. PTH stimulates the activity of osteoclasts and osteocytes, and inhibits the action of osteoblasts. The PTH increases the ruffled borders of the osteoclasts, which contributes to the increase in resorptive activity and also increases the number of osteoclasts

present on the bone surface. The increased activity of the two bone cells causes calcium and phosphate to be released into the circulatory system.

PTH also acts on the kidneys by causing them to retain calcium ions in the circulation and increase the excretion of phosphate ions in the urine. Indirectly, PTH stimulates the absorption of calcium from the ingested foods in the small intestine by affecting the action of the kidneys to synthesize vitamin D.

As mentioned, some vitamin D is obtained from the diet. Within the liver, vitamin D is broken down to hydroxycholecalciferol, which is transported in the circulatory system or stored in tissues. In the presence of PTH in the kidneys, the hydroxycholecalciferol is synthesized into the active form of vitamin D, a derivative of vitamin D_3 called calcitrol, which affects the absorption of calcium ions from the small intestine (Cormack, 1991).

The oxyphil cells are less abundant and larger than chief cells, but have a smaller nucleus. They are interspersed among the chief cells. The oxyphils appear at puberty, so they are believed to be undeveloped chief cells with no secretory activity; however, their function is not clear.

Tetany

A pathological occurrence associated with the parathyroid glands is tetany. When performing surgery on the thyroid gland or removing the parathyroid

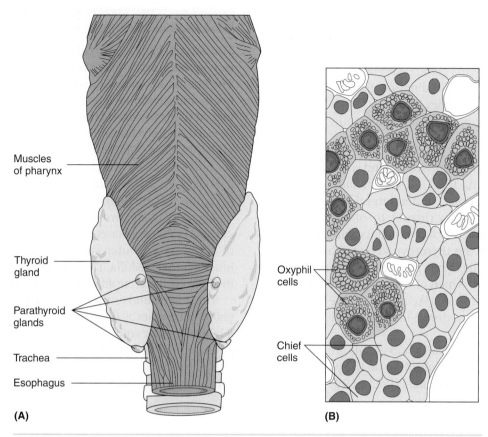

FIGURE 18-8   **The parathyroid glands. (A) Position and (B) their cellular components**

glands, at least one parathyroid gland must be left in place in order to ensure the secretion of calcium and maintain the proper circulating level. If all four glands are removed, the patient will experience hypoparathyroidism, which causes hypocalcemia, thus producing the neuromuscular symptoms of tetany.

Tetany is manifested by severe muscle cramps, convulsions, twitching of the muscles, and extreme flexion of the wrist and ankle joints, which can cause damage to the nerves, ligaments, tendons, and muscles of the joints, and even cause fractures. It is a result of a low level of calcium in the circulation whereby the skeletal muscles become overstimulated. Tetany can also be extremely life-threatening by causing severe laryngospasms that close off the airway. The patient is treated by intubating to maintain an open airway, IV administration of calcium gluconate to increase the calcium level in the circulation, sedatives, and anticonvulsant drugs. Since all four glands have been removed, the patient will have to maintain a daily drug therapy of oral calcium and vitamin D supplements for the rest of their life to avoid episodes of tetany.

During surgery, if all four parathyroid glands must be removed, the surgeon will implant as many as possible in one of the anterior muscles of the forearm. The blood supply to the muscle will supply the glands to keep them viable and they will continue to secrete PTH.

Blood Supply

The arterial blood supply to the parathyroid glands is from the inferior thyroid artery. A very small branch from the inferior thyroid artery supplies the inferior parathyroid gland. The posterior branch of the superior thyroid artery also sends out a branch, a small parathyroid artery, to the superior parathyroid gland (Skandalakis et al., 2000).

Locating Parathyroid Glands During Surgery

The key to finding the parathyroid glands is using the anatomic point at which the inferior thyroid artery enters the thyroid gland (Skandalakis et. al., 2000). The superior parathyroid glands often lie approximately $\frac{1}{2}$ inch above the point of entrance of the artery and the inferior parathyroid glands approximately $\frac{1}{2}$ inch below. If initially the inferior glands are not found, it is better to search a little higher than lower on the thyroid gland (Skandalakis et al., 2000). The best method for finding the glands is to palpate using the tip of the index finger.

Other strategies for finding the parathyroid glands include:

1. The inferior parathyroid gland is usually located first (Grant, 1997). It can be found in one of three locations: posterolateral surface of the lower lobe of the thyroid; tip of the superior or cervical portion of the thymus gland; or next to or within the thyrothymic ligament. The thyrothymic ligament is an extension of the thymus gland, which attaches to the lower lobe of the thyroid gland (Wells, 1997). The ligament is used as an anatomic landmark in locating the inferior gland.

2. The superior parathyroid glands are usually located with a globule of fat on the posterior border of the thyroid gland (Wells, 1997).

ADRENAL GLANDS

The adrenal glands, also called the suprarenal glands, rest on the superior pole of each kidney (Figure 18-9). The glands are enclosed with the kidneys in Gerota's fascia and surrounded by adipose tissue. They are attached to the fascia and the fascia is firmly attached to the abdominal wall and diaphragm to anchor the glands in place. A layer of connective tissue separates the outer capsule of the glands from the kidneys (Skandalakis et al., 2000). They are shaped somewhat like pyramids and are highly vascular structures. The medial borders of the two glands are approximately 4.5 cm apart (Skandalakis et al., 2000). The glands consist of three layers: outer capsule, adrenal cortex, and inner adrenal medulla. The adrenal cortex and adrenal medulla each secrete different hormones.

The cortex makes up the majority of the adrenal gland. It consists of three layers of tightly knit epithelial layers: outer zona glomerulosa, middle zona fasciculata, and inner zona reticularis.

The medulla, on the other hand, consists of irregularly shaped cells that are arranged around cap-

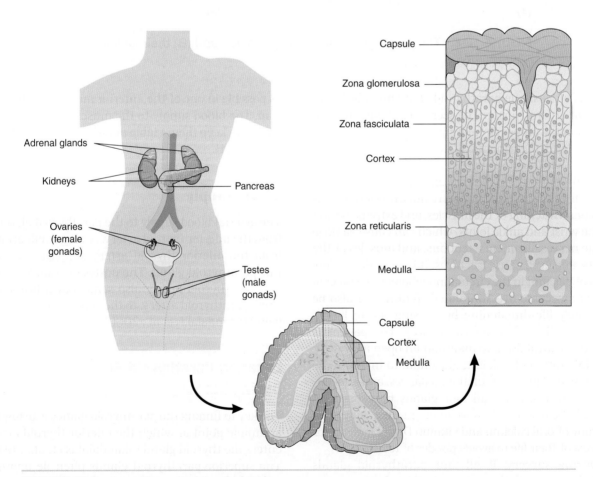

FIGURE 18-9 Location of adrenal glands

illaries. The cells of the medulla are actually postganglionic neurons and preganglionic autonomic nerve fibers that extend from the cells to the central nervous system.

Hormones Produced by the Adrenal Cortex

The cells within the adrenal cortex produce several hormones collectively referred to as corticosteroids. The corticosteroids synthesized by the adrenal cortex are the glucocorticoids and mineralocorticoids. The principal glucocorticoids are cortisol and corticosterone. The only mineralocorticoid of any significance is aldosterone.

Overall, the glucocorticoids are the cause of three primary actions:

1. They cause body cells to shift from carbohydrate catabolism to fat catabolism.
2. They aid in maintaining normal blood pressure.
3. They increase the breakdown of proteins to amino acids.

The secretion of the glucocorticoids increases during periods of stress, in particular stress caused by anxiety or severe injury. The hormones that will be discussed are aldosterone and cortisol.

Aldosterone

The cells in the zona glomerulosa are responsible for synthesizing aldosterone, which regulates the level of mineral electrolytes including potassium and sodium in the circulation. Aldosterone acts on the kidneys to decrease the level of sodium ions that are excreted and increase the level of postassium ions that are excreted. The regulation of the release of aldosterone is through the renin–angiotensin system.

The juxtaglomerular cells in the kidneys are stimulated by changes in the blood pressure and sodium ion level in the circulation. If either of these lower, the cells release the enzyme called renin. Renin breaks down the blood protein called angiotensinogen and this releases a peptide called angiotensin I. A second type of enzyme called angiotensin-converting enzyme, which is located in the lungs, changes angiotensin I to angiotensin II, which is released into the bloodstream. When angiotensin II enters the cortex, it stimulates the cells to release aldosterone.

By causing the kidneys to conserve sodium ions, aldosterone indirectly affects the retention of water, which helps to maintain the level of sodium ions in the bloodstream and blood volume. Additionally, angiotensin II is a strong vasoconstrictor that aids in maintaining the blood pressure.

Cortisol

Cortisol, also called hydrocortisone, affects the metabolism of glucose. It is synthesized in the zona fasciculata. Other actions of cortisol include:

1. Induces sodium ion retention by the kidneys.
2. Induces potassium ion excretion by the kidneys.
3. Stimulates the release of fatty acids from adipose tissue to be used as a source of energy and thereby decreases the use of glucose as the primary source of energy.
4. Stimulates gluconeogenesis by the liver cells, producing glucose from noncarbohydrate sources to increase the circulating level of glucose. The noncarbohydrate sources include circulating glycerol and amino acids.

Cortisol aids in maintaining the normal level of blood glucose concentration, in particular between meals. A negative feedback mechanism regulates the secretion of cortisol. The hypothalamus secretes corticotrophin-releasing hormone (CRH) into the hypophyseal portal veins. The veins transport CRH to the anterior lobe of the pituitary gland, which is then stimulated to secrete ACTH into the circulatory system. ACTH is transported to the adrenal cortex and stimulates the cortex to release cortisol. In turn, cortisol inhibits the secretion of CRH and ACTH; therefore, when the levels of those two substances decrease the secretion of cortisol decreases.

Cortisol occurs naturally in the body and is commercially produced for pharmacological purposes. It is used to treat autoimmune disorders, asthma, allergies, and given to patients who have undergone an organ transplantation procedure. However, the use of cortisol must be carefully monitored. It is a very powerful drug that can have toxic effects and cause various other pathological conditions, such as affecting bone growth in children and inhibiting cell division in developing body structures. Overall, commercially produced cortisol is used to treat the symptoms of inflammation. The actions of commercial cortisol include:

1. Inhibits the synthesis of prostaglandins
2. Inhibits edema by decreasing the permeability of capillaries, which prevents fluids from leaking into the surrounding tissues
3. Inhibits leukocyte migration
4. Aids in preventing the release of tissue-damaging enzymes from the lysosomal membranes

Hormones Produced by the Adrenal Medulla

The cells of the medulla that secrete hormones are called **chromaffin cells**. They synthesize and secrete the hormones epinephrine (adrenaline) and norepinephrine. These two hormones are amines, referred to as catecholamines.

The steps for the synthesis of the two hormones are as follows:

1. The enzyme tyrosine hydroxylase is located in the chromaffin cells. The enzyme converts tyrosine into an amino acid called dopa.
2. A second enzyme, dopa decarboxylase, converts dopa to dopamine.
3. A third enzyme, dopamine betahydroxylase, converts dopamine to norepinephrine.
4. A last enzyme, phenylethanolamine N-methyltransferase, converts norepinephrine to epinephrine.

Not all of the norepinephrine is converted to epinephrine; a small percentage is left unconverted. The two hormones are stored in vesicles called chromaffin granules.

The two hormones are very strong and their effects include:

1. Increase the heart rate.
2. Increase the blood pressure by vasoconstriction.
3. Increase the breathing rate.
4. Decrease the activity of the gastrointestinal system.
5. Increase the force of the contractions of the heart.
6. Relax the muscles of the throat.

These effects are known as the fight or flight response.

Epinephrine is commercially produced. It is used to treat anaphylaxis, laryngospasms, and bronchospasms, and to increase the effectiveness of local anesthetic drugs. Epinephrine is an emergency drug used to treat anaphylaxis. For example, individuals who are allergic to bee stings should carry a syringe containing epinephrine, which they can obtain by prescription. If stung, the tissues of the throat can swell due to the anaphylactic reaction and shut off the airway. Since epinephrine relaxes the muscle of the throat and increases the breathing rate, the administration of the drug is the first line of treatment.

Epinephrine is mixed with local anesthetic drugs, for example, xylocaine. Xylocaine with epinephrine is commercially purchased for use in the medical profession. For surgical purposes, the local anesthetic will be injected into an area in which the patient requires minor surgery, such as the removal of a small piece of tissue for examination by the pathologist. Since epinephrine is a vasoconstrictor, the vessels in the area of the surgical wound will bleed less. In addition, the local anesthetic will last longer since the vessels are constricted and cannot transport the local anesthetic away from the area as quickly as if they were not constricted.

Blood Supply

Remember the following important tip when surgery is performed on the adrenal glands: along with the thyroid gland, these glands have the greatest blood supply per gram of tissue (Skandalakis et al., 2000), and so they are highly vascular. Therefore, the surgical technologist should make sure she or he has plenty of hemostatic clamps for placement on bleeding vessels, a large supply of suture ties for tying off the bleeding vessels, and suture with needles for the same purpose as the suture ties. In addition, some surgeons prefer to have two sets of electrocautery (bovie). One bovie is for the primary surgeon and the other for the surgical assistant to keep up with the control of hemorrhage.

The arterial blood supply to the glands is as follows (Skandalakis et al., 2000):

1. One or more inferior adrenal arteries that branch from the renal artery
2. Six or more arteries that branch from the inferior phrenic arteries
3. Middle adrenal artery that branches from the aorta at or near the level of the origin of the superior mesenteric artery

These arteries branch extensively prior to entering the adrenal gland and form several arteries that penetrate over the entire surface of the adrenal gland capsule.

The venous drainage does not follow the course of the arteries and is much simpler in organization. One vein drains the adrenal gland and exits at the hilum of the gland. The left vein travels downward on the anterior surface of the adrenal gland; it joins the left inferior phrenic vein and the left renal vein. The right vein travels obliquely to join the posterior of the inferior vena cava.

PANCREAS

Refer to Chapter 15 for detailed information concerning the anatomic structure of the pancreas, its anatomic location, its functions as part of the digestive

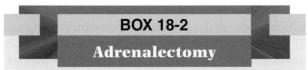

BOX 18-2
Adrenalectomy

An adrenalectomy is the surgical removal of an adrenal gland. It is most often performed due to a tumor of the gland, which is the cause of pheochromocytoma or Cushing's syndrome. The procedure can be performed endoscopically or as an open procedure.

The patient will be placed in the lateral position with the affected side up. The skin incision will be a flank incision. The retroperitoneal space is exposed and Gerota's fascia incised. The adipose tissue is separated from the kidney and adrenal gland, and the kidney is gently retracted downward. The layer of tissue separating the adrenal gland and kidney is incised to free up the gland. The gland can now be slightly rotated to expose the primary blood vessels. The adrenal artery is clamped, divided, and ligated first; then the same procedure is performed on the adrenal vein. Any other fibrous tissue attachments are incised and the adrenal gland is removed.

The wound is gently irrigated, bleeding is controlled, and a drain may be placed in the adrenal fossa. Gerota's fascia is sutured closed over the superior pole of the kidney and the rest of the wound is closed in layers.

gen from glucose and inhibits the conversion of amino acids into glucose. Insulin also aids in facilitating the diffusion of glucose into cells that contain insulin receptors, such as the cells of the heart, skeletal muscles, and adipose tissue. The actions of insulin include the following:

1. Decreases level of circulating glucose
2. Stimulates the transport of amino acids into cells
3. Increases the synthesis of protein
4. Stimulates the adipose cells to store fat

A negative feedback mechanism also controls the secretion of insulin. In addition, parasympathetic stimulation of the pancreas supplements the secretion of insulin and glucagons. When the circulating level of glucose is high, insulin is secreted and enters the liver. By stimulating the liver to form glycogen and promote the transport of glucose into muscle and adipose cells, insulin prevents too high of a level of circulating glucose, which could lead to hyperglycemia if left unchecked. When the glucose level lowers, the secretion of insulin decreases.

Neurons also use glucose for the synthesis of ATP. The neurons acquire glucose by diffusion, which is

system, and its blood supply. The focus of this section is on the endocrine function of the gland. The endocrine portion of the pancreas comprises groups of cells called **islets of Langerhans**, which are most numerous in the tail of the pancreas and contain four types of amino acid–derived hormone-secreting cells: alpha cells (α) that secrete glucagons; beta cells (β) that secrete insulin; delta cells (δ) that secrete somatostatin; and F cells that secrete pancreatic polypeptide (Cormack, 2001). The beta cells are the most common and the F cells are rare (Cormack, 2001).

Glucagon is a protein secreted from the alpha cells that travels to the liver. It stimulates the liver to break down glycogen into glucose, referred to as glycogenolysis, and convert amino acids into glucose, referred to as gluconeogenesis. Glucagon also causes the breakdown of fats into glycerol and fatty acids.

Glucagon is regulated through a negative feedback mechanism. A low level of circulating glucose stimulates the release of glucagons from the pancreas. Once the circulating level of glucose returns to normal, the secretion of glucagon decreases. This prevents hypoglycemia from occurring when the glucose level is low.

Insulin is also a protein, the action of which is opposite to that of glucagon. When insulin enters the liver, the hormone stimulates the organ to synthesize glyco-

BOX 18-3
Pancreatectomy

A pancreatectomy is the removal of the pancreas. It is primarily performed for the treatment of a cancerous tumor. The patient is placed in the supine position and the skin incision will be either a left subcostal or midline incision. If additional procedures will be performed, which is usually the case when removing the pancreas due to a tumor, most likely the incision will be midline.

The pancreas is exposed once the lesser omentum is incised and retracted. In addition, the hepatic flexure of the colon must be incised. The pancreas is examined and palpated by the surgeon to determine the size of the pathology and the extent of the resection to be performed. A large, long curved clamp will be placed across the pancreas distal to the area of resection. Using the scalpel, the surgeon divides the pancreas.

The posterior blood vessels are clamped, divided, and ligated. The pancreas is freed from its attachments to the spleen, and the tail and body of the pancreas are removed. Any remaining portion of the pancreas is sutured closed at the end of the stump.

The pancreatic duct is identified and anastomosed end-to-side to the jejunum with the use of suture. The wound is irrigated, bleeding is controlled, and the abdomen is closed in layers.

dependent on the level of circulating glucose and not necessarily on the availability of insulin. Therefore, the neurons are aware of changes in the level of circulating glucose and the normal functioning of the neurons is dependent on a normal level of glucose.

Therefore, insulin and glucagon function in somewhat of an antagonistic fashion to maintain the normal level of blood glucose concentration. But this antagonistic relation relies on the two hormones working together to maintain homeostasis. An individual who has the metabolic disorder called diabetes mellitus experiences insulin deficiency, which leads to hyperglycemia and is also associated with the loss of glucose through the urine called glycosuria. In some instances, the individual is treated by self-administration of insulin shots.

Somatostatin, a peptide hormone also called growth hormone–inhibiting hormone, regulates the metabolism of glucose by inhibiting the secretions of insulin and glucagon. It also inhibits the release of other hormones including pancreatic polypeptide, thyrotropin, cholecystokinin, and adrenocorticotropic hormone. Pancreatic polypeptide inhibits the action of pancreatic enzyme secretion, emptying of the bile from the gallbladder, and peristalsis of the intestine, which decreases the level of nutrients that are absorbed.

PINEAL GLAND

The pineal gland is a spherical structure located between the cerebral hemispheres, attached by a short stalk of tissue to the roof of the third ventricle

(Cormack, 2001). It is a very small endocrine gland, which produces the hormone melatonin. The capsule of the gland is pia-derived tissue and extending into it are trabeculae that subdivide the gland into lobules. The secretory cells are called **pinealocytes**, which have a large round nucleus and cytoplasmic extensions that end in club-shaped tips (Cormack, 2001). Between the cells are many capillary vessels.

The pinealocytes synthesize and secrete melatonin. Melatonin is affected by daylight and darkness. When light enters the eyes, nerve impulses from the retinas travel to the hypothalamus. From there the impulses enter the reticular formation and travel down into the spinal cord. Within the spinal cord, the impulses travel through the sympathetic nerve fibers back to the pineal gland in the brain. In response to the impulses that are relaying information to the pineal gland that light is entering from the environment, the secretion of melatonin is decreased. In response to a decrease or absence of light, the nerve impulses from the retinas decrease and the secretion of melatonin increases.

Melatonin also inhibits the secretion of gonadotropins from the anterior lobe of the pituitary gland, thereby inhibiting gonadal growth and function.

THYMUS

The thymus will be briefly discussed; for additional detailed information refer to Chapter 13. The thymus is primarily a lymphoid gland, but it does secrete a group of hormones called **thymic hormones (thymosins)**. The gland is located within the superior portion of the mediastinum, posterior to the sternum

IMPLICATIONS FOR THE SURGICAL TECHNOLOGIST

The challenge to the surgical technologist when assisting with procedures that involve glands of the endocrine system is the diversity of location of the glands. For example, the thyroid and parathyroid glands are located in the neck region; the pituitary and pineal glands are structures of the brain; and the adrenal glands rest on the kidneys. Therefore, the surgical technologist must have knowledge of the anatomy and physiology of the neck, nervous system, and genitourinary system in order to assist general surgeons when operating within the neck, assist during neurosurgery, and assist general surgeons who will enlist the help of a urologist when operating on the adrenal gland.

This challenge emphasizes the broad knowledge that surgical technologists must possess in order to properly function when assisting with surgery involving any body system. The surgical technologist could very well, in one day, be assigned to an operating room in which several separate operations are performed, each involving a differing body system. For example, the first operation of the day could be a thyroidectomy, so the surgical technologist must draw on their knowledge of the anatomy and physiology of the neck, which has several key anatomic structures. The next operation could be removal of a tumor of the pituitary gland, so now the surgical technologist must switch gears and be thinking about the nervous system and the delicate instrumentation and equipment needed for the procedure, and so forth. The importance of the role of the surgical technologist for the surgical team and the reliance the surgeon has on the abilities of the surgical technologist to assist him or her on a daily basis cannot be overemphasized.

Case Study 2

A patient is examined by a physician and presents with the following signs and symptoms: abnormal accumulation of fat in the face, back, and chest; weak muscles; hypertension; and hyperglycemia. The patient is diagnosed with an excessive production of glucocorticoids by the adrenal glands. Answer the following questions based on the case study:

1. What is causing the excessive production of the glucocorticoids?

2. What is the name given to this condition?

3. What surgical procedure is commonly performed to remove the tumor?

4. In what bone is the pituitary gland located?

5. What is the name of the depression in the bone in which the pituitary gland is located?

6. There are two initial incisions from which the surgeon can choose to begin the approach to the pituitary gland—name one of the incisions.

and between the lungs. During childhood the thymus is large and very active, but with the onset of puberty and on into old age it diminishes in size and function.

The thymic hormones support the production and differentiation of T-cell lymphocytes. The gland is characterized by three layers: the connective tissue capsule, the outer cortex, and the inner medulla. The cortex consists of epithelial cells and densely packed differentiating T cells. The epithelial cells are the source of three thymic hormones: thymosin, thymulin, and thymopoietin (Cormack, 2001).

The thymus is subdivided into a loose network of lobules by inward extensions of the capsule. The blood is supplied by capillaries that travel into the cortex from arterioles at the border of the gland. Interestingly, as opposed to lymph nodes, which are supplied by afferent lymphatics and efferent lymphatics, the thymus is supplied only by efferent lymphatics to transport lymph and lymphocytes away from the gland (Cormack, 2001).

CHAPTER SUMMARY

- The endocrine system consists of endocrine glands, which secrete hormones.

- Hormones regulate metabolic processes within the body.

- Hormones are classified as steroids, proteins, amines, peptides, or glycoproteins.

- Hormones act on specific cells by connecting to the binding site of the receptor cell. Within the cell, the steroid hormones combine with protein receptors, which activate genes resulting in the synthesis of specific proteins and causing changes in the metabolic processes of the body.

- Proteins, peptides, and amines are nonsteroid hormones.

- To effect changes, these hormones must use a first messenger and second messenger to activate the protein molecules and cause changes within the cells of the body.

- The most common second messenger is cyclic adenosine monophosphate (cAMP).

- TSH, ACTH, FSH, ADH, LH, PTH, and calcitonin rely on cAMP.

- Hormonal secretions are controlled by the nervous system, hypothalamus, or glandular responses.

- A negative feedback system involves a hormone reaching its optimum level, which signals to the endocrine gland to decrease the secretion of the hormone.

- The pituitary gland is located in the sella turcica within the sphenoid bone at the base of the brain.

- It consists of two lobes: anterior and posterior.

- The anterior lobe secretes the following hormones: TSH, ACTH, GH, PRL, and LH.

- The posterior lobe secretes OT and ADH.

- The hypophysioportal circulation is responsible for the transfer of hormones from the hypothalamus to the anterior lobe.

- The anterior lobe contains the following secretory cells: corticotrophs, gonadotophs, somatotrophs, mammatrophs, and thyrotrophs.
- ACTH controls the secretion of hormones from the cortex of the adrenal glands.
- FSH and LH are called gonadotropins, since they affect the gonads. They become active when an individual enters puberty.
- GH stimulates cells to divide at a faster rate, decreases the use of carbohydrates by the cells, increases the use of fats by the cells, and increases the rate of protein synthesis.
- PRL stimulates the production of milk in the mammary glands.
- TSH controls the secretion of hormones from the thyroid gland.
- Hormones travel to the posterior lobe by way of axons from the hypothalamic cells; they travel through the pituitary stalk and into the posterior lobe. The hormones are released from vesicles at the ends of axons in response to hypothalamic nerve impulses.
- ADH causes a decrease in the level of urine formation by acting on the kidneys to decrease the water volume that is excreted in the urine. The hypothalamus regulates the secretion of ADH.
- Oxytocin initiates the contractions of the uterus to begin the process of labor; causes contractions of the myometrium after the infant is born to aid in constricting blood vessels and to expel the placenta; and aids in the process of breast feeding.
- The thyroid gland consists of two lobes: the isthmus and occasionally a third lobe called the pyramid.
- The gland is contained in the inner connective tissue true capsule and outer surgical capsule.
- It consists of thyroid follicles that are lined by simple cuboidal epithelial cells. The follicles contain thyroglobulin. Thyroglobulin combines with iodine to be stored in the follicles.
- The other cells of the gland are the parafollicular cells (C cells).
- The three hormones synthesized by the gland are thyroxine, triiodothyronine, and calcitonin.
- Thyroxine and triiodothyronine levels are controlled by TSH. The actions of the two hormones include: increase rate of protein synthesis, aid in breakdown of lipids, aid in development and maturation of the nervous system, and increase the rate at which cells release energy from carbohydrates.

- The follicular cells require iodides to synthesize thyroxin and triiodothyronine.
- Thyroxine is more abundant in the body than triiodothyronine, but triiodothyronine is more potent.
- The C cells are located throughout the thyroid gland. The cells contain the hormone calcitonin.
- Calcitonin lowers the concentrations of calcium and phosphate ions by decreasing the rate at which the two substances are released from bone. The target cells of calcitonin are the osteoclasts.
- The strap muscles are the sternohyoid, sternothyroid, and omohyoid.
- The broad, thin muscle first encountered in the neck is the platysma.
- The arterial blood to the thyroid is supplied by the superior and inferior thyroid arteries and the thyroid ima artery. The superior thyroid artery is the first branch from the external carotid artery.
- The venous drainage consists of a plexus of vessels within the gland and on the surface. It is drained by the superior thyroid vein, middle thyroid vein, and inferior thyroid vein.
- The laryngeal nerves that must be preserved during surgery are the right and left recurrent laryngeal nerves and the superior laryngeal nerve.
- There are four parathyroid glands located on the posterior border of the thyroid gland; one pair is located inferiorly and the other pair superiorly.
- The parathyroid glands are small, ovoid yellowish brown structures.
- PTH is secreted by the glands.
- There are two types of cells in the glands: chief cells, which secrete PTH, and oxyphil cells, the function of which is not clearly understood.
- PTH is an antagonist to calcitonin. PTH increases the level of calcium ions and decreases the level of phosphate ions. PTH stimulates the activity of osteoclasts and osteocytes, and inhibits the action of osteoblasts.
- PTH acts on the kidneys to retain calcium ions to be returned to the circulation and increase the excretion of phosphate ions.
- Tetany is a pathology that occurs if all four parathyroid glands are injured or removed during surgery.
- The arterial blood supply to the parathyroid glands is from the inferior thyroid artery: a branch from the inferior thyroid artery supplies the inferior parathyroid glands, and a branch from the supe-

rior thyroid artery supplies the superior parathyroid glands.

- The key to finding the parathyroid glands during surgery is to use the point at which the inferior thyroid artery enters the thyroid gland. The thyrothymic ligament is another anatomic structure used to locate the glands.

- The adrenal glands rest on the superior poles of the kidneys. They are enclosed with the kidneys in Gerota's fascia.

- The glands consist of three layers: the capsule, adrenal cortex, and adrenal medulla.

- The cortex consists of three layers: the zona glomerulosa, zona fasciculata, and zona reticularis.

- The cells of the medulla are postganglionic neurons and preganglionic autonomic nerve fibers, which extend to the central nervous system.

- The cells of the adrenal cortex produce several hormones, classified as corticosteroids. There are two subdivisions of the corticosteroids: glucocorticoids and mineralocorticoids. The primary glucocorticoids are cortisol and corticosterone; the only mineralocorticoid that is of any importance is aldosterone.

- Glucocorticoids cause body cells to shift from carbohydrate catabolism to fat catabolism, aid in maintaining normal blood pressure, and increase breakdown of proteins to amino acids.

- Aldosterone regulates the level of mineral electrolytes such as potassium and sodium in the circulation. It acts on the kidneys to decrease the level of sodium ions that are excreted and increase the level of potassium ions that are excreted. The regulation of the secretion of aldosterone is by the renin–angiotensin system.

- Cortisol affects the metabolism of glucose, induces sodium ion retention by the kidneys, induces potassium ion excretion by the kidneys, stimulates the release of fatty acids from adipose tissue, and stimulates gluconeogenesis by the liver cells. It maintains the normal level of blood glucose concentration.

- Cortisol is commercially produced to treat inflammation, autoimmune disorders, asthma, and allergies, and is given to patients who have undergone organ transplantation.

- Commercial cortisol inhibits synthesis of prostaglandins, inhibits edema by decreasing permeability of capillaries, inhibits leukocytic migration, and aids in preventing release of enzymes that damage tissue.

- The cells of the medulla are chromaffin cells. They synthesize and secrete epinephrine and norepinephrine.

- Both hormones increase the heart rate, cause vasoconstriction to raise blood pressure, increase the breathing rate, decrease activity of the GI system, increase the force of contractions of the heart, and relax the muscles of the throat.

- Epinephrine is commercially produced. It is used to treat anaphylaxis and individuals who have sustained a heart attack, and is mixed with local anesthetic drugs.

- The thyroid gland is highly vascular. Its arterial blood supply is: inferior adrenal glands that branch from renal artery, branches of the inferior phrenic arteries, and middle adrenal artery.

- One vein drains the adrenal gland. The left vein joins the left renal vein and the right vein joins the inferior vena cava.

- The endocrine portion of the pancreas comprises the islets of Langerhans, which contain four types of hormone-secreting cells: alpha cells, which secrete glucagon; beta cells, which secrete insulin; delta cells, which secrete somatostatin; and F cells, which secrete pancreatic polypeptide. Beta cells are the most common.

- Glucagon stimulates the liver to break down glycogen into glucose and convert amino acids into glucose. This prevents hypoglycemia.

- Insulin is the antagonist to glucagons. It stimulates the liver to synthesize glycogen from glucose and inhibits the conversion of amino acids to glucose. Insulin prevents hyperglycemia.

- Diabetes mellitus is an insulin deficiency and is treated by self-administration of insulin shots.

- Somatostatin regulates the metabolism of glucose by inhibiting the secretion of insulin and glucagons. It also inhibits the release of other hormones.

- Pancreatic polypeptide inhibits the action of pancreatic enzyme secretion, emptying of bile from the gallbladder, and peristalsis of the intestines.

- The pineal gland is a round structure located between the cerebral hemispheres and attached to the roof of the third ventricle.

- It produces the hormone melatonin. The secretory cells are pinealocytes.

- The secretion of melatonin is affected by the presence of light. When light enters the eyes and the impulses reach the pineal gland, the secretion of melatonin decreases. In response to a decrease in light, the secretion increases.

- Melatonin also inhibits the secretion of gonadotropins.

- The thymus secretes a group of hormones called thymic hormones.

- The thymus is located posterior to the sternum in the upper portion of the mediastinum between the lungs.

- The thymus is highly active during childhood, but with the onset of puberty and on in to old age, it diminishes in function and size.

- Thymic hormones aid in the production and differentiation of T-cell lymphocytes.

- It has three tissue layers: the capsule, cortex, and medulla.

- The cortex consists of epithelial cells that are the source of three thymic hormones: thymosin, thymulin, and thymopoietin.

- Its blood supply is capillaries that travel into the cortex from arterioles.

- The thymus is supplied only by efferent lymphatics, which transport lymph and lymphocytes away from the gland.

- The challenge to the surgical technologist is the diversity of location of the glands and the various body systems that are involved.

CRITICAL THINKING QUESTIONS

1. What is the difference between an endocrine gland and an exocrine gland?
2. A patient enters the emergency department with the following symptoms: excess sweating, tachycardia, anxiety, tremor, severe headache, and pain in the epigastric region. An MRI reveals a tumor of the adrenal gland. What is the name of the tumor? What is the treatment? What is causing the symptoms?
3. When performing thyroid surgery, how would the surgeon most likely incise/separate the strap muscles to view the thyroid gland?
4. Melatonin is commercially produced and at one time was thought to be the answer to treating many disorders. However, the substance is now thought to aid in the treatment of only one disorder and could be a factor in affecting another disorder. Name those disorders and the role of melatonin.
5. A surgeon will be performing a minor surgical procedure in which a piece of tissue will be removed. She orders the local anesthetic Marcaine with epinephrine. Why does the surgeon want epinephrine?

REFERENCES

Cormack, D. H. (2001). *Essential histology* (2nd ed.). Philadelphia: Lippincott Williams & Wilkins.

Grant, C. S. (1997). Surgical anatomy of the thyroid, parathyroid, and adrenal glands. In L. M. Nyhus, R. J. Baker, & J. E. Fischer (Eds.), *Mastery of surgery* (3rd ed., Vol. 1, pp. 475–485). Boston: Little, Brown.

Gray, H. (1991). *Anatomy, descriptive and surgical*. St. Louis: Mosby-Year Book.

Shier, D., Butler, J., & Lewis, R. (2002). *Hole's human anatomy & physiology* (9th ed.). Boston: McGraw-Hill.

Skandalakis, J., Skandalakis, P. N., & Skandalakis, L. J. (2000). *Surgical anatomy and technique* (2nd ed.). New York: Springer-Verlag.

Wells, S. A. (1997). Total thyroidectomy, lymph node dissection for cancer. In L. M. Nyhus, R. J. Baker, & J. E. Fischer (Eds.), *Mastery of surgery* (3rd ed., Vol. 1, pp. 496–507). Boston: Little, Brown.

GLOSSARY

caused by hyperventilation or metabolic alkalosis can result from an excess intake or retention of bicarbonate, or loss of gastric acid due to vomiting.

Alleles: A variation of genes that occupy the corresponding space or loci on chromosomes. Each allele encodes for a particular inherited characteristic. An individual who has two identical alleles is said to be homozygous for that particular gene. An individual with two different alleles is said to be heterozygous; in this case, one of the genes will be dominant and the other recessive.

Allograft: Also called homograft; skin or tissue taken from the same species used as a temporary covering of burned areas.

All-or-none response: Refers to the fact that once a nerve pulse is generated through depolarization, the impulse never varies in strength.

Alveolar gland: Glands that secrete and transport milk to the nipple of the breast with an opening to the outside of the breast.

Alveolar processes: Located in the maxilla or mandible; the sockets for the teeth are located within the alveolar processes.

Alveoli (singular, alveolus): The smallest structures of the lungs, they are grapelike clusters located at the end of terminal bronchioles responsible for the exchange of gases.

Amphiarthrosis: A type of slightly movable joint; the joint has very little movement due to the slight flexibility of the fibrous cartilage that connects the bones.

Amphipathic molecule: A molecule that contains a hydrophobic and hydrophilic end with stretches of both hydrophilic and hydrophobic amino acids, but each end is able to display its own characteristics of solubility.

Ampulla of Vater: The slightly dilated area of the duodenum formed by the joining of the duct of Wirsung and common bile duct where they open into the duodenum.

Anaerobic threshold: Also referred to as lactic acid threshold; the outcome of the anaerobic phase of cellular respiration in which there is an increase in the level of lactic acid in the circulatory system.

Anal canal: The seventh portion of the colon; it begins at the rectum and ends at the opening of the anus; the mucous membrane of the anal canal is arranged into longitudinal folds called anal columns, that contain arteries and veins.

Anal sinuses: Small depressions located just superior to the anal valves that can become compacted with fecal matter leading to the formation of abscesses.

Anaphase: Third step of mitosis in which the DNA is equally divided between the two halves of the dividing cell.

Anatomic position: The position in which the human body is standing erect facing forward with arms at the sides, palms of the hands forward, and feet facing forward.

Anatomy: The study of the structure and morphology of the body and its systems.

Androgens: Medical term that refers to the group of male sex hormones.

Anemia: Blood disease that is caused by factors that destroy erthrocytes.

Angina pectoris: A substernal or retrosternal pain that occurs when the myocardial oxygen demand exceeds the supply.

Angiography: Diagnostic procedure in which a contrast solution is injected through a special type of catheter to provide an outline of the vascular system using x-ray; it still establishes the standard for the diagnosis and evaluation of vascular disease.

Angiotensinogen: Blood protein that is produced in the liver and is a precursor of angiotensin.

Antagonist: Muscle that resists the prime mover's action and works to cause action in the opposite direction.

Anterior cruciate ligament: One of two cruciate ligaments of the knee; prevents the femur from sliding posteriorly on the tibia, limits the medial rotation of the femur when the leg is in a fixed position with the foot planted, and prevents hyperextension of the knee.

Anterior superior iliac spine: A bony projection on the anterior edge of the iliac crest that serves as an important anatomic landmark when surgery is performed, since it is easily palpated.

Anterior: ventral; toward the front.

Antibodies: Glycoproteins produced by B lymphocytes that bind to the receptor site of the specific antigen that stimulated their production.

Anticodon: A sequence of three nucleotides (triplet) in tRNA. The anticodon is a triplet complementary to a triplet on the mRNA. The anticodon pairs with a specific codon of mRNA during protein synthesis, which indicates a specific amino acid.

Antidiuretic hormone (ADH): Hormone secreted by the posterior pituitary gland when the water level in the body is too low; causes the distal convoluted tubules and collecting tubules in the kidneys to increase the reabsorption of water from the renal filtrate, thereby increasing the water level, and aids in maintaining normal blood volume and blood pressure.

Antigen: Also called immunogen; any foreign substance that enters the body and stimulates the production of antibodies.

Antigen–antibody complex: Combination of an antibody with an antigen; the combination activates complement to lyse the invading bacterial cells, neutralize toxins, and increase phagocytosis.

Antigenic determinants: Sites on antigens to which antibodies or lymphocytes can bind.

Antiserum: Serum that contains specific antibodies; antiserum that contains antibodies against toxoids is called an antitoxin.

Anus: The opening of the anal canal through which feces pass; two sphincter muscles are located around the anus, the internal sphincter, which is an involuntary smooth muscle, and the external sphincter muscle, which is composed of voluntary skeletal muscle that the individual can control to inhibit defecation.

Aplastic anemia: The lack of production of erythrocytes.

Apneustic center: Located within the posterior portion of the pons, it is a collection of nerve tissue that controls the inspiratory rate of respiration.

Apocrine sweat glands: Located in the axillary and genital regions, they are activated during times of stress and exercise.

Aponeuroses (singular, aponeurosis): a special type of fascia that binds muscle to muscle; it is a strong sheet of fibrous connective tissue; an example is the aponeuroses of the external abdominal oblique muscle.

Appendicular skeleton: Includes bones of the pectoral girdle, upper extremities, pelvic girdle, and lower extremities.

Appendix: Short blind tube that is connected to the end of the cecum and held in place by a fold of peritoneum called the mesoappendix that attaches to the cecum; the appendix has no known function; it often becomes inflamed and infected and must be surgically removed, a procedure called an appendectomy.

Aqueous humor: Watery fluid contained in the anterior chamber that aids in maintaining the shape of the anterior portion of the eye.

Arterial embolism: A blood clot, piece of fat, air, or portion of a tumor that circulates through the cardiovascular system until it becomes lodged in smaller vessels, blocking the flow of blood to an extremity or body organ.

Arteries: Blood vessels that carry oxygenated blood away from the heart.

Arterioles: Small artery vessels.

Articulation: Refers to where the ends of two bones meet to form a joint.

Artificial active acquired immunity: Type of acquired immunity gained by vaccination; the vaccine contains a sufficient number of pathogens to cause the individual to form antibodies to that particular pathogen.

Artificial passive acquired immunity: Immunity acquired by transferring antibodies from an immune person to a susceptible person.

Ascending colon: The second portion of the colon; it begins at the ileocecal valve, traveling in a superior direction along the right side of the abdominal cavity and ending at the hepatic flexure.

Astrocyte: A type of neuroglial cell shaped like a star that serves as part of the blood–brain barrier to prevent particular substances from entering the brain.

Atheroma: The lesions associated with atherosclerosis that consist of a soft central region composed of lipids and cellular debris covered by a layer of fibrous tissue that contributes to narrowing of the lumen of an arterial vessel.

Atherosclerosis: Pathological condition that involves the formation of atheroma in the intima of medium and large arteries.

Atherosclerosis: The abnormal buildup of cholesterol inside an artery causing blockage of the blood flow.

Atlas: The first cervical vertebra; it supports the head.

Atom: The smallest division of an element; it is composed of neutrons, electrons, and protons.

Atomic number: The number of protons within the nucleus of an atom and equals the number of orbiting electrons; the number of protons in an element is constant.

Atria (singular, atrium): The two upper chambers of the heart that receive blood from the veins of the body.

Atrial natriuretic hormone (ANH): Hormone secreted by the atria of the heart that is an antagonist to aldosterone; decreases the reabsorption of sodium ions from the renal filtrate into the circulatory system; therefore, the sodium ions remain in the renal filtrate including water and excreted with the urine, which lowers the blood pressure and blood volume.

Atrioventricular node: Located in the septum between the two atria, it receives the impulse fired by the sinoatrial node that provides the conduction pathway between the atria and ventricles.

Atrioventricular orifice: An opening between the atrium and ventricle on each side of the heart.

Attenuation: The laboratory process of weakening a pathogen by causing genetic changes; it can be used as a vaccine called an attenuated vaccine.

Auerbach's plexus: Also called the myenteric plexus; an autonomic nerve network contained in the tunica muscularis layer of the intestine; parasympathetic impulses increase peristalsis and sympathetic impulses decrease peristalsis.

Auricle: The outer, visible portion of the ear that is located on each side of the head.

Autologous graft: Also called autograft; skin that is taken from a patient to be transferred to the recipient site on the same patient.

Autologous transfusion: Blood that is donated by the patient prior to their surgical procedure and that can be used for transfusion purposes.

Autonomic nervous system (ANS): Subdivision of the PNS; connects the CNS to the visceral organs via the cranial and spinal nerves to initiate involuntary responses.

Autosomes: Chromosomes that do not carry the X or Y genes and therefore are not sex chromosomes. There are 22 pairs in the human. They are involved in transmitting genetic traits other than those that are sex-linked.

Axis: The second cervical vertebra.

Axon: The extension of a neuron that transmits impulses away from the cell; a neuron has only one axon.

B

Ball-and-socket joint: A joint that consists of a bone that has a ball-shaped head at one end that articulates with a bone that has a cup-shaped socket; this type of joint allows for the widest range of motion.

Bartholin's duct: Single duct formed by Wharton's duct from the submandibular gland and Riviniani ducts of the sublingual glands.

Bartholin's glands: Also called the vestibular glands. Ducts are located on each side of the vaginal orifice that open into the vestibule; they are mucus-secreting glands that serve to lubricate the vaginal opening.

Basal body: Similar to a centriole except it is located at the base of a cilium or flagellum.

Basal ganglia: Collection of gray matter located within the white matter of the cerebral hemispheres that acts in conjunction with the cerebellum to coordinate body movement.

Base: Chemical compound that decreases the concentration of hydrogen ions by accepting them in solution.

Basement membrane: Also called the basement lamina; a thin layer of tissue that binds the underlying connective tissue layer to the upper tissue layers.

Basophil: Type of leukocyte that secretes heparin and histamine in response to chronic inflammation and healing from an infection.

Bile: Viscous, yellowish-green-colored liquid that contains cholesterol, bile pigments, and bile salts; the bile salts are the only substance in bile that have a digestive function; bile is produced by the hepatocytes in the liver.

Bipolar neuron: Neuron with one dendrite and one axon that functions as a receptor cell in special sense organs.

Blood pressure gradient: The difference between the mean blood pressure within the aorta and the mean blood pressure within the venae cavae as they enter the right atrium of the heart.

Blood pressure: The force that blood exerts against the internal walls of blood vessels.

Blood salvage: The collection and reinfusion of a patient's blood during surgery.

Brainstem: Connects the diencephalon to the spinal cord and consists of the medulla oblongata, pons, and midbrain.

Bronchioles: The smallest branches of the bronchi inside the lungs; they enter the lobules of the lung.

Buccal cavity: Medical term for the mouth.

Bundle of His: The electrical connection between the atria and ventricles that receives the impulse from the atrioventricular node.

Bursae (singular, bursa): Small fluid-filled sacs located between the tendons and bony prominences of a joint that contain synovial fluid to cushion and aid in the movement of tendons.

C

Calciferol: A form of vitamin D that increases the absorption of calcium and phosphate in the small intestine.

Calculi: Medical term that refers to stones such as kidney stones or bladder stones.

Calorie: The amount of heat required to raise the temperature of 1 gram of water by 1° Celsius.

Calyces (singular, calyx): Funnel-shaped structures that surround the papillae of the renal pyramids; they are formed by the expansion of the ureter upon entry into the kidney; there are two calyces: major and minor; the minor calyces empty into the two or three major calyces, which drain into the common renal pelvis; the calyces serve at the collection point of urine.

Canaliculi: Also called haversian canaliculus; they are tiny passages that radiate from the lacunae of the bone to the haversian canals providing an avenue for diffusion of nutrients and wastes.

Cancellous bone: Also called spongy bone; located at the ends of bone and lines the medullary marrow cavity, which consists of interspersed columns of bony substance called trabeculae with spaces between the columns.

Capillaries: Microscopic blood vessels the walls of which are only one cell thick in order to facilitate the exchange of nutrients and wastes between the blood and tissue fluid.

Capitulum: Located at the distal end of the humerus on the lateral side, it articulates with the radius at the elbow joint.

Carbohydrate: Molecules composed of chains of carbon atoms with hydrogen and oxygen atoms attached; they are the molecules from which all other biomolecules are derived.

Cardiac aneurysm: Abnormal bulging or ballooning of the ventricular wall due to an abnormal increase of ventricular pressure.

Cardiac cycle: All events that occur during a single heartbeat, including relaxation and contraction of the atria and ventricles.

Cardiac muscle: Located only in the heart, it is responsible for contracting and relaxing to pump the blood through the chambers of heart and into the blood vessels; it is the only muscle tissue in the body that has striations but is composed of smooth muscle.

Cardiac output: The amount of blood ejected from the left ventricle into the aorta or right ventricle into the pulmonary artery.

Cardiac sphincter: The point at which the esophagus joins to the superior end of the stomach.

Cardiovascular system: Subdivision of the circulatory system that consists of the heart, coronary arteries, and great vessels.

Carpals: The bones of the wrist joint.

Cecum: The first portion of the colon located in the lower right quadrant of the abdomen; the ileocecal valve is located at the superior portion of the cecum and indicates the joining of the ileum to the colon.

Cell-mediated immunity (CMI): Immunity that consists of T cells that work with B cells to control the cause of chronic infections.

Cellular respiration: Process of oxidizing food molecules such as glucose to carbon dioxide and water. The energy that is released is captured in the form of ATP for use by cells.

Central nervous system (CNS): Subdivision of the nervous system that consists of the brain and spinal cord.

Central venous pressure: The measure of the venous blood pressure within the right atrium.

Centriole: Type of organelle comprising cylindrical structures that consist of groups of microtubules and aid in organizing the assembly of microtubules during cell division.

Centromere: Middle area on a chromosome where the two strands of a chromosome are joined.

Cerebellum: Second-largest structure of the brain, located posterior to the medulla oblongata and inferior to the cerebrum's occipital lobe; functions include coordinating skeletal muscle movement and partially responsible for learning new motor tasks.

Cerebral cortex: A layer of neurons on the surface of the brain that is approximately 2–4 mm thick; the neurons have specialized functions depending on their location on the surface of the brain.

Cerebrum: The largest portion of the brain, divided into a right and left hemisphere and covered with gyri that are separated by sulci and fissures; functions include sensory integration and contralateral motor control.

Cerumen: The yellowish substance secreted by the ceruminous glands located in the dermis of the auditory canal of the ear; also referred to as ear wax.

Ceruminous glands: Type of sebaceous glands located in the dermis of the auditory canal of the ear; they secrete cerumen.

Chemoreceptor: Sensory receptor that is sensitive to changes in chemical concentration.

Chemotaxis: The chemical attraction of phagocytes to microbes due to chemicals released from injured tissue cells, peptides, and other microbial products.

Chief cells: Also called principal cells. Polyhedral-shaped cells located within the parathyroid glands that contain clear cytoplasm and a centrally located nucleus. The cells secrete parathyroid hormone.

Cholesterol: Type of fat ingested with foods such as eggs, meat, and cheese that is important in the manufacturing of body cells and synthesis of certain kinds of hormones.

Chordae tendineae: Fibrous chords attached to the tricuspid valve on the ventricular side that prevent the cusps of the valve from folding back into the atrium.

Chorion: Formed by a layer of cells and the trophoblast, it is the outermost embryonic membrane that eventually produces the placenta and is present until birth as the outer layer of the two layers that contain the amniotic fluid and fetus.

Chorionic villi: The tiny hairlike structures that form on the surface of the chorion that aid in forming the placenta.

Choroid coat: A vascular structure of the eye that forms the posterior portion of the middle tunic and lines the internal portion of the sclera; the vessels within the choroid provide nourishment to the posterior segment of the retina and contain the melanocytes that produce melanin.

Chromaffin cell: Special type of cells located in the medulla of the adrenal gland that synthesize and secrete the two catecholamines, epinephrine and norepinephrine.

Chromatin: Material within the cell nucleus from which the chromosomes are formed and contained. The chromatin consists of strands of DNA attached to a protein base and occurs in two different forms: euchromatin and heterochromatin. During cell division the chromatin condenses and forms the chromosomes.

Chromosomes: Threadlike structure located in the nucleus of a cell that transmit genetic information. Each chromosome consists of a coiled double-strand of deoxyribonucleic acid (DNA). The genes are located in a linear pattern along the length of each DNA strand.

Chronic obstructive pulmonary disease (COPD): Chronic airway obstruction that is secondary to emphysema, asthma, chronic bronchitis, or other respiratory disorders characterized by the inability to perform strenuous work or exercise that gradually worsens as the disease progresses.

Chylomicrons: The combination of cholesterol and protein that is absorbed and transported by the lacteals to the major lymph vessels.

Chymification: Medical term that refers to the process of breaking down food within the stomach.

Cilia: Short, hairlike structures that move in wavelike fashion to move fluids or materials past immobile cells, for example, the cilia that line the respiratory tract in humans.

Ciliary body: The thickest portion of the middle tunic of the eye that forms a ring around the anterior of the eye; consists of the ciliary processes and muscle that contract and relax to alter the shape of the lens.

Circulatory system: Body system that consists of the cardiovascular system and peripheral vascular system.

Circumcision: Surgical removal of the prepuce, which is more commonly known as the foreskin.

Citric acid: A six-carbon molecule that is broken down during the Krebs cycle to release carbon molecules and hydrogen ions.

Claudication: Severe pain in the muscles of the lower leg caused by poor circulation.

Clavicle: Commonly referred to as the collarbone; a long, slender curved bone that aids in keeping the shoulder joint in place and braces the movable scapula.

Cochlea: The structure of the inner ear that houses the organ of Corti.

Collecting tubule: Tubules that receive the urine from the distal convoluted tubules; several collecting tubules join to form a papillary duct that transfers the urine to the calyx.

Colloidal osmotic pressure: Process that helps to prevent edema and maintains normal blood pressure by keeping fluids within the vascular system.

Colon: Large-diameter tube that begins on the right side of the abdominal cavity traveling upward, across to the left, and downward, and ends at the anus; divided into the cecum, ascending colon, transverse colon, descending colon, sigmoid colon, rectum, and anal canal; the colon has four tunics: serosa, muscular, submucosa, and mucosa; functions include absorption of water to condense the feces, production of vitamin K by the bacteria within the organ, and expulsion of the feces.

Common bile duct: Formed by the joining of the cystic duct and common hepatic duct, and eventually the duct of Wirsung joins the duct to connect to the duodenum in order to transfer bile.

Common hepatic duct: The duct formed by the two hepatic ducts that exit the liver; it joins the cystic duct of the gallbladder to form the common bile duct; serves for the transfer of bile from the liver to the gallbladder and duodenum.

Compartment syndrome: The abnormal accumulation of fluid within a fascial compartment that increases the internal pressure, thereby inhibiting the blood flow to thereby tissues and causing ischemia and placing pressure on the nerves.

Complement: Group of 25–30 enzymatic serum proteins located in the blood plasma that are inactive until needed during an antibody–antigen reaction; it is a nonspecific body defense mechanism that increases the inflammatory response, assists in the lysis of an antigen, aids in neutralizing microbial toxins, and aids in chemotaxis.

Complement cascade: The process in which complement aids in the lysis of bacterial cells through a complex biochemical process that causes an accumulation of fluid in the bacterial cells until the cell ruptures.

Compound gland: A classification of multicellular gland that is a multilobed gland with a branched duct arising from each lobe.

Compound: Substance that can be broken down into two or more other substances by chemical means.

Condyle: Bony projection on the surface of a bone located at the epiphysis that articulates with another bone; serves as a site for the attachment of ligaments.

Condyloid joint: Formed by the end of one bone articulating with the fossa of another bone and allows movement in only one plane with limited lateral movement.

Cones: One to two types of photoreceptors located in the sensory layer of the retina that provide the ability to see colors and sharp images.

Conjunctiva: A thin, transparent mucous membrane composed of stratified columnar epithelium that lines the inner surface of the eyelids.

Cornea: The outer tunic located on the anterior portion of the eye; it is a transparent structure that focuses the light rays the enter.

Coronal plane: Frontal plane; imaginary line that divides the body into anterior and posterior sections that are at a right angle to the sagittal plane.

Coronary artery bypass grafting: Surgical procedure that involves harvesting and attaching a vein, such as the saphenous vein from the leg, to the affected coronary artery and attaching it to the aorta, thereby bypassing the affected coronary artery.

Coronary artherosclerotic heart disease: Type of coronary artery disease characterized by narrowing of the lumen of a coronary artery due to the buildup of atheroma.

Coronoid process: One of the divisions of the rami of the mandible; it is situated anterior to the mandibular condyle; the processes serve as points of attachment for muscles used when chewing.

Cortical bone: Also called compact bone; the hard, dense tissue that surrounds the bone marrow cavity and comprises the majority of bone tissue.

Costal cartilages: The cartilages that join the first seven pairs of ribs—referred to as the true ribs—to the sternum.

Cranial cavity: Division of the dorsal cavity that contains the brain.

Cross section: Imaginary line that divides the body transversely at a right angle to the long axis of the body organ.

Cross-bridges: Twisted protein strands that make up the myosin molecule in skeletal muscle tissue and project outward toward the actin myofilaments; the actin molecule contains a binding site for attachment of the cross-bridges.

Crossing over: The exchange of sections of paternal and maternal chromatids, forming chromatids with new combinations of genetic material during the first meiotic prophase stage.

Crown: Portion of the tooth located above the gum.

Cystic artery: Artery that supplies the gallbladder.

Cystic duct: Duct that exits the gallbladder and serves to transfer bile to the gallbladder; it joins the common hepatic duct to form the common bile duct to transfer bile away from the gallbladder.

Cytoplasm: The substance of a cell other than the nucleus that lies within the cytoplasmic membrane.

Cytoplasmic membrane: The membrane that surrounds a cell and contains the contents of the cell.

D

Dead space: Abnormal pockets of space between tissue layers in which fluid or air can accumulate, causing a delay in wound healing and contributing to the development of a postoperative infection due to the growth of bacteria within the space.

Deciduous teeth: Medical term for the temporary or baby teeth.

Deglutition: Medical term for swallowing.

Dehiscence: Abnormal partial or total separation of a layer or layers of tissue after closure with suture or staples; usually occurs between the 5th and 10th postoperative days.

Deltoid tuberosity: Bony prominence located on the lateral side of the midshaft of the humerus that serves as the site of insertion for the deltoid muscle.

Dendrite: An extension of a neuron that receives information; neurons may have one or more dendrites.

Dental pulp: Highly vascular soft substance located within the pulp cavity of a tooth; the pulp cavity contains the blood vessels and nerves that supply the tooth.

Dentin: Bonelike substance that encloses the pulp cavity of the tooth and is the layer underneath the enamel layer of the crown.

Depolarization: When a neuron is stimulated causing the inside of the cell to become more positive than the outside.

Descending colon: Fourth portion of the colon; it begins at the splenic flexure, travels downward along the left side of the abdominal cavity, and ends at the sigmoid colon; primary support of the descending colon comes from direct attachment to the posterior abdominal wall.

Detrusor muscle: The inner smooth muscle layer that surrounds the bladder; when the muscle contracts it pushes on the bladder forcing the urine into the urethra.

Diaphragm: Musculofibrous structure that separates the thoracic cavity from the abdominal cavity. It contains the openings for the aorta, esophagus, and inferior vena cava. The diaphragm aids respiration by its up-and-down movements.

Diaphragm: Specialized muscle that separates the thoracic cavity from the abdominopelvic cavity and is essential during breathing.

Diaphysis: The shaft or middle portion of a long bone.

Diarthrosis: A type of freely movable joint that allows the most movement of any type of joint; the articular ends of the joint are covered by a thin layer of articular cartilage that protects the ends from wear and tear, and reduces friction during movement.

Diastole: The relaxation of the heart.

Diencephalon: Composed of gray matter nuclei, located between the midbrain and cerebrum; the structures that make up the diencephalons are the thalamus, hypothalamus, posterior pituitary gland, and pineal gland.

Differential white blood cell count: Test conducted in the laboratory to determine the percentage of each type of leukocyte that is present in a sample of 100 leukocytes.

Digestion: The chemical and mechanical breakdown of food into simpler chemical substances that can be used by the cells of the body.

Digestive system: Body system that includes the mouth, teeth, tongue, salivary glands, pharynx, esophagus, stomach, liver, gallbladder, biliary duct system, pancreas, small intestine, and colon. Responsible for breaking down food particles into forms that can be used by the body cells for energy.

Disaccharide: Two-sugar (carbohydrate) units.

Distal: Away from the origin; opposite of proximal.

Doppler probe: Ultrasonic instrument used to identify and assess the vascular status of peripheral arteries and veins by magnifying the sound of the blood moving through the vessel.

Dorsal cavity: Division of the body that contains the cranial and spinal cavities.

Douglas' cul-de-sac: Also called the rectouterine pouch; thin layer of tissue located in the superior portion of the vagina separates it from the rectum; it is formed by the broad ligament.

Duct of Santorini: The second duct that occasionally occurs and exits from the duct of Wirsung and opens separately onto the duodenum, superior to the ampulla of Vater.

Duct of Wirsung: Also called the pancreatic duct; a large duct that travels the length of the pancreas through which the pancreatic juice travels to the duodenum.

Ductus arteriosus: Vessel in the fetus that connects the pulmonary artery with the descending thoracic aorta, thereby bypassing the lungs.

Ductus venosus: A continuation of the umbilical vein in the fetus that serves to shunt blood from the placenta to the inferior vena cava.

Ductus venosus vessel: Vessel in the fetus that bypasses the liver and connects to the inferior vena cava. It carries oxygenated blood from the placenta to the fetal circulation.

Dynamic equilibrium: The ability of an individual to adjust to movements away or toward the body's center of gravity by changing the base of his or her support.

Dysphagia: Medical term for difficulty in swallowing.

Dysuria: Medical term for painful urination, usually due to a urinary tract infection or calculi.

E

Eccrine sweat gland: Also called merocrine sweat gland; located all over the body, they release their fluid by exocytosis and play an important role in the maintenance of normal body temperature.

Edema: Also referred to as lymphedema; the abnormal accumulation of lymph fluid, in particular in the extremities.

Effector: A component of a closed-system mechanism for the maintenance of homeostasis; the effector is a body organ or substance such as an enzyme that produces an effect such as a chemical reaction.

Ejaculatory duct: Formed by the joining of the vas deferens and seminal vesicle, the duct passes through the prostate gland and becomes the urethra; responsible for transporting the sperm cells contained in the semen.

Electrolyte: Compound that disassociates into positive and negative ions in a solution and can conduct an electric current.

Electromyography (EMG): Diagnostic tool used to record the electrical activity in a skeletal muscle; the recording is called an electromyogram; useful in diagnosing neuromuscular pathologies.

Electron: Negatively charged particle that has a specific mass and spin; very small in size.

Element: One of several basic substances that cannot be broken down by chemical means; all matter is composed of fundamental elements.

Embryo: The stage of development of a fetus that begins from the time of implantation of the fertilized ovum in the uterus to the end of the eighth week. The stage is characterized by rapid growth, development of the external features, and development of the primary organ systems.

Emphysema: The abnormal, irreversible enlargement of the alveoli due to the destruction of the alveolar walls resulting in the decreased elastic recoil of the alveoli; often occurs in conjunction with COPD.

Enamel: The hardest and most compact substance of the body; it forms the outer layer of the tooth.

Encapsulated nerve endings: Category of afferent nerve in which there are several types that are mechanoreceptors, which relay the sensations of touch and pressure to the hypothalamus for interpretation.

Endarterectomy: The surgical excision of atheromatous tunica intima of an artery in order to restore the lumen of the vessel to its normal diameter.

Endochondral ossification: The development of the long bones of the embryonic skeleton by the differentiation of mesenchymal cells into chondroblasts that synthesize the bone matrix.

Endocrine gland: Body glands that produce and secrete their substances into tissue fluid or the circulatory system.

Endocrine system: Body system that consists of the pituitary gland, thyroid, parathyroid glands, thymus, adrenal glands, testes, and ovaries; glands are responsible for the secretion of hormones.

Endomysium: A thin layer of connective tissue that surrounds each muscle fiber in a fascicle.

Endoplasmic reticulum: Type of organelle that is a network of tubules enclosed in a cytoplasmic membrane in the cytoplasm of cells. It is the site of synthesis of proteins and lipids and transport of these substances within the cell.

Endosteum: A fibrous layer of tissue that lines the medullary cavity.

Energy: The ability to do work or activity; forms include light, electricity, sound, and heat, which all produce changes in matter.

Eosinophil: Type of leukocyte that becomes active in the presence of infections, infestations, and allergies.

Ependymal cell: Ciliated cell that aids in moving cerebrospinal fluid through the central nervous system; other types produce cerebrospinal fluid within the ventricles.

Epicondyle: Bony projection on the surface of a bone located superior to the condyle.

Epicondyles: Located just superior to the two condyles of the humerus, they serve as attachments for the ligaments and muscles of the elbow joint.

Epigastric region: Located in the superior middle region of the abdomen.

Epiglottis: Cartilage-like structure that closes over the opening of the larynx during swallowing to prevent food and liquid from entering the larynx and trachea; it is supported by the elastic cartilage called epiglottic cartilage.

Epimysium: A thin layer of connective tissue that encloses a skeletal muscle.

Epimysium: Connective tissue layer that intimately encloses a skeletal muscle.

Epineurium: A thin layer of dense connective tissue that encloses an entire nerve.

Epiphyseal disk: Also called epiphyseal plate; an area of the long bone that is a transverse disk of hyaline cartilage that forms between the junction of the diaphysis and epiphysis; it marks the area of bone growth until the diaphysis and epiphysis join together indicating the bone has reached its full length and maturity.

Epiphyses (singular, epiphysis): The ends of a long bone.

Epispadias: Congenital deformity in which the urethral opening is located on the dorsal surface of the penis, proximal to the glans, or in females, a fissure of the upper wall of the urethra; surgical repair is necessary to locate the opening in the normal anatomic position.

Erythrocyte: Medical term for red blood cell; it is responsible for transporting oxygen from the lungs to the tissues and aids in transporting carbon dioxide from the tissues to the lungs.

Erythropoiesis: The medical term referring to the synthesis of erythrocytes.

Erythropoietin: Hormone secreted in reaction to a person experiencing hypoxia; it acts on the red bone marrow to increase the production of erythrocytes, which will increase the oxygen-carrying level of the blood in order to resolve the hypoxic state.

Eschar: The blackened tissue that forms due to a third-degree burn that destroys all of the layers of the skin; it consists primarily of collagen.

Esophageal hiatus: The opening in the diaphragm for the esophagus.

Esophagus: Muscular tube that begins at the laryngopharynx and ends at the cardiac sphincter of the stomach; it provides the passageway for food to the stomach.

Estrogen: Group of female hormones that promote the development of female secondary sex characteristics; aid in the preparation of the female genital tract for fertilization, implantation, and nutrition of the embryo. The ovaries are the primary source of estrogen.

Ethmoid bone: One of eight cranial bones; located anterior to the sphenoid bone that consists of two lateral masses of bone joined in the midline by the cribriform plates that form a portion of the nasal cavity; the lateral portions of the bone are called the superior nasal concha and middle nasal concha, which support the mucous membranes of the nasal cavity; in addition a triangular process called the crista galli projects into the cranial cavity and serves as the site of attachment of the meningeal membranes.

Euchromatin: A type of chromatin that is active in gene expression during cell division; it is abundant in active, transcribing cells and undergoes constant condensing and uncoiling during each phase of cell division.

Eukaryotic: Eukaryocyte; a cell with a true nucleus; the nuclear materials are bound by a nuclear membrane.

Eustachian tube: Tubular structure that connects the middle ear to the nasopharynx and serves to equalize air pressure within the middle ear with that of the external atmosphere.

Excision: Removal of tissue and body organs.

Exocrine gland: Body glands that produce and secrete their substances into ducts.

External auditory meatus: An opening located in each temporal bone for the ear canal.

External nares: Openings in the nose through which air is inhaled and exhaled.

External respiration: Refers to the exchange of gases between the air that has been inhaled into the alveoli and the blood in the pulmonary capillaries.

Extracellular fluid (ECF): The body's water, which is located in the plasma, tissue fluid, synovial fluid, serous fluid, aqueous fluid, and cerebrospinal fluid.

Extracorporeal circulation: The term used to refer to the function of the pump oxygenator or heart–lung machine; the oxygenation of blood (the function of the lungs) and pumping of the blood (function of the heart).

F

Fascial compartment: Formed by deep fascia, a compartment is an individual or group of muscles that is tightly surrounded by fascia walling it off from the body; the majority of compartments are located in the extremities.

Facial nerve: Pair of sensory and motor cranial nerves that arise from the brainstem and divide into six branches that innervate the scalp, eyelids, muscles of facial expression, jaw, and cheeks; specifically innervates the orbicularis oris muscle that surrounds the mouth.

Facilitated diffusion: Type of molecular transfer in which energy is not required, but does involve a protein that binds to the molecule for transport across the cell membrane.

Fascia: Type of fibrous connective tissue that varies in thickness and density, of which there are three types: deep, subcutaneous, and subserous.

Fascicles: The bundles of muscle fibers surrounded by the perimysium.

Fasciculi: Small bundles of muscle wrapped by a layer of connective tissue called the perimysium.

Fasciotomy: Surgical procedure performed to treat compartment syndrome in which a series of small incisions is made in the region of fluid accumulation to allow it to escape and reduce the pressure in the fascial compartment.

Fast-twitch fibers: One of two categories of muscle fibers that rapidly contract, but fatigue much sooner than slow-twitch fibers; as compared to slow-twitch fibers they contain less myoglobin, fewer mitochondria, and the blood supply is not as great.

Fibroblast: Large, elongated flattened cell and the most common cell type of connective tissue; it gives rise to several types of precursor cells such as the osteoblast and chondroblast.

Fibrous pericardium: One of two layers of the pericardium; it attaches to the large vessels of the heart, posterior portion of the sternum, vertebral column, and central portion of the diaphragm, but not to the heart itself.

Fibrous pericardium: Outer membranous layer of the pericardial sac.

Fibula: One of two bones of the lower leg located on the lateral side; a long, slender bone that is not as strong as the tibia and thus it does not serve as a weight-bearing bone; serves primarily as a site for the attachment of ligaments and muscles of the lower leg.

Filtration: Process by which water is moved from one compartment of the body to another. For example, the blood vessels represent one type of compartment; the water inside the vessels is plasma and the process of filtration within the capillaries forces some of the plasma into the extracellular tissue spaces.

Fimbriae: Hairlike extensions located along the edge of the opening of the fallopian tube that serve to guide the zygote into the tube; one fimbriae, called the ovarian fimbria, is longer than the others and extends and connects to the ovary.

Flagella: Long, thin, appendages that move in whiplike fashion to provide mobility to a cell.

Flat bone: Category of bone, so named due to the bone being flat; examples include cranial bones, sternum, and ribs.

Fontanels: Commonly referred to as soft spots, they represent the areas of the bones of the cranium of an infant that have not matured and completed their growth; fibrous connective tissue is located between the bones.

Foramen magnum: The large opening in the occipital bone of the cranium through which the nerve fibers of the brain pass through to become the spinal cord.

Foramen ovale: An opening in the interatrial septum of the fetus that provides a passageway for blood from the right atrium to the left atrium, thus bypassing the lungs.

Foramen: Opening in a bone or tissue.

Fossa: Slight depression on the end of a bone.

Free nerve endings: Category of afferent nerves that lie next to hair follicles and are mechanoreceptors, which allow the person to be receptive to the movement of hair.

Friable: Easily torn, shattered, or crushed.

Frontal bone: One of eight cranial bones that forms the anterior portion of the skull superior to the eyes; forms the roof of the nasal cavity and roofs of the bony eye sockets and contains the two frontal sinuses.

G

Gallbladder: Pear-shaped organ located on the inferior surface of the right lobe of the liver that is divided into a fundus, body, and neck; functions include storage of bile, concentration of the bile by reabsorbing water, and release the bile for entrance into the duodenum.

Gastric glands: Tube-shaped structures located in the mucous membrane of the stomach and containing small openings at their ends called gastric pits; the glands contain three kinds of secretory cells: mucous cells, also called goblet cells; chief cells, also called peptic cells; and parietal cells, also called oxyntic cells.

Gastric juice: The combined secretions of the secretory cells of the stomach; consists of mucus, pepsinogen, and hydrochloric acid.

Gastrophrenic ligament: Fold of peritoneum that extends from the diaphragm to the cardia portion of the stomach to aid in keeping the stomach in anatomic position.

Genes: The structures located on the chromosomes that carry and transfer genetic material and information. The gene is a particular nucleic acid sequence within a DNA molecule that occupies a precise space on a chromosome.

Genitourinary system: Also called the urinary system. Body system that consists of the two kidneys, two ureters, urinary bladder, and urethra. Responsible for the removal of wastes from the blood and forming urine to remove the wastes and excess fluid.

Genome: The complete makeup of genes in each cell of an organism. Research is focusing on mapping the entire genome of humans.

Genotype: The complete genetic makeup of an organism determined by the location of the genes on the chromosomes.

Gerota's fascia: Also called renal fascia; the concave bed of adipose tissue on which each kidney rests and serves to cushion, support, and hold the kidneys in place.

Gingiva: The gum tissue of the mouth that lies over unerupted teeth and around the necks of erupted teeth.

Glans penis: The conical tip of the penis formed by the corpus spongiosum; the meatus of the urethra is located at the distal tip.

Glenoid cavity: Also called the glenoid fossa; depression in the scapula that serves as the socket for the rounded head of the humerus to form the shoulder joint.

Gliding joint: A joint in which the articulating surfaces of both bones are slightly curved or flat and allow twisting and side-to-side movements.

Glomerular filtration rate (GFR): The amount of urine formed by the kidneys in one minute.

Glomerular filtration: The filtration of blood that flows through the glomeruli and becomes renal filtrate; it involves plasma, waste products, and small protein particles being forced out of the glomeruli by the blood pressure and into Bowman's capsule to form the renal filtrate.

Glycolysis: The breakdown of glucose to pyruvic acid during cellular respiration.

Goblet cell: Specialized type of cell located between the columnar epithelial cells of the duodenum that produces and secretes mucus to lubricate the intestinal wall.

Goblet cells: Specialized epithelial cells that line the mucous membrane of the respiratory, gastrointestinal, and genitourinary tracts and secrete mucus.

Golgi apparatus: Type of organelle located next to the nucleus composed of stacks of flattened membranous sacs; serves as site for refining proteins synthesized by the endoplasmic reticulum and packages them into vesicles.

Golgi tendon organ: Sensory impulses from these receptors produce an inhibiting reflex for muscle contraction; located in tendons at the point of their attachment to a muscle.

Granular leukocyte: One of two types of leukocytes that have multilobed nuclei.

Granulocytes: One of two categories of leukocytes; when stained and placed under a light microscope the leukocytes can be seen to contain large granules in the cytoplasm; the three types of granulocytes are neutrophils, eosinophils, and basophils.

Gray matter: An area that contains a collection of a large number of cell bodies.

Greater curvature: Inferior border of the stomach.

Greater omentum: An extension of the peritoneum that is attached to the greater curvature of the stomach and the first part of the duodenum; it drapes over the small intestine and transverse colon.

Greater trochanter: Bony prominence located laterally on the femur and serves as the point of insertion for the iliopsoas muscle.

Greater tubercle: Bony prominence located on the lateral side of the humeral head that serves for the insertion of the tendons of the supraspinatus, infraspinatus, and teres minor muscles.

Group translocation: Type of molecular transfer that requires energy; a protein specifically binds the target molecule and during transport across the cell membrane a chemical modification takes place; the substance is now chemically different as it enters the cell.

H

Hartmann's pouch: The area of the neck of the gallbladder that becomes enlarged due to the collection of gallstones forming a pouch.

Haustrae: Series of pouches in the colon formed by the layer of longitudinal muscle fibers that are separated by bands called tenia coli, which extend the length of the colon.

Haversian canal: Tiny longitudinal canals in bone tissue that contain blood vessels, connective tissue, a nerve, and possibly a lymphatic vessel.

Haversian system: A canal within the compact bone that travels in a longitudinal direction and contains a venule, nerve, and arteriole. The system consists of the lamellae, haversian canal, tiny passages called haversian canaliculi that connect to the larger haversian canals, and Volkmann's canals, which also connect with the haversian canals and contain small blood vessels. There are hundreds of haversian systems in compact bone.

Hematopoiesis: Also referred to as hemopoiesis; the medical term that refers to the formation of blood cells.

Hematuria: Medical term for blood in the urine, usually due to a urinary tract infection or calculi.

Hemodilution: The removal of blood preoperatively; the patient is immediately given IV fluids to compensate for the removed blood; postoperatively the blood is reinfused.

Hemoglobin: Protein located within erthrocytes that gives blood its red color and transports oxygen molecules from the lungs to the cells of the tissues.

Hemopneumothorax: The abnormal accumulation of blood and air in the pleural space, usually due to traumatic injury.

Hemorrhagic anemia: Type of anemia due to hemorrhage caused by trauma or internal bleeding.

Hemostasis: The medical term that refers to inhibiting or stopping the escape of blood from a blood vessel either through natural processes or artificial means.

Hepatic ducts: Two large right and left ducts of the liver formed by the bile canals that exit each lobule of the liver; the two ducts join to form the common hepatic duct, which exits the liver.

Hepatic flexure: Anatomic landmark where the ascending colon ends and the transverse colon begins.

Hepatocytes: The cells of the liver that are the functional units of the liver that produce bile.

Herniation: A pathological occurrence involving the protrusion of a body organ or tissue through an abnormal opening in the muscle or other tissue.

Hesselbach's triangle: Anatomic triangle formed inferiorly by the epigastric artery, laterally by the rectus abdominus muscle, bounded by the inguinal ligament; used to identify direct hernias.

Heterochromatin: A type of chromatin that is inactive in gene expression and remains condensed throughout the cell cycle and is seen in resting cells.

Hiatal hernia: An abnormal weakening of the esophageal hiatus that allows the superior portion of the stomach to protrude into the thoracic cavity resulting in the reflux of gastric juices into the esophagus, causing irritation of the inner lining, damage to the cells, and dysphagia.

Hinge joint: The joint is formed by the convex surface of one bone end articulating with the concave surface of the other bone allowing for extension and contraction.

Histamine: Chemical located in the mast cells in connective tissue, platelet cells, and basophils that is released from injured cells and causes vasodilation.

Histiocyte: Also called macrophage; a phagocytic type of cell that is a part of the immune system.

Homeostasis: Coordination of all the functions of the body systems to maintain a normal internal environment.

Hormone: Substance that chemically affects the metabolism and functioning of the body.

Human immunodeficiency virus (HIV): The virus that is the cause of acquired immunodeficiency syndrome (AIDS). The target cells of the virus are CD4 T lymphocytes and macrophages. The natural immune defense system of the body is suppressed leaving the individual prone to a variety of infections. HIV is subdivided into two related types: HIV-1, the predominant pathogen worldwide, and HIV-2, which is endemic in West Africa.

Human leukocyte antigen: Any one of genetic markers within the major histocompatibility complex used for DNA analysis to determine tissue compatibility for transplantation.

Human leukocyte antigens (HLA): Genetic marker on the surface of white blood cells; it is identified by a test called tissue typing that is important for patients who could be receiving a donor organ.

Humerus: The upper arm bone that extends from the scapula to the elbow and forms part of the shoulder and elbow joints; the proximal end is a smooth, rounded ball that fits into the glenoid fossa of the scapula to form the shoulder joint.

Humoral antibodies: Antibodies produced by lymphocytes due to the presence of specific pathogens that are located in the lymph fluid and plasma.

Humoral immunity: Refers to the immunity provided by circulating antibodies produced by B cells.

Hyoid bone: Located in the neck between the mandible and larynx, it functions to support the tongue and serves as the site of attachment of the muscles that aid in tongue movement during swallowing; it is the only bone of the body that does not articulate with or connect to another bone.

Hypochondriac regions (right and left): Located on each side of the epigastric region of the abdomen.

Hypogastric region: Located in the lower middle region of the abdomen below the umbilical region.

Hypophysioportal circulation: A plexus of veins that transport blood and hormones from the hypothalamus to the adenohypophysis.

Hypospadias: Congenital deformity in which the urethral opening is located on the ventral surface of the penis or, in females, within the vagina; surgical repair is necessary to locate the opening in the normal anatomic position.

Hypothalamus: Consists of a collection of nuclei located inferior to the thalamus; functions, among many, include coordination of the activities of the autonomic system, secretion of neurosecretory substances that stimulate the anterior pituitary gland, and regulation of emotional and behavior patterns through connections with the limbic system.

I

Ileocecal valve: Located where the jejunum connects to the cecum of the colon; allows for the transfer of digested contents into the colon.

Iliac crest: The edge of the ilium that flares outward and serves as a primary source for obtaining bone for bone grafts.

Iliac regions (right and left): Located on each side of the hypogastric region of the abdomen.

Ilium: The largest of the three bones that form the majority of the pelvis.

Immunoglobulin (Ig): The class of proteins that antibodies belong to; immunoglobulins are also located in the lymph fluid, tears, saliva, and colostrum.

Incision: Also called surgical incision; intentional cut through intact tissue in order to expose the underlying tissue and body structures.

Incus: Also called the anvil; one of three small ossicles located in the middle ear that aids in transmitting sound waves; it articulates with the body of the stapes.

Inferior nasal conchae: Two scroll-shaped bones that attach to the lateral walls of the nasal cavity, which support the mucous membranes of the nasal cavity.

Inferior: Caudal; below, underneath, or toward the feet

Inorganic compound: Chemical compound made of molecules that do not contain the element carbon or derivatives.

Insertion: The end of the muscle that attaches to the movable end of a bone.

Inspiration center: Located within the medulla of the brainstem, it is responsible for producing the rhythmic impulses that travel along the nerve routes to the respiratory muscles to stimulate contraction, thereby causing inhalation.

Integumentary system: Body system that contains the skin, sweat glands, sebaceous glands, hair, and nails; several functions including protecting tissues and structures located underneath the skin, regulation of body temperature, cutaneous and pressure sensations, and first line of defense against microbial invasion.

Intercostal muscles: The muscles located between the ribs divided into two categories: external intercostal muscles and internal intercostal muscles. The intercostal muscles are innervated by the intercostal nerves.

Interleukin-1 (IL-1): A protein produced by leukocytes with several immune system functions including activation of resting T cells and endothelial and macrophage cells, mediation of inflammation, stimulation of the liver to store iron, and stimulation of synthesis of lymphokines.

Internal respiration: Refers to the exchange of gases between the systemic capillaries and tissue cells of the body.

Internal urethral sphincter: Involuntary sphincter formed by the detrusor muscle located around the opening of the urethra in the neck region of the bladder.

Interphase: Last step of mitosis in which the new cell begins all the processes of maintaining viability. This stage lasts until the cell begins mitosis.

Intervertebral disks: The fibrocartilage located between the vertebrae that are connected by ligaments and serve as a cushion for the vertebral bones.

Intracellular fluid (ICF): The water that is within the cells of the body. Approximately 60% of the body's water is ICF.

Intracoronary thrombolysis: Procedure that involves the injection of the enzyme streptokinase into the coronary artery to disolve blockages caused by thrombi.

Ion: A positively or negatively charged atom; make it possible for compounds to recombine into different compounds.

Ionization: The gain or loss of electrons.

Iris: The colored portion of the eyeball that lies between the cornea and lens in order to divide the space between the two structures into the anterior chamber and posterior chamber.

Irregular bone: Category of bone, so named due to the shape of the bone; examples include bones of the face and cranium.

Ischial spine: A bony pointed projection superior to the ischial tuberosity on the lower edge of the ischium that can be felt during a diagnostic digital vaginal examination and is used as a guide in determining the pelvic size.

Ischial tuberosity: Bony prominence located on the lower edge of the ischium that serves for the attachment of ligaments and leg muscles, and aids in supporting the weight of the body when seated.

Ischium: One of three bones of the pelvis; it forms the inferior portion and is L-shaped.

Islets of Langerhans: Groups of cells within the pancreas that perform the endocrine functions by producing insulin, glucagons, and pancreatic polypeptide. The hormones are secreted directly into the bloodstream and aid in the regulation of carbohydrate metabolism. The islets are located throughout the pancreas and consist of three primary types of cells: beta cells, which secrete insulin; alpha cells, which secrete glucagons; and pancreatic peptide cells, which secrete pancreatic polypeptide.

Isotope: One or more forms of an element that will have the same number of protons and electrons, but the number of neutrons varies.

J

Juxtaglomerular apparatus: Composed of juxtaglomerular cells and the macula densa next to the glomerulus in the kidney, the apparatus is important in the regulation of the secretion of renin.

K

Karyotype: A chart that diagrams the chromosomes of an individual or species, arranged in pairs according to size.

Keratinized: Epithelial cells that have lost their moisture and are composed of the protein called keratin.

Keratinocytes: Stratified squamous keratinized epithelial cells of which the epidermal layer of the skin is composed.

Ketoacidosis: Type of acidosis caused by an accumulation of ketones in the body, resulting in the widespread breakdown of fats due to an abnormal carbohydrate metabolism. Frequently a complication of diabetes mellitus.

Kidney: Reddish-brown-colored organ shaped like a kidney bean located on each side of the vertebral column that serves to filter impurities from the blood and form urine for excretion from the body; it is divided into three sections: cortex, medulla, and pelvis; on the medial side of the kidney is the hilum where the renal artery enters and the renal vein and ureter exits.

Kinetic energy: Energy of motion.

Kinins: Chemical located in plasma that causes vasodilation, increases the permeability of blood vessels, and aids in attracting neutrophils to injured tissue.

Krebs cycle: Also called the citric cycle or tricarboxylic acid cycle. Takes place in the mitochondria to oxidize molecules to yield energy and CO_2.

Kupffer cells: Large fixed cells within the liver that remove bacteria, dead erythocytes, and dead leukocytes by the process of phagocytosis.

L

Labyrinths: Also called the inner ear, consists of a series of canals and chambers located in the temporal bone.

Lacrimal bones: Two bones located in the medial wall of each bony eye socket that serve to hold the lacrimal ducts in place.

Lacteal: Lymphatic capillary located in each villi of the small intestine that is responsible for absorbing fats.

Lacteals: Specialized type of lymph capillaries located in the villi of the small intestine responsible for absorbing fat-soluble nutrients as an end product of digestion.

Lactiferous duct: A duct that carries milk from the lobes of each breast to the nipple and has an opening to the outside of the body.

Lacuna: A space in compact bone that contains an osteocyte.

Lacunae: Cavities within cartilage that contain chondrocytes and are surrounded by matrix; also found in bone in which the osteocyte resides.

Lamellae: Bone matrix that is deposited in thin circular, concentric patterns around haversian canals.

Lamellae: The concentric rings of compact bone that comprises the osteon.

Langerhans cell: Mobile phagocytic cells located in the epidermis the functions of which include attacking cancerous cells, traveling to the lymph nodes where lymphocytes detect the pathogen thus beginning the immune response, and the skin's primary antigen-presenting cells for helper T cells.

Larynx: Commonly referred to as the voice box; flexible, tubular structure that contains the vocal cords, it connects the pharynx to the trachea and functions as part of the passageway for air. It consists of three single cartilages, thyroid, cricoid, and epiglottic, and three paired cartilages, arytenoids, corniculate, cuneiform; the cartilages are held together by ligaments and voluntary muscle.

Lateral malleolus: Large bony prominence located on the lateral distal end of the fibula that articulates with the talus bone to form a portion of the ankle joint.

Lateral: Toward the side of the body, away from the midline.

Left lower quadrant: Abdominal quadrant located on the lower left side of the abdomen.

Left upper quadrant: Abdominal quadrant located on the upper left side of the abdomen.

Lens: Round, transparent structure of the eye that is located posterior to the iris that has suspensory ligaments attached to its edges to pull the lens outward, causing it to be flat in shape.

Lesser curvature: The superior border of the stomach.

Lesser omentum: An extension of the peritoneum that covers the ventral and dorsal surfaces of the stomach and the first part of the duodenum; it extends from the surface of the liver to the diaphragm, covering the end of the esophagus, and aids in holding the stomach in place.

Lesser trochanter: Bony prominence located on the medial side of the femur and inferior to the greater trochanter.

Lesser tubercle: Bony prominence located on the anterior side of the humeral head that serves as the site of insertion of the subscapularis tendon.

Leukocyte: Medical term for a white blood cell that functions to protect the body against infection and disease.

Leydig cells: The testicular interstitial cells that produce the androgens.

Ligament of Treitz: Important surgical landmark when performing abdominal surgery that marks the end of the duodenum and the beginning of the jejunum; referred to as a suspensory ligament, it arises from the diaphragm and attaches to the upper surface of the duodenojejunal junction.

Ligaments: Fibrous tissue composed of collagenous bundles that are slightly elastic and more flexible than tendons and connect bone to bone to form joints.

Limbic system: A ring of gray matter nuclei located on the inner border of the cerebrum that forms a border around the brainstem; functions include providing ability to distinguish between favorable or unfavorable stimuli, memory formation, and emotional expression.

Lingual frenulum: Membranous fold of tissue that connects the tongue to the midline of the floor of the mouth.

Lingual tonsils: Specialized lymph tissue located at the base of the tongue that forms a rounded projection containing the opening leading to a cavity surrounded by lymphoid tissue.

Lipids: Simple fats composed of chains of molecules called triglycerides.

Liver: The second-largest organ of the body; it is divided into two unequal right and left lobes by the falciform ligament; the liver has numerous functions associated with the digestive system including the formation and secretion of bile, protein metabolism, carbohydrate metabolism, storage of vitamins, and synthesization cholesterol, lipoproteins, and phospholipids.

Lobules: The small lobes or compartments of the lung segments that represent the basic units of the lung.

Long bone: Category of bone, so named due to the length of the bone; examples include the humerus, femur, and phalanges.

Lower esophageal sphincter (LES): Circular layer of muscle fibers at the cardiac sphincter of the stomach that contracts to close the entrance to the stomach and relaxes to allow food to enter the stomach.

Lumbar regions (right and left): Located on each side of the umbilical region of the abdomen.

Lungs: The organs of respiration located on each side of the sternum in the thoracic cavity that consist of spongy, elastic tissue. The right lung is divided into three lobes and the left lung into two lobes. The lungs are conical in shape with a top rounded portion called the apex and a concave base that rests on the convex surface of the diaphragm.

Lymph capillaries: The smallest vessels of the lymph system, they extend into the interstitial spaces forming networks that travel parallel to the blood capillaries.

Lymph fluid: The interstitial fluid formed from plasma that enters and travels through the lymph vessels.

Lymph nodes: Groups of lymphatic tissue located throughout the lymph circulatory pathway that serve to filter bacteria and other foreign material as the lymph fluid passes through.

Lymph nodules: Groups of lymphatic tissue, but the nodules are larger than lymph nodes; they are a collection of lymph cells located beneath the layer of mucous membranes and strategically located near body openings in order to destroy bacteria before they can reach the blood circulatory system.

Lymphadenitis: Inflammation of the lymph nodes.

Lymphatic afferent vessels: Lymphatic vessels that transport lymph fluid to a lymph node.

Lymphatic efferent vessels: Lymphatic vessels that exit from a lymph node.

Lymphatic system: Also called the immune system; composed of the lymph fluid, lymph nodes, lymphatic vessels, spleen, and thymus gland. Responsible for the drainage of excess interstitial fluid and absorbing fats, and aiding in preventing disease and infection of the body.

Lymphocytes: One of two types of agranuloctyes; they are not phagocytic, but play an important role during the humoral immune response and cell-mediated immune response.

Lysosome: Type of organelle that digests waste materials and food within the cell; the lysosome is bound by a cytoplasmic membrane that contains the digestive enzymes.

M

Macromolecule: A large molecule that is a biological building block; four groups: carbohydrates, proteins, lipids, and nucleic acids.

Macula lutea: A yellowish spot located in the central region of the retina; it is the region of the retina that is the area of highest visual acuity and contains only cones.

Major histocompatibility complex (MHC): A group of proteins located on the outer membrane of a cell that aids in identifying self and nonself cells.

Malleus: Also called the hammer; one of three small ossicles located in the middle ear that aids in transmitting sound waves; the handle of the malleus is connected to the tympanic membrane and its head articulates with the body of the incus.

Mandible: The bone of the lower jaw shaped like a horseshoe that flattens on each side and projects upward to form the rami; the superior border of the mandible contains the sockets for the lower teeth.

Mandibular condyle: One of the divisions of the rami of the mandible that articulates with the glenoid fossae of the temporal bones to form the temporomandibular joint (TMJ).

Mandibular foramen: Opening located on the medial side of the mandible, inferior to the rami, that allows blood vessels and a nerve to travel through to supply the roots of the lower teeth; serves as the site where dentists inject local anesthetic agents in order to block the nerve impulses.

Mandibular fossa: A slight depression in each temporal bone that articulates with the condyles of the mandible to form the temporomandibular joints.

Marsupialization: Surgical procedure in which a closed cavity is converted into an open cavity to treat an infection and is allowed to heal from the bottom upward.

Mast cell: Located in connective tissue, these cells are usually located near blood vessels and secrete heparin, histamine, serotonin, and bradykinin in response to injury, infection, and allergic reaction.

Mastication: Medical term for the action of chewing food.

Mastoid process: Rounded bone processes on each temporal bone located just inferior to the external auditory meatus that serve as sites of attachment of neck muscles.

Matrix: Nonliving material that may be liquid, semisolid, or solid.

Matter: Objects that have mass and fill space.

Maxillary bones: Two bones of the upper jaw that form a portion of the anterior hard palate, floors of the bony eye sockets, floor of the nasal cavity, and contain the sockets for the upper teeth; the maxillae contain the maxillary sinuses.

Meatus: The opening of the urethra at the tip of the penis.

Medial malleolus: The large bony prominence located on the medial side of the tibia.

Medial: Toward the middle of the body; imaginary midline that divides the body into equal right and left halves.

Mediastinum: Space located between the two lungs, separating them.

Medullary canal: Also called the medullary cavity; the canal that is located in the middle of bones and runs the length of the bone.

Meibomian glands: The large sebaceous glands located in the eyelids.

Meiosis: The division of a sex cell (egg and sperm cells) as it matures resulting in sex cells that have half the number of chromosomes (23).

Meissner's corpuscle: Receptor that aids in detecting light touch or texture of items.

Meissner's plexus: Autonomic nerve network located in the tunical submucosal layer of the intestine that innervates the layer; parasympathetic impulses increase the release of digestive secretions and sympathetic impulses decrease the release of secretions.

Membrane excitability: The process in which nerve cells generate electrical impulses.

Memory cells: Type of B cell that can be stimulated to produce antibodies when the body is exposed to an antigen that had previously invaded.

Meninges: Thin membranes that line the cranial and spinal cavities.

Meninges: Three thin layers of protective tissue that cover the brain and spinal cord.

Menisci (singular, meniscus): Two C-shaped fibrocartilages located in the knee joint that separate the ends of the femoral and tibial bones and serve to keep the bones from rubbing against each other and as a cushion.

Menopause: The period of a female's life marked by the cessation of the menstrual cycle due to the few remaining ovarian follicles that can respond to gonadotropins. The follicles will not mature, thus ovulation does not occur, causing the level of estrogens to decrease. Many females going through menopause experience hot flashes, which are vasomotor symptoms.

Mesencephalon: Also called the midbrain; it is a section of the brainstem located between the diencephalons and the pons; it contains tracts of white matter and gray matter nuclei. Functions include serving as a reflex center for the eye, head, and neck movements; subconscious muscle movement; muscular movements.

Mesentery: A folded extension of the peritoneum that invests the abdominal organs to aid in keeping them in normal anatomic position; it attaches the small intestine and colon to the posterior abdominal wall.

Mesentery: Fold of the peritoneal layer that invests the intestines and attaches them to the posterior abdominal wall for support.

Mesocolon: Three folds of peritoneal tissue that connect the colon to the posterior abdominal wall; the three folds are the ascending mesocolon, transverse mesocolon, and descending mesocolon.

Messenger RNA (mRNA): A copy of half of a DNA gene that carries information from DNA to the ribosomes. mRNA contains codons, which are encoded into amino acids during the translation process.

Metacarpals: The five bones located in the palm of the hand that are cylindrical in shape; articulate proximally with the carpal bones and distally with the phalanges.

Metaphase: Second step of mitosis in which the centromeres are attached to microtubules and the chromosomes are aligned together.

Metastasis: The transport of cancerous cells, most often by lymphatic vessels, to other sites in the body.

Metatarsals: The five bones of the foot that articulate with the tarsals; the heads form the ball of the foot, and the distal ends articulate with the proximal phalanges of each toe.

Microglial cell: Protect the neurons by phagocytosis.

Microtubules: Tiny fibers made of chained proteins that extend from each half of the cells and attach at the centromere.

Midsagittal plane: Median plane; imaginary line that vertically divides the body into equal left and right portions.

Mitochondria: Referred to as the powerhouse of the cell, these organelles are the major energy production center in eukaryotes. They function in cellular metabolism and respiration through the conversion of the potential energy of food molecules into ATP.

Mitosis: The process of eukaryotic cell division.

Mitral valve: Also called the bicuspid valve; one of two atrioventricular orifices located between the left atrium and left ventricle.

Molecular pump: Certain enzymes that provide a chemical pump, which requires energy in the form of ATP to move substances through the cytoplasmic membrane during active transport.

Molecule: Group of atoms joined by chemical bonds, created by electron attraction and interaction.

Monocytes: One of two types of agranulocytes that mature into macrophages when they enter the bloodstream in response to an infection.

Mononuclear phagocytic system: Consists of monocytes, macrophages, and endothelial cells that remove the products of the fibrin network formed during coagulation.

Monosaccharide: Single-sugar (carbohydrate) unit.

Motor end plate: The membrane of the muscle fiber at the myoneural junction, which contains a large number of nuclei and mitochondria.

Motor neurons: Neurons that extend from the spinal cord and stimulate skeletal muscle fibers to contract.

Motor unit: The motor neuron and muscle fibers that are connected to the branches of the axon of a motor neuron.

Mucus: A thick, viscous fluid secreted by specialized epithelial cells of the mucous membranes that keep membranes lubricated.

Multipolar neuron: Neuron with multiple dendrites and only one axon.

Multiunit smooth muscles: One of two types of smooth muscle that do not function as a unit as compared to visceral smooth muscle; they are separate independent units that work separately; located in the walls of blood vessels and irises of the eyes.

Muscle sense: Movements of the body that individuals are not aware of, such as walking and jumping, and that do not require constant attention.

Muscle spindle: When a muscle is stretched, the fibers inside the spindle send impulses to the cerebrum and cerebellum via the spinal cord for perception of limb position and coordination of muscle contraction; located near the origin of the tendons that connect the muscle to bone.

Myelin sheath: Also called the neurilemma; the insulating material that covers an axon.

Myocardial infarction: Medical term for heart attack that results in the death of heart muscle tissue.

Myocardial ischemia: The lack of oxygen to the heart muscle.

Myofibril: The threadlike strands that comprise a skeletal muscle fiber and are the major component of muscle contraction and relaxation.

Myofilament: The very thin filament that comprises a myofibril.

Myogenic: The contraction of the cardiac muscle, referring to the spontaneous, involuntary rhythmic activity of the muscle.

Myoglobin: Pigment that aids in providing oxygen to skeletal muscles by binding to oxygen molecules and temporarily storing the oxygen in the muscle tissue;

the pigment is responsible for giving skeletal muscle its reddish-brown color.

Myogram: The recording of a contraction of a muscle caused by electrical stimulation in the lab setting.

Myoneural junction: Also called the neuromuscular junction; the region where an axon of a motor neuron and muscle fiber come into contact.

Myosin: One of two kinds of protein myofilaments; it is the thick filament that makes up half of the proteins that occur in skeletal muscle tissue and contributes to the striations in the skeletal muscle.

N

Nasal bones: Two long, rectangular bones that join at the midline to form the bridge of the nose and serve as the site of attachment of the cartilage that comprises the majority of the nose.

Nasal cavities: The two inner portions of the nose formed by the external nares and separated by the nasal septum.

Nasal conchae: Also called the turbinates; three bones with a scroll-like appearance that project medially from the lateral wall of each nasal cavity that are highly vascular. The three conchae are the superior, middle, and inferior conchae.

Nasal mucosa: The lining of the nasal cavities, which consists of ciliated epithelium that contains goblet cells that produce mucus.

Nasal septum: The middle portion of the nose composed of the vomer and ethmoid bones that separates the nasal cavities.

Natural active acquired immunity: Type of acquired immunity stimulated by a specific infection; antibodies are produced by the stimulated lymphocytes that may provide partial or total resistance to reinfection by the pathogen.

Natural passive acquired immunity: Immunity acquired by antibodies present in the bloodstream of a pregnant female crossing the placenta to the fetus.

Neck: Portion of the tooth where the crown meets the root.

Negative-feedback mechanism: The body's response to a stimulus by reversing the effects of the stimulus.

Nephron: The functional unit of the kidney of which there are approximately 1 million in each kidney; it is here that urine is formed; each nephron consists of a renal corpuscle and renal tubule.

Nervous system: Body system that consists of the brain, spinal cord, cranial nerves, and peripheral nerves. Functions include sensory and motor reactions, and integrative including memory.

Neuroglial cell: Specialized cell that insulates, supports, and protects the neuron.

Neurons: The specialized cells that make up nerve tissue found in the brain and spinal cord and peripheral nerves; they transmit information from one cell to another.

Neurotransmitters: Chemicals that are stored in the synaptic vesicles of the axon of a motor neuron that are involved in the process of contraction; the primary neurotransmitter of motor neurons is acetylcholine.

Neutron: A particle located in the nucleus of atoms that has no electric charge and contributes to the atomic mass; approximately the same size as a proton.

Neutrophil: Type of leukocyte that ingests and destroys bacteria through the process of phagocytosis.

Nissl bodies: Ribosomes attached to the endoplasmic reticulum that synthesize significant amounts of protein with a neuron.

Nitrogenous bases: Cyclic molecules that consist of carbon and nitrogen in the ring structure.

Nociceptor: Pain receptor that consists of free nerve endings that are stimulated when tissues are damaged.

Nodes of Ranvier: Gaps in the myelin sheath that allow ions to easily flow from the extracellular fluid to the axons.

Normal ranges: The ranges in which the body systems of the body properly function.

Nuclear envelope: The membrane that surrounds the nucleus within a cell.

Nuclear pores: Small openings in the nuclear envelope that allow specific materials to pass in to and out of the nucleus.

Nucleic acids: Long chain compounds that form the genetic material of the cell and direct the synthesis of protein within the cell.

Nucleolus: Small, dense structures located in the cytoplasm of a cell that contain ribosomes, RNA, DNA, and proteins and are essential in the formation of ribosomes that synthesize cell protein.

Nucleotides: A compound that consists of a phosphate group, pentose sugar, and nitrogenous base; chains of nucleotides form DNA and RNA.

Nyctalopia: Night blindness.

O

Occipital bone: One of eight cranial bones; it forms the back and base of the skull; it contains the large opening called the foramen magnum; it is joined to the parietal bone at the lamboidal suture.

Occipital condyles: Two rounded processes located on each side of the foramen magnum that articulate with the first vertebra of the vertebral column.

Olecranon process: Two bony prominences located at the proximal end of the ulna just inferior to the articulation with the humerus that serve as attachment for the tendon of the triceps brachii muscle.

Olfactory organ: The organ of smell located in the roof of each nasal cavity called the olfactory area; contains the olfactory receptor cells, which are a type of neuron responsible for the detection of smells and communicating the information to the brain.

Oligodendroglial cell: Similar to astrocytes, but smaller and provide support by forming a rigid connection between neurons; they and produce myelin.

Omentum: Double fold of peritoneum that hangs loosely downward covering the intestines.

Oogenesis: The formation of eggs by meiosis that takes place in the ovaries of females.

Opsonins: Antibody molecules that secrete a serum protein that coats a bacterial cell and promotes the attachment of phagocytes to the pathogens; the process is called opsonization.

Optic chiasma: The area where the optic nerve of each eye crosses at the base of the brain just anterior to the pituitary gland.

Organelle: Highly specialized cellular structure that carries out a specific cellular activity.

Organic compound: Chemical compounds that contain carbon and have a carbon–hydrogen bond.

Origin: The end of the muscle that attaches to the immovable end of a bone.

Osmosis: The process that involves the diffusion of water through semipermeable cell membranes from an area of greater concentration to an area of lesser concentration. The movement aids in keeping the water and electrolyte levels normal within the body.

Ossification: Also referred to as osteogenesis; refers to the development of bone.

Osteoclast: Multinucleated cell that rests in recesses of bone called Howship's lacunae; functions in the development, growth, and repair of bone including breakdown and resorption.

Osteoblast: Basophilic cell that synthesizes collagen and glycoprotein to form the bone matrix; large, polygonal-shaped cell that cannot divide and eventually develops into an osteocyte.

Osteocyte: Basophilic cell responsible for maintaining the bone matrix; in the fetus represents the last stage of bone maturation; the cells lie in the lacunae of compact bone.

Osteon: The basic structural substance of compact bone.

Osteoprogenitor cell: Stem cells of skeletal tissue.

Ovarian follicles: Slight recess in an ovary that contains liquid and follicular cells that surround an ovum.

Oxygen debt: The quantity of oxygen that lungs take up during recovery from exercise that is in excess of the quantity that is normally needed during rest or pre-exercise; represents the gaining of oxygen that was depleted during the period that oxygen uptake was inadequate during exercise to sustain aerobic metabolism.

P

Pacinian corpuscle: Composed of connective tissue and cells that detect deep pressure and vibrations.

Palate: The roof of the mouth; divided into the hard palate located in the anterior portion and the posterior soft palate.

Palatine bones: Two bones located inferior to the maxillae that form the posterior portion of the hard palate of the mouth, floor of the nasal cavity, and lateral walls of the nasal cavity.

Palatine tonsils: Specialized lymph tissue located on each side of the pharynx covered by mucous membrane and containing numerous lymph follicles; this is the tissue often surgically removed due to chronic infections.

Pancreas: Body organ that performs both endocrine and exocrine functions; divided into three portions: head, body, and tail; the acinar cells of the organ perform the exocrine function by producing pancreatic juice, which consists of enzymes that break down fats, proteins, carbohydrates, and nucleic acids.

Papillae: Small projections located on the surface of the tongue that contain the taste buds, which detect sweet, sour, bitter, and salt.

Parafollicular cells: Also referred to as C cells. The cells are located between the thyroid follicles and secrete the hormone calcitonin.

Paranasal sinuses: Air-filled cavities located in the cranium that affect the tone of the voice and reduce the weight of the skull due to the air within the cavities.

Paransal sinuses: Four sinuses, maxillae, frontal, sphenoid, and ethmoid, that are lined with ciliated epithelium; functions include transporting mucus into the nasal cavity, making the skull lighter in order to hold the head up for long periods, and providing resonance to the voice.

Parasympathetic division: Subdivision of the ANS that calms the body, conserves energy, and restores homeostatic balance.

Parietal bones: Two of the eight cranial bones; they form part of each side and roof of the crainium; the two bones join at the midline by the sagittal suture and with the frontal bone at the coronal suture.

Parietal layer: Serous membrane that forms the inner lining of the abdominal and thoracic cavities.

Parietal pericardium: Middle membranous layer of the pericardial sac.

Parietal peritoneum: Layer of the peritoneal membrane that lines the wall of the abdominopelvic cavity.

Parietal pleura: Layer of the pleural membrane that lines the wall of the thoracic cavity.

Passive diffusion: Type of molecular transfer in which there is no transport protein and energy is not required.

Patella: Medical term for the kneecap; a flat, irregularly shaped bone that is contained within the quadriceps tendon on the anterior of the knee joint.

Patellar ligament: Thick, large, flat, strong ligament attached to the anterior of the patella and distally to the tibial tuberosity.

Pathophysiology: The study of diseases and disorders of the body.

Pelvic cavity: Subdivision of the abdominopelvic cavity that contains the sigmoid, rectum, urinary bladder, and internal reproductive organs.

Pelvis: The large bowl-shaped bone of the lower trunk that consists of the sacrum, coccyx, and pelvic girdle; it provides support for the upper and lower trunks of the body, serves for attachments of muscles of the femur, and aids in protecting internal pelvic organs.

Pepsin: The enzyme that is responsible for beginning the process of digestion of protein in the stomach; within the stomach pepsinogen comes into contact with hydrochloric acid and is converted to pepsin.

Peptide: Molecular chain of two or more amino acids joined by peptide bonds.

Perception: Conscious awareness of a sensation after interpretation by the brain.

Percutaneous transluminal coronary angioplasty: The procedure in which a balloon-tipped catheter is inserted into a coronary artery; the balloon is inflated, pressing the atheroma against the artery wall and opening up the artery to allow the normal flow of blood.

Pericardial sac: A membrane that encloses the heart to provide protection and cushioning.

Pericardium: A thin membranous sac that encloses the heart to provide protection and prevent it from rubbing against the thoracic wall.

Pericytes: The undifferentiated cells located in the endothelial layer of capillaries and venules that can produce smooth muscle cells.

Perimysium: Inward extensions of the epimysium that continue between the bundles of muscle fibers dividing the muscle tissue into sections.

Peripheral nervous system (PNS): Subdivision of the nervous system that consists of the nerves that connect the portions of the body to the CNS.

Peripheral vascular system: Subdivision of the circulatory system that consists of the arteries, veins, and capillaries outside of the heart.

Peristalsis: The rhythmic wavelike motion of smooth muscle that represents the coordinated contractions and relaxations of the longitudinal and circular layers of the muscle.

Peritoneal space: The space between the parietal peritoneum and visceral peritoneum that contains serous fluid.

Peritoneum: A thin serous membrane that lines the abdominal wall of the body and is reflected over the viscera; divided into the parietal peritoneum, which lines the abdominal cavity, and the visceral peritoneum, which forms the outer serosal layer of the abdominal organs. A thin space, called the peritoneal space, exists between the mesentery and peritoneum and contains serous fluid.

Permanent teeth: Also called the secondary teeth; the teeth that enter after deciduous teeth fall out and remain with the adult for the rest of their life.

Pernicious anemia: The failure of erythrocytes to mature due to the absence of an intrinsic factor secreted by the stomach.

Peyer's patches: Specialized group of lymphatic nodules that form a single layer within the mucous membrane of the ileum opposite the mesentery, but their function is unknown.

pH scale: Scale used to measure acidity and alkalinity; ranges 0–14 with 0–7 being acidic and 8–14 being alkaline.

Phagocytosis: The process used by phagocytes of surrounding and ingesting a foreign particle or microbe; it is considered part of the body's second line of defense.

Phagosome: The sac that is the end result of the process of phagocytosis where the sides of the pseudopod of the phagocyte meet to completely surround the pathogen.

Phalanges: The small bones located in the fingers and toes.

Pharynx: Commonly referred to as the throat; tubular structure that extends from the base of the skull to the esophagus; it is the only structure that serves as a passageway for the respiratory and digestive tracts; it is divided into three portions: nasopharynx, oropharynx, and laryngopharynx; the digestive role of the pharynx is to begin the process of swallowing.

Phleborheography: Diagnostic process used to diagnose deep vein thrombosis.

Phospholipid: A class of compounds found in living cells that contain phosphoric acid, fatty acids, and a nitrogenous base.

Photopigments: Colored proteins located in rods and cones that change their structure in response to the absorption of light and initiate the events that cause receptor potential.

Physiology: The study of the functions of the body.

Pinealocytes: The secretory cells of the pineal gland, which contain a large round nucleus and cytoplasmic extensions. The cells are responsible for the synthesis and secretion of melatonin.

Pivot joint: This type of joint allows only a rotational movement around a central axis, such as the radius rotating around the ulna.

Placenta: A saclike structure formed from the chorion that surrounds the fetus. It is through this membrane that nutrients and oxygen are exchanged from the maternal blood to the embryo's blood, and waste products and carbon dioxide are exchanged from the embryo's blood into the maternal blood for removal.

Plasma: The straw-colored fluid portion of blood in which blood cells and platelets are suspended.

Plethysmography: Diagnostic instrument used to determine the variations in the amount of blood flow through an extremity.

Pleura: The serous membranes of the thoracic cavity.

Pleural cavity: The space within the thorax that contains the lungs and pleural membranes.

Pleural membranes: Delicate serous membranes divided into the visceral pleura, which covers the lungs, and parietal pleura, which lines the thoracic cavity. Between the two pleura is the narrow pleural, which contains serous fluid.

Pluripotent cell: Stem cells located in the red bone marrow from which blood cells originate.

Pneumotaxic center: Located in the pons, impulses from the center interrupt the signals to the apneustic center to aid in exhalation.

Podocytes: A specialized type of epithelial cells contained in the parietal layer of the Bowman's capsule; they extend branches that attach to the glomerular capillaries to form one of the several types of filtering devices in the kidney.

Polycythemia: Clonal stem cell disorder that results in an abnormal increase in the number of circulating erythrocytes.

Polymer: Also called polysaccharide; long chains of sugar (carbohydrate) units.

Polypeptide: Long chain of amino acids joined by peptide bonds.

Positive-feedback mechanism: Mechanism used by a body system in which the input increases or accelerates the body's response.

Posterior cruciate ligament: One of two cruciate ligaments of the knee, which prevents the femur from sliding anteriorly onto the tibia.

Posterior: Dorsal; toward the back.

Potential energy: Energy that an object has stored due to its position as related to a zero position.

Presbyopia: Near-sightedness; the lens of the eye decreases in elasticity, thereby decreasing accommodation making it more difficult to view objects at a close range.

Primary bronchi: The two tubular structures that are a bifurcation of the trachea in the mediastinal space, which enter each lung at the hilum and further divide inside the lungs.

Prime mover: Refers to the muscle that contracts or flexes.

Primitive heart tube: The tube that represents the fusion of the two endocardial tubes and is the beginning of the development of the heart in the fetus.

Primordial follicles: Undeveloped cells that develop during the early stages of embryonic development and are precursors of the oogonia or spermatogonia; they develop outside the gonads and migrate to the embryonic ovaries and testes to mature.

Progesterones: Group of female hormones that affect the cycles of the uterus, affect the mammary glands, and aid in regulating the secretion of gonadotropins; the ovaries are the primary source of progesterone.

Projection: The process used by the brain to send the sensation back to the point of origin so the individual can identify the area of stimulation.

Prokaryotic: A cell that lacks a true nucleus and does not have a nuclear membrane.

Prolactin: Hormone secreted by the anterior pituitary gland into the circulatory system. In combination with other hormones, it stimulates the development and growth of the mammary glands. Along with glucorticoids, it is necessary for the initiation of milk production in the breasts and sustaining the milk production.

Prophase: First step of mitosis in which the chromosomal DNA is distributed between the two halves of the cell.

Prostaglandins: Chemicals released by injured cells that increase the action of histamine and kinins and aid in phagocytosis.

Protease inhibitor (PI): Class of antiretroviral drugs that inhibit HIV protease, thereby interfering with HIV maturation and replication; drugs include saquinavir, ritonavir, and indinavir. PIs are used in combination with reverse transcriptase inhibitors.

Protein: One of a large group of naturally occurring complex organic nitrogenous compounds; composed of amino acids.

Proton: Positively charged particle located in the nucleus of atoms contributing to the atomic mass; the number of protons equals the atomic number of the element.

Proximal: Closer to the origin.

Puberty: Stage of life that usually begins between the ages of 12 and 15 years in which the female and male physically mature; the ability to reproduce begins and the secondary sex characteristics develop.

Pubis: One of three bones of the pelvis, it forms the anteromedial portion; the ischium and pubis join to form the large obturator foramen.

Pulmonary edema: The abnormal accumulation of fluid in the extravascular spaces and/or alveoli of the lungs.

Pulmonary surfactant: A thin, filmy layer of fluid released by the lamellar bodies within the type II pneumocytes; the fluid covers the alveoli to reduce the surface tension forces and aid in the expansion of the alveoli.

Pump oxygenator: Also called the heart–lung machine; used during open heart surgical procedures to divert the blood around the heart to the rest of the body; the machine assumes the roles of the heart and lungs during the procedure.

Purkinje fibers: Receive the impulse from the bundle of His and spread the action potential to the apex of the left ventricle and upward to the ventricular myocardium resulting in ventricular contraction.

Pyruvate: Molecule that is important during the Krebs cycle made during glycolysis from glucose and broken down into two carbon molecules within the mitochondria, thus releasing carbon dioxide.

R

Radial tuberosity: Bony prominence located just inferior to the head of the radius that serves as the point of attachment for the tendon of the biceps brachii muscle.

Radius: One of two bones of the forearm; it extends from the elbow to the wrist and rotates around the ulna upon movement; in the anatomic position, the radius lies on the thumb side of the hand.

Reactive hyperemia: A reaction of the blood vessels in the skin or body organ that is an increase in the amount of blood in an area of the body where circulation has been reestablished after a period of occlusion.

Rectum: Sixth portion of the colon; it begins at the sigmoid colon and ends at the anal canal; it descends in an anteroposterior curve called the sacral flexure, passing into the pelvic cavity to join the anal canal.

Recurrent laryngeal nerve: Branch of the vagus nerve that innervates all of the muscles of the larynx except the cricothyroid. If injured during surgery, it can result in temporary or permanent hoarseness of the voice.

Red bone marrow: Semisolid tissue that functions in the production of erythrocytes, leukocytes, and platelets.

Referred pain: Pain that occurs other than at its origin.

Reflex: Involuntary reflex to an external response.

Refraction: The bending of light rays as they enter the eye.

Renal columns: Extensions of cortical substance from the renal cortex into the medulla that are located on the lateral margins of individual lobes of the kidney; thus each lobe consists of a renal pyramid and renal columns.

Renal corpuscle: Portion of the nephron in the kidney that consists of the glomerulus and Bowman's capsule, which lie in the cortex of the kidney; the glomerulus is a network of capillary vessels and Bowman's capsule is an extension of the end of a renal tubule and surrounds the glomerulus.

Renal filtrate: Fluid contained within the small space that exists between the two layers of Bowman's capsule; it is formed in the glomerulus and eventually becomes urine.

Renal pyramid: Wedge-shaped structures located in the renal medulla that contribute the division of the kidney into several lobes, thereby making the kidney multilobar; the superior portion of each renal pyramid tapers to form several renal papillae.

Renal tubule: The second portion of a nephron in the kidney; it is a continuation of Bowman's capsule and is subdivided into the proximal convoluted tubule, loop of Henle, and distal convoluted tubule.

Renin–angiotensin mechanism: Body mechanism that aids in increasing the blood pressure; the end result of the mechanism is the production of angiotensin II, which causes vasoconstriction and stimulates the increase in the secretion of the hormone aldosterone.

Repolarization: The process by which the neuron returns to its resting potential.

Reproductive system: Subdivided into the male and female reproductive system. Responsible for producing and maintaining the spermatozoa in the male and the ova of the female.

Resistance: Hindrance of blood flow within the cardiovascular system due to the friction of blood against the walls of a vessel.

Respiratory system: Body system that includes the nasal cavity, pharynx, larynx, trachea, bronchii, bronchioles, alveoli, and lungs. Responsible for the exchange of oxygen and carbon dioxide between the blood and inhaled air.

Resting potential: The electrical component of neurons in which the inside of the cell has a negative charge and the outside has a positive charge.

Reticuloendothelial system (RES): Nonspecific system that refers to the collection of phagocytic cells that line the sinusoids of the spleen, lymph nodes, bone marrow, intestines, liver, and brain the function of which is to remove and destroy foreign debris, microbes, excess cellular secretions, dead leukocytes, and dead erythrocytes.

Retina: The complex structure that is part of the inner tunic of the eye and contains the photoreceptors and vitamin A; it prevents light from being reflected back into the eye.

Retrocecal: Term used to describe when the appendix is located upward and inward behind the cecum, making it difficult to remove during an appendectomy.

Retroperitoneum: Also called the retroperitoneal space; the area located posterior to the parietal peritoneum, extending from the diaphragm to the pelvis; the three regions are the anterior pararenal, perirenal, and posterior pararenal.

Retroviruses: A family of RNA viruses distinguished by the possession of a viral reverse transcriptase that transcribes viral RNA into provirus DNA, which is integrated into the host cell's genome; two subfamilies: oncoretroviruses and lentiviruses. HIV belongs to a family of retroviruses.

Rh factor: Named after the Rhesus monkey, it is a protein within the blood; when identified the individual is said to be either Rh− or Rh+.

Ribosome: Type of organelle that is the site of protein synthesis, where RNA is translated into protein; they either float freely in the cytoplasm of the cell or are bound to the endoplasmic reticulum.

Right lower quadrant: Abdominal quadrant located on the lower right side of the abdomen.

Right upper quadrant: Abdominal quadrant located on the upper right side of the abdomen.

Riviniani ducts: Excretory ducts of the sublingual gland.

Rods: One of two types of photoreceptors located in the sensory layer of the retina; they are important for the visualization of shades of gray in dim light and visualizing general shapes.

Root canal: Tubular extensions located in the root of a tooth that extend upward and contain the vessels that enter the tooth.

Root: Portion of the tooth located in the alveolar process of the jaw.

Rotator cuff: Consists of four muscles—supraspinatus, subscapularis, teres minor, and infraspinatus—that form a cuff around the shoulder joint to stabilize and allow for a range of motions.

Rough endoplasmic reticulum (Rough ER): Endoplasmic reticulum that has ribosomes attached.

Rugae: Thick folds formed by the mucosal and submucosal layer in the stomach that smooth out when the stomach is full and allow the stomach to expand.

Rule of Nines: A diagnostic method of estimating how much surface of the body has been burned; the areas of the body are subdivided into 9% or multiples of 9% of the body surface area.

S

Sacroiliac joint: The area that joins the sacrum to the ilium of the pelvic girdle and consists of fibrocartilage.

Sacroiliac joint: The area where the posterior side of the ilium connects to the sacrum of the pelvis.

Saddle joint: The articulating ends of both bones have concave and convex surfaces in which the surface of one bone fits into the same surface of the other bone, allowing movement in many planes.

Sagittal plane: Imaginary line that vertically divides the body into unequal left and right halves.

Salivary glands: Three pairs of glands—parotid, submandibular, and sublingual—that produce the saliva in the mouth.

Salt: A compound formed by the chemical reaction of an acid and base.

Sarcolemma: The thin cell membrane that surrounds the cells of the smooth muscle tissue and contains the sarcoplasm.

Sarcolemma: Thin membrane that covers each skeletal muscle fiber and is electrically polarized.

Sarcomeres: The functioning units of a myofibril that occur as repeating sections along the length of a myofibril, joined end to end.

Sarcoplasm: Semifluid cytoplasm of skeletal muscle cells that contains the nuclei and mitochondria.

Sarcoplasm: The cytoplasm of the cells of smooth muscle tissue.

Sarcoplasmic reticulum: A complex network of tubules and sacs that surround each myofibril in skeletal muscle tissue; it regulates the calcium ion concentration within the myofibrils.

Scapula: Commonly referred to as the shoulder blade; a flat, broad triangular bone located in the upper region of the back and containing the glenoid fossa that serves as the socket for the head of the humerus to form the shoulder joint.

Schwann cell: Also called the neurolemmocytes; the cells that produce the fatty substance that makes up the myelin sheath.

Sclera: The tough, white portion of the eye that provides protection, gives the eyeball its shape, and serves as the site of attachment for the extrinsic muscles.

Sellick's maneuver: Also called cricoid pressure; the thumb and forefinger are used to apply external pressure to the cricoid cartilage of the larynx causing slight blockage of the esophagus. The procedure is performed just prior to induction of general anesthesia to reduce the risk of aspiration by the patient.

Sensation: Feeling that occurs when the brain receives sensory impulses from the peripheral nervous system.

Sensor: A component of a closed-system mechanism for the maintenance of homeostasis; the sensor reacts to physical stimuli such as a change in temperature.

Sensory adaptation: Process when receptors are continuously stimulated causing sensory impulses to be delivered at a decreasing rate until the receptors do not send any receptors at all.

Seroma: The accumulation of serum within tissue or organ that can eventually form fibrous tissue.

Serous pericardium: One of two layers of the pericardium that is subdivided into the epicardium and parietal layer.

Sesamoid bone: Also called round bone; so named due to the round shape of the bone; an example includes the patella.

Sex chromosomes: Chromosomes that carries the X and Y genes, and therefore is involved in transmitting sex-linked genetic traits. Humans have only one pair of sex chromosomes, numbered 23.

Short bone: Category of bone, so named due to the length of the bone; examples include carpal bones and tarsal bones.

Sigmoid colon: Fifth portion of the colon; it derives its name from its S shape beginning at the end of the descending colon and ending at the rectum; it contains the sigmoid flexure, which is the narrowest region of the colon; it is the most frequent site of colon cancer and volvulus.

Simple gland: A classification of multicellular gland that communicates with the surface through an unbranched duct.

Sinoatrial node: The electrical pacemaker of the heart located in the right atrial wall that fires an electrical impulse that stimulates the cardiac muscle fibers to contract.

Skeletal muscle: Also called voluntary or striated muscle; attached to bones, they contract and extend to aid in movement of the body.

Skeletal muscles: Also called voluntary muscles; the muscles that attach to bones and are consciously moved.

Skeletal system: Body system that consists of the bones, muscles, ligaments, cartilage, and tendons; functions include supporting and giving shape to the body, and movement of the body.

Sliding filament theory: The theory used to explain the contraction and relaxation of a skeletal muscle, referring to the sliding action of the actin and myosin filaments past one another when a muscle contracts.

Slow-twitch fibers: Also called red fibers; one of two categories of muscle fibers that can sustain contractions for a long period of time without fatigue setting in; the fibers contain myoglobin.

Small intestine: Long, convoluted tube where the processes of digestion and absorption primarily occur; begins at the pyloric sphincter of the stomach and ends where it joins to the cecum of the colon at the ileocecal valve; divided into three sections: duodenum, jejunum, and ileum; the layers of the small intestine wall are, from outside to inside: serosa, muscular, submucosa, and mucosa.

Smooth endoplasmic reticulum (Smooth ER): Endoplasmic reticulum that does not have ribosomes attached.

Smooth muscle: Also called involuntary muscle; muscle that that is located in the wall of the stomach, intestines, urinary bladder, blood vessels, and uterus that is not under the control of the individual and does not contain striations.

Smooth muscle: Also called involuntary or nonstriated muscle; one of the layers of the wall of the intestinal tract and blood vessels.

Somatic cell: Any cells of the tissues of the body that contain the diploid number of chromosomes, distinguished from the egg and sperm cells, which contain the haploid number.

Somatic nervous system (SNS): Subdivision of the PNS; responsible for connecting the CNS to the skin and skeletal muscles via the cranial and spinal nerves to initiate voluntary movements.

Somatic sense: Sense that involves receptors associated with the skin, muscles, joints, and visceral organs.

Spermatic cord: Enclosed structure that descends from the deep inguinal ring to the testis, containing arteries, veins, nerves, lymphatics, and the vas deferens for each testis.

Spermatids: Male germ cell that is produced from a spermatocyte and becomes a mature spermatozoon during the last stages of spermatogenesis.

Spermatogenesis: The formation of sperm cells by meiosis that takes place in the testicles of males.

Spermatogonia: Male cell that eventually produces spermatocytes during spermatogenesis.

Spermatozoa: Mature male germ cell that develops in the seminiferous tubules of the testis and is responsible for fertilizing the female egg.

Sphenoid bone: One of eight cranial bones; it is butterfly-shaped, located in the anterior portion of the skull, and forms part of the base and sides of the cranium, and floors and sides of the bony eye sockets; it also contains the indentation called the sella turcica, which contains the pituitary gland and two sphenoidal sinuses.

Sphenoidal sinuses: Two sinuses contained within the sphenoid bone of the cranium that lie next to each other and travel downward into the nasal cavity.

Sphincter of Oddi: The opening of the ampulla of Vater that consists of a circular band of smooth muscle that surrounds the sphincter to aid in the release of pancreatic juice into the duodenum.

Spinal cavity: Division of the dorsal cavity formed by the vertebrae that contains the spinal cord.

Spindle: Formed during the late prophase step of mitosis; composed of microtubules that extend from the centrosomes and connect the with one another.

Spleen: Vascular body organ located in the upper left quadrant of the abdomen that contains lymphoid nodules and serves to filter blood.

Splenectomy: Surgical removal of the spleen.

Splenic flexure: Anatomic landmark where the transverse colon ends and the descending colon begins.

Stapes: Also called the stirrup; one of three small ossicles located in the middle ear; it aids in transmitting sound waves and rests on the oval window of the inner ear.

Static equilibrium: The ability of an individual to adjust to movements away or toward the body's center of gravity while maintaining a base of support.

Steno's duct: The excretory duct of the parotid gland.

Sternum: Also called the breastbone; located along the midline in the anterior portion of the rib cage, it is a flat, elongated bone that is divided into the upper manubrium, body, and lower xiphoid process.

Stomach: Large muscular pouch located below the diaphragm that is the primary organ of digestion; divided into four regions: cardiac, fundus, body, and pyloric.

Stratum basale: A subdivision of the stratum germinativum that connects the epidermis to the basement membrane.

Stratum corneum: Upper, last layer of the epidermis; it consists of dead cells.

Stratum germinativum: Deepest layer of the epidermis.

Stratum granulosum: Layer of the epidermis that lies above the stratum spinosum.

Stratum lucidum: Layer of the epidermis that lies above the stratum spinosum.

Stratum spinosum: Layer of the epidermis that lies above the stratum germinativum.

Stress incontinence: Type of incontinence most often experienced by females, in which the bladder area and muscles are stressed due to sitting, laughing, and exercise and urine leaks from the bladder. The condition results from a change in the base of the bladder and distortion of the urethrovesical angle caused by childbirth or aging. Surgery is performed to correct the condition.

Stretch receptors: Also called proprioceptors; located within muscles, they sense changes in the length of a muscle as it stretches and send the sensory impulses to the brain where they are interpreted.

Striations: The alternating light and dark bands found in skeletal muscles.

Subcutaneous layer (hypodermis): Layer of tissue beneath the dermis consisting of loose areolar connective tissue and adipose tissue that connects the dermis to the underlying structures; purposes include providing insulation from the cold and protecting internal body organs and bony prominences.

Sudoriferous glands: Sweat glands; tubular gland with a base that is coiled and a duct that transports the sweat to the skin surface.

Superior laryngeal nerve: Innervates the pharynx, larynx, and cricothyroid muscle. If injured during surgery or traumatic injury, it can result in the loss of the high pitch tone of the voice.

Superior: Cephalad; above or toward the head.

Surgical neck: The area of the humerus just inferior to the anatomic neck so named due to the common occurrence of fractures in that region.

Suture lines: The serrated connections between the bones of the cranium that become more stable over time; examples include coronal suture, frontal suture, and sagittal suture.

Sympathetic division: Subdivision of the ANS that initiates the fight or flight response.

Symphysis pubis: A disk of fibrocartilage that connects the two pubic bones of the pelvis and serves as a cushion between them.

Synapse: The area between the terminal branches of an axon and the ends of a branched dendrite.

Synaptic cleft: The small gap between the axon of a motor neuron and the motor end plate of the muscle fiber.

Synaptic cleft: The small space between the terminal branch of an axon and the end of a dendrite branch.

Synaptic vesicles: The distal end of the axon of a motor neuron that contains many mitochondria and tiny vesicles that store neurotransmitters.

Synarthrosis: A type of immovable joint in which the joints are very close together and separated only by a thin layer of cartilage.

Synergist: Muscles that contract and assist the muscle that is the prime mover.

Synovial joint: Another term that refers to diarthroses; the joint capsule is located at the articulation and consists of two layers; the outer layer is connective tissue and the second layer is the synovial membrane that secretes synovial fluid, which acts as a lubricant to reduce friction during movement.

Synovial membrane: Also called synovium; a highly, vascularized connective tissue membrane that lines the capsule of a bone joint and produces synovial fluid.

Systole: The contraction of the heart.

T

Target tissue: The group of cells that are specifically affected by a hormone.

Tarsal bones: The seven bones of the ankle joint: talus, calcaneus, navicular, cuboid, medial cuneiform, middle cuneiform, and lateral cuneiform.

Taste buds: The organs of taste that are located primarily on the surface of the tongue, located within the papillae.

Telophase: Fourth phase of mitosis in which a nucleus forms in each half, a new nuclear membrane forms around the DNA of each cell, a new cell membrane is formed dividing the cell in two, and the two cells break away from each other.

Temporal bones: Two of the eight cranial bones; they form a portion of the sides and base of the skull and join the parietal bones at the squamosal suture.

Tendinitis: Inflammation of a tendon.

Tendons: Dense fibrous connective tissue composed of parallel fibers; connects muscle to bone.

Tenosynovitis: Inflammation of the tenosynovium.

Tenosynovium: Connective tissue sheath that keeps the parallel fibers of tendons held together to form the tough, inelastic, cordlike tendon structure.

Tension pneumothorax: The abnormal accumulation of air in the pleural space resulting in a positive pleural pressure that causes the lung to collapse, leaving a space for the heart, great vessels, trachea, and esophagus to shift to the opposite side of the chest, which is referred to as mediastinal shift.

Thoracic cavity: Subdivision of the ventral cavity that contains the esophagus, thymus gland, trachea, lungs, heart, and great vessels.

Thoracic duct: One of the major lymph ducts formed by the joining of the lymph vessels from the lower portion of the body; it joins the left subclavian vein and drains lymph from the intestinal, lumbar, left subclavian, bronchomediastinal and left jugular trunks.

Thrombin: Enzyme that is a necessary component of the body's natural coagulation process; it reacts with fibrinogen to form fibrin.

Thrombocyte: Medical term for platelets, which are important in the process of blood coagulation.

Thymic hormones: Also called thymosins. The hormones aid in the production and differentiation of T-cell lymphocytes.

Thymosin: An immunologic hormone produced by the thymus gland that is active through puberty and decreases in amount thereafter.

Thymus gland: Gland that consists of two lobes located in the mediastinal region extending superiorly to the inferior edge of the thyroid gland and inferiorly to the fourth costal cartilage; it is responsible for the production of T cells and is highly active through puberty then greatly diminishes in size and function.

Thyroglobulin: A glycoprotein that combines with iodine to be stored in the thyroid follicles and is available for later use to synthesize and secrete thyroid hormone.

Tibia: Commonly referred to as the shin bone; one of the two bones of the lower leg, located on the medial side.

Tibial tuberosity: Bony prominence located just inferior to the condyles of the proximal tibia that provides attachment for the patellar ligament.

Tissue: Collection of a group of cells that have a similar function.

Tongue: Muscular structure located on the floor of the mouth that is essential for speech, swallowing, and taste.

Tonus: Also called muscle tone; the low level of sustained continuous partial contraction within muscle fibers.

Toxoid vaccine: Vaccine prepared from extotoxins that are inactivated by chemicals or heat and injected to cause the formation of antibodies that neutralize the exotoxins secreted by the pathogens; used to prevent diphtheria and tetanus.

Trabeculae: The bony substance that comprises the columns within cancellous bone.

Trachea: Commonly called the windpipe; flexible tubular structure that extends from the larynx to the bifurcation of the bronchi. It consists of 20 C-shaped rings of cartilage held together by muscle and fibroelastic connective tissue.

Transfer RNA (tRNA): Type of RNA that carries the anticodon that specifies a particular amino acid. The anticodons are the bases for the codons or triplets on the mRNA. The tRNA translates the mRNA codon into the specific protein.

Translation inhibitory protein (TIP): Protein produced by healthy cells that blocks the translation of viral RNA, thereby inhibiting the spread of an infection and protecting the surrounding cells.

Transverse colon: The third portion of the colon; it begins at the hepatic flexure, travels across the top of the abdominal cavity, and ends at the splenic flexure; it is attached to the undersurface of the diaphragm by the phrenocolic ligament, and the transverse mesocolon attaches the posterior side to the spine.

Transverse plane: Horizontal plane; imaginary line that divides the body into superior and inferior portions, equal or unequal.

Transverse process: Located between the pedicles and lamina of a vertebra and serves as a point of attachment for the ligaments and muscles of the vertebral column.

Triad: Consists of two cisternae and transverse tubules and indicates the region where myosin and actin myofilaments overlap in skeletal muscle tissue; transverse tubules are attached to the surface of the sarcoplasmic reticulum and contain extracellular fluid; each transverse tubule is located between two cisternae, which serve as reservoirs for extracellular fluid.

Triangle of Calot: Anatomic triangle formed by the cystic duct, common hepatic duct, and inferior border of the liver used to locate the cystic artery.

Tricuspid valve: The valve of the tricuspid, which is one of two atrioventricular orifices that open between the right atrium and right ventricle.

Triglyceride: A molecule that consists of a molecule of glycerol and fatty acids joined to the carbons contained by the glycerol by covalent ester or ether bonds.

Trigone of bladder: Anatomic landmark formed by the two ureteral openings into the bladder and the urethral opening.

Triplet: A code for one amino acid.

Trochanter: A large bony process that serves as a site for the attachment of muscles.

Trochlea: Located at the distal end of the humerus on the medial side, it articulates with the ulna.

Tropomyosin: One of two proteins that are part of the actin myofilaments in skeletal muscle tissue; it is a thin rod-shaped strand located within the longitudinal grooves of the actin helix and acts together with the other protein, troponin, to regulate the interactions of myosin and actin during muscle contractions.

Troponin: One of two proteins that are part of the actin myofilaments in skeletal muscle tissue; it holds the protein tropomyosin in position within the actin helix and works with tropomyosin to regulate the interactions of myosin and actin during muscle contractions.

Tubal pregnancy: Pregnancy that occurs within the fallopian tube; the fertilized ovum fails to travel to the uterus and develops in the fallopian tube. Eventually, due to the small diameter of the fallopian tube, the embryo breaks through the wall of the fallopian tube.

Tubular reabsorption: The reabsorption and secretion of renal filtrate and water; reabsorption occurs between the renal tubules and peritubular capillaries; the four processes of reabsorption are active transport, passive transport, pinocytosis, and osmosis.

Tunica adventitia: Outer layer of the wall of an artery.

Tunica intima: Inner layer of the wall of an artery.

Tunica media: Middle layer of the wall of an artery.

Tunics: The tissue layers or coats of the intestinal wall; the layers from inside to outside are tunica mucosa, tunica submucosa, tunica muscularis, and serosa, also called serous layer.

Twitch: A single contraction of a muscle.

U

Ulna: One of two bones of the forearm; the proximal end articulates with the humerus at the trochlear notch and the distal end articulates with the radius at the ulnar notch.

Umbilical region: Located in the central middle region of the abdomen below the epigastric region.

Unipolar: A neuron with only one extension from the cell body that serves as both the axon and peripheral dendrite.

Urea: Amino acids broken down by the liver and excreted in the urine as the nitrogenous waste product.

Ureter: Long tube with a very small diameter that exits from the hilum of the kidney and conducts urine from the kidney to the bladder.

Urethra: Tube connected to the urinary bladder with an opening to the outside of the body that transports urine from the bladder to the outside of the body.

Urinary bladder: Hollow, muscular organ located in the anterior of the pelvis that serves for the collection and retention of urine until an individual urinates.

Urinary tract infection (UTI): An infection of the urethra or urinary bladder, most often a bacterial infection. Females are more prone to developing UTIs than males due to the location of the urethral opening, shortness of the tube, and straightness of the tube.

Urocanic acid: Specialized molecules that suppress the immune response to UV-damaged cells in order to provide the damaged cells of the skin the opportunity to repair themselves.

Uvula: Cone-shaped extension of the soft palate located in the posterior of the mouth; during swallowing the muscles draw the soft palate and uvula upward to close the opening between the nasal cavity and the pharynx.

V

Vacuole: Membranous sacs that form when a portion of the cell membrane invaginates and pinches off, taking with it a piece of substance from outside the cell to the inside.

Vagus nerve: Nerve that innervates the pharynx and larynx.

Valence electrons: Electrons orbiting on the outermost level that determine how an element will react during a chemical reaction.

Vasoconstriction: The contraction of the smooth muscle fibers in the tunica media of an artery, resulting in the narrowing of the lumen of the vessel.

Vasodilation: The relaxation of the smooth muscle fibers in the tunica media of an artery resulting in an increase in the diameter of the lumen of the vessel.

Vasopressin: Also called antidiuretic hormone (ADH). It decreases the production of urine by increasing the reabsorption of water by the renal tubules. It is released due to a decrease in blood volume or an increase in the concentration of sodium in the circulatory system. ADH also contracts the smooth muscle layer in blood vessels to aid in raising the blood pressure.

Veins: Large blood vessels that transport nonoxygenated blood back to the heart.

Ventral cavity: Division of the body that contains the thoracic and abdominopelvic cavities.

Ventricle: One of four cavities in the brain that produce and contain cerebrospinal fluid.

Ventricles: The two lower chambers of the heart that pump blood into the arteries leading away from the heart.

Venules: Small veins.

Vertebrae: The bones of the vertebral column that are separated by fibrocartilage called intervertebral disks.

Vertebral canal: Also called the vertebral foramen; the opening or passageway through the vertebral column that contains the spinal cord.

Vertebral column: Begins at the foramen magnum and extends posteriorly to the pelvis; it supports the head and trunk, forms the vertebral canal, and is flexible to allow body movement.

Vesical trigone: Anatomic landmark formed by the two openings of the ureters and opening of the urethra; located on the floor of the bladder, it contains no rugae, and therefore it does not expand.

Vesicle: Small membrane-bound sacs that contain the proteins synthesized by the endoplasmic reticulum and refined by the Golgi apparatus.

Villi: Minute projections located on the inner lining of the small intestine that increase the surface area of the epithelium for absorption of nutrients by projecting into the lumen of the small intestine in order to make contact with digestive contents.

Viscera: Internal organs enclosed within a body cavity.

Visceral layer: Serous membrane that covers the organs of the abdomen and thorax.

Visceral pericardium: Inner membranous layer of the pericardial sac that covers the surface of the heart.

Visceral peritoneum: Layer of the peritoneal membrane that covers the organs of the abdominopelvic cavity.

Visceral pleura: Layer of the pleural membrane that covers the lungs.

Visceral smooth muscle: One of two types of smooth muscle; it is the most common type located in the walls of hollow body organs.

Vitamins: Coenzymes that are necessary for growth and normal body functions; they must be obtained from the diet or vitamin supplements; a deficiency in a certain type of vitamin can result in a specific disease or disorder of the body.

Vitreous humor: The jellylike substance contained in the posterior cavity that contributes to maintaining normal intraocular pressure and prevents the eyeball from collapsing.

Vocal cords: Elastic fibers that are centrally located in the larynx and situated on either side of the glottis, the opening between the cords. The cords are responsible for producing speech.

Volvulus: The abnormal twisting of the bowel upon itself, causing an intestinal obstruction and preventing the flow of blood to that portion of the bowel.

Vomer bone: Thin, flat bone located in the midline of the nasal cavity; it connects to the ethmoid bone to form the nasal septum.

W

Wharton's duct: The excretory duct of the submandibular gland.

White matter: An area that is a collection of bundles of axons, leading away from the cell bodies through the brain that transmit impulses between specific locations in the brain.

X

Xenograft: Skin or tissue taken from another species used as a temporary covering of burned areas.

Z

Zygomatic bones: Two bones that form the lateral walls and floors of the bony eye sockets, and the cheek prominences; each bone has a temporal process that joins the zygomatic process to form the zygomatic arch.

INDEX

C

U

V

W

Y

Z